GLOBAL PRAISE FOR
TRANSFORMING NURSING THROUGH KNOWLEDGE

"A timely publication for all healthcare professionals that will advance the movement from tradition to evidence-based practice, education, and policy. It is a welcome resource for nursing and healthcare faculty and students for teaching and understanding theory, application, and lived experiences related to guideline development, implementation science, and evaluation. The book achieves the goals of education, inspiration, and motivation for evidence-based healthcare in a global context."

–Cynthia Baker, PhD, RN
Executive Director
Canadian Association of Schools of Nursing

"The Registered Nurses' Association of Ontario (RNAO) is known for its robust capacity to create Best Practice Guidelines (BPG) that have enhanced clinical practice and outcomes around the world. In addition to its deep contribution to quality improvement through BPGs, RNAO is an international leader in cutting-edge implementation science. Implementation is recognized as an inherently difficult element for improving care, and we are extremely proud to support RNAO's expertise and unwavering commitment to innovation and excellence."

–Bob Bell, MDCM, MSc, FRCSC, FACS, FRCE (hon)
Professor of Surgery, University of Toronto
Deputy Minister
Ministry of Health and Long-Term Care, Ontario, Canada

"This book is titled Transforming Nursing Through Knowledge, *but it's also about transforming knowledge through nursing. It offers a pragmatic and 'can-do' approach to spreading knowledge that combines the discipline of evidence, the rigor of implementation science, the contagion of social movement thinking, and the energy of shared purpose. Anyone with a passion for knowledge management should read this book, way beyond the field of nursing."*

–Helen Bevan
Chief Transformation Officer
National Health Service (NHS), Horizons, England

"Thoughtful, compelling, and inspiring! This book is an extraordinary tool for those seeking to optimize practice and patient outcomes. It is also a must-read for faculty and policymakers wanting to learn and teach how evidence-based practice can be scaled up into a national and global revolution. Through theoretical underpinnings and lived experiences in a variety of global contexts, readers will gain an in-depth understanding of how to get started, move forward, and achieve outstanding results."

–Janet Davidson, OC, BScN, MHSA, LLD(hon)
Chair, Board of Directors
Canadian Institute for Health Information

"Ensuring that nursing care is informed by the best evidence and addressing the barriers and facilitators to implementation of best practice are critical in optimizing health outcomes. Transforming Nursing Through Knowledge provides a road map for knowledge utilization and will be a useful resource for both novice and expert practitioners."

–Patricia M. Davidson, PhD, RN
Dean and Professor
Johns Hopkins School of Nursing, USA

"The Registered Nurses' Association of Ontario has been at the forefront of defining and promoting evidence-based nursing in Canada and worldwide for more than 2 decades. This book provides an excellent summary of the theoretical underpinnings and practical experiences of the Best Practice Guidelines and Best Practice Spotlight Organizations programs. The concepts and ideas are relevant to anyone interested in improving healthcare to improve patient outcomes. Highly recommended!"

–Jeremy M. Grimshaw, MBChB, PhD, FCAHS
Senior Scientist, Ottawa Hospital Research Institute
Professor, Department of Medicine, University of Ottawa
Canada Research Chair in Health Knowledge Transfer and Uptake

"Grinspun and Bajnok have done a brilliant job mapping how to create evidence-based cultures. The book is a masterpiece for health systems anywhere in the world—from policymakers to executives to clinicians. It provides rigorous methodology for all components of clinical Best Practice Guidelines development, implementation, and evaluation. Equally important, it highlights how professional nursing associations and unions positively partner to achieve better health for all."

–Vickie Kaminski, MBA, RN
Chief Executive, SA Health, South Australia

"This publication is a testimony to the monumental contribution RNAO has made over the past decade to develop and implement best practice guidelines. It is an impressive text that shares the story across the full spectrum—from conception to operationalization in various contexts around the world. Clinicians, educators, administrators, students, and policymakers will find this user-friendly text a go-to resource in bridging the gap between evidence and practice and evidence and policy—and how to make both a reality. Transforming Nursing Through Knowledge will inspire nursing and other healthcare professionals to be change agents that shape a future of enhanced care and outcomes for the public we serve."

–Hester C. Klopper, PhD, MBA, HonsDNurse, FANSA, FAAN, ASSAF
Deputy Vice Chancellor: Strategy and Internationalisation
Stellenbosch University, South Africa
Editor-in-Chief, *International Journal of Africa Nursing Sciences*

"Grinspun and Bajnok have crafted an inspiring book that shows what you can achieve when you think big and deliver consistently. Together with their collaborators, they have built an initiative on three strong pillars: guideline development, implementation science, and outcomes evaluation. The authors have scaled up this initiative across sectors within a health system and across health systems. They have shown that a professional association can, with the right leadership, drive improvements in practice and work environments."

–John N. Lavis, PhD, MD
Professor, Director, McMaster Health Forum
Codirector, WHO Collaborating Centre for Evidence-Informed Policy
Canada Research Chair in Evidence-Informed Health Systems

"This work is recommended both for those who start their first steps into evidence-based practice and those scientists dedicated to implementation science and knowledge management. It begins with a necessary chapter dedicated to banishing the erroneous caring-competence debate. Subsequently, it includes a thorough description of the RNAO guidelines, illustrating the parallel evolution they have followed in developing new methods such as GRADE. The core of the manual is comprehensive content dedicated to guidelines implementation, often forgotten in other works. That is one of the book's greatest strengths, especially the Best Practice Spotlight Organizations (BPSO) and their extension to undergraduate education."

–José Miguel Morales Asencio, PhD, RN
Head of the Department of Nursing
Professor of Research and Evidence Based Health Care
Faculty of Health Sciences, University of Málaga
Málaga, Spain

"Bold, visionary, and pragmatic, Grinspun and Bajnok's book is a detailed account of what is globally known as one of the most robust evidence-based practice programs. Transforming Nursing Through Knowledge *is also a practical tool for anyone intent on bringing rigorous evidence and passion to optimize health outcomes for patients, save money in the health system, and make policy changes happen. Simply put: a gift!"*

–Chris Power, BScN, MHSA, CHE
Chief Executive Officer
Canadian Patient Safety Institute

"The development of RNAO's Best Practice Guidelines has been one of the most important achievements for better medical care and an optimized healthcare system. The guidelines help us move away from the old 'this is how I have always done it' to a new 'this is how I should do it,' transforming care through robust evidence-based knowledge. I congratulate and endorse Doris Grinspun and Irmajean Bajnok for their invaluable contribution to the integral management of our patients."

–Ricardo Schwartz, MD
Surgeon Oncologist
President, Chilean Society of Mastology

"A powerful, detailed, and compelling masterpiece that provides a visionary yet practical road map on how to move evidence from a theoretical concept to a global movement that improves outcomes for patients, health professionals, health organizations, and policymakers. Grinspun, Bajnok, and the tremendous team of writers assembled for this book make it a go-to resource for all who want to transform healthcare through robust use of evidence."

–Judith Shamian, PhD, MPH, RN, DSc(hon), LLD(hon), FAAN
NQuIRE, Founding Chair
International Council of Nurses (ICN) President Emerita

"I am so impressed by such a great publication on the power of nursing knowledge. This book generously shares with us the essence of the Registered Nurses' Association of Ontario Best Practice Guidelines Program. Filled with robust theoretical underpinnings applied to vivid examples and real cases in the field, this book will guide and direct nurses and other healthcare professionals eager to improve health outcomes to conduct implementation research for more effective nursing and public health."

–Hongcai Shang, MD, PhD
Director, Key Laboratory of Chinese Internal Medicine of Ministry of Education
Beijing University of Chinese Medicine

"On behalf of Health Standards Organization (HSO) and Accreditation Canada (AC), we commend the Registered Nurses' Association of Ontario (RNAO) on the publication of Transforming Nursing Through Knowledge. *Consistent with HSO's and AC's approach to people-centred best practices, the RNAO continues to make important progress in the area of evidence-based resources, helping to improve quality, safety, and efficiency so healthcare organizations, providers, clinicians, and learners can deliver the best possible care and service."*

–Leslee J. Thompson
CEO, Health Standards Organization and Accreditation Canada

TRANSFORMING
NURSING
THROUGH
KNOWLEDGE

Best Practices for Guideline Development, Implementation Science, and Evaluation

DORIS GRINSPUN, PhD, MSN, BScN, RN, LLD(hon), Dr(hc), O.ONT
IRMAJEAN BAJNOK, PhD, MScN, BScN, RN

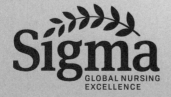

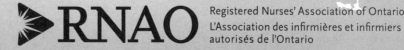

Registered Nurses' Association of Ontario
L'Association des infirmières et infirmiers
autorisés de l'Ontario

Speaking out for nursing. Speaking out for health.

The Sigma Theta Tau International Honor Society of Nursing (Sigma) is a nonprofit organization whose mission is advancing world health and celebrating nursing excellence in scholarship, leadership, and service. Founded in 1922, Sigma has more than 135,000 active members in over 90 countries and territories. Members include practicing nurses, instructors, researchers, policymakers, entrepreneurs, and others. Sigma's more than 530 chapters are located at more than 700 institutions of higher education throughout Armenia, Australia, Botswana, Brazil, Canada, Colombia, England, Ghana, Hong Kong, Japan, Jordan, Kenya, Lebanon, Malawi, Mexico, the Netherlands, Pakistan, Philippines, Portugal, Singapore, South Africa, South Korea, Swaziland, Sweden, Taiwan, Tanzania, Thailand, the United States, and Wales. Learn more at www.sigmanursing.org.

Sigma Theta Tau International
550 West North Street
Indianapolis, IN, USA 46202

To order additional books, buy in bulk, or order for corporate use, contact Sigma Marketplace at 888.654.4968/US and Canada or +1.317.634.8171 (outside US and Canada).

To request a review copy for course adoption, email solutions@sigmanursing.org or call 888.654.4968/US and Canada or +1.317.634.8171 (outside US and Canada).

To request author information, or for speaker or other media requests, contact Sigma Marketing at 888.634.7575 (US and Canada) or +1.317.634.8171 (outside US and Canada).

ISBN:	9781945157639
EPUB ISBN:	9781945157646
PDF ISBN:	9781945157653
MOBI ISBN:	9781945157660

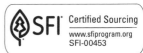

SFI label applies to text stock

Library of Congress Cataloging-in-Publication data

Names: Grinspun, Doris, author. | Bajnok, Irmajean, author. | Sigma
  Theta Tau International, issuing body.
Title: Transforming nursing through knowledge : best practices for guideline
  development, implementation science, and evaluation / Doris Grinspun,
  Irmajean Bajnok.
Description: Indianapolis, IN : Sigma Theta Tau International, [2018] |
  Includes bibliographical references.
Identifiers: LCCN 2018008029 (print) | LCCN 2018008923 (ebook) | ISBN
  9781945157646 (epub ebook) | ISBN 9781945157653 (PDF ebook) | ISBN
  9781945157660 (Amazon/Mobi ebook) | ISBN 9781945157639 (pbk.) | ISBN
  9781945157646 (EPUB) | ISBN 9781945157653 (PDF) | ISBN 9781945157660 (MOBI)
Subjects: | MESH: Evidence-Based Nursing--standards | Practice Guidelines as
  Topic
Classification: LCC RT41 (ebook) | LCC RT41 (print) | NLM WY 100.7 | DDC
  610.73--dc23
LC record available at https://lccn.loc.gov/2018008029

First Printing, 2018

Publisher: Dustin Sullivan	**Managing Editor:** Carla Hall
Acquisitions Editor: Emily Hatch	**Development and Project Editor:** Kezia Endsley
Editorial Coordinator: Paula Jeffers	**Copy Editor:** Erin Geile
Cover Designer: Rebecca Batchelor	**Proofreaders:** Gill Editorial Services, Todd Lothery
Interior Design/Page Layout: Rebecca Batchelor	**Indexer:** Joy Dean Lee

DEDICATIONS

This book is dedicated to:

- Nurses in all roles and other health professionals for their unwavering commitment and passion for excellence in care

- Healthcare organizations in all sectors and academic institutions that strive to create practice and learning environments that optimize evidence uptake

- Students in the health professions who will benefit from this book to continue building on the legacy of evidence-based practice

- Governments and other stakeholders who aim to improve health system effectiveness and optimal outcomes for all

- Members of the public, who place their trust in nurses, and whose health and well-being are the focus of our work

Together we must ensure our health system is based on the best evidence possible to build healthy communities for today and tomorrow.

ACKNOWLEDGMENTS

We acknowledge the staff of the Registered Nurses' Association of Ontario (RNAO), present and past, who have contributed their expertise and unwavering commitment to develop and give voice to the Best Practice Guidelines Program. Special thanks to the Government of Ontario for recognizing RNAO's capacity to lead this ground-breaking program and achieve outcomes beyond our dreams. Our Expert Panels and stakeholder reviewers, who have generously volunteered their time and knowledge to create rigorous evidence-based guidelines and related tools, deserve our deepest appreciation.

Recognition is extended to our local and international advisory councils who have contributed knowledge and sage advice. We applaud our Best Practice Spotlight Organizations (BPSO) and their Champions for giving life to this global movement through leadership and purposeful action across the spectrum from direct care to the boardroom. Endless gratitude to RNAO's board of directors, assembly of representatives, and all the association's members for being proud ambassadors of this leading-edge work.

We are indebted to the author teams of each chapter, who have brilliantly showcased the theories and their lived experiences presented in this book. Heartfelt gratitude goes to Josephine Mo for her exquisite competence and countless hours in coordinating communications and fine editing of this book. The Sigma editorial team, especially Carla Hall and Emily Hatch, have enriched this book and our lives. Their expertise, can-do attitude, and kindness make Sigma a publisher of choice and a dream team to work with—we will be forever grateful to you. We deeply thank our families, who have been part of this journey from the beginning, understanding the importance of excellence in nursing and our dedication to this work. Finally, we warmly thank each other for the journey we have traveled together. Building this groundbreaking global movement has been important, fulfilling, and fun. Producing this book is the icing on the cake.

ABOUT THE AUTHORS

DORIS GRINSPUN, PhD, MSN, BScN, RN, LLD(hon), Dr(hc), O.ONT

Doris Grinspun is Chief Executive Officer of the Registered Nurses' Association of Ontario (RNAO), the professional association representing registered nurses, nurse practitioners. and nursing students in the province of Ontario, Canada's largest jurisdiction. RNAO's mandate is to advance healthy public policy and the role of registered nurses and nurse practitioners. Grinspun assumed this position in 1996. She is the founder and visionary of RNAO's internationally renowned Best Practice Guidelines Program and a leading figure in Canadian and international health and nursing policy.

From 1990 to 1996, Grinspun served as Director of Nursing at Mount Sinai Hospital in Toronto. She has also worked in practice and administrative capacities in Israel and the United States. Grinspun, who was born in Chile, has an RN diploma from Hadassah School of Nursing in Jerusalem, Israel; a baccalaureate degree in nursing and organizational behavior from Tel Aviv University, Israel; a master of science in nursing from the University of Michigan in Ann Arbor, Michigan, USA; and a PhD from the Department of Sociology at York University in Toronto, Ontario, Canada.

Grinspun is Adjunct Professor in the Faculty of Nursing at the University of Toronto, Adjunct Professor at the University of Ottawa School of Nursing, and Associate Fellow of the Centre for Research on Latin America and the Caribbean (CERLAC) at York University. Grinspun was a member of the board of directors of Sigma Theta Tau International Honor Society of Nursing (Sigma) from 2013–2017. She has served on several Sigma task forces and committees and is a proud Virginia Henderson Fellow.

For over 2 decades, Grinspun has led many international programs in Latin and Central America, China, Australia, and Europe. Having published and spoken extensively in Canada and abroad, she is a forceful advocate of Canada's universal health system and the contribution of registered nurses and nurse practitioners to its success. Her expertise is in the areas of health, healthcare, and nursing.

Grinspun appears frequently in the media, advancing nursing, health and social policy, and evidence-based practice. She has been featured in major media outlets and publications for her bold, compelling, and visionary leadership. Examples include *North of the City* (Ontario, 2004); *National Review of Medicine* (Canada, 2004); *GP Provincial Profile* (Ontario, 2005); *Pace International* (Australia, 2005); *Factor Hispano* (2006); *Nursing Economic$* (USA, 2010); *Jewish Tribune* (Canada, 2013); *El Pais* (Spain, 2014); *La Vanguardia* (Spain, 2012, 2014); and numerous newspapers in Chile, Peru, and Spain in 2016, 2017, and 2018.

Throughout her career, Grinspun has received numerous professional and scholarly awards. In 2003, she was invested by the government of Ontario with the Order of Ontario, in recognition of the highest level of individual excellence and achievement in any field. In 2010, the Canadian Hispanic Business Association named her one of the 10 Most Influential Hispanic Canadians. In 2011, Grinspun was conferred the degree of doctor of laws honoris causa by the University of Ontario Institute of Technology. In 2012, she received the Nursing Leadership Award from Sigma's Lambda Pi at-Large Chapter. Also in 2012, Grinspun was the recipient of the Nursing Leadership Award from the Canadian College of Health Leaders. In 2013, she received the Queen's Diamond Jubilee Medal. In 2017, she was conferred the Lampara Florencia Nightingale (Lamp of Florence Nightingale) by the Colegio de Enfermeros de Peru (College of Nurses of Peru). Also in 2017, she was declared Distinguished Visitor Municipalidad de Tacna, Peru, and conferred with Tacna's City Medal. In February 2018, Grinspun was the first nurse ever to be bestowed a doctor honoris causa by the Universitat de Lleida - Spain.

IRMAJEAN BAJNOK, PhD, MScN, BScN, RN

Irmajean Bajnok is former Director of RNAO's International Affairs and Best Practice Guidelines Centre (IABPG). In this capacity from 2007 to 2016, she oversaw the development, dissemination, implementation support activities, and evaluation of the RNAO Best Practice Guidelines (BPG) in both clinical and healthy work environment areas. She initiated and led the development of the groundbreaking Healthy Work Environment Best Practice Guidelines, which expanded to incorporate both system- and organizational-related BPGs. Bajnok shaped the Healthy Work Environment BPGs to address the central issues of leadership, teamwork, professionalism, workload and staffing, and cultural diversity as well as ongoing critical work environment and system challenges. She played a lead role in the many strategies developed to support and evaluate implementation of evidence-based practice locally, provincially, and internationally through the RNAO BPGs.

Born in Saskatchewan, Bajnok earned her RN diploma from Winnipeg General Hospital and a BScN from the University of Alberta. She has a master's in nursing and a PhD in epidemiology from Western University.

Bajnok is recognized as a leader in implementation science. In her roles with RNAO, she developed a number of creative approaches to support knowledge translation locally, nationally, and globally. Bajnok played a pivotal role in implementing and sustaining RNAO clinical and healthy work environment best practices through RNAO's Champion Network, Best Practice Spotlight Organization Designation, Nursing Order Sets, and BPG-related learning institutes. She also had a defining role in her work as Codirector of the Nursing Best Practice Research Centre (NBPRC) and as Coeditor of the *Diabetic Foot Canada* open-access online journal.

Promotion of evidence-based cultures has been a passion for Bajnok as she travelled extensively in Canada and internationally, working with healthcare professionals and organizations to advance evidence-based nursing practice cultures as part of RNAO's Best Practice Spotlight Organization Designation and the Best Practice Champions Network. In her tenure as Director of the IABPG Centre, the BPSO Designation—widely recognized as an effective organizational-level knowledge-translation strategy—was augmented to include a new category of Academic BPSOs, now boasting worldwide uptake. Bajnok was also instrumental in expanding the BPSO Designation both provincially and internationally, such that it now extends to 12 countries and continues to grow.

Bajnok holds a university appointment at the University of Ottawa as Adjunct Professor in the School of Nursing, Faculty of Health Science.

Prior to joining the RNAO team, Bajnok had an extensive and successful career in practice, academia, and administration, including professorial roles at the University of Western Ontario and Ryerson University, where she served as Director of the nursing program from 1982–1988 and led faculty in development of the nursing undergraduate degree program, the first basic degree program at Ryerson. Her practice roles spanned acute care as a Practice Director at Mount Sinai Hospital in Toronto and home care as the Director of Professional Practice at VON Toronto, Canada. She was the founding Director of the WHO Collaborating Centre at Mount Sinai Hospital and served as the founding Executive Director of the Development of Women's Health Professionals Program in Pakistan, a multipartnership program with the Aga Khan University, McMaster University, and the governments of Canada and of Pakistan.

Bajnok is a Past President of the Registered Nurses' Association of Ontario (1977–1979), a former member of the Council of the College of Nurses of Ontario (1998–2004), and a former Sigma committee member (November 2015–November 2017).

CONTRIBUTING AUTHORS

Sonia Abad Vasquez, MA, BScN, RN
Former Chief of Nursing, Clínica las Condes—BPSO Direct-Service

Sonia Abad Vasquez was Chief of Nursing at the Clínica las Condes from 2012 to 2017. She was responsible for administrative management and human capital management, training of high-level teams, and implementation of evidence-based nursing as a measure to ensure quality care and person-centered care in the institution. Abad Vasquez graduated as an RN and a midwife from the Universidad Católica de Chile. She has a master's in administration and management in health from the Universidad de los Andes and is currently pursuing a master's in nursing management from the European University of Madrid. She has participated in various programs for health executives, including observership in different hospitals in Latin America, Europe, and the US. Abad Vazquez is a highly regarded teacher in postgraduate programs, congresses, and seminars. She has more than eight years of clinical experience in critical patient care, as well as strong leadership in administration and management working with interprofessional teams and advancing leading practices in ambulatory care and emergency services.

Laura Albornos-Muñoz, BSc
Researcher, Nursing and Healthcare Research Unit (Investén-isciii)
Instituto de Salud Carlos III—BPSO Host

Laura Albornos-Muñoz holds a bachelor of science from the University of Valladolid. Since 2010, she has worked as a researcher at the Spanish Centre for Evidence-Based Nursing and Healthcare of the Nursing Research Unit (Investén-isciii). She has been a member of the scientific committee for numerous international conferences. Albornos-Muñoz has experience in healthcare methodology and has been involved in national and European research projects related to evidence-based implementation, especially in falls prevention and health promotion. Other projects include active ageing and healthcare from programs such as FP7, CIP, National Agency and Thematic Network in elderly and frailty (RETICEF).

Barbara Bell, MN, BScN, RN, CHE
Former Chief Nursing Executive and Health Professions Officer
West Park Healthcare Centre—BPSO Direct-Service

Barbara Bell is Vice President, Quality and Safety, at the Central Local Health Integration Network. She is a former Chief Nursing Executive and Health Professions Officer at West Park Healthcare Centre in Toronto. Over the course of 19 years at West Park, she held a number of positions and provided leadership to a range of areas: professional practice, clinical decision support, research administration, quality, risk management, health records, ethics, and privacy. She championed West Park's ongoing commitment to the implementation of Best Practice Guidelines and launched Practice Development.

Alejandra Belmar Valdebenito, BScN
BPSO Lead, Clínica Las Condes—BPSO Direct-Service

Alejandra Belmar Valdebenito is a registered nurse at the Clínica Las Condes (CLC) in Santiago, Chile. She has a baccalaureate degree from Universidad de Los Andes in Santiago; diploma in critical care of adult patients; diploma in management and infection control; and postgraduate degree in administration and management of clinical services. Belmar Valdebenito is completing a master of epidemiology at the Universidad de los Andes. She is an expert in caring for critical patients, having worked in the adult intensive care unit of CLC from 2010 to 2015. In 2015, Belmar Valdebenito was appointed Program Manager and BPSO lead, responsible for implementation and supervision of the BPSO Designation in Clínica las Condes and RNAO Best Practice Guidelines, coordination of annual international nursing conferences, and implementation of nursing research projects. She is currently in training to become an RNAO certified trainer.

Rob Bonner
Director, Operations and Strategy, Australian Nursing and Midwifery Federation (ANMF) (SA Branch)—BPSO Host

Rob Bonner is Director, Operations & Strategy for the Australian Nursing and Midwifery Federation (SA Branch). His role includes leadership of the South Australia Branch's industrial, education, and membership programs. Bonner led a national research team that established an evidence-based methodology for staffing and skills mix in resident aged care. He is a member of the Australian Industry & Skills Committee, which provides advice to state and Australian governments through the COAG Ministerial Council and regulates training packages for all industry sectors. He is also a member of the SA Training & Skills Commission, which provides advice to the SA Government on workforce, training and skills matters and regulates areas of apprenticeships and traineeships. Bonner also serves on the Steering Committee of the Rosemary Bryant AO Research Centre, in collaboration with ANMF (SA Branch) and the University of South Australia, and he is a member of the board of the Rosemary Bryant AO Foundation. In the health and community services sector, Bonner has a long history of active thought and change leadership in areas such as health workforce, translation of evidence into practice, career structures, workloads and their management, and information systems and their support of clinical practice.

Mariam Botros, DCh, IIWCC, CDE, Wounds Care Fellowship, University of Toronto
Executive Director, Wounds Canada

Mariam Botros is Executive Director of Wounds Canada. She is a chiropodist at Women's College Hospital Wound Healing clinic and a Clinical Director of Diabetic Foot Canada. She is Codirector of the International Interprofessional Wound Care Course (IIWCC) at the University of Toronto. Botros has lectured on programs internationally in the area of diabetic foot complications and amputation prevention. She brings both practical and professional experience to her effective approach to leadership. This is gained from roles as an executive director, healthcare practitioner, healthcare educator, researcher, and faculty member for many well-recognized organizations.

Sonya Canzian, MHSc, RN, CNN(C), Executive Vice President Clinical Programs,
Chief Nurse and Health Disciplines Executive, St. Michael's Hospital—BPSO Direct-Service

A registered nurse, Sonya Canzian joined St. Michael's Hospital in 1990. Since then, she has held progressively senior positions in critical care, education, and administration. Canzian is responsible for operational management of the trauma/neurosurgery, mobility, heart and vascular, critical care, specialized complex care, and cancer services programs. She is also accountable for nursing and health disciplines professional practice, education, and research. Cross-appointed to the University of Toronto and a Lecturer in the critical care program at George Brown College, she also acts as a Canadian Nurses Association mentor for neuroscience nursing certification and National Director and Instructor for the Advanced Trauma Care for Nurses course for the Society of Trauma Nurses. Canzian holds a master's in health science from Charles Sturt University in Australia.

Olga L. Cortés, PhD, MSc, CCN, RN
Associated Researcher, Research Department and Nursing Department at Fundación
Cardioinfantil-Instituto de Cardiología, Bogotá, Colombia—BPSO Direct-Service

Olga L. Cortés is a graduate student in the master's and PhD program at McMaster University, Hamilton, Ontario. She was trained as an intensive care nurse and is now a Research Associate at the Cardioinfantil Foundation Institute of Cardiology (FCI-IC). Her primary interest is in assessing the impact of nursing interventions such as early mobilization and prevention of complications associated with prolonged bed rest in hospitalized adults and the elderly with chronic conditions. She is a leader in nursing research in conducting randomized controlled clinical trials and conducting systematic reviews and meta-analysis. Cortés leads the PENFUP study on the impact assessment of the use of hydrocolloid dressings in prevention of pressure ulcers in high-risk adults and the PAMP Phase II study on the evaluation of the impact of walking versus scheduled noncardiac surgery in mobilization during hospitalization. She has contributed to the implementation of the RNAO Best Practice Guidelines at the FCI-IC.

Lucia Costantini, PhD, RN
Associate Director, RNAO

Lucia Costantini assumed the position of Associate Director for Guideline Development, Research and Evaluation at the RNAO International Affairs and Best Practice Guidelines Centre (IABPG) in January 2018. Prior to that, she was a Program Manager in the IABPG Centre. She received a diploma in nursing from Mohawk College in 1998. From there, she entered clinical practice, gaining invaluable experience working in surgical and critical care areas. While working at the bedside, Costantini continued her education and completed a bachelor of science in nursing from Ryerson University in 2000. Postgraduation, she shifted her clinical focus toward working with adults receiving acute and chronic hemodialysis. She returned to Ryerson University and completed a master of nursing in 2006. Other clinical practice experiences included Education Coordinator for the renal program and the independent dialysis program. Costantini completed her doctoral studies at McMaster University in June 2016. In her doctoral dissertation, she developed and evaluated an instrument that measures self-management for adults with multiple comorbidities receiving in-center and home hemodialysis; she also examined psychological distress and coping strategies in this population.

Elizabeth Dabars, AM
Adjunct Associate Professor, CEO/Secretary, ANMF (SA Branch)—BPSO Host

Adjunct Associate Professor Elizabeth Dabars, AM, is the CEO/Secretary of the ANMF (SA Branch), representing more than 20,000 members across South Australia and taking pride in the fact that membership has grown by 90% since she came to office in March 2008. She holds qualifications in nursing, education, leadership, management, and law, and she worked as a Solicitor at Duncan Basheer Hannon immediately prior to taking up her current role. Her academic status is held with Flinders University, becoming a member (AM) in the General Division of the Order of Australia in June 2014 in recognition of her significant service to medical administration, particularly to nursing and midwifery, and to community and mental health organizations.

Tracey DasGupta, MN, RN
Director of Interprofessional Practice, Sunnybrook Health Sciences Centre—
BPSO Direct-Service

Tracey DasGupta is Director of Interprofessional Practice at Sunnybrook Health Sciences Centre and an Adjunct Lecturer at the Bloomberg Faculty of Nursing at the University of Toronto. She has been passionate about healthcare, quality of life, leadership, and interprofessional collaboration since becoming a nurse in 1991. She has fulfilled direct-care roles along the continuum of care and has had the opportunity to continue to grow in leadership roles such as educator, professional practice leader, and director of nursing practice. In her current role, she is providing leadership for interprofessional care and best practice implementation. She believes that in life, it is important to find something worth pursuing and then to pursue it with passion.

Barbara Davies, PhD, RN, FCAHS
Professor, Retired, University of Ottawa, Ontario, Canada

Barbara Davies has taught research methods in undergraduate and graduate programs. She was Codirector of the Nursing Best Practice Research Unit/Centre for 9 years and Vice Dean of Research for the Faculty of Health Sciences. She received a Premier's Research Excellence Award from the Ministry of Enterprise, Opportunity and Innovation of Ontario, Canada. She is a Fellow of the Canadian Academy of Health Sciences. Her research program aims to increase the translation and uptake of evidence into practice for front-line healthcare workers, decision makers, and consumers. She is actively involved in the development, implementation, evaluation, and sustainability of best practice guidelines in nursing and healthcare. She was Cochair of the development panel for the *RNAO Toolkit: Implementation of Best Practice Guidelines*. She recently published *Reading Research: A User-Friendly Guide for Health Professionals*, Sixth Edition, with Elsevier.

Maribel Esparza-Bohórquez, MSc, BScN, RN
Chief of Nursing Division, Fundación Oftalmológica de Santander (FOSCAL)
BPSO Direct-Service

Maribel Esparza-Bohórquez has been Chief Nurse of FOSCAL since 2005. She holds a BScN degree from the Universidad Industrial de Santander. She has a certificate in education and health audits from the Universidad Autonóma de Bucaramanga in Bucaramanga, Colombia. Esparza-Bohórquez has a master's in nursing with specialization in management from the Universidad Nacional de Colombia. She holds a position with the departmental court of nursing ethics of the North Oriental region in Colombia and is an RNAO-certified BPSO orientation trainer.

Olga Lucía Gómez Díaz, MA(Ed), RN
Director of the Nursing Department at Universidad Autonóma de Bucaramanga
BPSO Direct-Academic

Olga Lucia Gómez Díaz is a registered nurse leader with many years of experience in practice, administration, education, and research. She is the inaugural Director of the nursing program at Universidad Autónoma de Bucaramanga (UNAB), a position she has held since 2008. At UNAB, she has worked with her team in leading the development of the nursing curriculum. Prior to that, she worked as Coordinator and Consultant of the nursing department at Fundación Oftalmológica de Santander. She works closely with health educators in research groups in the medicine, nursing, and psychology fields at UNAB. She has received several awards, including the National Anthropology Award, and awards of Nursing Excellence granted by Universidad Industrial de Santander and Colciencias.

Esther González-María, PhD, MSc, RN
Knowledge transfer, Nursing and Healthcare Research Unit (Investén-isciii)
Instituto de Salud Carlos III—BPSO Host

Esther González-María has formal education in nursing from the Universidad Autónoma of Madrid (1985). She obtained a maîtrise en sciences at the University of Montreal (1993) and a PhD in nursing care research from the Universidad de Murcia (2015). González-María is a member of a Thematic Network on Healthy Ageing and Frailty (CIBERFES), and she has participated in large national and international research projects. She is a reviewer of several scientific international nursing journals. Her main focuses of research are 1) enhancing evidence-based practice and knowledge transfer in nursing clinical practice; 2) factors influencing knowledge translation; 3) measurement of nursing process and nursing staffing characteristics and the impact of nursing on patient outcomes; and 4) nursing-sensitive indicators.

Lina Maria Granados Oliveros, MSc, RN
Hospitalization Coordinator, CLINICA FOSCAL—BPSO Direct-Service

Lina Maria Granados Oliveros is a registered nurse at FOSCAL. She holds a baccalaureate degree from the Universidad Industrial de Santander; a master's in nursing with emphasis in the perinatal maternal area of the Universidad Nacional of Colombia; and a magistrate of the northeast regional departmental court of nursing.

Valerie Grdisa, PhD, MS, BScN, RN
Director, International Affairs and Best Practice Guidelines (IABPG) Centre, RNAO

Valerie Grdisa is Director of the IABPG Centre at RNAO, a position she assumed in November 2016. She brings with her 3 decades of relevant experience as a clinician (registered nurse and nurse practitioner), health services administrator, faculty and academic administrator, consultant, and senior government official. Throughout her career, she has implemented the RNAO BPGs into both service provider organizations and academic institutions. In her government role, she was Senior Nursing Advisor in Alberta, Canada, where she worked closely with ministers of health, the deputy minister, and her assistant deputy colleagues on a wide range of projects, including development of the health system blueprint and an integrated health human resources strategy. Grdisa holds a bachelor of science in nursing from the University of Toronto, a master of science from the State University of New York, and a doctorate of philosophy in health services and policy research from McMaster University, specializing in measuring system integration. She is an Adjunct Professor in the Faculty of Health Sciences at the University of Lethbridge and with the University of Calgary's nursing faculty. Grdisa has been a proud and active RNAO member since the 1990s.

Guo Hailing, RN
Associate Professor, Director of Nursing, and BPSO Sponsor, DongZhiMen Hospital
BPSO Direct-Service, affiliated with Beijing University of Chinese Medicine

Guo Hailing is Associate Professor of Nursing; Master Supervisor; Director of the nursing department of DongZhiMen Hospital affiliated with Beijing University of Chinese Medicine; and sponsor of the Best Practice Spotlight Organization (BPSO) at DongZhiMen Hospital. She holds a number of positions, including Executive Director of the Institute of National Higher Education of Traditional Chinese Medicine (TCM), council member of the nursing branch of the China Hospital Research Institute, Vice Chairperson of the nursing specialized committee of the Beijing association of integrated Chinese and Western medicine, Vice Chairperson of the nursing specialized committee of Beijing TCM association, Project Leader of key specialties of Beijing TCM administration, and leader of the Beijing training base (DongZhiMen hospital) of TCM nursing personnel. She is also Associate Editor of the textbook *Clinical Nutriology* for the adult nursing education program in higher institutions of TCM. She has led and participated in eight research projects, published 15 articles, and applied for two national patents. She is also an editorial board member of *Chinese Journal of Modern Nursing*.

Barbara Heatley O'Neil, MAdEd, BScN
President, O'Neil Co-Active Coaching Group
Former Chief Nursing Executive, Chief of Interprofessional Practice and
Organizational Development
Bluewater Health—BPSO Direct-Service

Barbara Heatley O'Neil has held various leadership positions in the acute care sector. She obtained her bachelor of science in nursing from the University of Windsor. In 2008, she became Chief Nursing Executive and Chief of Interprofessional Practice and Organizational Development at Bluewater Health, where she led the initiative to become a Registered Nurses' Association of Ontario Best Practice Spotlight Organization (BPSO). With an interest in organizational culture, O'Neil completed her master of adult education (St. Francis Xavier University). She is a teacher of appreciative inquiry and is a Myers-Briggs Type Indicator Practitioner. She is writing a book about servant leadership. O'Neil retired from Bluewater Health in March 2016 and began her second career as President and Executive Leadership Coach at O'Neil Co-Active Coaching Group. She describes this as legacy work, where coaching, knowledge, complex influencing strategies, writing, and leadership combine to help others become successful. She believes that leadership requires kindness, a positive attitude, and courage.

Edith Ho, GradDipBus(AdminMgmt), BNg, RN
Professional Officer, Australian Nursing and Midwifery Federation (ANMF)

Edith Ho is a registered nurse who has worked in different clinical settings overseas and in Australia and has held senior nursing informatics, management, and leadership roles in acute care nursing. She completed a graduate diploma in business administration, a bachelor of nursing, and postgraduate studies in medical imaging and acute care nursing. As a professional officer at the ANMF (SA Branch), Ho plays a significant role on the Australian BPSO Project Team, supporting the Australian BPSO sites in BPG implementation. She is the Australian BPSO NQuIRE Manager. In that position, she utilizes her nursing informatics experience and management knowledge, leads the program evaluation, and validates data definitions, calculation, and applications. Ho also guides the review of the evaluation methodology and its related clinical and quality outcomes.

Carol Holmes, MN, RN, GNC(C)
Former Program Manager, Long-Term Care Best Practices Program, RNAO

Carol Holmes recently retired after 43 years in nursing. Her professional experience spans nursing clinical practice, education, leadership, and administration. While working in academic teaching hospitals, she led the development, implementation, and evaluation of evidence-based programs that resulted in positive outcomes for older adults. In the role of Program Manager with the Long-Term Care Best Practices Program from April 2014 to May 2017, Holmes led a team of 16 registered nurses providing implementation expertise to Ontario long-term care homes to systematically integrate RNAO's clinical and Healthy Work Environment Best Practice Guidelines. She co-led development of the Long-Term Care Best Practice Spotlight Organization and led the development of key resources supporting knowledge transfer and capacity building. Holmes is a registered nurse with undergraduate and graduate nursing degrees from the University of Toronto. She has advanced clinical knowledge in the care of older adults and has been a Canadian Nurses Association certified gerontological nurse for 18 years.

Jennifer Hurley, MHSM, RN, RM
Manager, Professional Programs, Australian Nursing and Midwifery Federation (SA Branch)—BPSO Host

Jennifer Hurley is a registered nurse and midwife who has worked in a diverse range of leadership, clinical, informatics, and management roles across the acute, sub-acute, and community sector at state and national levels. As part of her current role as Manager, Professional Program, at the ANMF (SA Branch) and Manager of the Australian Best Practice Spotlight Organization Program, Hurley has led the establishment and implementation of the internationally recognized Registered Nurses' Association of Ontario BPSO Program in Australia—transferring the latest evidence into practice within SA Health sites. The BPSO Program is recognized as an enabler of nurses and midwives, leading the way with its bottom-up approach. Hurley has also had an integral role in the development of the SA Public Sector Safe Staffing model and the development and implementation of the supporting business rules that provide the framework for the ongoing development, monitoring, review, and management of this new staffing model. In her current role at ANMF (SA Branch), she supports the recognition and advancement of the essential role of nurses, midwives, and personal care assistants in the provision of health and aged care at a state level. Hurley represents members in a wide range of issues impacting the nursing and midwifery professions—and ultimately the health and well-being of the community.

Suman Iqbal, MSN/MHA, RN, CON(C)
Senior Manager, Long-Term Care (LTC) Best Practices Program, RNAO

Suman Iqbal is Senior Manager, Long-Term Care (LTC) Best Practices Program, at the Registered Nurses' Association of Ontario (RNAO), a position she has held since 2017. The primary functions of the role are to advance province-wide implementation and evaluation of Best Practice Guidelines (BPG) in the LTC sector by leading, coordinating, and developing program-based projects, resources, and activities. Prior to that, Iqbal was the LTC Best Practice Coordinator for Provincial Projects, where she led the review and development of the *LTC Best Practices Toolkit*, Second Edition, and the Nursing Orientation e-Resource. Iqbal is a registered nurse with a combined master of science in nursing and master of health administration from the University of Phoenix. She has over 30 years of experience in delivering person-centered care in acute care oncology and long-term care settings in various roles, including senior leadership. She has successfully established, led, and sustained positive change through best practice implementation and quality-improvement initiatives in long-term care and acute care, including Best Practice Spotlight Organization (BPSO) predesignation activities.

Sheila John, MScN, BScN, RN
Senior Manager, Mental Health & Addiction and Tobacco Intervention Initiative, RNAO

Sheila John is a registered nurse who is currently Senior Manager for Mental Health and Addiction and the Tobacco Intervention Initiative in the International Affairs and Best Practice Guidelines Centre at RNAO. She obtained her undergraduate nursing degree from Ryerson University and her master of science in nursing degree from D'Youville College in New York. John's work has primarily focused on mental health through roles as a Clinical Practice Leader at Rouge Valley Health System, Instructor for Durham College, and direct-care nurse at Trillium Health Partners. Her current role at RNAO involves overseeing the successful Mental Health and Addiction program and the Tobacco Intervention Initiative. John has managed the Tobacco Intervention Initiative during her 9 years at RNAO and is pleased to have added the Mental Health and Addiction program to her portfolio. She was also the guideline development lead for the BPG Integrating Tobacco Interventions into Daily Practice.

Zhao Junqiang, BScN, RN
BUCM School of Nursing—BPSO Direct-Academic

Zhao Junqiang is an MSN candidate, a member of Beijing University of Chinese Medicine Joanna Briggs Institute Centre of Excellence, and a member of the Beijing University of Chinese Medicine Best Practice Spotlight Organization (BPSO). Research interests include knowledge transfer and sustainability of guideline utilization. He has published 18 articles and participated in seven national, provincial, or university projects.

Bahar Karimi, MN, MHSc (HA), RN, CHE
Director of Resident Services, St. Peter's Residence at Chedoke-Thrive Group—
LTC-BPSO Direct-Service

Bahar Karimi is a health system leader with a history of progressive leadership that spans working as a personal support worker to a senior executive leader. She is passionate about leadership, teaching, politics, and the profession of nursing. She feels strongly that her calling as a nurse is to empower vulnerable and marginalized populations. She has been involved with multiple teams and professional and community organizations as a way to give back to society. Currently, Karimi is Director of Resident Services at St. Peter's Residence at Chedoke-Thrive Group, a 210-bed, nonprofit, long-term care facility in Hamilton. A strong nursing advocate, she is also a member of RNAO and President of the Hamilton Chapter Executive Team. Karimi was the RNAO liaison through St. Peter's BPSO candidacy process when the organization went through a significant culture shift toward evidence-based practice, demonstrating exceptional growth and strong commitment toward implementation of RNAO BPGs and contributing to many practice changes within the organization.

Nancy Lefebre, MScN, BScN, CHE, Extra Fellow, FCCHL
Chief Clinical Executive and Senior Vice President, Saint Elizabeth Health Care—
BPSO Direct-Service

Nancy Lefebre is responsible for advancing Saint Elizabeth's shared value strategy, positioning the organization as a leader in social innovation and impact. Her special interests include end-of-life care, knowledge mobilization, and community partnerships. In her quest to ensure that a strong evidence base underpins healthcare practices, Lefebre has established a strong clinical team and collaborative research center. One of the first nursing leaders in Canada to complete the Executive Training for Research Application (EXTRA) Fellowship program, Lefebre brings to Saint Elizabeth more than 25 years of experience in the North American healthcare sector, with a focus on community care. She is an Adjunct Lecturer at the Lawrence S. Bloomberg Faculty of Nursing, University of Toronto, and a former President of the Academy of Canadian Nurses.

Yan Lijiao, MS, RN
BUCM School of Nursing—BPSO Direct-Academic

Yan Lijiao was born in Hunan Province, China. She earned her master's degree from Beijing University of Chinese Medicine in 2014 and worked as a nurse in the University of Hong Kong-Shenzhen Hospital in 2014 and 2015. She now works at Beijing University School of Nursing and has been the BPSO Lead at Beijing University of Chinese Medicine since 2016. Her research field is evidence-based nursing. Since 2012, as the Principal Investigator involved in two school-level projects and as a participant involved in 10 projects, Lijiao has published six academic papers in Chinese core journals as the first author. The papers include one systematic review protocol registered in PROSPERO (international prospective register of systematic reviews) and one systematic review. She has been the second author on two academic papers, both systematic reviews published in clinical otolaryngology.

Monique Lloyd, PhD, RN
Principal Consultant, MAL Consulting

Monique Lloyd is a Research Consultant with extensive experience in and broad knowledge of nursing effectiveness and outcomes research. She has a strong interest in methods to synthesize and report nursing research, particularly approaches to increase the rigor and integrity of synthesis methods to ensure accurate and valid interpretation of the evidence. From 2011 to 2015, Lloyd was RNAO's Associate Director of Guideline Development, Research and Evaluation, overseeing the research processes of guidelines in development and revision. During her tenure, she led the transition from outsourcing guidelines' systematic reviews to a centralized, in-house research program. Lloyd also led the development and launch of NQuIRE (Nursing Quality Indicators for Research and Evaluation), an international quality measurement program evaluating the outcomes of RNAO Best Practice Guideline implementation.

Anne-Marie Malek, BN, MHSA, RN, CHE
President & CEO, West Park Healthcare Centre—BPSO Direct-Service

Anne-Marie Malek is President and Chief Executive Officer of West Park Healthcare Centre in Toronto. West Park provides a spectrum of post-acute services, including specialized rehabilitation, community living, complex continuing care, long-term care, primary care, and community outreach services. Malek has led several transformational change initiatives within the Healthcare Centre, driven its capital and strategic renewal, and assumed a lead role in the development of an LHIN-level population health strategy. Under her leadership, West Park was designated a Founding Best Practice Spotlight Organization of the RNAO. She has served on the boards of the Regional Geriatric Program of Toronto, the Public Services Health and Safety Association, and the West Park Family Health Team. She holds an Adjunct Lecturer appointment at the Institute of Health Policy, Management and Evaluation at the University of Toronto.

JoAnne MacDonald, PhD, MN, RN
Associate Professor, Rankin School of Nursing, St. Francis Xavier University—BPSO Direct-Academic

JoAnne MacDonald, PhD (University of Ottawa), MN (Dalhousie University), RN, is an Associate Professor with St. Francis Xavier University Rankin School of Nursing. She practiced in community/public health and maternity nursing for 22 years before joining St. Francis Xavier in 2008. She has taught community/public health nursing, research methods, healthcare trends and issues, nursing leadership, and health promotion. MacDonald is currently involved in a series of Best Practice Guideline research projects aimed at evaluating the integration of Best Practice Guidelines in undergraduate curriculum, the development of educational indicators to monitor the impact of Best Practice Guideline use in undergraduate curriculum, and the establishment of academe and health service provider partnerships to enhance evidence-based practice. MacDonald served as Curriculum Chair of the St. Francis Xavier University School of Nursing and as the Rankin School of Nursing Academic Best Practice Spotlight Organization lead.

Heather McConnell, MA(Ed), BScN, RN
Associate Director, Guideline Implementation and Knowledge Transfer, RNAO

Heather McConnell is Associate Director, Guideline Implementation and Knowledge Transfer, at the Registered Nurses' Association of Ontario, a position she has held since 2007. In this role, she leads a multifaceted implementation program to support the uptake of evidence in practice. This includes a range of strategies directed toward individual, organization, and systems levels. McConnell is a senior member of the Nursing Best Practice Research Centre (NBPRC). From 2001 to 2007, she was an RNAO Program Manager. Over her career, she has worked in a variety of settings, including academia, acute care, oncology, and home healthcare. Her clinical management experience includes direct-care and middle management in the home health sector, where she provided leadership to support evidence-based home health nursing services.

Susan McNeill, MPH, RN
Manager, Implementation Science, RNAO

Susan McNeill is a master's-prepared nurse who has a passion for dignified, quality care. She has a background in clinical nursing, program development, education, and population health promotion. She has practiced nursing in Canada, New York, and Bangladesh. Joining the Registered Nurses' Association of Ontario in 2012, McNeill has been the guideline development lead for three evidence-based Best Practice Guidelines: *Preventing and Addressing Abuse and Neglect of Older Adults: Person-Centred, Collaborative, System-Wide Approaches*; *Delirium, Dementia, and Depression in Older Adults: Assessment and Care* (2nd ed.); and *Preventing Falls and Reducing Injuries From Falls* (3rd ed.). She collaborates with the Canadian Patient Safety Institute as the Falls Intervention Lead. Her current role at the RNAO is focused on supporting the uptake of best practices through implementation science.

Sabrina Merali, MN, RN
Program Manager—Mental Health and Addiction Initiative, RNAO

Sabrina Merali has been Program Manager for the Mental Health and Addiction Initiative at the Registered Nurses' Association of Ontario International Affairs and Best Practice Guidelines Centre since 2012. She is a registered nurse with an honors bachelor's degree in health sciences, specializing in rural health, from the University of Western Ontario. Merali also obtained her bachelor of science in nursing and master of nursing from the University of Toronto, specializing in community health. She has experience in acute care and public healthcare systems, working in chronic disease management and prevention roles. Her roles included supporting clients pre- and post-transplantation, providing 1:1 counselling, working with diverse populations to promote health, utilizing community development and engagement techniques to foster supportive environments conducive to health, focusing on social determinants of health, and project management on community-wide implementation projects.

Josephine Mo, BA(hon)
Executive Assistant to the CEO and BPSO Latin America Program Coordinator, RNAO

Josephine Mo joined the RNAO team in 2011. From 2011 to 2013, she was Project Coordinator in the International Affairs and Best Practice Guidelines Program. In 2013, Mo assumed the position of Executive Assistant to CEO Doris Grinspun and Coordinator of the Latin America BPSO Program at RNAO. Driven by a spirit of inquiry and a desire to make a positive impact, she earned her bachelor of arts with honours in sociology and has established her career in the nonprofit sector. She is committed to the work of RNAO, an organization that speaks out for quality nursing and equitable healthcare with values, evidence, and courage. In addition to providing comprehensive administrative support to the CEO, she coordinates the implementation, research, evaluation, and spread of Best Practice Guidelines by academic and healthcare organizations in Latin America through the Best Practice Spotlight Organizations (BPSO) Program. In her role, Mo has also contributed to numerous submissions and events that advance the role of nurses and leverage their expertise to shape healthy public policy.

Teresa Moreno-Casbas, PhD, MSc, RN, FEAN
Director of the Spanish Nursing and Healthcare Research Unit (Investén-isciii), Instituto de Salud Carlos III; Head, BPSO Host in Spain—BPSO Host

Teresa Moreno-Casbas is the founding and current Director of the Nursing and Healthcare Research Unit (Investén-isciii) located at the Instituto de Salud Carlos III. She is also head of the BPSO Host in Spain. She obtained her RN degree in 1981 at the Universidad de Valladolid, a maîtrise en sciences at the University of Montreal in 1993, and a PhD in epidemiology and public health in 2007 at the Universidad Rey Juan Carlos. Her postdoctoral work at the University of Toronto focused on healthcare policy, promoting safe care for nurses and patients nationally and internationally. In 2012, in recognition of her expertise and substantive leadership and contributions to nursing scholarship, research, and practice in Spain and internationally, Moreno-Casbas was invested as a FEAN. She is a reviewer of national and international research proposals and of several scientific international nursing journals, and she is research leader of a Thematic Network on Healthy Ageing and Frailty (CIBERFES). She also has led several national and European-funded projects. Moreno-Casbas' program of research focuses on three objectives: 1) efficiency of healthcare services provided to elderly and frail people by nurses; 2) measurement of nursing process and nursing staffing characteristics and the impact of nursing on patient outcomes; and 3) enhancing evidence-based practice and knowledge transfer in nursing clinical practice and factors influencing knowledge translation.

Lynn Anne Mulrooney, PhD, MPH, RN
Senior Policy Analyst, RNAO

Lynn Anne Mulrooney is Senior Policy Analyst at the Registered Nurses' Association of Ontario (RNAO), a position she assumed in 2005. She has had the privilege of working as a staff nurse in Toronto, a community health nurse in Dene and Inuit communities in the Northwest Territories and Nunavut, and a community health nurse/relief worker in Ethiopia and Somalia. Mulrooney has a master of public health degree and a PhD in political science from the University of Hawaii at Manoa. Her work at RNAO includes public policy research and political action on health equity, social determinants of health, mental health, addiction, and human rights. She holds an Adjunct Lecturer appointment at the Lawrence S. Bloomberg Faculty of Nursing, University of Toronto.

Shanoja Naik, PhD, MPhil, MSc, BEd, BSc
Data Scientist/Statistician, RNAO

Shanoja Naik has been the Data Scientist/Statistician at the Registered Nurses' Association of Ontario since January 2017. Over the past 15 years, she has worked in various roles as scientist, researcher, manager (data analytics), and statistician/analyst in government, corporate, and academic settings. In addition, she held faculty roles at University of Waterloo and Trent University in Ontario, Canada, and Centre for Mathematical Sciences, Kerala, India. In 2010, Naik conferred her doctorate degree in statistics from Mahatma Gandhi University, India, focused on time series modeling, in her thesis titled *Pathway Distributions and Autoregressive Modeling*. She has several publications focused on various topics within vast specialty areas, including survival modeling, credit risk analysis, statistical mechanics, time series modeling, market research, and population studies [*Lifetime Data Analysis* (2017), *Axioms* (2016), *Indian Journal of Statistics* (2015), *Statistics and Probability Letters* (2014), *Statistical Papers* (2012), and others.]. In 2008, she was honoured by the United Nations for her contribution in methodological statistics. Naik has a master of philosophy in statistics specialized in multivariate analysis and least absolute value deviations; a master of science in statistics (thesis: *Uniformly Minimum Variance Unbiased Estimation and Applications*); a bachelor of science in statistics (top rank); and a bachelor of education in mathematics with interest in adult education and psychology from the Education and Training Department, University of Kerala, India.

Beth O'Leary, PMP
Program Manager, Senior-Friendly Strategy & Best Practice Implementation, Sunnybrook Health Sciences Centre—BPSO Direct-Service

Prior to joining the Sunnybrook team, O'Leary had a number of rehabilitation consulting and leadership roles with the Workplace Health, Safety & Compensation Commission in New Brunswick. As well, she undertook case management and rehabilitation consulting roles with insurer and legal representatives in Ontario, managing care for individuals catastrophically injured in motor vehicle accidents, especially those with acquired brain injury. More recently, O'Leary has been involved in project management at Sunnybrook, leading clinical unit/program/corporate initiatives addressing RNAO best practice implementation and a senior-friendly strategy.

Yaw O. Owusu, PhD, MS, MSc, BSc
Former Associate Director, Evaluation & Monitoring, RNAO

Yaw O. Owusu was Associate Director (2015 to December 2017), Evaluation and Monitoring within the International Affairs and Best Practice Guidelines Centre at the Registered Nurses' Association of Ontario (RNAO). He has a PhD in health policy with a specialization in health economics from the Centre for Health Economics and Policy Analysis (CHEPA) at McMaster University, Hamilton, Ontario. He has a strong appreciation of large data systems, evidence-based policy, and health economic analysis. With robust expertise in these areas, Owusu has been invited to present to varied audiences, including policymakers, executive leaders, and fellow researchers. In 2013, he was recognized with the Ontario Health Human Resource Research Network (OHHRRN) Award.

Tasha Penney, MN, RN
Former Implementation Manager, Mental Health and Addiction Initiative, RNAO

Tasha Penney is former Implementation Manager for the Mental Health and Addiction Initiative at the Registered Nurses' Association of Ontario, a position she assumed in 2017. Her portfolio includes overseeing the development of evidence-based resources and the implementation and dissemination activities aimed at increasing nurses' capacity in the area of mental health and substance use. From 2013 to 2017, she was Manager of Research overseeing the development process of all systematic reviews conducted by the research team, leading the development of BPG, as well as managing RNAO's Advanced Clinical Practice Fellowship (ACPF) program. She is a member of the Nursing Best Practice Research Centre (NBPRC) and Sigma Theta Tau International Honor Society of Nursing (Lambda Pi at-Large Chapter). Penney completed a master of nursing at Ryerson University with a specialization in the health and well-being of communities. She has extensive clinical experience working with marginalized and vulnerable populations with major mental illness. She is currently leading the development of RNAO's Supervised Injection Services BPG, which is scheduled for release in 2018.

Holly Quinn, MHS, BScN, RN
National Director: Clinical/Quality; Chief Nursing Officer, Bayshore HealthCare Ltd.—BPSO Direct-Service

Holly Quinn has contributed to the health and well-being of Canadians through a variety of nursing roles within the acute and home care sectors over a 40-year span. She attained her nursing diploma from George Brown College, St. Michael's Campus, followed by her BScN from Laurentian University and her master's in health studies from Athabasca University. Quinn currently works for Bayshore HealthCare Ltd. as Chief Nursing Officer and National Director: Clinical/Quality, where her passion for a culture of clinical excellence, innovation, transformation, and engagement has supported excellence in client care and healthy work environments for regulated and unregulated care professionals.

Karen L. Ray, MSc, RN
Manager of Knowledge Translation, Saint Elizabeth Health Care—BPSO Direct-Service

Karen L. Ray leads, directs, and supports the creation, dissemination, exchange, and management of knowledge by participating in research activities and putting evidence into practice. Her leadership has been a key part of enabling and putting into practice Saint Elizabeth's activities as an RNAO Best Practice Spotlight Organization. This includes working with the clinical practice team to implement and evaluate guidelines, participating in RNAO sustainability activities, and acting as a mentor for numerous fellowships.

Michelle Rey, PhD, MSc, BSc
Senior Manager in Clinical Programs, Centre for Addictions and Mental Health

Michelle Rey was the Associate Director, Evidence and Guideline Development, at RNAO from 2015 to 2017. She oversaw the research and evidence development teams and the methodology for guideline development. In addition, she oversaw the inception of RNAO's patient and public engagement initiative. Prior to joining RNAO, Rey was Clinical Manager at Cancer Care Ontario, where she led the national engagement in the review of cancer drug-funding sustainability. She was Research Director at the Ivey International Centre for Health Innovation at Western University, where she led development of the research strategy and execution of health innovation research projects. Rey was Interim Director, Performance Measurement & Reporting, at Health Quality Ontario, where she was the lead, and the Ontario Primary Care Performance Measurement Initiative. She has a PhD in medical genetics from the University of Toronto and master and bachelor of science degrees in biochemistry from Queens University. Rey is currently a Senior Manager in Clinical Programs at the Centre for Addictions and Mental Health.

Tian Runxi, MSN, RN
Chief Head Nurse, DongZhiMen Hospital, Affiliated to Beijing University of Chinese Medicine—BPSO Direct-Service

Tian Runxi was born in Beijing, China. She graduated from Beijing University of Chinese Medicine in 2013. She is the Chief Head Nurse and BPSO Lead in DongZhiMen Hospital. She also works as the Adjunct Teacher of Beijing University of Chinese Medicine. She is a member of the Nursing Education Research Association of the Higher Education Association of Chinese medicine, the youth council of the nursing administration branch of Beijing Nursing Association, and the youth council of the nursing branch of the Chinese medical association. She has led two research projects and published eight first-author academic papers. She has also applied for two patents. Her research interests are evidence-based nursing, clinical nursing, and nursing education.

Aracelly Serna Restrepo, BScN
Head of the Nursing Department at the Cardioinfantil Foundation Cardiology Institute (FCI-IC)—BPSO Direct-Service

Aracelly Serna Restrepo is a registered nurse leader who graduated from the University of Caldas. She obtained a certificate in health human resources management and organizational development from the University of Rosario. She also is a faculty member for graduate studies in administration and business of the University of Rosario. She has been at the helm of FCI-IC since 2010.

Shirlee M. Sharkey, CHE, MHSc, BScN, BA
President & CEO, Saint Elizabeth Health Care—BPSO Direct-Service

Shirlee M. Sharkey's background as a registered nurse with experience in a variety of healthcare settings has infused her 2 1/2 decades of leadership of Saint Elizabeth to influence and guide her staff and the health system. Her vision of the possibilities in the home care space allowed her to nurture and grow Saint Elizabeth into a national healthcare enterprise delivering direct care, virtual services, consultancy, and research support. Sharkey serves on numerous boards and panels ranging from health to education and was one of the early Presidents of the Canadian Home Care Association. She is an Adjunct Professor at the Faculty of Nursing, University of Toronto, and has a cross appointment at the Institute of Health Policy Management and Evaluation, University of Toronto. Under Sharkey's leadership, Saint Elizabeth was among the first healthcare organizations that partnered with the RNAO to develop and implement nursing Best Practice Guidelines and to achieve designation as a Best Practice Spotlight Organization.

Ronald Gary Sibbald, MD, BSc, FRCPC (Med, Derm)
MACP, FAAD, MEd, FAPWCA, DSc(hon)

Ronald Gary Sibbald is a dermatologist and internist with a special interest in wound care and education. He is a Professor of Medicine and Public Health at the University of Toronto and an international wound care key opinion leader (educator, clinician, and clinical researcher). Sibbald is co-founder of the Canadian Association of Wound Care and former Director of the Wound Healing Clinic, Women's College Hospital. He is also Past President of the World Union of Wound Healing Societies (2012–2016). In 1999, he co-developed the International Interprofessional Wound Care Course and has been the Director for 31 courses worldwide. He has over 200 publications and is Coeditor and chapter author of the *Chronic Wound Care 5* textbook. Sibbald received the Queen Elizabeth II Diamond Jubilee medal in 2013 and honorary doctor of science from Excelsior College in 2014. Sibbald was a Cochair of the RNAO Assessment and Management of Pressure Injuries BPG, published in 2016.

Amalia Silva-Galleguillos, MSc, RN
BPSO Leader, Nursing Department, University of Chile—BPSO Host-Academia

Amalia Silva-Galleguillos is a doctoral candidate at the Universidad Complutense de Madrid. She holds a master's in international public health; a master's in research in healthcare; a diploma in competence-based education; a diploma in nursing in medical-surgical emergency care; a diploma in teaching of biomedical sciences; training in evidence-based nursing from the Institute for Johns Hopkins Nursing; and a degree in nursing-obstetrics. She currently is an Associate Professor in the Department of Nursing, University of Chile, with more than 23 years of experience in pre- and post-graduate teaching and curriculum development. Silva-Galleguillos is also the National Coordinator for the Pan American Health Organization (PAHO) Evidence-Based Nursing Network and Director of the Journal of the Nursing Department, University of Chile. She has served in various positions of senior academic management at the University of Chile, and for 4 years, she was in charge of the Commission of the National Examination of Nursing as part of the Chilean Association of Education in Nursing. Silva-Galleguillos is a RNAO-certified BPSO orientation trainer.

Kyle Smith, BSc
Database/web developer, RNAO

Kyle Smith is a Database/Web Developer at the Registered Nurses' Association of Ontario (RNAO) and is Lead Developer of the Nursing Quality Indicators for Reporting and Evaluation (NQuIRE) system. He began working at RNAO in March 2013 and took over the development of the NQuIRE system. Over the next 5 years, he has added many new features to the system, including custom reports, a custom data import module, and user training videos. Smith also works on other projects at RNAO, including the BPSO database. Prior to working at RNAO, he worked in the bioinformatics and software quality assurance fields. He holds a bachelor of science degree from McMaster University and a bioinformatics certificate from Seneca College.

Janet E. Squires, PhD, RN
Associate Professor, Scientist, University of Ottawa, Ottawa Hospital Research Institute

Janet E. Squires' research is focused on improving knowledge translation by healthcare professionals. Her current research centers on the design, implementation, and evaluation of theory-informed and context-optimized interventions to increase healthcare professionals' use of research and research-based behaviours as a strategy to contribute to improved patient and system outcomes. Her research program has four main foci: 1) exploring organizational context and its role in knowledge translation; 2) designing and testing theory-informed interventions to change healthcare professionals' behaviours; 3) measurement and survey design/psychometrics; and 4) systematic reviews. She is currently involved in several nationally funded projects examining the role of context in knowledge translation and developing and testing interventions to change behaviour of healthcare professionals (e.g., increasing organ donation in adult hospitals, improving hand hygiene practice in adult hospitals, improving pain practices in paediatric hospitals, and improving resident outcomes in nursing homes).

Althea Stewart-Pyne, MHSc, RN
Program Manager, Healthy Work Environment, RNAO

Althea Stewart-Pyne is a master's-prepared registered nurse and a graduate of York University. Since 2009, she has led the development of the Healthy Work Environment Best Practice Guidelines at the

Registered Nurses' Association of Ontario's International Affairs and Best Practice Guidelines (IAB-PG). These guidelines are positioned as evidence-based resources to transfer knowledge to healthcare professionals. Stewart-Pyne promotes an evidence-based approach to optimize health delivery through partnerships across the care continuum. A strategic thinker with proven health system leadership competencies and skills, she has over 25 years of experience in healthcare management and demonstrated achievements in hospital and community health. Stewart-Pyne is passionate about her leadership role in creating healthy work environments that improve the quality of working life for nurses.

Ru Taggar, MN, RN
Vice President, Quality and Patient Safety, Chief Nursing and Health Professions Executive, Sunnybrook Health Sciences Centre—BPSO Direct-Service

Ru Taggar is Vice President, Quality & Patient Safety, Chief Nursing and Health Professions Executive at Sunnybrook Health Sciences Centre. He is also Vice President, Trauma, Emergency & Critical Care, including Burns and Neurosurgery and the Women & Babies' Program. Through this role, Taggar has led the development of the hospital's Enterprise Risk Management Program, the Quality Improvement Plan, and the hospital-wide Patient Centred Care and Interprofessional Care strategies. Most recently, she oversaw the development of Sunnybrook's first quality strategic plan. She holds an Adjunct Clinical appointment at the Lawrence Bloomberg Faculty of Nursing, University of Toronto. She is also a guest lecturer in the Master's of Quality & Patient Safety Program through the university's HPME Program. Taggar is Cochair of the Toronto Academic Health Science Network (TAHSN) Practice Committee and is a member of TAHSN's Health Analytics Advisory Committee. She is also a board member of the Regional Geriatric Program (RGP).

Carol Timmings, MEd (Admin), BNSc, RN
Director, Child Health and Development and Chief Nursing Officer, Toronto Public Health—BPSO Direct-Service

Carol Timmings is Director, Child Health and Development, and CNO with Toronto Public Health. She holds a bachelor of nursing science degree and a master of education degree in policy and administration, both from Queen's University. As Chief Nursing Officer with Toronto Public Health, Timmings is also responsible for nursing human resource planning, quality nursing practice, and enhancing nursing contributions to organizational effectiveness related to improved health outcomes at individual, group, and population levels. She is President of the Registered Nurses' Association of Ontario (RNAO) for the April 2016 to April 2018 term. She is also a member of the advisory board for the National Collaborating Centre for Determinants of Health. In 2010, Timmings received the Association of Local Public Health Agencies Distinguished Service Award in recognition of her outstanding leadership and contributions to public health in Ontario. OPHA also honoured her in 2015 with a Lifetime Membership Award in recognition of her outstanding leadership and contributions to the association.

Gurjit Kaur Toor, MPH, BScN, RN
Evaluation Manager, RNAO

Gurjit Kaur Toor is Evaluation Manager in the International Affairs and Best Practice Guideline Centre (IABPG) at the Registered Nurses' Association of Ontario (RNAO), a position she has held since 2017. From 2015 to 2017, she was RNAO's Data Quality Analyst. She works closely with the Best Practice Spotlight Organizations (BPSO) to evaluate the impact of their guideline implementation efforts. Toor provides education and training for nurses to evaluate evidence-based practice changes, develop resources for guideline evaluation, and use the Nursing Quality Indicators for Reporting and Evaluation (NQuIRE) data system. She also leads the continuous data quality improvements for NQuIRE and provides consultation on both implementation and evaluation measures, including NQuIRE indicators. Toor has a master of public health (MPH) in epidemiology from the University of Toronto and graduated with distinction from McMaster University with her bachelor of science in nursing. She also has a bachelor of science from McGill University. She draws from a breadth of clinical experiences in acute care and public health and is passionate about building evaluation capacity and bringing the evaluator out in every nurse.

Tazim Virani, PhD, RN
Senior Lead Strategic Initiatives
Saint Elizabeth Health Care—BPSO Direct-Service

Tazim Virani has over 30 years of experience working in clinical, management, research, and education spheres, largely with healthcare systems in Canada. She was the founding Director of the RNAO's Nursing Best Practice Guidelines Program for its first 8 years (1998 to 2007), as well as the Codirector of the Nursing Best Practice Research Unit for the same period. Under her leadership, many of the BPG Program's building blocks were established including the first 30 clinical Best Practice Guidelines, the Best Practice Champions Network, and the Best Practice Spotlight Organization Designation, as well as numerous research studies. Virani was a recipient of the RNAO Best Practice Doctoral Fellowship to study the sustainability of Best Practice Guidelines at the organizational level. She continues to champion evidence-based practice at all levels from direct care to system policy. Currently, she is focusing on innovations to transform healthcare.

Leeann Whitney, MAEd, BScN, RN
Executive Director, North Bay Nurse Practitioner-Led Clinic—BPSO Direct-Service

Leeann Whitney, BScN (Laurentian University), MAEd (Central Michigan University), is the Executive Director at the North Bay Nurse Practitioner-Led Clinic (NBNPLC) in North Bay, Ontario. She has an extensive background in nursing including acute care, nursing education, public health, and nursing administration. Whitney was instrumental in the NBNPLC's achievement of RNAO Best Practice Spotlight Organization in 2015. She is maintaining a membership with RNAO, CNO, and the Community Health Nurses Interest Group. Whitney currently teaches casually at Nipissing University, North Bay, Ontario, where she has taught courses in nursing informatics, community health nursing, nursing theory, leadership, and current nursing issues. She is very proud of the work RNAO has achieved in advancing the profession of nursing.

Rita Wilson, MEd, MN, RN
eHealth Program Manager, RNAO

Rita Wilson is the eHealth Program Manager at RNAO, a position she assumed in 2011. Her passion for technology and nursing fuels her drive to optimize patient safety and health outcomes by developing and disseminating technological solutions that foster evidence-based practice. Wilson is also leading the cutting-edge work on development of nursing order sets (NOS) to complement RNAO's Best Practice Guidelines. RNAO's NOS are designed to translate knowledge into practice as they are embedded into electronic health information systems.

Hao Yufang, PhD
Professor, BUCM School of Nursing—BPSO-Direct, Academic

Hao Yufang is Dean of the School of Nursing at the Beijing University of Chinese Medicine. She is an academic leader; Consultant of the Beijing University of Chinese Medicine Centre for Evidence-Based Nursing, a Joanna Briggs Institute Centre of Excellence; BPSO sponsor; member of the nursing education steering committee of the Ministry of Education; and chair of the Nursing Education Research Association of the Chinese Higher Medical Education Academy of Chinese Medicine. Her research interests include nursing education, Chinese medicine nursing, and evidence-based nursing.

TABLE OF CONTENTS

UNIT 4 INSPIRING AND MANAGING IMPLEMENTATION ON A GLOBAL SCALE 285

FOREWORD

Transforming Nursing Through Knowledge: Best Practices for Guideline Development, Implementation Science, and Evaluation by Doris Grinspun and Irmajean Bajnok is a one-of-a-kind book. Not only does it provide the best methods for creating evidence-based guidelines, but it describes the most effective strategies for implementing them in a variety of healthcare and academic settings.

Although a wealth of studies document the positive outcomes associated with evidence-based care, translation of evidence into clinical practice still occurs at a snail's pace because of multiple barriers that continue to exist in healthcare systems throughout the world. How to overcome these barriers in implementing evidence-based guidelines is a highlight of this book. Grinspun and Bajnok have a wealth of expertise in guideline development, implementation, and evaluation that is exquisitely shared in this book.

This book is a must-read because it is based on solid guidelines produced by the Registered Nurses' Association of Ontario (RNAO) and real-world implementation of these guidelines by organizations throughout Canada and the world. It provides the lived experience of healthcare and academic organizations, allowing readers to gain keen insight into what works best in translating evidence into practice to ultimately improve healthcare quality and patient outcomes.

Unique to this book is its emphasis on using technology to ease and speed the implementation of evidence-based guidelines into practice and its focus on using evidence to drive health policy. Stephen R. Covey, the famous American motivational speaker, said, "To know but not to do is really not to know." Therefore, I encourage everyone who reads this book to take action on its terrific content and rapidly put the knowledge gained into practice—as all people throughout the world deserve the best care.

–Bernadette Mazurek Melnyk, PhD, RN, CRNP, FAANP, FNAP, FAAN
Vice President for Health Promotion
University Chief Wellness Officer
Dean and Professor, College of Nursing
Professor of Pediatrics and Psychiatry, College of Medicine
Executive Director, the Helene Fuld Health Trust National Institute for
Evidence-Based Practice in Nursing and Healthcare
The Ohio State University, Ohio, USA

INTRODUCTION

This book was born out of a deep desire to share our expertise in developing a world-class, evidence-based practice (EBP) program that has achieved exceptional results through the use of best practice guidelines (BPG), transforming the practice of nurses and enriching the lives of patients in Ontario, Canada, and abroad. The book will be of interest to those who wish to learn from the evolution of a successful large-scale global program focused on advancing EBP—evidence to education, evidence to clinical practice, evidence to work environments, and evidence to policy—to bring about deep individual, organizational, and health system change. It will also be of interest to researchers, faculty, staff development educators, and students, who will benefit from the theoretical components related to all aspects of guideline development, implementation science, and outcomes evaluation. It will inspire healthcare organizations in any sector and invite them to join in this phenomenal movement to optimize their patients' and organizational outcomes.

The goal of this book is to share the extraordinary yet purposeful evolution of the RNAO Best Practice Guidelines (BPG) Program, from its inception in 1998 to its central position in international nursing and health services today. This purposeful evolution is present in the conceptualization and programmatic approach, as well as within and across all three pillars of the program from guideline development, to implementation, to evaluation.

From conceptual and programmatic underpinnings to lived experiences of faculty, students, nurse executives, direct nurses, and other health professionals, the book in its transparency leaves no stone unturned so others can gain from our expertise and learnings. It provides the reader with the latest in guideline development, implementation science, and evaluation at scale; and it expands current thinking about health system change. The book showcases exemplars in academic and service organizations all over the world, conquering context and language differences, to make teaching and clinical practice the best they can be. Several chapters focus on the lived experience of using BPGs in academia and service organizations in powerful ways to make EBP a reality. These chapters can be used as a guide to those aiming to advance evidence-based teaching and practice.

The special features in each chapter will be meaningful to all readers, in particular nursing students and the academic and staff development nurse educator audience. These features include:

- Learning objectives

- Critical thinking/reflection questions

- Key messages highlighted for quick review

- Short segments of voices from the field reflecting quotes or comments from BPG developers, users, and evaluators

- Case studies

Clinicians and administrators preparing for adoption of evidence-based practice will find this book beneficial as a source of knowledge and inspiration. In particular, the examples of how organizations have prepared their work environment and taken steps to initiate and sustain practice and culture change will energize those seeking similar transformation. The wealth of knowledge embodied in this book will inform both faculty and students about guideline development, implementation science, monitoring, and evaluation.

The book will be a guide to faculty aiming to enhance the curriculum and student learning through integration of BPGs. It will also appeal to researchers interested in guideline development, implementation and evaluation, and the links between evidence-based guidelines, evidence-based practice, and evidence-based policy.

Policy experts will value success stories on how to optimize knowledge transfer and evidence uptake at the health system level, and how to create evidence-based cultures and sustained practice change using best evidence in healthcare settings. Researchers and health system planners will be intrigued by our experience using both conventional and social-movement approaches to envision, plan, deliver, and sustain in strength and fidelity a large-scale health system change within and outside one country's borders.

It is recommended that *Transforming Nursing Through Knowledge* be included as a textbook in undergraduate and graduate nursing curricula, and as a reference in other nursing and clinical courses, as well as research, leadership, management, program development, policy, and evaluation courses. It is designed to be a "go to" book for healthcare organizations, chief transformational officers, health executives including nurses, and all professionals interested in creating evidence-based cultures: how to get started, move forward, and achieve results. Finally, it can serve as an important reference for those in the quality improvement, patient safety, risk management, policy development, and evaluation fields.

The book contains an introductory chapter in Unit 0, followed by 16 chapters divided into five units, addressing the three pillars of guideline development, implementation, and evaluation. In particular, Unit 1 focuses on guideline development, Units 2, 3, and 4 address key aspects of guideline implementation, and Unit 5 is devoted to guideline evaluation. Each unit progresses from theoretical chapters to chapters that address application and lived experiences. The book ends with a closing chapter in Unit 6 that brings to the reader the urgent need for nurses and other health professionals to leverage evidence-based practice and evidence-based policy to drive healthy public policy.

The introductory chapter in Unit 0, *Setting the Stage*, recounts the inspiring beginning that reflects the conceptual underpinnings of the RNAO BPG Program—embedded in a strong philosophy of knowledge-based caring. It then details the purposeful evolution and social movement approach to the program in each of the three pillars. This chapter concludes with a discussion of the elements, in particular collective identity, that have made this program such a resounding success. The chapters in Unit 1, *Guideline Development: First Pillar for Success*, provide seminal knowledge about guideline development and its importance, addressing both clinical practice and healthy work environment guidelines. The reader learns about RNAO's groundbreaking work in each of these areas, which are foundational to the full expression of the BPG Program.

The chapters in Unit 2, *Implementation Science: Second Pillar for Success*, provide a wealth of information beginning with the theory of implementation science, and addressing how RNAO has used technology to enable and extend BPG use, and the many supports at the micro, meso, and macro levels that move implementation from a science to action. In this unit, we also share extraordinary knowledge-translation methods, including the most popular one at the organizational meso level—the Best Practice Spotlight Organization (BPSO) Designation. Service and academic BPSOs share in their own words case studies, stories, quotes, and lessons learned. The chapters in Unit 3, *Scaling Up, Scaling Out, and Scaling Deep: System-Wide Implementation*, provide several successful examples of RNAO's approaches to BPG Program scaling at broad regional, provincial, and national levels, reflecting program adaptations to ensure both fit to context and fidelity to philosophy and program parameters.

The chapters in Unit 4, *Inspiring and Managing Implementation on a Global Scale*, illustrate how spread has extended to the world stage, where BPSOs are acknowledged as the means to ignite the passion of direct-care nurses and students, the support of administrators and faculty, the engagement of other healthcare professions including senior executives in service and academia, and the interest of the public, to enhance the quality of care and teaching for the benefit of patients globally. Unique viewpoints and experiences about evidence-based education and clinical practice in combination with culture and context from BPSOs in China, Chile, Colombia, and Spain make the unit distinctive in its transparency and display of raw passion for this work.

The chapters in Unit 5, *Evaluating Outcomes, Proving Results: Third Pillar for Success*, demonstrate the brilliance of NQuIRE as a comprehensive international data system of indictors that measures the outcomes of BPG implementation. NQuIRE is both validating and challenging our understanding of BPG use and its impact in nursing and healthcare. A specific application of NQuIRE data shows both the value of this data system in monitoring, measurement, and evaluation as well as the influence of evidence-based practice on economic outcomes. Included here is the experience in Australia of showing the clinical and economic outcomes of using BPGs through the BPSO movement.

The closing chapter in Unit 6, *Next Steps: From Practice to Policy*, is an urgent call for nurses to become a body politic to heighten the profession's contribution to the public as evidence-based experts. It presents conceptually and through the use of two powerful case studies how a nursing organization works, as a collective and in partnership with others, to leverage evidence-based practice and evidence-based policy to drive healthy public policy for all.

UNIT 0: SETTING THE STAGE

Chapter 1, by Grinspun, provides the conceptual and programmatic underpinnings of the BPG Program led by RNAO. It highlights a broad conceptualization of caring that encompasses the cognitive, physical, and relational dimensions of nursing practice. It explains why the focus on nursing knowledge, broadly defined in this way, is so important for patient, healthcare organizations, academic institutions, and health system outcomes. It underscores the value add of a program specifically designed to develop, disseminate, and support nurses to implement evidence-based knowledge in their day-to-day practice. Moving from theory and concepts to the programmatic and institutional background, the chapter then recounts the 2-decade history of RNAO's BPG Program, focusing on its origins, goals, design, scientific basis, purposeful evolution, and social movement thinking that drive its success. It points to the uniqueness of the BPG Program that focuses on: 1) guideline development; 2) dissemination, implementation, and sustainability; and 3) monitoring and evaluation. It showcases the nursing and broader context in Ontario, Canada that makes this program possible and its extraordinary national and international expansion from its inception to date. The final section highlights the seven key factors that have made this program the success it is today and expands on the concept of collective identity.

UNIT 1: GUIDELINE DEVELOPMENT—FIRST PILLAR FOR SUCCESS

Chapter 2, by Rey, Grinspun, Costantini, and Lloyd, provides an overview of guideline development and the importance of robust evidence-based guidelines in healthcare today. RNAO's seven-step, rigorous guideline development process (that is consistent with the AGREE II Standards) is highlighted, with attention to the overall purpose of each step of guideline development and the ongoing attention to quality improvement. Aspects of the development process featured are the enhanced systematic review, the modified-Delphi process used for building recommendations, and the progression of RNAO's application of GRADE (Grading of Recommendations Assessment, Development and Evaluation) to mark the quality of evidence and strength of the recommendations. The chapter provides answers to key challenges in guideline development such as timelines, resources, keeping guidelines current, and teaming up with experts to achieve maximum results.

Chapter 3, by Bajnok and Stewart-Pyne, identifies the strong links between work environments and uptake of EBP, clinical BPGs, and clinical excellence. Highlighted are RNAO's impetus behind the initiation of Healthy Work Environment Best Practice Guidelines (HWE BPGs) and the model of healthy work environments that guided the processes. The chapter also outlines the participatory processes used to identify and evaluate the early foundational BPGs and how these have been implemented in workplaces in all sectors. The chapter provides an overview of the outcomes of HWE BPG implementation, including enhanced provider satisfaction and sustained uptake of clinical practice guidelines, leading to better client and organizational outcomes. Concluding the chapter is a case study outlining HWE BPG implementation and resulting organizational changes that impacted successful clinical BPG uptake.

UNIT 2: IMPLEMENTATION SCIENCE: SECOND PILLAR FOR SUCCESS

Chapter 4, by Grinspun, McConnell, Virani, and Squires, provides the foundation for RNAO's groundbreaking work in BPG implementation at the micro, meso, and macro levels. Each of RNAO's signature implementation strategies is highlighted with a brief history along with key evidence based in implementation science that was used to shape and support the strategy. Discussed are the RNAO Champion Network; the RNAO Learning Institutes including the BPG Institute; and RNAO's popular Implementation Toolkit and Educator's Resource. These tools synthesize best evidence and related recommendations to direct guideline implementation in both service and academia. Finally, the Best Practice Spotlight Organization (BPSO) Designation is briefly outlined (to be discussed in detail in Chapter 6), as well as system-level implementation strategies, with both regional and national reach (discussed in detail in Chapter 10). Future perspectives close the chapter and address such areas as patient engagement, technology, deimplementation, and how RNAO is building a research collaboratory to contribute to implementation science through on-the-ground participatory research.

Chapter 5, by Wilson and Bajnok, showcases RNAO's technology-related resources to support evidence-based practice. The chapter highlights RNAO's contribution to nursing and eHealth and to advancing the nursing profession's full engagement in eHealth. From this beginning, key resources are discussed that showcase technology as an enabler of evidence-based practice. These resources include RNAO's BPG App that is accessed around the world by thousands of students, faculty, nurses, and other health professionals; RNAO's evidence-based nursing order sets, including samples that outline key features and their coding to the international classification of nursing practice (ICNP); and RNAO's BPG on supporting clinician and patient involvement in design and adoption of technology in healthcare.

Chapter 6, by Bajnok, Grinspun, McConnell, and Davies, focuses on the BPSO Designation and how its vision is being realized through the key implementation supports for the BPSOs. Detailed in the chapter is a discussion of the formal BPSO Agreement and how it defines and strengthens the BPSO Designation, leading to full engagement, commitment to achieve deliverables, sustained BPG implementation, and evaluation of results. It discusses the purpose and impact of the BPSO Orientation Program, coaching model, capacity building, implementation, evaluation, and reporting requirements. The elements of the RNAO Implementation Toolkit and how they are incorporated into the BPSO Designation to inform a structured implementation methodology are briefly outlined. The important roles of peer BPSOs and Designated BPSO Mentors in knowledge translation and building a collective identity are presented. Concluding the chapter is a view of the future in relation to dynamic sustainment and fidelity in the BPSO Designation.

Chapter 7, by Sharkey, Lefebre, Ray, Malek, Bell, Taggar, O'Leary, and DasGupta, launches the first in-depth discussion of BPSOs and their lived experiences. The chapter features three BPSOs: a home healthcare organization, a complex continuing care organization, and an acute care organization, representing both the "pioneer" BPSOs, and those who followed. Each BPSO speaks from the perspectives of their motivation to become a BPSO, unique successes and challenges, how the BPSO Designation shaped their current work culture, and what has enabled them to sustain and expand their work some 5 to 15 years later. Lastly, the chapter provides insights into how these leaders and leading organizations plan to take their BPSO work into the future.

In Chapter 8, by Timmings, O'Neil, Whitney, Quinn, and Canzian, five BPSOs from across all sectors (and ranging from early to more recent cohorts) tell their powerful stories. The BPSOs discuss why they chose to join the BPSO movement, how they got started, what their successes and challenges were, what the overall organizational impact was, and how the BPSO Designation defines their organization today. Plan to be amazed at how the BPSO Designation has transformed practice in a public health unit; defined and broadened primary care in a Nurse Practitioner-Led Clinic; contributed to national dissemination of evidence-based practice in a home healthcare organization; supported a community hospital in achieving a person-centered care cultural revolution; and finally how an acute care setting implemented numerous BPGs to create a "tsunami of evidence-based practice" across the entire organization.

Chapter 9, by MacDonald, Silva-Galleguillos, Gómez Díaz, and Bajnok, presents a world-view of BPSOs in academia through collective experiences of academic BPSOs in Canada, Chile, and Colombia. The chapter commences with a brief history of RNAO's early work in academia. Of particular focus here are the development of the Educator's Resource to support BPG integration in the curriculum and faculty's use of BPGs that led to the formal academic BPSO Designation popular around the world today. Also included is an overview of how academic BPSOs shape their undergraduate and graduate nursing curricula to integrate RNAO BPGs and evidence-based practice. Readers will appreciate gaining a perspective on the different BPG-integration approaches used globally and the discussion of their impact on curricula, faculty, students, and healthcare organization partners.

UNIT 3: SCALING UP, SCALING OUT, AND SCALING DEEP: SYSTEM-WIDE IMPLEMENTATION

Chapter 10, by McConnell, Merali, John, McNeill, and Bajnok, outlines factors that influence successful scaling up, out, and deep at micro, meso, and macro levels. Three case studies are presented that relate to specific RNAO projects based on selected BPGs in the areas of mental health and addiction, smoking cessation, and falls prevention. This chapter charts the work of each initiative. It describes how critical BPG-related health outcomes in each of the above areas have been impacted at regional, provincial, and national levels, across a variety of sectors, through maximizing system-wide engagement. Successful scaling strategies used in each project are highlighted, demonstrating the strategic focus of RNAO on different aspects of scaling from increasing exposure to influencing policy to impacting culture.

Chapter 11, by Holmes, Iqbal, Karimi, McConnell, and Bajnok, describes the Long-Term Care (LTC) Best Practices Program and its 15-year history. Key resources, including the LTC coordinators as BPG implementation facilitators, web-based tools used around the world, and an active Champion program, are featured. This chapter also showcases the development and phenomenal success of the LTC BPSO Designation—boasting growth to over 50 organizations in just three years. Central to the chapter is an illustration of the scaling approaches used to shape the BPSO Designation to fit the long-term care culture while maintaining program fidelity.

UNIT 4: INSPIRING AND MANAGING IMPLEMENTATION ON A GLOBAL SCALE

Chapter 12, by Bajnok, Grinspun, and Grdisa, addresses the overall impact of the BPSO Designation and how this has and will increasingly influence nursing and healthcare worldwide. Focal in the chapter is the use of Rogers' diffusion theory to document factors that have influenced the phenomenal spread of RNAO BPGs and the BPSO Designation globally. The BPSO Direct and Host Models are examined, delineating their role in facilitating the management and sustainment of this broad spread. Also explained are pivotal approaches to BPSO quality assurance and fidelity, such as the BPSO Orientation Program, audit and feedback process, and training-of-trainers model. These approaches all support effective global spread, while ensuring consistency and engaging local and international BPSO partners. The chapter wraps up with a futuristic view of the BPSO Designation and emerging new directions necessary as the BPSO Designation continues to go viral.

Chapter 13, by Moreno-Casbas, González-María, and Albornos-Muñoz, showcases the birth of RNAO's international focus, beginning in Spain with the translation of all RNAO BPGs into Spanish, extending to development of the BPSO Host Model to support this long-distance BPSO, and resulting in designation of their first Spanish BPSOs, three years later. The chapter also features the growth of Spain's BPSO Designation, which in five years has expanded to 81 organizations in a variety of sectors and academia, all across the country. RNAO's social movement philosophy and purposeful evolution of the BPG program are evident in discussions of Spain's strong contribution to NQuIRE's development and BPG impact evaluation, as well as key implementation science and evaluation lessons learned. These have been shared with and have benefitted all BPSOs, contributing greatly to the collective identity in the BPSO Designation.

Chapter 14, by Yufang, Hailing, Lijiao, Runxi, and Junqiang, documents the exciting work in RNAO's partnership with China related to establishment of a service and an academic BPSO. Attention is drawn to the widespread and transformative impact of the BPSO Designation in these BPSO organizations, other centers in China, and the nursing profession. The chapter presents the themes of Champion building, knowledge transfer, scope of practice changes, and role of the BPSO Lead in creating success in BPG implementation in BPSOs. The integration of traditional Chinese medicine and traditional Chinese nursing within the BPSO model is central to its success and is highlighted as an aspect of dynamic sustainability.

Chapter 15 by Serna Restrepo, Esparza-Bohórquez, Abad Vasquez, Cortés, Granados Oliveros, Belmar Valdebenito, Mo, and Grinspun, exposes the unique approaches to the BPSO Designation in Latin America, incorporating the use of a rapidly growing BPSO Consortium that crosses borders, and full participation in NQuIRE to inform quality improvement and sustain effective results. The consortium has nurtured robust visibility and collective identity that brings together RNAO's BPSOs in the Latin American cultural context and has resulted in inspiring levels of support from the writers of this chapter to 20 new BPSOs that have joined the BPSO movement in recent years. This peer support is evident through capacity building, ongoing mentorship and generous sharing of learnings, including the sponsorship of a national conference that rotates amongst BPSOs in these countries. The chapter showcases the approaches and achievements of three BPSOs from their beginnings with guidelines selection, to their implementation strategies, to results in patient outcomes.

UNIT 5: EVALUATING OUTCOMES, PROVING RESULTS: THIRD PILLAR FOR SUCCESS

Chapter 16, by Grdisa, Grinspun, Toor, Owusu, Naik, and Smith, traces the history of NQuIRE—Nursing Quality Indicators for Reporting and Evaluation—from its conception stage through to the early beginning as a database system. The chapter also highlights the current state of NQuIRE poised to produce comparative reports and the Nursing Trends Report, and to be a source of data for practitioners, quality improvement and patient safety leaders, administrators, researchers, and policymakers. Descriptions of the NQuIRE vision, purpose, and infrastructure are provided. Examples of structure, process, and outcome indicators are shared and linked to demonstrate the impact of BPG use around the world. Key sections emphasize NQuIRE support for BPSOs, capacity building, ensuring data quality as conceptualized through the Data Quality Framework, and future directions, including dissemination of NQuIRE-driven findings in Evidence Boosters and the Nursing Trends Report.

Chapter 17, by Bonner, Hurley, Ho, and Dabars, discusses the work of the Australian Nursing and Midwifery Federation (ANMF) (SA branch) in its role as a BPSO Host supporting four multisite BPSOs Direct in South Australia. The chapter chronicles the progress of the BPSO Designation with the initial stages of gaining government support, recruiting and selecting BPSOs, capacity building, and the Host's role in providing support to the BPSOs. Prominent in the chapter is discussion of ANMF's full participation in NQuIRE and its link to determining financial outcomes. In this regard, the role of RNAO BPG recommendations and related NQuIRE structure, process, and outcome indicators are highlighted as they apply to cost benefit analysis of BPG implementation. The methodology and related tools used to demonstrate the impact of BPSOs for clients, providers, organizations, and healthcare dollars are a primary focus of this chapter.

UNIT 6: NEXT STEPS: FROM PRACTICE TO POLICY

Chapter 18, by Grinspun, Botros, Mulrooney, Mo, Sibbald, and Penney, addresses the link between evidence-based practice and evidence-based policy and how to connect one with the other to achieve healthy public policy. It shares a larger story about how a professional nursing organization can become a transformative social force and an effective policy advocacy machine that is respected and influential in a key jurisdiction—Ontario, Canada's largest province—as well as nationally and internationally. It describes how a group of nurses, who 2 decades ago were mostly spectators and watched policy processes unfold, is now a leading contributor to and formulator of policy. This success story has lessons for nursing organizations anywhere that want to become policy and politically relevant. It demonstrates how one can build on nurses' clinical work and expertise to the policy frameworks and social contexts that shape how nurses' work is enabled or blocked. The chapter provides two detailed case studies of how nurses' evidence-based work affects patients' health outcomes and how they can leverage evidence and advocacy to affect health system policy changes that ultimately feed back into practice and better healthcare and health for all.

1

TRANSFORMING NURSING THROUGH KNOWLEDGE: THE CONCEPTUAL AND PROGRAMMATIC UNDERPINNINGS OF RNAO'S BPG PROGRAM

Doris Grinspun, PhD, MSN, BScN, RN, LLD(hon), Dr(hc), O.ONT

LEARNING OBJECTIVES

After reading this chapter, you will be able to:

- Understand the conceptual and programmatic underpinnings of the Registered Nurses' Association of Ontario's (RNAO) Best Practice Guidelines (BPG) Program

- Define the term *Best Practice Guideline* and outline the benefits of BPGs

- Describe two artificial dichotomies in nursing and how they have influenced the nursing profession and the BPG Program

- Identify the three pillars of the BPG Program and how they inter-relate

- Learn the concepts of *scaling up, scaling out, and scaling deep*

- Discuss the factors that have secured the success of RNAO's BPG Program

- Explain the concept of *collective identity* and the role it plays in shaping and sustaining evidence-based practice cultures and BPG uptake

INTRODUCTION

"Unless we are making progress in our nursing every year, every month, every week, take my word for it we are going back."

—Florence Nightingale

This chapter shares the conceptual and programmatic underpinnings of the Best Practice Guidelines (BPG) Program led by the Registered Nurses' Association of Ontario (RNAO), the professional association of nurses in Canada's largest province. BPGs are "systematically developed statements to assist practitioner and client decisions about appropriate healthcare for specific circumstances" (Field & Lohr, 1990, p. 8). RNAO's BPGs are based on the best evidence and include recommendations for nurses, other health professionals, administrators, educators, and policymakers to improve clinical and work-environment outcomes. BPGs offer an evaluation of the quality of the relevant scientific literature and an assessment of the likely benefits and harms of a particular intervention. This information enables healthcare providers to select the best care for patients based on their preferences. RNAO's BPG Program is comprehensive and multifaceted, including guideline development, active support for implementation, and an international data system for outcome evaluation.

The chapter is organized in four main sections. The first section highlights the conceptual underpinnings for the BPG Program. It underscores a paradigmatic change in nursing to diminish unnecessary dichotomies artificially created by our profession, such as those between caring versus competence, caring versus curing, and emotional versus cognitive work. Instead, it embraces a broad conceptualization that encompasses the cognitive, physical, and relational dimensions of nursing practice, all equally important and all requiring competence and expertise. It explains why the focus on nursing knowledge, broadly defined in this way, is so important for patient, organizational, and health system outcomes, as well as the value added from a program specifically designed to develop, disseminate, and support nurses in using evidence-based knowledge in their day-to-day practice. This section also highlights the dual responsibility of individual nurses and their work environments for delivering safe, quality care.

The second section shifts the discussion from theory and concepts to the programmatic and institutional background. It recounts the 2-decade history of RNAO's BPG Program and focuses on its origins, goals, design, and evolution. It draws attention to the uniqueness of the BPG Program that focuses on: 1) guideline development; 2) dissemination, implementation, and sustainability; and 3) monitoring and evaluation. It highlights the nursing and broader context in Ontario, Canada that makes this Program possible and its extraordinary local, national, and international expansion from its inception in 1998 to date.

The third section of this chapter explores the factors that have made this Program the success it is today, drawing out lessons for others. The seven factors of focus are: location, comprehensiveness, robustness, proven results, accessibility, leading edge, and collective identity.

Finally, in the last section we explore what the next steps for RNAO's BPG Program might be, connected as they are to the local and global needs of the nursing community and the people we serve.

THE VISION: A PARADIGMATIC CHANGE IN NURSING

This book and the BPG Program it describes focus on nursing knowledge. In particular, we answer the questions: Why is evidence-based practice not commonplace in healthcare today? Why is evidence-based practice central to advance nursing care? And how does it affect patient, organizational, and health-system outcomes? Readers may think it is a given that all health professionals' practice is based on the best available evidence and question why we should focus an entire programmatic effort and this book on nursing knowledge. The simple answer is that this is not the case, and, in fact, practicing according to the latest research and evidence requires a dedicated academic, professional, and organizational effort to make it happen. It does not happen by default. The sole purpose of the BPG Program is to assist nurses, other health professionals, and the organizations and health systems in which they work to advance in this direction. To grasp the full vision of the BPG Program and why it is needed, let's first engage in an analytical discussion on what "caring" in nursing is.

"Caring" is a critical concept in the practice of nursing. Although at first glance it would appear that its meaning is obvious and shared by everyone, on closer look that simplicity disappears and a number of questions arise. Is caring a human trait or a competence? Is caring intuition or learned knowledge? Is it emotional and relational work, or is it also cognitive and physical work? Is caring the moral responsibility of each individual nurse, or a collective responsibility? As we will see, clarifying these questions, and sharpening our understanding of what nursing caring is, stands at the core of this RNAO program focused on advancing nursing knowledge.

This chapter addresses these and other critical issues in nursing that explain why RNAO—a professional association for registered nurses, nurse practitioners, and nursing students in Ontario, Canada—decided to embark on a large-scale program focused on evidence-based practice (EBP).

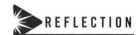 **REFLECTION**

How pervasive is evidence-based practice in healthcare? In nursing? In your workplace, is your practice—and others' practices—based on evidence? If yes, what tools do you use? If not, why?

WHAT IS CARING?

Nursing is firmly rooted in an ethos of caring and care. Considered vital to nursing, it is not a surprise that care and caring are foundational to many nursing theories and to nursing education (Benner, 1994; Bishop & Scudder, 1991; Boykin & Schoenhofer, 1993; Gadow, 1985; Leininger, 1980; Watson, 1985, 2005). The perception of nursing as a "caring profession" is also consistently expressed by members of the public (Young-Mason, 1997), by the media (Picard, 2000), and by policy analysts and policymakers (Decter, 2000).

Definitions of care and caring are diverse. The terms have been variously defined as: moral ideals (Gadow, 1985; Watson, 1999), nurturing activities (Leininger, 1978; Swanson, 1991), essential to nursing practice (Weiss, 1988), a way of practicing (Swanson, 1999), a human trait (Griffin, 1983; Ray, 1989; Roach, 1987), an effect (Forest, 1989), and an experience (Boykin & Schoenhofer, 1993).

Caring, a foundational concept for nursing, has at times been criticized as a "soft script" that has not served nurses or patients well (Buresh & Gordon, 2003; Gordon, 1997). Some argue that nurses have traditionally been socialized to follow a "virtue script" emphasizing acts of compassion over knowledge and skill, which has served neither the profession nor the patients well (Gordon, 2005; Nelson & Gordon, 2006). Grinspun's (2010) ethnographic study on the social construction of nursing caring found that the virtue script reinforces behaviour patterns to the detriment of nurses and patients, resulting in a discourse that emphasizes emotional support and minimizes cognitive effort, competence, and expertise.

What follows are two conceptual dichotomies that help explain why RNAO embarked on an evidence-based practice program.

THE CARING-COMPETENCE DICHOTOMY

Halldórsdóttir (1997) points out that the "artificial dichotomy between caring and competence that has emerged in some of the existing scholarly work is most unfortunate, given that nursing is a practical science in which competence is primary, especially from a patient's perspective" (p. 105). She argues that promoting nursing as both an art and a science requires competence and caring as essential ingredients. The patients she interviewed consistently emphasized competence as an essential professional caring component and stated that caring without competence is of little value. At the same time, professional competence does not mean becoming less human. Halldórsdóttir's interviewees explicitly emphasize the human aspects of nursing care: showing genuine concern and respect for individual patients, accepting patients as they are, and acknowledging pain and suffering. Her central message is that "patients do not see caring and competence as dichotomous; rather, they perceive them as two elements that have to go hand in hand to be of any value to professional caring" (Halldórsdóttir, 1997, p. 110). Calman's (2006) conclusions are similar, with patients viewing knowledge and technical skills as threshold competencies that are necessary but not completely sufficient. In a like manner, Liu, Mok, and Wong (2006) report that nursing caring as perceived by Chinese cancer patients includes qualified professional knowledge; attitudes and skills in oncology; and useful informational, emotional, and practical support. This view is reinforced by Grinspun's (2010) doctoral dissertation in which a central finding is that "caring is not only a relational or emotional process, but also one involving intellectual and physical effort" (p. 12).

Knowledge as a foundational concept in nursing is an implicit expectation for patients and at times for nurses themselves. Indeed, research shows that the public and patients assume nurses are always competent, and even if some were to question it, their ability to assess such competence is often nonexistent—especially in terms of clinical knowledge and technical skills. Calman (2006) suggests that most patients take technical and clinical competence for granted, assuming that hospitals are concerned about hiring competent nurses. If true, this addresses the conflicting evidence concerning what patients value. Calman (2006) writes that the literature on the subject has advocated either interpersonal or technical skill. His study indicates that both interpersonal and technical skill are important as the foundation of competent practice, but that patients may not highlight this because it is seen as in the domain of nurses and not patients, and it is assumed to be always present (Calman, 2006: p. 722).

Rejecting a caring-competence dichotomy is a step in the right direction, but one that requires conceptual distinctions between caring (defined in the narrow sense of affect and love) and competence (defined in the narrow sense of physical and cognitive work). Such distinctions are problematic in several ways. First it implies inborn capabilities for relational caring. Second, it implies that the physical and cognitive work of nurses are not ways of caring. To avoid this artificial dichotomy, it is necessary to conceptualize two dimensions of caring work: 1) caring broadly encompasses all practice domains, and 2) competence in all practice domains is required for effective caring encounters to take place.

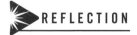 **REFLECTION**

How have you experienced the caring-competence dichotomy in your nursing education and/or practice?

In our BPG Program, we envision that all domains of nursing practice—whether emotional or clinical—require competence, and that facilitating access to evidence serves to advance competence and expertise.

THE CARING-CURING DICHOTOMY

Another problematic and, again, artificially created dichotomy is that of the caring-curing paradigm. Moland (2006) argues that a narrow definition of caring puts nurses in a lower position to physicians, who are charged with curing—a role based on scientific knowledge and technical expertise. This reflects poorly on nurses' moral integrity, contributes to their self-deprecation as knowledge workers, and reduces opportunities for physicians to see them as such (Moland, 2006).

A caring-curing dichotomy poses significant challenges for nurses wanting workplace equality since it assumes that one health professional uses the heart to provide comfort, while the other uses the brain to address clinical problems. Consistent with this image, one profession commands love from patients and the other respect. It is unfortunate to encounter interactions where nurses are discussing clinical situations with physician counterparts and observe them present their expertise in the form of suggestions rather than assertions of knowledge (Grinspun, 2010).

RNAO's BPG Program is envisioned as facilitating access to rigorous evidence for all domains of nursing practice including health promotion (e.g., prevention of child obesity), disease prevention (e.g., smoking cessation), and curative aspects of clinical care where nurses play a leading role (e.g., wound care for persons with diabetes).

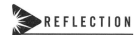

REFLECTION

What roles do nurses themselves play in perpetuating or dispelling views associated with the caring-curing dichotomy? How can we all help each other be more vigilant in dispelling this dichotomy?

REDEFINING CARING AS COGNITIVE, PHYSICAL, AND RELATIONAL WORK

Partial definitions of nurses' caring work as mainly emotional and relational work, compounded by interprofessional hierarchies and organizational structures that to this date venerate (or fear) physicians over all other health professions, have detrimental consequences for patients and the health system as a whole. The most harmful consequence (and by no means the only one) is the silencing of nurses' knowledge (Grinspun, 2010: p. 193). The human tragedy and suffering that result from silencing nursing knowledge is palpable and devastating (Grinspun, 2010: p. 269); it was, for example, in full display in the court case of a paediatric cardiac surgeon who was held responsible for the deaths of twelve infants in a Canadian hospital in Manitoba. The hearing transcripts indicate that the hospital administrators described staff nurses as "emotional" when they repeatedly expressed concerns about clinical malpractices and the excessive number of deaths associated with the male surgeon. The investigators concluded that the experiences and observations of nursing staff throughout 1994 led them to voice serious and legitimate concerns, but they were ignored (Manitoba Health, 2001; Sinclair, 2001).

Indeed, nurses' knowledge and nurses' ability to contribute their knowledge to advance excellence in clinical care are strongly influenced by status and power (Grinspun, 2007, 2010). The delegitimizing of nursing knowledge as "intuition" is a case in point. One can often hear nurses describe a "gut feeling," a "hunch," or "intuition," when what they are actually describing is a sophisticated process of rapid cognition. Rapid cognition is "expert knowledge that allows nurses to grasp patterns across multiple patients and clinical scenarios and correctly apply them to new clinical situations. Rapid cognition requires advanced clinical knowledge, pattern recognition, and patient-specific knowledge gained through relationship continuity" (Grinspun, 2010, p. 178). Labelling such a sophisticated cognitive process as "intuition" belittles nursing knowledge and harms patients who may not get the full benefit of this disempowered knowledge.

The BPG Program powers a conceptualization of nursing caring practice that encompasses cognitive caring (e.g., clinical knowledge, care planning), physical caring (e.g., bathing), and relational caring (e.g., communication, touch, presence, compassion). In this way, the Best Practice Guidelines support excellence in nursing care and serve, also, as a megaphone for nurses to speak about their practice.

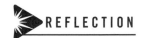

REFLECTION

Why is it important for nurses and for patients that we view caring from a perspective of cognitive, physical, and relational work rather than mainly an emotional response?

CARING: AN INDIVIDUAL AND COLLECTIVE RESPONSIBILITY

The work of nurses with patients—in all its domains—takes place within the social organization of a particular workplace—be that a primary care clinic, hospital unit, a patient's home, a long-term care home, a school, or anywhere else that nurses work. Thus, understanding the work environment of nurses and shaping it in a way that advances good nursing care is paramount to good nursing outcomes.

Understanding nurses' caring work as a labour process that, like other human services, is historically and socially constructed under specific conditions, values, and power relations is paramount to enable nurses to deliver safe and quality services (Grinspun, 2010). For example, much has been written about the detrimental impact on patient outcomes that results from reducing the number of registered nurses (RN) in hospital care (Aiken et al., 2001; Aiken, Clarke, Sloane, Sochalski, & Silber, 2002; Aiken, Clarke, Sloane, Lake, & Cheney, 2008; Aiken et al., 2016; Kane, Shamliyan, Mueller, Duval, & Wilt, 2007; Needleman, Buerhaus, Mattke, Stewart, & Zelevinsky, 2002; Needleman, Buerhaus, Stewart, Zelevinsky, & Mattke, 2006; RNAO, 2017a), yet the replacement of RNs with less-qualified personnel continues in Canada and elsewhere. Others have written about the impact of organizational models of care delivery, arguing that models that promote continuity of care and avoid care fragmentation—such as primary nursing—are preferred (Grinspun, 2010; Meyer, Wang, Li, Thomson, & O'Brien-Pallas, 2009; RNAO, 2006). Such models, however, come into sharp contradiction with cost-driven recommendations made by business consultants, who often promote organizational models that move away from an all-RN staff and emphasize a skill mix with larger proportions of less-educated personnel using RNs in mainly a coordinating capacity (Cummings, 2006; Urden & Walston, 2001).

This perspective, which emphasizes the importance of workplace social relations, assumes that enacting caring practices for patients—whether emotional, physical, or cognitive—is a collective responsibility involving important labour processes that can advance or hinder optimal care. Understanding the labour processes of nurses' work helps us address the systemic and structural enablers and blockages that affect their care. Indeed, "nurses' caring work is socially constructed in the context of their day-to-day private and working lives and impacted by cultural, socio-political and economic realities" (Grinspun, 2010, p. 11).

Such is the reason behind the three main areas of best-practice recommendations provided in each guideline: 1) practice recommendations, or what nurses need to do to optimize patient outcomes; 2) education recommendations, or what nurses need to know to deliver optimal nursing care; and 3) organization and policy recommendations, or what organizations need to do to optimize the uptake of knowledge and the ability to enact that knowledge in daily practice. RNAO has further acknowledged the centrality of work environments by augmenting the clinical BPGs with work environment BPGs. Chapter 2 focuses on clinical guidelines, and Chapter 3 focuses on work environment BPGs.

Shifting from the conceptual underpinnings of the BPG Program, we will now move to the context that made this Program possible and facilitated its evolution.

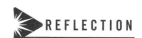 **REFLECTION**

How do organizational contexts and power relations impact the practice of nurses? Have you experienced such impacts in your work and/or school?

ORIGINS AND EVOLUTION OF RNAO'S BEST PRACTICE GUIDELINES PROGRAM

During 1996 and 1997, there was widespread disruption in Ontario's hospital system as a result of restructuring and layoffs of nurses. RNAO took on a leading role during this difficult period, which led to a positive engagement with government. In 1997, the Ontario government passed the *Expanded Nursing Services for Patients Act*. In March 1998, following RNAO's *Putting Out the Healthcare Fire* report (RNAO, 1998) and meetings with Ontario's Premier and Minister of Health, the government announced at RNAO's Annual General Meeting in April of 1998 the establishment of the Ontario Nursing Task Force to enhance the quality of patient care through the effective use of nursing resources (RNAO, 2013). Its 1999 report, *Good Nursing, Good Health: An Investment for the 21st Century*, recommended several strategies designed to help Ontario retain and attract nurses, improve working conditions for nurses, and ensure nurses have the knowledge and skills they need to provide care in an increasingly complex environment (Ontario Ministry of Health and Long-Term Care—Nursing Task Force, 1999). One of the report's recommendations was to establish clinical models in practice environments to allow nurses to gain expertise in clinical areas and be recognized for these additional skills. RNAO leveraged this recommendation to submit a proposal for funding a program on evidence-based guidelines.

REGISTERED NURSES' ASSOCIATION OF ONTARIO (CANADA)

The Registered Nurses' Association of Ontario (RNAO) is the professional association representing registered nurses, nurse practitioners, and nursing students in Ontario. Since 1925, RNAO has advocated for healthy public policy, promoted excellence in nursing practice, increased nurses' contribution to shaping the healthcare system, and influenced decisions that affect nurses and the public they serve.

RNAO's strategic directions are:

- Engaging with registered nurses, nurse practitioners, and nursing students to stimulate membership

- Influencing public policy that strengthens Medicare (Canada's universal publicly funded and administered healthcare system) and impacts on the determinants of health

- Advancing the role and image of nurses as members of a vital, knowledge-driven, caring profession, and as significant contributors to health

- Speaking out on emerging issues that impact nurses and the nursing profession, health, and health services (RNAO, n.d.-a)

RNAO had the capability and experience to lead this initiative on behalf of the nursing community. We had already gained experience creating nursing guidelines based on the best available evidence (Grinspun, Librado, & Góngora, 2005). RNAO also had the social and professional networks required to disseminate the guidelines across Ontario and Canada. RNAO's initial proposal recommended that the guidelines be developed in areas where nursing has an impact on health and clinical outcomes so they could benefit a significant number of people. We reminded government that poll after poll shows the Canadian public considers nursing the most trustworthy of all occupations and that BPGs are a critical tool to support nurses in their day-to-day practice. Indeed, BPGs serve to augment the public's deep trust for nurses by strengthening nurses' clinical and organizational knowledge. In 1998, Ontario's Minister of Health Elizabeth Witmer saw the potential of BPGs, and in 1999 she allocated multi-year funding to RNAO to create a dedicated program for BPG development and implementation.

PURPOSE, GOALS, AND OBJECTIVES OF THE BPG PROGRAM

The BPG Program was officially launched in 1999 by RNAO in partnership with the Ontario Ministry of Health and Long-Term Care (MOHLTC). The purpose of the Program from its inception has been to support Ontario nurses—registered nurses (RN), nurse practitioners (NP), and registered practical nurses (RPN/LPN)—by providing them with Best Practice Guidelines (BPG) for client care. We envisioned this would advance nurses' opportunities to assert their clinical and relational competence and expertise based on the most relevant evidence. This emboldened capacity would inspire action at the individual level of each nurse and nursing student, and, by extension, to the collective levels of service and academic organizations, and influence the broad spectrum of health policy. In doing so, nurses would optimize their contribution to patients, organizations, and health system outcomes.

The goals of the Program are to:

- Improve the consistency and quality of nursing care across the province of Ontario

- Increase access to quality nursing services

- Disseminate resources as broadly as possible so that maximum benefits are achieved for clients, nurses, and the health system

The Program objectives are to:

- Develop, implement, and evaluate three nursing BPGs per year

- Review and revise the BPGs every 5 years

- Develop and implement effective dissemination and implementation mechanisms to secure uptake and sustainability of BPGs

- Evaluate the development, dissemination, and implementation processes, as well as the outcomes associated with the BPGs

BPG PROGRAM: DESIGN AND PURPOSEFUL EVOLUTION

We recognized early on that the traditional tightly planned, and often top-down, approach used by health managers would not produce the type of social engagement needed to deliver substantive and sustained clinical, organizational, and health system change through the BPG Program. Our approach needed to be multifaceted and include magnetic processes that would attract nurses to mobilize their internal commitment and energy to become the drivers for change. In a manner consistent with RNAO's overall approach to working with our members, the BPG Program emulates a grassroots movement—one that both creates and delivers the changes proposed by the clinical guidelines. The end goal of this movement has been, by design, consistent and clear: to advance evidence-based practice and improve patient, organization, and health system outcomes. A secondary goal, one we have not shied away from, is to position nursing and nurses as knowledge professionals and robust contributors to health outcomes.

An important feature of the BPG Program has been its purposeful evolution, both as a comprehensive Program and in each of its components. *Purposeful evolution* means that we make conscious and intentional decisions about slowing down or accelerating growth and expansion; thus, we decided early on that needs from the field and readiness at RNAO would drive the growth and evolution of the Program. This purposeful evolution enables us to ensure a dynamic, evergreen Program that is responsive to the needs of Ontario's health system, patients, and nurses. This has also enabled us to evolve the Program and move beyond the borders of the province of Ontario, embracing both the Canadian and global community—something we did not envision in 1999. At this time, we are fully cognizant of the opportunities with the international expansion of the Program, as well as the potential challenges such growth entails. The positive outcomes of this purposefully (by design) evolutionary approach, discussed in detail in Chapter 12, are evident as well in each of the other chapters of this book. Figure 1.1 shows the BPG Program model with its three pillars.

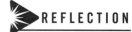

REFLECTION

What advantages are there to having the guideline development, implementation, and evaluation pillars all part of the same program? Do you see any disadvantages? If yes, how could they be overcome?

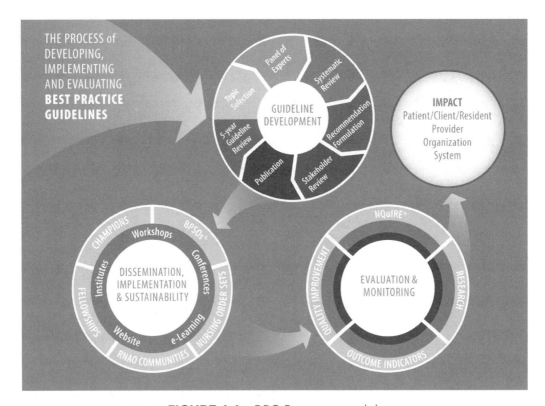

FIGURE 1.1 BPG Program model.

KEY FEATURES OF RNAO'S BPG PROGRAM

The key features of the Program are highlighted in this section, and a detailed account of each main component follows in later chapters of this book.

BPG DEVELOPMENT

The first four BPGs were developed by the end of 2000, pilot tested in 2001, and publicly launched and published in 2002 (Scarrow, 2008). In 2003, we decided that in addition to evidence-based guidelines that advance the clinical practice of nurses, there was an urgent need for evidence-based guidelines to enrich work environments. By 2003, RNAO had issued 17 clinical guidelines and an evidence-based "toolkit" for organizations to implement guidelines (JPNC Implementation Monitoring Subcommittee, 2003). The speed of progress continued sharply in response to demands from the field. By 2008, there were 31 clinical guidelines and six healthy workplace BPGs produced and in use all over Ontario and across Canada (Scarrow, 2008).

To ensure currency of the evidence, we began slowing down new guidelines' production to produce the next generation of the existing guidelines. In 2017, the BPG Program counted 41 clinical guidelines, as well as 12 Healthy Work Environment Best Practice Guidelines (e.g., prevention of violence in the workplace) and/or health system guidelines (e.g., transitions of care). RNAO's unwavering commitment to maintaining a rigorous guideline revision cycle has resulted in a trusted and dependable relationship between RNAO and its guidelines users and funders. The focus of Chapter 2 is the development of our clinical practice BPGs.

BEST PRACTICE GUIDELINE DISSEMINATION, IMPLEMENTATION, AND SUSTAINABILITY

RNAO's plans from the outset included broad dissemination of the evidence-based guidelines and active support for their implementation. The implementation works at three levels singularly and/or collectively: the micro level of individual nurses, meso level of service and academic organizations, and macro level of health systems. The goal is to ensure effective, sustained, and scalable implementation of BPGs in both clinical and management practices. Today, RNAO leads what is likely the most robust and expansive implementation program for evidence-based practice for nurses anywhere in the world, and is amongst the strongest in any healthcare field. This is the result of a zealous approach dedicated to implementation science combined with constant attention to learning from and responding to in-the-field needs. The BPG Program has purposefully evolved over time, both in its depth and breadth of understanding, as well as its ability to mobilize evidence-based knowledge.

The work of Moore, Riddell, and Vocisano (2015) discusses social entrepreneurship program expansion in three ways: 1) *scaling up*, or expanding coverage; 2) *scaling out*, or altering the policies, laws, and standards; and 3) *scaling deep*, or changing the norms. They argue that to maximize the benefits from implementation efforts, all three aspects of scaling are important. Adapting these concepts to RNAO's Program, we engage in scaling up when BPGs are disseminated widely within an organization; scaling out, when they are disseminated to other organizations or to the health system; and scaling deep, when uptake and sustainability have occurred and an evidence-based culture has been achieved. Scaling deep can occur within an organization or across the health system, especially through policy impact. We use these concepts to briefly describe the evolution of RNAO's BPG implementation.

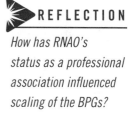

REFLECTION

How has RNAO's status as a professional association influenced scaling of the BPGs?

SCALING UP: DISSEMINATION AND UPTAKE

The focus of scaling up is on wide dissemination and uptake of BPGs within an organization. Our first broad dissemination initiative was the development of *Champions*. We began to train individual nurses as BPG Champions in 2002 to facilitate BPG uptake in their workplaces. By 2003 we had 278 champions in all sectors of Ontario's healthcare system (JPNC Implementation Monitoring Subcommittee, 2003). At first, all the Champions were direct care RNs; over the years the role has evolved to include all nurses and other health professionals in all roles. From the outset and to this day, these are individuals selected by their organizations (and in many organizations, selected by their peers) and/or who volunteer for this role. Such a bottom-up approach helps ensure role sustainability. Champions are passionate about evidence-based practice and improving people's care and health. They raise awareness of BPGs, support understanding, and influence their uptake amongst workplace peers. In 2002, with already hundreds of Champions trained, we launched the *Champions Network* to foster active engagement and knowledge exchange amongst Champions and between them and RNAO.

Now, through this program, over 50,000 volunteer champions access tools and strategies such as in-person workshops, teleconferences, webinars, and online modules. Details of this program are discussed in Chapter 4. The program has expanded to include Certified BPSO Orientation Trainers and Certified BPSO Auditors. These new roles are discussed in Chapter 12.

The next evolution of the BPG Program was the creation of *Best Practice Spotlight Organizations* (or BPSOs) to support healthcare organizations in systematically implementing guidelines. BPSOs were first launched in 2003 in Ontario. We worked with the first seven healthcare organizations to jointly co-create a structured approach for organizations to use BPGs and evaluate their impact (RNAO, 2004). Designation as a BPSO involves a competitive application process and is reserved for healthcare and academic organizations that are selected to sign a formal 3-year agreement to implement multiple BPGs. The criteria here have also purposefully evolved. For example, the request for proposals (RFP) requirement for the first three BPSO cohorts in Ontario was to implement a minimum of three clinical BPGs of their choice. The RFP requirement for cohorts four and five was to implement a minimum of five BPGs of their choice. Starting with cohort six (the current one at time of writing), the RFP stipulates two BPGs of their choice and three common to their healthcare sector (public health, primary care, hospital, home care, nursing home, etc.). Currently with 550 BPSOs worldwide, as illustrated in Figure 1.2, the global BPSO network, such an approach allows for robust data to fuel evaluation and comparison of outcomes in like organizations. BPSOs have a choice to renew their agreement following successful completion of their first 3-year agreement. Each renewal is for 2 additional years during which they commit to ongoing spread of existing guidelines, uptake of two new guidelines, and evaluation of their impact on outcomes.

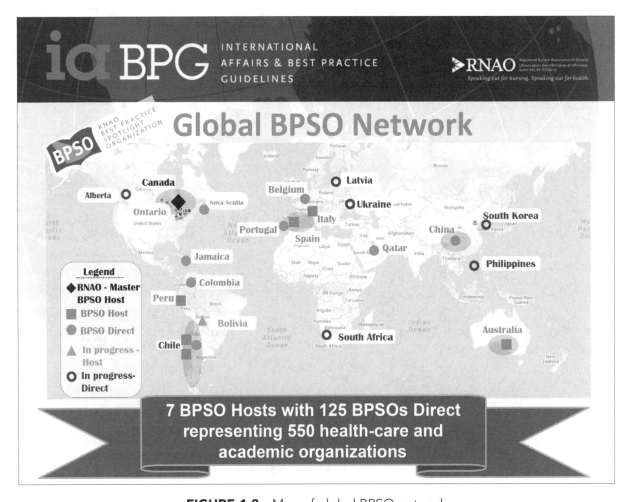

FIGURE 1.2 Map of global BPSO network.

BPSO MODELS

The Best Practice Spotlight Organization (BPSO) Designation is an opportunity for health service and academic organizations to formally partner with RNAO over a 3-year period. Following this period, the partnership is renewed biennially. The goal of the partnership is to create evidence-based practice cultures through systematic implementation and outcomes evaluation of multiple RNAO BPGs.

There are two BPSO models for service and academic organizations considering applying to achieve their BPSO Designation:

- The *BPSO Direct Model*—Best suited for single organizations wishing to apply to RNAO to engage in the 3-year partnership. These organizations work directly with RNAO to meet the BPSO requirements designation. In Ontario, health organizations that are part of this program are BPSO Direct.

- The *BPSO Host Model*—Best suited for organizations that have the capacity to run, on behalf of RNAO, the full BPSO Designation program for a group of health and/or academic institutions within a country, region, or community. In this model, the BPSO Host enters into a formal agreement with RNAO to deliver and oversee the RNAO BPSO Designation in the country or region where it is located. The BPSO Host is responsible for selecting the BPSO Direct organizations; providing orientation, education, and support; monitoring progress; and evaluating outcomes. The BPSO Host submits regular reports to RNAO. The BPSO Host acts as the liaison between RNAO and the BPSOs in the specific country, region, or community—ensuring full consistency and systematic deployment of all aspects of the RNAO BPG Program, including: guideline implementation, evaluation, sustainability, spread, scaling-up, and scaling-out.

RNAO supports BPSO Hosts and BPSO Direct Organizations outside of Ontario with materials, methodology, and ongoing mentorship—free of charge. In turn, BPSOs do not receive funding from RNAO and must secure the resources to fully manage the BPSO.

In 2010, the BPG Program opened its doors internationally when the government of Spain approached RNAO—first to collaborate in translating the guidelines into Spanish and subsequently to support the creation of a network of BPSOs in that country. This was an important opportunity; Spain is a country with over 46 million people and 164,385 nurses (in 2015). The translation of RNAO's BPGs into Spanish has been critical to opening access to RNAO's BPGs to the world's millions of Spanish-speaking nurses and other health professionals. It also led to envisioning a model that would enable expansion and sustainability of the BPSO Designation at home and abroad; with this the BPSO Host—which coordinates a network of BPSOs—was born. These important developments and their outcomes to date are highlighted in Chapters 12 and 13.

Expanding nationally and internationally was an important leap in RNAO's BPG Program, and the results are impressive. In 2014 RNAO had 370 BPSO sites across Ontario, Quebec, Nova Scotia, and outside Canada; today we have 550. Chapter 6 details the work of BPSOs. We envisioned BPSOs as living labs that would enable us to demonstrate how nursing care, based on evidence contained in RNAO's

BPGs, improves patients' health as well as organizational and health system outcomes. Chapters 7, 8, 9, 11, 13, 14, 15, and 17 discuss the experiences of BPSOs in their own voices and show a vision that is now a lived reality.

BPSOs have proven to be a powerful mechanism to spread and sustain the use of RNAO's BPGs and very effective in enabling a sense of collective identity amongst the participants, a concept I will return to later on in this chapter. They have also nurtured a culture of evidence-based practice in healthcare organizations (Bajnok, Grinspun, Lloyd, & McConnell, 2015; Grinspun, 2011). Its success has been acknowledged both in Canada (Health Council of Canada, 2012) and internationally (WHO, 2015).

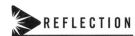

REFLECTION

How does a common language in nursing, derived from use of RNAO's BPGs, shape the profession and its impact worldwide?

SCALING OUT NATIONALLY AND INTERNATIONALLY

The Program has also evolved in its breadth, and many Ontario-born programs have been scaled out to the national and international levels. For example, recognizing the expertise of RNAO, the Canadian Patient Safety Institute (CPSI) approached RNAO to act as a national lead agency on falls prevention and to develop a resource on *Falls Prevention/Injury Reduction Getting Started Kit*. Over the past 10 years, based on the highly popular BPG on falls widely used in all sectors, RNAO has partnered with CPSI on a number of falls-related *Safer Healthcare Now!* programs—National Collaborative for the Prevention of Falls in Long-Term Care (2008–2009), Falls Virtual Collaborative (2010–2011), and Falls Facilitated Learning Series (2011–2012)—and it has developed a highly beneficial resource on sustainability of falls-prevention programs. RNAO co-hosted all these national activities with CPSI, drawing on lessons obtained from the Long-Term Care (LTC) Best Practices Program initiated in Ontario in 2005, which has led to improved quality of care for residents and the facilitation of an evidence-based practice culture amongst direct care staff through the implementation of BPGs in LTC homes. Chapter 10 provides details on the scaling initiatives, including RNAO's work with CPSI as their falls lead, leveraging RNAO's BPG on falls. In Chapter 11, the Long-Term Care Best Practices Program is outlined in full, describing both its key success and effective scaling components.

APPLYING TECHNOLOGY-ENABLED TOOLS

The BPG Program recognized from the outset the value of technology-enabled tools to support nursing practice. A first of its kind, it created evidence-based practice "nursing order sets" derived from the practice recommendations of RNAO's BPGs. It also developed an *eHealth Toolkit* (RNAO, 2009). More recently, it launched the *Adopting eHealth Solutions: Implementation Strategies BPG* (RNAO, 2017b) with funding from Canada Health Infoway, an independent, federally funded, not-for-profit organization tasked with accelerating the adoption of digital health solutions across Canada (Punch, 2017). These tools, detailed in Chapter 5, are designed to facilitate the translation of evidence into nursing practice, using technology.

Through such eHealth innovations, and in particular the nursing order sets, RNAO has earned the accreditation—one of only 15 centers in the world, and the first in North America—as a Research & Development Centre working under the International Classification for Nursing Practice (ICNP) (International Council of Nurses, 2013). The accreditation recognizes RNAO's ongoing contribution to the International Council of Nurses' (ICN) eHealth Program through the development of ICNP codes derived from RNAO's nursing order sets and BPG outcome measures.

RNAO's nursing order sets are evidence-based interventions and clinical decision support resources derived from RNAO's clinical BPGs (RNAO, n.d.-b). They enable the integration of the best available evidence into daily clinical practice using technology to facilitate access at the point-of-care. Nursing order sets support the evaluation of BPG implementation by providing a mechanism to link specific interventions to corresponding evidence-based indicators. Each intervention statement is aligned with the ICNP terminology language to support the standardized collection and exchange of nursing information globally.

Another BPG spawning example is the Pan-Canadian *Prevention of Abuse and Neglect of Older Adults* Best Practice Guideline Initiative, which is focused on recognizing, managing, and preventing the abuse and neglect of older adults throughout various healthcare institutions and community settings in Canada. Funded by the Government of Canada's New Horizons for Seniors Program, this initiative includes development of an evidence-based BPG by RNAO; a strategy for dissemination, implementation, and evaluation; practice tools; an e-learning program; and plain-language resources for the public. The initiative builds on the success of a collaborative project between RNAO and the Canadian Nurses Association (CNA), also funded by the federal government, which launched the Prevention of Elder Abuse Centres of Excellence (PEACE) in 2010 in 10 long-term care homes across the country.

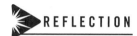

REFLECTION

What impact has the integration of evidence-based practice and technology in RNAO's implementation resources had on the uptake of both?

Similarly, the Nursing Best Practice Smoking Cessation Initiative started in Ontario and then expanded across the country in partnership with CNA with funding from Health Canada. It tackles the leading preventable cause of premature death, disease, and disability, based on evidence suggesting that even minimal intervention by healthcare professionals can dramatically reduce rates of smoking. With a focus on knowledge transfer, mobilization of networks, and increased use of existing services and programs, the goal of this national initiative is to strengthen nurses' capacity to help their clients by implementing smoking cessation strategies and techniques in their daily practice. By 2013, the Initiative had formally reached 350 organizations and established over 2,600 Smoking Cessation Best Practice Champions across Canada. This program is detailed in Chapter 10.

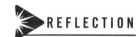

REFLECTION

What factors have been pivotal to the success of several provincial and national initiatives that have been based on the BPGs?

Although the BPG Program is based in Ontario, it is deeply significant across Canada and internationally. As evidence of this, BPGs have been translated into French, Spanish, Chinese, Japanese, German, and Italian. Moreover, some 30 of RNAO's clinical BPGs are available on the National Guideline Clearinghouse (NGC), a website established by the Agency for Healthcare Research and Quality (AHRQ), part of the U.S. Department of Health and Human Services. Chapters 13, 14, 15, and 17 share some experiences of BPSO international partners.

SCALING DEEP: TRANSFORMING VALUES AT THE INDIVIDUAL, ORGANIZATIONAL, AND HEALTH SYSTEM LEVELS

Its location within a professional nursing association enriches the BPG Program because it provides a large voluntary membership of RNs, NPs, and nursing students ready to adopt and test the BPGs. Thus, identifying an initial base of early adopters and a testing ground for BPGs was never an issue for RNAO. RNAO's network of professional links to other nursing and non-nursing associations has also benefited the Program. As you will read in Chapter 18, non-nursing partners see the benefits of RNAO's expertise in guideline development and implementation, as well as its powerful impact in health, healthcare, and nursing policy. Being part of a large professional association also means having expert staff. RNAO is organized in seven departments, each with extensive expertise in their fields: Executive Office; Membership and Services; International Affairs and Best Practice Guidelines (IABPG—the department responsible for the BPG Program); Nursing and Health Policy; Communications; Information Management and Technology; and Finance and Administration.

RNAO's work is always strategic, analytical, and actionable. Thus, while one often hears about the need to leverage nurses' expertise into the policy arena (Cohen et al., 1996; Ellenbecker et al., 2017), RNAO acts on this mandate and brings about deep individual, institutional, and broad health system changes in both practice and policy. The BPG Program has been central to RNAO's policy work in areas of nursing practice and work environment. In turn, RNAO policy work has influenced the development of specific BPGs. An example of the latter is a BPG being developed at the time of writing related to nursing care in supervised injection services; more on this in Chapter 18.

Various chapters in this book reflect on deep practice and policy changes that are taking place within BPSOs. For example, Chapter 14 describes changes in scope of practice at a large BPSO hospital in China resulting from nurses' added expertise in wound care using RNAO's guideline. These nurses in China have internalized guideline knowledge and speak with pride about being BPSO Champions, assuming the role with seriousness and sophistication. Chapter 15 describes improvements in human and material resources when nurses give proof that mattresses modified based on BPG descriptions were bringing positive results, causing the hospital administration to approve funding to change all mattresses. In Chapter 17, the Australian Nursing and Midwifery Federation (SA Branch) influences policy by showing the value added of expert clinical nurses using BPGs.

Chapter 18 displays RNAO's capacity to leverage BPGs into policy gains and vice versa. It focuses on the important augmentation of the BPG Program and the richness that ensues when evidence-based clinical knowledge meets evidence-based policy and advocacy knowledge. If pursued vigorously, the outcome is the collective good of our health systems and the people we serve. Scaling deep often leads to the formation of collective identity, which is one of the most impactful outcomes of the BPG Program.

MONITORING, EVALUATION, AND RESEARCH

The next step in the purposeful evolution of the BPG Program was devising a system to monitor and evaluate the impacts of RNAO's BPGs in organizations that implemented them. The impacts can span the whole spectrum of outcomes, from provider and patient to organizational to health system performance. For this purpose, RNAO partnered with BPSOs in Canada and abroad to understand their needs and capacity, leading to the launch of another first-of-its-kind—a comprehensive and free of charge international data system available to all BPSOs. The *Nursing Quality Indicators for Reporting and Evaluation* (NQuIRE) project consists of a database, an online data-entry system, a data dictionary—including a set of organization-level structural indicators and a set of process and outcome indicators for each BPG—as well as data collection and reporting processes (RNAO, n.d.-c).

Through NQuIRE, RNAO collects, analyzes, and reports quality-indicator data submitted by health-care service and academic BPSOs. NQuIRE supports BPSOs in making effective practice improvements by providing organizational and comparative data on BPG-directed nursing care processes and resulting clinical outcomes. With NQuIRE data, BPSOs are able to track their progress, identify areas for improvement, highlight areas for further investment, and advance quality improvement to optimize clinical, organizational, and health system outcomes. By monitoring, evaluating, and reporting quality improvements in nursing care across the globe, NQuIRE is producing BPSO-validated and endorsed quality indicators that will contribute to sustainability and enhance our understanding of the full impact of evidence-based nursing practice on healthcare quality and health outcomes. Chapter 16 details the progress and outcomes available through NQuIRE, and its utility for particular BPSOs is described in various chapters.

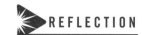

REFLECTION

How do you think such a robust and comprehensive system for evaluation of BPG use will impact the Program and those who adopt the BPGs?

THE BPG PROGRAM: FROM LOCAL IMPACT TO SEISMIC TRANSFORMATION OF NURSING PRACTICE GLOBALLY

Funded by Ontario's Ministry of Health and Long-Term Care, and independently run, the BPG Program attracted from its inception broad provincial interest in the then-emerging field of clinical guideline development. In the early 1990s, McMaster University had launched its evidence-based curriculum for medicine in Ontario (Guyatt, 1991), and RNAO took the lead in nursing's movement into evidence-based practice. The delivery of the first four guidelines quickly demonstrated RNAO's capacity to develop quality products. Guidelines, however, could have remained on library shelves if it had not been for the parallel and rich program RNAO developed to advance the uptake and utilization of the guidelines in day-to-day clinical practice. This groundbreaking pillar of the BPG Program cemented its place as a leader in implementation science. Already in 2005, RNAO was featured internationally as a robust clinical guideline program (Jordan, 2005) and sought after for its expertise in both guideline development and knowledge translation. While evaluation was a component of the Program from the outset, the systematic evaluation of BPG impacts on patient outcomes evolved through the years from independent evaluations by its implementers to co-creation of the NQuIRE quality indicators system described above and in Chapter 16.

The BPG Program has achieved remarkable accomplishments and demonstrated vast capacity for rapid expansion and innovation since its start in 1999. Developing RNAO's vision and evolving it purposefully throughout the years has greatly contributed to its success. RNAO has guided the Program from inception to maturity in an organic way, informed at the macro level by theories about diffusion of innovation and large-scale system change (Edwards, Rowan, Marck, & Grinspun, 2011; Moore et al., 2015; Rogers, 1962, 2003) and social movements literature (Melucci, 1980, 1989, 1996); at the meso level by knowledge-transfer scholarly work (Curran, Grimshaw, Hayden, & Campbell, 2011; Grimshaw, Eccles, Lavis, Hill, & Squires, 2012; Sales, Smith, Curran, & Kochevar, 2006; Shekelle, Woolf, Eccles, & Grimshaw, 1999; Straus, Tetroe, & Graham, 2013), and field experience from nurses and organizations—especially our BPSO partners.

At the core of these perspectives is a deep respect, understanding, and accounting for local context and both top-down and bottom-up dynamics. Instead of delivering on a vision fully set by RNAO for others to follow, we chose a beginning path for a program that would advance evidence-based practice in nursing. This path has subsequently been shaped, modified, and adapted, based on new evidence and the evolving socio-political context, to remain responsive to the needs of Ontario, Canada and the world. For example, while other clinical guidelines programs have plans for guideline development decided years in advance, RNAO's flexible approach allows it to respond to evolving provincial and national priorities such as it did when moving ahead with the development of a guideline for Supervised Injection Services (discussed in Chapter 18), or partnering for the eHealth BPG mentioned earlier. Similarly, our implementation plans evolved to embrace national and international nursing organizations in response to their interest in participation. Undoubtedly, central characteristics of this winning vision have been to be good listeners, responsive to context, and committed to shared ownership. Although RNAO has led the effort, the reality of the BPG Program today has been collectively shaped by multiple actors engaged at all levels of the Program.

LARGE-SCALE BPG PROGRAM SPREAD: SUCCESS FACTORS

Multiple factors have contributed to the large-scale spread of the BPG Program and advancing it from producing localized systemic change to leading a seismic transformation of nursing care worldwide. Each chapter that follows highlights various contributing factors that are important. Stepping back and reflecting on the 20 years that have passed since launching the Program, seven broad features of the Program appear central to its success:

1. **Location**—The BPG Program is enriched by being located within a professional nursing association. At the structural level, RNAO's membership-driven association means that there are already thousands of nurses on board, eager to uptake the knowledge contained in the BPGs, apply it to their work, and bring it to patients and to their organizations. It also means that a large group of nurses in all roles and sectors have knowledge needs for which they would like evidence-based answers. The fact that RNAO is composed of a large staff of experts in policy, communications, and information technology means a constant attentiveness to support the BPG Program in succeeding.

2. **Comprehensiveness**—The Program offers nurses, healthcare organizations, academic institutions, and health systems—anywhere in the world—a "full package" inclusive of guidelines, implementation, and evaluation mechanisms to advance evidence-based practice. These are rigorous guidelines that meet international standards. Users can also rely on a solid and well-supported approach to implementation. The last component of the package is a system to evaluate impacts on patients, healthcare organizations, and health systems. As such, it is the only program of its kind for nurses and other health professionals that includes guideline development, implementation, and evaluation.

3. **Robustness**—There is a commitment to outstanding quality for each component of the Program. As a result, in the development pillar, RNAO's BPGs are included in major databases for meeting international standards. In the implementation pillar, BPGs are integrated locally, nationally, and internationally in nursing program curriculum and in day-to-day practice in all

academic and service BPSOs, as well as in many non-BPSOs. The evaluation pillar, while still young, is already delivering with a high degree of maturity, as evidenced through numerous published articles from RNAO and most importantly from BPSOs locally and globally.

4. **Proven results**—The Program in its distinct components produces results. This is why Canada's Council of the Federation selected several BPGs from RNAO for national implementation. Most importantly, as you read through this book, you too will marvel at the results experienced using the Program in various healthcare sectors in Ontario and Canada, as well as in Australia, Belgium, Chile, China, Colombia, Italy, Jamaica, Peru, Portugal, Qatar, and Spain.

5. **Accessibility**—The Program is open-access and free of charge, starting from the BPGs that are freely accessible for download from the RNAO website. This is in keeping with a philosophy that knowledge is to be shared for the collective good, not for private enrichment.

6. **Leading-edge**—The Program is not static; it is always informed by the evidence and in touch with the experience in the field. Indeed, the desire to be responsive to the field inspires us to explore different solutions and bring crucial innovations to the Program (e.g., BPSO Hosts).

7. **Collective identity**—This last point, collective identity, warrants added attention because it is a concept not often discussed in the evidence-based practice or diffusion of innovations literature. It is a concept we borrow from the social sciences and in particular from theoretical perspectives and research about social movements. This is the result of a purposeful and effective methodology of authentic engagement led by RNAO.

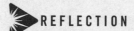 **REFLECTION**

In thinking about the factors attributed to the success of the BPG Program, do you agree? What others would you add?

THE BPG PROGRAM AS A COLLECTIVE IDENTITY

Collective identity is a concept first developed by Alberto Melucci in 1989. Melucci's *collective identity* is "an interactive and shared definition produced by several interacting individuals who are concerned with the orientation of their action as well as the field of opportunities and constraints in which their action takes place" (1989, p. 34). Unsatisfied with the gap between theories on how collective actions form and how individuals find motivation, Melucci (1989) defines an intermediate process, in which individuals recognize that they share certain orientations in common and on that basis decide to act together. For him, collective identity is a process negotiated over time and characterized by three dimensions: a "cognitive definition," which entails a common framework, goals, means, and environments of action; "active relationship" amongst participants; and "emotional investment" amongst the participants (Melucci, 1989). Melucci's definition of collective identity is highly relevant to understand the success of RNAO's BPG Program.

Using social theory concepts represents a sharp departure from traditional approaches to healthcare transformations. Typically, health system change relies heavily on a set of top-down directives with fully planned phases or steps designed to "manage the change" and strategies aimed at getting rank and file employees to "buy into the change." Bates, Robert, and Bevan (2004) discuss the limitations of traditional approaches and explore the potential of social movement theory to understand large-scale health system transformations in the United Kingdom's National Health System. Their conclusion is that "the components of a social movements and a programmatic approach to large scale organizational change are not necessarily mutually exclusive and may represent the next phase of healthcare improvement" (Bates, Robert, & Bevan, 2004, p. 65).

Consistent with Melucci's (1989) work, RNAO's BPG Program orientation has been geared toward shared ownership and a nurturing of collective identity amongst participants and stakeholders at all levels. Our work with the BPSOs emphasizes a transparent, engaging, and motivational approach that encourages identification with and active participation in all pillars of the Program, as the reader will experience throughout this book. From its inception, we readily connected with enrolled clinicians, organizational and health system administrators, educators, researchers, and policymakers to make them active participants in the process. As described in Chapter 2, in addition to RNAO's professional perspective, we included (and still include) other equally important voices such as Ontario's professional association for RPNs/LPNs. The message was that the BPG Program is a collective good for nurses and the people we serve.

The media and the public have been critical partners. Cementing nursing as a "knowledge profession" and nurses as knowledge workers has meant that anytime there is a clinical topic of import in a media outlet, we respond and reference RNAO's BPGs. Throughout the years, letters to the editor have focused on a myriad of topics including falls, staffing, and obesity (Bajnok, 2008, 2009; Virani, 2007). Since 2012, we augmented these "just in-time" responses to media with on-the-ground press conferences during Nursing Week, organized by BPSOs in partnership with RNAO. At these and other events, BPSO staff and patients display their evidence-based expertise and its positive impact (Zych, 2012).

A final component in this concerted effort to develop a collective identity around the BPG Program has been the link between evidence-based practice and evidence-based policy, a bidirectional effort that has produced impactful results on institutional policies and macro health system policy. These changes are discussed in Chapter 18 as a wrap-up to this book.

Today, RNAO's BPG Program plays a leading role in clinical and healthy work environment guideline development, implementation science, and outcome evaluation—provincially, nationally, and internationally. The Program enables organizations and health systems to focus on patient care and clinical excellence, using the latest research to inform practice and optimize outcomes. The BPG Program has helped advance government priorities, as well as patient, provider, organizational, and health system outcomes. It is recognized across the globe for its rigorous guideline development, transformational approaches that are contributing to implementation science, and robust evaluation methodology (Di Costanzo, 2013; Scarrow, 2008; WHO, 2015). Indeed, BPGs have become part of the nursing culture and lexicon in Ontario and all over Canada, and BPSOs constitute a galvanizing global movement in nursing, and one that creates a collective identity.

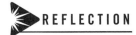

REFLECTION

Have you been involved in a project where you experienced collective identity? Can you describe how you felt? How critical is collective identity for sustained change?

LOOKING FORWARD TO THE FUTURE

RNAO BPGs are revolutionizing nursing through a focus on knowledge that optimizes the delivery of care anywhere in the world. These robust, evidence-based tools have captured the imagination of nurses in practice, administration, education, research, and policy. They have won the hearts and minds of nurses in all roles and especially of direct care nurses: in the community, hospitals, nursing homes, and just about everywhere nurses work. Nurses understand that BPGs are instrumental in moving the profession to a fully evidence-based practice, and that is where they want to go. The biggest success is that growing segments of the nursing community are joining in as BPSOs, sharing their excitement as they team up with RNAO and one another, taking ownership of the movement.

The future is rich with opportunities as the influence of the BPG Program continues to expand across all dimensions including new guidelines, more Champions, additional BPSOs, and expanded capacity to evaluate impact. At the service level, this means we can partner as regional networks, following on the BPSO consortium model that has already been established in Latin America, a model that nurtures rich learning and strong collective identity. Trained auditors and orientation facilitators from various countries will enable Program fidelity and sustainability, as well as further engender collective identity and build shared ownership. Academically, a new generation of students is already graduating à la BPG/BPSO, as both inquisitive professional nurses and change agents for evidence-based practice. Multiplied by thousands, in a few years they will have experienced and will contribute through their careers to a scaling deep of evidence-based values and culture.

Lastly, three important recent innovations are of vital importance to this ever-growing Program. The first engages BPSOs who continue to lead in the implementation pillar. Together with BPSOs, we have launched an *Implementation Research Collaboratory* that will enable us within a few years to identify *implementation indicators* to fully understand which are the most powerful and effective strategies to ensure uptake, sustainability, and fidelity of BPGs in service and academia. These will then be entered as formal indicators into NQuIRE, allowing us to continuously learn about implementation processes and their degree of success on evidence uptake and sustainability. The second innovation is the Evidence Boosters (EB) produced through the monitoring and evaluation pillar. Discussed and showcased in Chapters 11 and 16, EBs demonstrate the value and impact of BPG implementation in BPSOs. These EBs, which are already being produced, also serve as audit and feedback reports for nurses in all roles to showcase their work within their organizations. EBs will act as a springboard for "trending reports," from BPG launch to implementation to sustainability, which will contribute to an in-depth understanding of the economic impact of evidence-based nursing practice and healthy work environments. The third innovation involves demonstrable economic and business benefits. We are already exploring the creation of a nursing atlas on "the state of nursing care," such as falls for older persons, pressure injuries, and so on, telling the story of what excellence in nursing looks like around the globe and the impact it has on patients, organizations, and health system outcomes— clinically and financially.

Going forward, we must always keep front and center the people and communities we as nurses serve. The ultimate goal is for the public— individually and collectively—to receive the best possible care every time they come into contact with a nurse. They must always remain the real winners of this important effort.

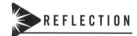

REFLECTION

How do the three innovations discussed here help RNAO's BPG Program and continue its profound impact on the profession, healthcare, and population health outcomes?

KEY MESSAGES

- The main purpose of the BPG Program is to assist nurses, other health professionals, and the organizations and health systems in which they work to embrace practice and education based on the best available evidence.

- Caring, a foundational concept for nursing, has at times been criticized as a "soft script" that has not served nurses or patients well. Advancing nursing as an art and a science requires competence in both.

- A caring-curing dichotomy poses significant challenges for nurses wanting workplace equality, especially with physicians, because it assumes that one health professional uses the heart to provide comfort and care, while the other uses the brain to cure clinical problems.

- The BPG Program powers a conceptualization of nursing caring practice that encompasses cognitive caring (e.g., clinical knowledge, care planning), physical caring (e.g., bathing), and relational caring (e.g., communication, touch, presence, compassion).

- RNAO's BPG Program facilitates access to rigorous evidence for all domains of nursing practice: cognitive, physical, and relational. Evidence also pertain to health promotion, disease prevention, and curative aspects of clinical care where nurses play a leading role.

- The BPG Program is based on scientific and nontraditional multifaceted strategies of social engagement, including magnetic approaches that attract nurses to mobilize knowledge, commitment, and energy, becoming drivers of sustained clinical, organizational, and health system change.

- As a result of a zealous approach dedicated to implementation science combined with constant attention to learning from and responding to in-the-field needs, RNAO leads what is likely the most robust and expansive implementation program for evidence-based practice for nurses anywhere in the world, and is amongst the strongest in the healthcare field.

- The location of the BPG Program within a professional nursing association has advanced its goals because it provides a large voluntary membership of nurses and nursing students ready to adopt and test the BPGs, identifying an initial base of early adopters.

- The BPG Program has been central to RNAO's policy work in areas of nursing practice (i.e., funding for offloading devices) and the work environment. In turn, RNAO policy work has influenced the development of specific BPGs (i.e., implementing supervised injection services).

- NQuIRE supports BPSOs in making effective practice improvements to optimize clinical, organizational, and health system outcomes by providing organizational and comparative data on BPG-directed nursing care processes and clinical/financial outcomes.

- Multiple factors have contributed to the large-scale spread of the BPG Program and advancing it from producing localized systemic change to leading a seismic transformation of nursing care worldwide. Central to it is the sense of collective identity.

- RNAO BPGs are revolutionizing nursing through a focus on knowledge that optimizes the delivery of care anywhere in the world. These robust, evidence-based tools have captured the imagination of nurses in practice, administration, education, research, and policy.

REFERENCES

Aiken, L. H., Clarke, S. P., Sloane, D. M., Sochalski, J. A., Busse, R., Clarke, H., . . . Shamian, J. (2001). Nurses' reports on hospital care in five countries: The ways in which nurses' work is structured have left nurses among the least satisfied workers, and the problem is getting worse. *Health Affairs, 20*(3), 43–53.

Aiken, L. H., Clarke, S. P., Sloane, D. M., Sochalski, J., & Silber, J. H. (2002). Hospital nurse staffing and patient mortality, nurse burnout, and job dissatisfaction. *JAMA: Journal of the American Medical Association, 288*(16), 1987–1993.

Aiken, L. H., Clarke, S. P., Sloane, D. M., Lake, E. T., & Cheney, T. (2008). Effects of hospital care environment on patient mortality and nurse outcomes. *Journal of Nursing Administration, 38*(5), 223–229.

Aiken, L. H., Sloane, D., Griffiths, P., Rafferty, A. M., Bruyneel, L., McHugh, M., . . . Sermeus, W. (2016). Nursing skill mix in European hospitals: Cross-sectional study of the association with mortality, patient ratings, and quality of care. *BMJ Quality & Safety, 26*, 559–568. doi: 10.1136/bmjqs-2016-005567

Bajnok, I. (2008, May 23). Healthy work environment Best Practice Guidelines [Letter to the editor]. *Welland Tribune.*

Bajnok, I. (2009, August 7). Falls in older adults and recommendations in RNAO's BPG [Letter to the editor]. *National Post.*

Bajnok, I., Grinspun, D., Lloyd, M., & McConnell, H. (2015). Leading quality improvement through Best Practice Guideline development, implementation, and measurement science. *Med UNAB, 17*(3), 155–162.

Bates, P., Robert, G., & Bevan, H. (2004). The next phase of healthcare improvement: What can we learn from social movements? *Quality & Safety in Health Care, 13*(1), 62–66.

Benner, P. E. (1994). *Interpretive phenomenology: Embodiment, caring, and ethics in health and illness.* Thousand Oaks, CA: Sage Publications.

Bishop, A. H., & Scudder, J. R. (1991). *Nursing: The practice of caring.* New York, NY: National League for Nursing Press.

Boykin, A., & Schoenhofer, S. O. B. (1993). *Nursing as caring: A model for transforming practice.* New York, NY: National League for Nursing.

Buresh, B., & Gordon, S. (2003). *From silence to voice: What nurses know and must communicate to the public.* Ithaca, NY: Cornell University Press.

Calman, L. (2006). Patients' views of nurses' competence. *Nurse Education Today, 26*(8), 719–725.

Cohen, S. S., Mason, D. J., Kovner, C., Leavitt, J. K., Pulcini, J., & Sochalski, J. (1996). Stages of nursing's political development: Where we've been and where we ought to go. *Nursing Outlook, 44*(6), 259–266.

Cummings, G. (2006). Hospital restructuring and nursing leadership: A journey from research question to research program. *Nursing Administration Quarterly, 30*(4), 321–329.

Curran, J. A., Grimshaw, J. M., Hayden, J. A., & Campbell, B. (2011). Knowledge translation research: The science of moving research into policy and practice. *Journal of Continuing Education in the Health Professions, 31*(3), 174–180.

Decter, M. B. (2000). *Four strong winds: Understanding the growing challenges to health care.* Toronto, ON: Stoddart.

Di Costanzo, M. (2013). Becoming a BPSO. *Registered Nurse Journal, 25*(2), 12–17.

Di Costanzo, M. (2014). Therefore, be it resolved that . . . *Registered Nurse Journal, 26*(4), 23–25.

Edwards, N., Rowan, M., Marck, P., & Grinspun, D. (2011). Understanding whole systems change in health care: The case of the nurse practitioners in Canada. *Policy, Politics, & Nursing, 12*(1), 4–17.

Ellenbecker, C. H., Fawcett, J., Jones, E. J., Mahoney, D., Rowlands, B., & Waddell, A. (2017). A staged approach to educating nurses in health policy. *Policy, Politics & Nursing Practice, 18*(1), 44–56.

Field, M., & Lohr, K. (1990). *Clinical practice guidelines: Directions for a new program.* Washington, DC: National Academies Press.

Forest, D. (1989). The experience of caring. *Journal of Advanced Nursing, 14*, 815–823.

Gadow, S. (1985). The nurse and patient: The caring relationship. In A. H. Bishop & J. R. Scudder (Eds.), *Caring, curing and coping: Nurse, physician, patient relationships* (pp. 31–43). Tuscaloosa, AL: The University of Alabama Press.

Gordon, S. (1997). *Life support: Three nurses on the front lines* (1st ed.). Boston, MA: Little Brown.

Gordon, S. (2005). *Nursing against the odds: How health care cost cutting, media stereotypes, and medical hubris undermine nurses and patient care.* Ithaca, NY: ILR Press, an imprint of Cornell University Press.

Griffin, A. P. (1983). A philosophical analysis of caring in nursing. *Journal of Advanced Nursing, 8*, 289–295.

Grimshaw, J. M., Eccles, M. P., Lavis, J. N., Hill, S. J., & Squires, J. E. (2012). Knowledge translation of research findings. *Implementation Science, 7*, 50. doi: 10.1186/1748-5908-7-50

Grinspun, D. (2007). Healthy workplaces: The case for shared clinical decision making and increased full-time employment. *Healthcare Papers, Vol. 7 Special Issue*, 69–75.

Grinspun, D. (2010). *The social construction of caring in nursing* (Doctoral dissertation). York University, Toronto, ON.

Grinspun, D. (2011). Guías de práctica clínica y entorno laboral basados en la evidencia elaboradas por la Registered Nurses' Association of Ontario (RNAO) (Evidence based clinical practice and work environment guidelines prepared by the RNAO). *Enferm. Clin., 21*, 1–2.

Grinspun, D., Librado, R., Góngora, A. (2005). Centros de excelencía en enfermería de rehabilitación: Un sueno a alcanzar. Centres of excellence in rehabilitation nursing services: A dream to be achieved. *Enfermería Global, 7*, 1–8.

Guyatt, G. H. (1991). Evidence-based medicine. *ACP J Club, 114*, A16. doi: 10.7326/ACPJC-1991-114-2-A16

Halldórsdóttir, S. (1997). Implications of the caring/competence dichotomy. In S. E. Thorne & V. E. Hayes (Eds.), *Nursing praxis: Knowledge and action* (pp. 105–124). Thousand Oaks, CA: Sage Publications.

Health Council of Canada. (2012). *Understanding clinical practice guidelines: A video series primer.* Retrieved from https://healthcouncilcanada.ca/files/CPG_Backgrounder_EN.pdf.pdf

International Council of Nurses (ICN). (2013). *RNAO-ICNP Research and Development Centre.* Retrieved from http://www.icn.ch/what-we-do/rnao-icnp-research-and-development-centre/

Jordan, Z. (2005, Oct/Dec). Turning challenges into opportunities. *PACEsetterS, 2*(4), 6–11.

JPNC Implementation Monitoring Subcommittee. (2003, November). *Good nursing, good health: The return on our investment—Progress report.* Toronto, ON: Queen's Printer for Ontario.

Kane, R. L., Shamliyan, T. A., Mueller, C., Duval, S., & Wilt, T. J. (2007). The association of registered nurse staffing levels and patient outcomes: Systematic review and meta-analysis. *Med Care, 45*(12), 1195–1204.

Leininger, M. M. (1978). *Transcultural nursing: Concepts, theories, and practices.* New York, NY: John Wiley & Sons.

Leininger, M. M. (1980). Caring: A central focus of nursing and health care services. *Nursing & Health Care, 1*(3), 135–176.

Liu, J. E., Mok, E., & Wong, T. (2006). Caring in nursing: Investigating the meaning of caring from the perspective of cancer patients in Beijing, China. *Journal of Clinical Nursing, 15*(2), 188–196.

Manitoba Health. (2001). *Report of the Review and Implementation Committee for the report of the Manitoba Pediatric Cardiac Surgery Inquest.* Winnipeg, MB: Ministry of Health, Government of Manitoba.

Melucci, A. (1980). The new social movements: A theoretical approach. *Social Science Information, 19*(2), 199–226.

Melucci, A. (1989). *Nomad of the present: Social movements and individual needs in contemporary society.* Philadelphia, PA: Temple University Press.

Melucci, A. (1996). *Challenging codes: Collective action in the information age.* Cambridge, UK: Cambridge University Press.

Meyer, R. M., Wang, S., Li, X., Thomson, D., & O'Brien-Pallas, L. (2009). Evaluation of a patient care delivery model: Patient outcomes in acute cardiac care. *Journal of Nursing Scholarship, 41*(4), 399–410.

Moland, L. L. (2006). Moral integrity and regret in nursing. In S. Nelson & S. Gordon (Eds.), *The complexities of care: Nursing reconsidered* (pp. 50–68). Ithaca, NY: ILR Press/Cornell University Press.

Moore, M., Riddell, D., & Vocisano, D. (2015). Scaling out, scaling up, scaling deep: Strategies of non-profits in advancing systemic social innovation. *Journal of Corporate Citizenship, Vol. 2015*(58), 67–84(18). https://doi.org/10.9774/GLEAF.4700.2015.ju.00009

Needleman, J., Buerhaus, P., Mattke, S., Stewart, M., & Zelevinsky, K. (2002). Nurse staffing levels and the quality of care in hospitals. *The New England Journal of Medicine, 346*(22), 1715–1722.

Needleman, J., Buerhaus, P. I., Stewart, M., Zelevinsky, K., & Mattke, S. (2006). Nurse staffing in hospitals: Is there a business case for quality? *Health Affairs (Millwood), 25*(1), 204–211.

Nelson, S., & Gordon, S. (2006). *The complexities of care: Nursing reconsidered.* Ithaca, NY: ILR Press/Cornell University Press.

Ontario Ministry of Health and Long-Term Care—Nursing Task Force. (1999, January). *Good nursing, good health: An investment for the 21st century* (Ministry report). Retrieved from http://www.health.gov.on.ca/en/common/ministry/publications/reports/nurserep99/nurse_rep.aspx

Picard, A. (2000). *Critical care: Canadian nurses speak for change.* Toronto, ON: HarperCollins.

Punch, D. (2017, February 3). *Upcoming guideline recommends eHealth strategies to improve health system.* Retrieved from http://rnao.ca/news/media-releases/2017/02/23/ehealth-improve-health

Ray, M. A. (1989). The theory of bureaucratic caring for nursing practice in the organizational culture. *Nursing Administration Quarterly, 13*(2), 31–42.

Registered Nurses' Association of Ontario (RNAO). (n.d.-a). *Mission and values.* Retrieved from http://rnao.ca/about/mission

Registered Nurses' Association of Ontario (RNAO). (n.d.-b). *Nursing order sets.* Retrieved from http://rnao.ca/ehealth/nursingordersets

Registered Nurses' Association of Ontario (RNAO). (n.d.-c). *Nursing Quality Indicators for Reporting and Evaluation (NQuIRE).* Retrieved from https://nquire.rnao.ca/

Registered Nurses' Association of Ontario (RNAO). (1998, March). *Putting Out the Health Care Fire: A Proposal to Reinvest in Nursing Care in Ontario. A report submitted to Premier Michael D. Harris.* Toronto, ON: Registered Nurses' Association of Ontario.

Registered Nurses' Association of Ontario (RNAO). (2004, January 13). *RNAO partners with seven health-care organizations to implement and evaluate nursing BPGs.* Retrieved from http://rnao.ca/news/media-releases/RNAO-partners-with-seven-health-care-organizations-to-implement-and-evaluate-nursing-BPGs

Registered Nurses' Association of Ontario (RNAO). (2006). *Client centred care* (Revised supplement). Toronto, ON: Registered Nurses' Association of Ontario.

Registered Nurses' Association of Ontario (RNAO). (2009). *About the eHealth Toolkit.* Retrieved from http://rnao.ca/ehealth/toolkit

Registered Nurses' Association of Ontario (RNAO). (2013, June). *RNAO's Proud Past.* Retrieved from http://rnao.ca/sites/rnao-ca/files/RNAOs_Proud_Past_-_June_2013.pdf

Registered Nurses' Association of Ontario (RNAO). (2017a). *70 years of RN effectiveness.* Retrieved from http://rnao.ca/bpg/initiatives/RNEffectiveness

Registered Nurses' Association of Ontario (RNAO). (2017b). *Adopting eHealth solutions: Implementation strategies.* Toronto, ON: Registered Nurses' Association of Ontario.

Roach, M. S. (1987). *The human act of caring: A blueprint for health professions.* Toronto, ON: Canadian Hospital Association.

Rogers, E. M. (1962). *Diffusion of innovations.* New York, NY: Free Press of Glencoe.

Rogers, E. M. (2003). *Diffusion of innovations* (5th ed.). New York, NY: Free Press.

Sales, A., Smith, J., Curran, G., & Kochevar, L. (2006). Models, strategies, and tools: Theory in implementing evidence-based findings into health care practice. *Journal of General Internal Medicine, 21*(Supplement 2), S43–S49.

Scarrow, J. (2008). Revolutionizing nursing practice. *Registered Nurse Journal, 20*(2), 12–17.

Shekelle, P. G., Woolf, S. H., Eccles, M., & Grimshaw, J. (1999). Developing guidelines. *BMJ, 318*(7183), 593–598.

Sinclair, M. (2001). *The report of the Manitoba Pediatric Cardiac Surgery Inquest: An inquiry into twelve deaths at the Winnipeg Health Sciences Centre in 1994 (Sinclair Report).* Winnipeg, MB: Provincial Court of Manitoba.

Straus, S., Tetroe, J., & Graham, I. (Eds.). (2013). *Knowledge translation in health care* (2nd ed.) Oxford, UK: Wiley-Blackwell.

Swanson, K. M. (1991). Empirical development of a middle range theory of caring. *Nursing Research, 40,* 161–166.

Swanson, K. M. (1999). What is known about caring in nursing science—A literary meta-analysis. In A. S. Hinshaw, S. Feetham, & J. L. F. Shaver (Eds.), *Handbook of clinical nursing research* (pp. 31–60). Thousand Oaks, CA: Sage Publications.

Urden, L. D., & Walston, S. L. (2001). Outcomes of hospital restructuring and reengineering—How is success or failure being measured? *Journal of Nursing Administration, 31*(4), 203–209.

Virani, T. (2007, April 10). Combatting obesity: MDs urge new checkup routine: Height, weight—and waistline. *The Globe and Mail.*

Watson, J. (1985). *Nursing: The philosophy and science of caring.* Boulder, CO: Colorado Associated University Press.

Watson, J. (1999). *Nursing: Human science and human care. A theory of nursing* (Reprint of 1988 ed.). New York, NY: National League for Nursing.

Watson, J. (2005). *Caring science as sacred science.* Philadelphia, PA: F.A. Davis Co.

Weiss, C. J. (1988). Gender-related perceptions of caring in the nurse-patient relationship. In M. M. Leininger (Ed.), *Care: The essence of nursing and health* (Rerelease of 1984 ed., pp. 161–182). Detroit, MI: Wayne State University.

WHO Regional Office for Europe. Copenhagen, Denmark. (2015). Spain BPSO Host. Nurses and Midwifes: A vital resource for Health. European compendium of good practices in nursing and midwifery towards Health 2020 goals. *SPAIN: Implementation of evidence-based guidelines to establish a network of centres committed to using best care practices* (pp. 40–42). Retrieved from http://www.euro.who.int/en/health-topics/Health-systems/nursing-and-midwifery/publications/2015/nurses-and-midwives-a-vital-resource-for-health.-european-compendium-of-good-practices-in-nursing-and-midwifery-towards-health-2020-goals

Young, L. (2011). There are 31 interest groups to choose from at RNAO: Which one appeals to you? *Registered Nurse Journal, 23*(5), 18–21.

Young-Mason, J. (1997). *The patient's voice: Experiences of illness.* Philadelphia, PA: F.A. Davis.

Zych, M. (2012, May 3). *Health-care professionals mark Nursing Week with a commitment to better patient care.* Retrieved from http://rnao.ca/news/media-releases/2012/05/03/health-care-professionals-mark-nursing-week-commitment-better-patient

GUIDELINE DEVELOPMENT: FIRST PILLAR FOR SUCCESS

2

THE ANATOMY OF A RIGOROUS BEST PRACTICE GUIDELINE DEVELOPMENT PROCESS

Michelle Rey, PhD, MSc, BSc
Doris Grinspun, PhD, MSN, BScN, RN, LLD(hon), Dr(hc), O.ONT
Lucia Costantini, PhD, RN
Monique Lloyd, PhD, RN

LEARNING OBJECTIVES

After reading this chapter, you will be able to:

- Understand the evolution of Best Practice Guidelines as useful knowledge tools in the delivery of evidence-based care

- Outline the qualities of an effective guideline, according to international guideline-development standards

- Describe the seven steps of RNAO's BPG development process and why each is important

- Discuss the elements of a systematic review that contribute to guideline rigor

- Determine the components of RNAO's BPG development process that serve to reduce bias

- Appreciate enhancements used and planned in the RNAO BPG development methodology, including application of GRADE frameworks

INTRODUCTION

This chapter describes the Registered Nurses' Association of Ontario's (RNAO) guideline development process, a pillar of the Best Practice Guideline (BPG) Program, which was introduced and described in Chapter 1. The process is delineated using RNAO's seven steps of rigorous guideline development, which adhere to international standards, and is depicted in Figure 2.1.

Included is a detailed overview of each step, with special emphasis on evidence synthesis through systematic reviews of peer-reviewed literature and the modified-Delphi consensus process used with the Expert Panel to refine evidence-based recommendations. The chapter outlines RNAO's emerging work in aligning methodologies with GRADE (Grading of Recommendations Assessment, Development and Evaluation), to evaluate the quality of evidence and strength of recommendations. RNAO's approach to ongoing process and outcome evaluation and continuous quality improvement with guideline development methods is also highlighted. The chapter provides answers to key challenges in guideline development such as timelines, resources, updating cycles, and engaging experts in effective and efficient processes to achieve maximum results.

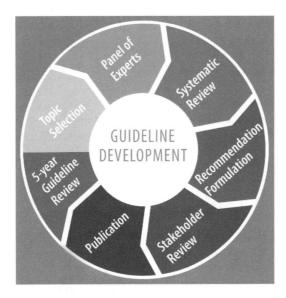

FIGURE 2.1 The guideline development pillar of the BPG Program showing steps in RNAO's BPG development process.

BEST PRACTICE GUIDELINES: WHY?

The importance of robust evidence-based clinical practice guidelines cannot be overestimated. Globally, governments and clinicians are aiming to improve healthcare and optimize outcomes through initiatives that support evidence-based clinical care. Despite this laudable goal, variations in clinical practice first described by Wennberg and Gittelsohn (1973, 1982) continue, and so do the problematic results (Institute of Medicine [IOM], 2011; Grinspun, Melnyk, & Fineout-Overholt, 2014; Melnyk et al., 2012). Yet, patients trust and rely on healthcare providers for quality care and assume that those providers have the knowledge and expertise to make the best health-related decisions.

An important tool to respond to this challenge is the availability, uptake, and consistent utilization of clinical practice guidelines and rigorously developed evidence-based recommendations. These guidelines aid healthcare providers, often faced with difficult decisions, overwhelming evidence, and considerable uncertainty, to make informed clinical decisions when treating patients. Best Practice Guidelines can aid clinicians and patients to determine the best options for a particular disease, condition, or health issue. Trustworthy guidelines are developed with the intent to improve healthcare quality while bolstering clinical, financial, and organization outcomes.

SCIENCE OF GUIDELINE DEVELOPMENT: SETTING THE STANDARDS

Previous approaches to guideline development focused on tradition (i.e., "we have always done it this way") or authority (i.e., the most senior or well-respected physician) (AGREE Collaboration, 2003). Today, guidelines are based on an appraisal of current evidence, resulting in statements (derived by consensus) on best practices in healthcare. In 2011, the Institute of Medicine (IOM) reported that the Guidelines International Network database held more than 3,700 clinical practice guidelines from 39 countries, with an additional 2,700 guidelines in the National Guideline Clearinghouse (NGC), part of the Agency for Healthcare Research and Quality (AHRQ) (IOM, 2011a). The large number of available clinical practice guidelines challenges users, including practitioners, to determine which guidelines are of high quality. The positive or negative impact of implementing guidelines may vary significantly based on their quality. Guidelines developed using evidence on benefits and harms of treatments or interventions have the potential to improve healthcare and health outcomes and decrease morbidity and mortality (Grimshaw et al., 2004; Melnyk et al., 2012). Low-quality guidelines may cause harm to patients and should be carefully appraised for validity and reliability of their information and supporting evidence (Shekelle et al., 2000).

This increase in the number of guideline developers, the inconsistencies in the methodology, and the variable quality of recommendations made it apparent that a set of standards was needed to strengthen trust in the guideline development process, the guidelines developed, and the outcomes associated with their implementation. Guideline users needed a mechanism to identify high-quality, trustworthy clinical practice guidelines to support health-related decision-making that enhanced healthcare quality and outcomes. Thus, guideline-development standards would help developers to create reliable guidelines that improve decision-making, quality, and outcomes.

TRUSTWORTHY GUIDELINES

In 2008, the IOM entered into a contract with the Secretary of the Department of Health and Human Services to identify "the best methods used in developing clinical practice guidelines [in order] to ensure that organizations developing such guidelines have information on approaches that are objective, scientifically valid, and consistent" (Institute of Medicine, 2011b, p.1/para. 2). The resulting IOM (2011) report, *Clinical Practice Guidelines We Can Trust*, provided a revised definition of an evidence-based clinical practice guideline, including recommendations on what a guideline should entail, and eight standards for guideline development. The IOM recommendations for trustworthy guidelines included (2011a) that they should:

- Be based on a systematic review of the existing evidence

- Be developed by a knowledgeable, multidisciplinary panel of experts and representatives from key affected groups

- Consider important patient subgroups and patient preferences, as appropriate

- Be based on an explicit and transparent process that minimizes distortions, biases, and conflicts of interest

- Provide a clear explanation of the logical relationships between alternative care options and health outcomes, and provide ratings of both the quality of evidence and the strength of recommendations and

- Be reconsidered and revised as appropriate when important new evidence warrants modification of recommendations

The eight standards for trustworthy guidelines proposed by the committee that were derived from these recommendations addressed the following (IOM, 2011a):

- Transparency

- Management of conflict of interest

- Guideline development group composition

- Clinical practice guideline–systematic review intersection

- Establishing evidence foundations for and rating strength of recommendations

- Articulation of recommendations

- External review

- Updating

More information on these standards is available from the Health and Medicine Division of the National Academies of Sciences, Engineering, and Medicine (formerly the IOM), http://www.nationalacademies.org/hmd/.

GUIDELINES 2.0

The findings of the IOM resulting in the Standards for Trustworthy Guidelines (2011), as well as many other reviews of guideline development methods, highlighted the need for a systematic review and documentation of the diverse processes for guideline development available to organizations (Qaseem et al., 2012; Schünemann et al., 2007; Woolf et al., 2012). Although many manuals for single organizations are available as a complement to the eight IOM standards, a comprehensive list of items to consider related to each of the standards on an international scale was not available. The Guideline International Network (GIN) Working Group systematically compiled and made available a comprehensive checklist of items and a portal for related resources for guideline developers to consider for all stages of the guideline enterprise (Schünemann et al., 2013). The result of this work, entitled Guidelines 2.0, was a comprehensive, 18-point list of topics to consider during development of guidelines (AGREE Collaboration, 2003), outlined on the following page:

1. Organization, Budget, Planning, and Training

2. Priority Setting

3. Guideline Group Membership

4. Establishing Guideline Group Processes

5. Identifying Target Audience and Topic Selection

6. Consumer and Stakeholder Involvement

7. Conflict of Interest Considerations

8. (PICO) Question Generation

9. Considering Importance of Outcomes and Interventions, Values, Preferences and Utilities

10. Deciding What Evidence to Include and Searching for Evidence

11. Summarizing Evidence and Considering Additional Information

12. Judging Quality, Strength, or Certainty of a Body of Evidence

13. Developing Recommendations and Determining Their Strength

14. Wording of Recommendations and of Considerations of Implementation, Feasibility, and Equity

15. Reporting and Peer Review

16. Dissemination and Implementation

17. Evaluation and Use

18. Updating

Consideration of these 18 topics is crucial when developing trustworthy guidelines, as well as when such guidelines are being implemented and/or evaluated.

HOW TO KNOW WHICH GUIDELINES ARE TRUSTWORTHY: APPRAISAL OF GUIDELINES

This section outlines the various tools developed to help one determine whether the proposed guidelines are trustworthy or not. It covers the AGREE II and NEATS tools.

AGREE II

The AGREE (Appraisal of Guidelines Research and Evaluation) tool was published in 2003 by a group of international guideline developers and researchers, the AGREE Collaboration. The AGREE Collaboration (2003) defined quality of guidelines as the confidence that the potential biases of guideline development have been addressed adequately and that the recommendations are both internally and externally valid, and are feasible for practice. The guideline appraisal process to determine quality includes judgments about the methods used for developing the guidelines, the components of the final recommendations, and the factors associated with implementation.

Common to many new assessment tools, ongoing development was required to improve its measurement properties, usefulness to a range of stakeholders, and ease of usage. The original four-point response scale for each item of the AGREE instrument did not comply with methodological standards of health measurement design. This noncompliance threatened the performance and reliability of the instrument (National Guidelines Clearinghouse, n.d.). Data on the usefulness of the AGREE items were not systematically obtained from different groups of users. As a result of these shortfalls, the tool was subsequently revised and tested for reliability and validity. It now comprises 23 items organized into the original six quality domains (Brouwers et al., 2010), which are addressed more fully in following sections.

One of the most significant changes in the AGREE II appraisal tool is inclusion of the statement "strengths and limitations of the body of evidence are clearly described" (Brouwers et al., 2010, p. 2) as a measurement item in the rigour of development domain. The domain of editorial independence was strengthened to encourage that the content of the guideline not be influenced by funding sources. Conflict of interest (COI) must be recorded and clearly addressed during the guideline development process.

The 23-item tool comprises six guideline quality-related domains (Brouwers et al., 2010):

- **Domain 1**—Scope and Purpose is concerned with the overall aim of the guideline, the specific health questions, and the target population (items 1–3).

- **Domain 2**—Stakeholder Involvement focuses on the extent to which the guideline was developed by the appropriate stakeholders and represents the views of its intended users (items 4–6).

- **Domain 3**—Rigour of Development relates to the process used to gather and synthesize the evidence as well as the methods to formulate the recommendations and to update them (items 7–14).

- **Domain 4**—Clarity of Presentation deals with the language, structure, and format of the guideline (items 15–17).

- **Domain 5**—Applicability pertains to the likely barriers and facilitators to implementation, strategies to improve uptake, and resource implications of applying the guideline (items 18–21).

- **Domain 6**—Editorial Independence is concerned with the formulation of recommendations not unduly biased with competing interests (items 22–23).

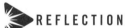

REFLECTION

What are some of the advantages of having and using international standards for guideline development, and why is this important?

Overall assessment includes the rating of the overall quality of the guideline and whether the guideline would be recommended for use in practice.

The AGREE II instrument is recognized as an international tool for the assessment of guidelines. A 10-year revision cycle was determined and updates were completed on September 2013; they did not result in further changes to the tool. Other AGREE appraisal tools and checklists have been created and will be discussed further in the section on aligning rigorous processes of evidence synthesis.

NEATS

The NGC has created a global repository for guidelines, and to ensure that only trustworthy and credible guidelines are housed within the repository, NGC aligned its inclusion criteria with IOM and GIN 2.0 standards. All submitted guidelines must include a systematic review published within the last 5 years. The guideline assessment results are posted on the NGC's website. For the purpose of assessing guidelines against the IOM standards, the NGC, in partnership with the AGREE Research Trust and others, created a new appraisal tool, the National Guideline Clearinghouse Extent Adherence to Trustworthy Standards (NEATS) Instrument. Each element of the eight standards and sub-standards is rated using a binary and five-point Likert scale ranging from lowest to highest adherence to the standard.

RNAO AND BEST PRACTICE GUIDELINES

RNAO Best Practice Guidelines (BPG) are systematically developed, evidence-based statements that include recommendations for nurses and the interprofessional clinical team, administrators, educators, policymakers, and patients and their families to improve outcomes on specific clinical, system, and healthy work environment topics. BPGs offer an evaluation of the quality of the relevant scientific literature and an assessment of the likely benefits and harms of a particular intervention, and present this information in specific recommendations for practitioners, organizations, educators, and policymakers. When appropriate, the BPG recommendations are targeted to be inclusive of and generalizable to all healthcare sectors (acute care, community, long-term care, complex continuing care, and rehabilitation). These recommendations enable healthcare providers to plan and deliver care for their patients based on best evidence, and aid those in education and organizational and health policy roles to use evidence in their curriculum and policy-related decision-making. BPGs should be used as a tool or template to enhance decision-making and support the provision of the best possible evidence-based care. Figure 2.2 graphically displays and explains the types of recommendations included in RNAO's clinical BPGs. These evidence-based recommendations influence practice at the individual and team level, as well as policy and education to ensure BPG uptake and sustained use.

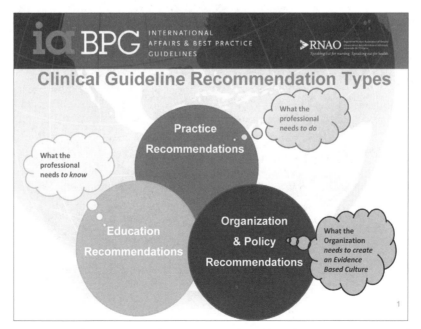

FIGURE 2.2   Types of recommendations in RNAO clinical Best Practice Guidelines.
© Registered Nurses' Association of Ontario (RNAO). All rights reserved.

Nurses, other healthcare professionals, and administrators who lead and facilitate practice changes say that RNAO's BPGs are invaluable resource tools for advancing evidence-based clinical practice, and for the development of policies, procedures, practice protocols, educational programs, assessment interventions, and documentation tools. Nurses who provide direct care say they benefit from reviewing the recommendations and seeing the evidence in support of the recommendations and the process that was used to develop the guidelines. As we discuss in Chapter 5, *Technology as an Enabler of Evidence-Based Practice*, RNAO's BPG recommendations for practice can be easily integrated into electronic health records. RNAO recommends that practice settings/environments adapt these guidelines in formats that are user-friendly for practitioners. There are currently 53 published guidelines, an Implementation Toolkit, and an Educator's Resource to support implementation. Additional new guidelines are being developed every year. The BPGs have been organized into themes representing key clinical areas of practice, and System and Healthy Work Environments, as shown in the circles in Figure 2.3 (RNAO Best Practice Guideline thematic organizing framework), with BPG covers from guidelines in that category as samples. To date, guidelines have been translated into French, Spanish, Italian, Chinese, German, and Japanese with a commitment to translating more materials on an ongoing basis.

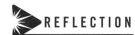

REFLECTION

How do you think recommendations in the three areas identified—practice, education, and policy—impact BPG use by individuals and the organization and uptake at a systems level?

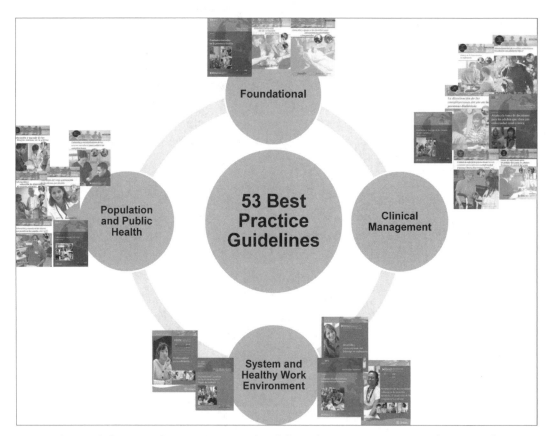

FIGURE 2.3 RNAO Best Practice Guideline thematic organizing framework.

RNAO FUNDING

Funding granted to the RNAO by the Ontario Ministry of Health and Long-Term Care supports the BPG Program Managers, project co-coordinators, and nursing research associates and expenses related to guideline development projects (i.e., Expert Panel meetings, health services librarian, and document retrieval) and the costs of printing and disseminating published guidelines. Expert Panel members are not remunerated for their time. The RNAO does not provide financial support to Expert Panel members to attend or present RNAO BPG work at conferences. Any and all monies from sales of hardcopy versions of Best Practice Guidelines are directed back into the program.

The time required to develop an RNAO BPG is approximately 14 months, including the completion of systematic reviews. See Appendix A at the end of this chapter for a detailed account of the timelines, actions, and outcomes during the 14-month process.

RNAO'S SEVEN-STEP GUIDELINE DEVELOPMENT PROCESS

RNAO's process for BPG development has been used for almost two decades and has proven to be a user-friendly, effective, and efficient methodology. Over the years, each step has been altered as necessary to be consistent with current international guideline-development standards and our own quality-improvement processes. The seven steps include topic selection, use of an Expert Panel, systematic literature review, recommendation formulation, stakeholder review, publication, and a 5-year guideline review that produces the next editions of existing guidelines. Each step is described fully in this section.

TOPIC SELECTION

Topics for RNAO Clinical Nursing BPGs are selected using a priority-identification matrix. Appendix B at the end of this chapter provides an example of a priority-identification matrix. The process includes a set of criteria to guide the systematic assessment of a selected list of suggested topics and feedback from a range of stakeholders provided through focus groups. A completed assessment of each topic, carried out by a team of reviewers, leads to an overall suggestion for guideline development. Any group or individual may propose a guideline topic to the RNAO through a variety of methods such as:

1. "Submit an Idea" on the RNAO website at www.rnao.ca

2. Writing to RNAO's CEO or director/associate directors of the IABPG Centre

3. A rapid review or environmental scan (i.e., scoping search for trends, hot topics, practice concerns)

4. A survey requesting individuals to rank identified topics on a five-point Likert scale

5. Report sources (e.g., coroner's inquest, government or related agency)

RNAO selects topics for guideline development annually. All topics submitted are identified, and a maximum of three priority topics are chosen based on the following systematic assessment criteria.

- Key priority areas identified by the Ontario Ministry of Health and Long-Term Care (MOHLTC)

- Request from major public health agency

- Coroner's inquest

- Within the scope of nursing practice (RN, NP, RPN/LPN), and applicable in a range of practice settings

- A multidisciplinary approach would be appropriate for BPG development

- Builds on a previously developed guideline or general topic area

- Potential for partnerships in BPG development with other agencies (i.e., Heart & Stroke; Canada Health Infoway)

- Perceived need for the guideline, as identified by those submitting the topic for consideration

- Evidence to support the guideline recommendations is available

- No other good quality guideline exists on the topic area

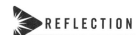

REFLECTION

What are the best ways to determine topics for guideline development, what criteria would you set for such a selection process, and why?

Upon reviewing all submissions based on the above criteria, a report is created outlining the first, second, and third choice of topics. The results are shared with the BPG team. Consensus is achieved on priority topics, and results are shared and submitted for approval to the chief executive officer (CEO) of RNAO, who reports the selected topics to the MOHLTC.

When a topic is selected for potential new guideline development, the assigned RNAO Best Practice Guideline Development Team Lead assembles a focus group of subject matter experts (SMEs) and key opinion leaders to discuss relevant content and identify the scope and purpose of the guideline. SMEs may become potential RNAO Expert Panel members.

The objectives of the focus group are to identify:

- The scope of the proposed guideline

- Current tools and resources

- Current research

- Gaps in the current literature or guidelines pertaining to the proposed guideline topic area

These individuals come together during a series of teleconferences hosted by the RNAO and communication via email and telephone. Structured, open-ended questions are posed to the group, and the information they share is transcribed and referenced throughout the BPG development process.

EXPERT PANEL

Composition of the Expert Panel

Nurses (RN, NP, and RPN) make up 50% of the RNAO Expert Panel; the second half are other health professionals (social workers, registered dieticians, physicians, physiotherapists, etc.) and persons and family members with lived experience in the defined topic area. Expert Panel composition whenever possible represents: 1) expertise on the subject matter in direct and advanced clinical practice, research, education, administration, and policy; 2) rural and urban work settings; and 3) the spectrum of health services including public health, primary care, acute care, home healthcare, and long-term care as appropriate to the guideline topic. Invitations for panel membership are extended to the Ontario Nurses' Association (labour union for RNs) and the Registered Practical Nurses Association of Ontario (professional association for RPNs) to ensure equitable representation from all nursing perspectives. Representatives from First Nations, Inuit, people with lived experience, and students are routinely sought for inclusion on the panel. The aim is to have equal representation from each of the four major groups (patients, direct-care clinicians, researchers/educators, and system-level representatives). The RNAO requests a letter of intent and resume from the Expert Panel member with an indication of support from his/her organization to ensure commitment from the individual and organization. All individuals involved in developing the guideline are acknowledged in the published guideline.

Early in the panel selection process, two panel cochairs are identified by the RNAO Best Practice Guideline Development Team Lead, one of whom must be a PhD-prepared nurse with content expertise on the chosen topic. The second cochair can be from a discipline other than nursing or a lived experience representative. These individuals assist with expert-panel selection and support effective functioning of the panel in the development process respective of milestone timelines. The panel cochairs ensure that all members of the Expert Panel are engaged in the guideline development process and all voices are heard and respected. The RNAO Best Practice Guideline Development Team Lead assigned to each BPG works with the panel cochairs to facilitate group meetings and progress through the BPG development process.

Responsibilities of the Expert Panel

A terms of reference (TOR) document is developed for each RNAO Expert Panel (see Appendix C at the end of this chapter). The TOR outlines RNAO's mandate and the IABPG Centre structure, key RNAO stakeholders who will be involved in the guideline, and the approach and plan for guideline development including timelines and deliverables. The TOR document is distributed to all panel candidates prior to their acceptance to participate as a member of the RNAO Expert Panel. Expert Panel members are required to declare any conflicts of interest.

The lifespan of each guideline development Expert Panel is approximately 14 months with a commitment to meet twice in person and via teleconferences as needed. Generally, the Expert Panel members' responsibilities include development of:

- **Practice Recommendations**—Statements of best practice based on the best available evidence and expert consensus.

- **Education Recommendations**—Statements of educational requirements and educational approaches/strategies for clinicians for the introduction and implementation of the BPG.

- **Organization and Policy Recommendations**—Statements of conditions required for the successful implementation of the BPG by a health service practice setting or academic organization. The conditions for success are largely the responsibility of the organization and impact local policy and procedures, although they may have implications for policy at a broader level.

- **Evaluation Criteria**—Indicators used for evaluating the BPG in the practice setting. These indicators include structure, process, and outcome indicators for organizations, nurses, and clients, as well as measures for economic cost and resource utilization.

- **Implementation Tools**—User-oriented tools to facilitate the implementation of the BPG recommendations, which are appended to the guideline. Tools may target staff nurses, nursing students, or other healthcare professionals.

- **Health Education Fact Sheets**—Plain language hand-outs that highlight key information from the guideline and are used by nurses and other healthcare professionals for educating patients, their families, and members of the public (see Appendix D at the end of this chapter).

- **Research Gaps and Implications**—Identification of gaps in the current evidence and suggestion of areas for future research inquiry.

SYSTEMATIC LITERATURE REVIEW

The first RNAO guideline was issued in 2001. At the time, the guidelines were produced using comprehensive literature reviews. From 2012 and onward, RNAO BPGs have been based on systematic reviews of the evidence. This approach is intended to create guidelines grounded in rigorous, systematic reviews, and ensures that recommendations are based on empirical evidence as opposed to clinical judgment. There may be instances in the absence of scientific evidence where recommendations are based on Expert Panel consensus.

A systematic review working subgroup is identified from within the Expert Panel membership on the bases of skill and interest. This subgroup is responsible for assisting with the development and submission of a manuscript of the systematic review completed to develop the new guideline. Specific responsibilities of this subgroup include outlining the process used for the systematic review, literature search parameters, types of studies (i.e., study design), and the associated reference list of included studies and findings. Members of the systematic review working subgroup are listed as authors on the submitted manuscript, with the participating IABPG Centre members assigned to guideline development (e.g., RNAO Best Practice Guideline Development Team Lead, Nursing Research Associate). The published systematic reviews (Almost et al., 2016; Harripaul-Yhap, Dusek, Pearce, & Lloyd, 2015; Hirst et al., 2016; Legere et al., 2017; Recalla et al., 2013; Sharma, Bamford, & Dodman, 2016; Suva et al., 2015; Wilding & Wagner , 2012; Ye et al., 2017) are substantive evidence-based resources frequently accessed by nurses and other stakeholders related to the topic area.

Identify scope, search terms, and databases

At the first guideline development meeting (i.e., Expert Panel Launch), the Expert Panel reviews the purpose and scope of the guideline, including any suggestions from the focus group(s). The purpose and scope are refined to describe specific objectives, research questions addressed by the guideline, and target audiences. Inclusion and exclusion criteria, search terms and key words, and search databases are identified during the first meeting to guide the literature search. A health sciences librarian is engaged to further develop the search strategy. Timelines for the guideline development and meeting schedule are finalized by the RNAO Best Practice Guideline Development Team Lead with the Expert Panel.

Use existing guidelines

Prior to the Expert Panel launch, the RNAO Best Practice Guideline Development Team Lead works with the Nursing Research Associates (NRA) to conduct a broad Internet search for existing guidelines on the defined topic area. An established list of evidence-based-practice websites and known guideline developers is searched using a set of preliminary search terms. This list of evidence-based-practice websites and known guideline developers is reviewed annually, and changes are made by the RNAO IABPG Centre based on recommendations by the RNAO Best Practice Guideline Development Team.

Retrieved guidelines are shortlisted using the established standard inclusion criteria, which include:

- Published in English language

- Developed within the timeframe identified by the Expert Panel

- Strictly on the topic area

- Evidence-based

- Available and accessible for retrieval

The guidelines are reviewed and independently appraised by two reviewers from the guideline development team using the Appraisal of Guidelines for Research and Evaluation Instrument (AGREE II) (www.agreetrust.org). The AGREE II Instrument evaluates the process of clinical practice guideline development and the quality of reporting. Guidelines of high quality are brought forward to the Expert Panel for consideration as evidence. Expert Panel members are instructed to:

1. Suggest any further guidelines not identified by the guideline development team

2. Review the guideline and consider the following questions:

   a. Are there any guidelines that replicate the identified topic? If so, does the existing guideline(s) include the same specific questions that the Expert Panel is interested in?

   b. If the guideline includes information that the Expert Panel is interested in but it seems outdated, should it be used but updated and/or expanded using findings from the literature search?

   c. If a guideline exists and its content answers one or more of the specific questions the Expert Panel is interested in, and uses current, evidence-based information, should it be included or endorsed in the development of the RNAO guideline content or recommendations?

   d. Given the content and questions asked in the existing guidelines being appraised, are there gaps that the RNAO guideline being developed can address? Gaps include: scope of questions, populations targeted, quality of evidence supporting the guideline, and whether the guideline includes recommendations specifically for nurses.

Guidelines selected for inclusion are used by the Expert Panel with the associated scientific literature and other resources as evidence for drafting guideline recommendations.

Frame clinical questions using PICO

Given the guidelines that exist and the knowledge gaps that remain, the Expert Panel develops specific research questions. Where appropriate, the research questions are structured using the PICO format (Fineout-Overholt & Johnston, 2005):

- **P**atients or population to which the question applies

- **I**ntervention (or diagnostic test, exposure, risk factor, etc.) being considered in relation to these patients

- **C**omparison(s) to be made between those receiving the intervention and another group that does not receive the intervention

- **O**utcome(s) to be used to establish the size of any effect caused by the intervention

Identify and select evidence

A search strategy and a literature search is conducted by a health sciences librarian based on the research questions and the inclusion criteria provided by the RNAO Expert Panel. All references are downloaded into a reference management database. The search strategy is documented at the RNAO home office for the purpose of transparency and future referral. The Expert Panel is asked to submit any potentially relevant research studies as hand-search articles. Identified studies are forwarded to the RNAO Best Practice Guideline Development Team Lead who then cross references these studies with the librarian's search results, using the same predefined inclusion and exclusion criteria.

RNAO employs six full-time master's-prepared nursing research associates (NRA) trained in systematic reviews. Two NRAs begin the literature review, guided by the following process for identifying and selecting the evidence, which follows the standard steps of a rigorous systematic review process:

- Two NRAs (a lead reviewer and a second reviewer) independently review article titles and abstracts to decide whether they should be included or excluded when compared to the inclusion criteria.

- The NRAs' "title and abstract" screening results are compared. A third reviewer acts as a tie-breaker to resolve any discrepancy where reviewers differ in their decision regarding inclusion of study.

- Full-text articles for studies selected to be included are retrieved. Two NRAs independently review the full-text articles to determine if they are relevant to the clinical research question. This stage is referred to as "relevance review." Discrepancies are resolved by a third reviewer.

- During the screening process, the lead reviewer tracks decisions regarding each study's inclusion and exclusion status, and reasons for these decisions. Decisions and rationale for inclusion and exclusion are recorded to maintain an audit trail.

This process is repeated for each clinical research question, resulting in several systematic reviews per guideline.

Evaluate evidence

Inter-rater reliability (McHugh, 2012) must be determined between the two NRAs prior to the quality appraisal and data extraction of the articles. Inter-rater reliability refers to the consistency of agreement in the quality-appraisal scores between the two NRAs. Inter-rater reliability or the kappa calculation should be greater than or equal to 80%. When inter-rater reliability is established, the lead reviewer and second reviewer quality appraise the articles using standardized appraisal tools (see Appendix E at the end of this chapter). The quality ratings of each article are documented by the NRAs in an electronic template. A final data table of studies and corresponding quality ratings is forwarded to the RNAO Best Practice Guideline Development Team Lead.

▶ REFLECTION

In what ways does a systematic review strengthen a BPG and give the user confidence in its recommendations? What are the disadvantages of incorporating a systematic review in the development process, if any?

Data extraction tables and final report

The NRAs develop data extraction tables for the research questions. These tables are used by the Guideline Development Lead to draft practice, education, and policy/organization recommendations for the guideline. The final report consists of narrative summaries and appendices of the data extraction tables, prepared by the NRAs. The systematic review manuscript incorporates the methodology of the review, written by the NRAs as the review progresses, in accordance with submission guidelines for the specific journal chosen by the working group.

FORMULATE GUIDELINE RECOMMENDATIONS

Levels of evidence

Each guideline recommendation is assigned a level of evidence based on the type of research study conducted that produced the recommendation (see Appendix F at the end of this chapter).

Consensus building for practice, education, and organization/policy recommendations

After the Guideline Development Lead drafts recommendations and evidence summaries, the Expert Panel will review the documents and reach consensus on the recommendations for inclusion in the guideline. RNAO has chosen to use the modified-Delphi technique to support consensus-building of recommendations for the guideline.

Modified-Delphi process

The Delphi technique has been in use in many fields including science and technology, war prevention, space progress, public policy, education, and health since the 1950s, and it was first officially published in 1963 (Dalkey & Helmer, 1963). The Delphi technique is a forecasting approach that is based on the outcomes of several sets of questions, the results of which are combined and shared in another iteration for response by a panel of experts until consensus is reached. However, there are a number of variations that occur, and in these cases the technique is referred to as the modified Delphi. The modified-Delphi approach has been used in healthcare to develop recommendations and guidelines as an alternative to conventional meetings, avoiding problems arising from powerful personalities, group pressures, and the effects of status.

The hierarchical structure of the health professions, where more junior practitioners may be reluctant to challenge the opinion of their seniors, has led to the Delphi technique being increasingly employed in nursing and similar research (Williams & Webb, 1994). The structure and sense of direction of the technique provides focus and avoids entropic and often counterproductive discussions and digressions common in face-to-face group discussions. A modified-Delphi approach is frequently used for recommendation development and other stakeholder-engagement activities. Through a collaborative review, individual feedback, and discussion of the draft recommendations, current evidence, and evidence gaps, the Expert Panel determines the final set of recommendations, as depicted in Figure 2.4.

Recommendation Build Process

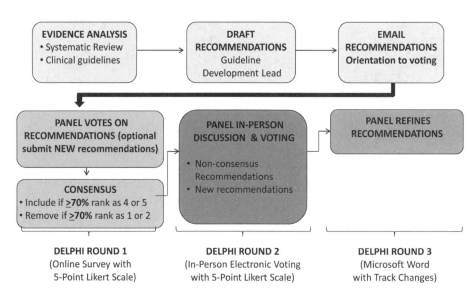

FIGURE 2.4   RNAO's BPG recommendation build process using the modified-Delphi technique.
© Registered Nurses' Association of Ontario (RNAO). All rights reserved.

Research gaps and future implications

Guideline recommendations may be based on qualitative and quantitative research evidence and/or expert opinion. In the process of reviewing the evidence, the guideline development Expert Panel identifies gaps in the research literature pertinent to the guideline topic area. When considering the research gaps, the Expert Panel may identify priority research areas and list them in the BPG. The list, though not exhaustive, is an attempt to identify and prioritize some of the significant knowledge gaps in the area.

STAKEHOLDER REVIEW

As a component of the guideline development process, the RNAO is committed to obtaining feedback from healthcare providers in a wide range of practice settings, knowledgeable administrators, funders of healthcare services, and stakeholder associations throughout Canada and internationally. Once the recommendations are complete, the draft guideline is submitted to a set of external stakeholders for review and feedback. An acknowledgement of the reviewers is provided in every guideline.

Composition of stakeholders

Stakeholder reviewers may be individuals with expertise in the relevant area of the guideline or people involved in implementing the guidelines or affected by their implementation (e.g., direct-care nurses, nursing students, physicians, interprofessional team, nurse executives, etc.).

RNAO finds stakeholder reviewers in a variety of ways. RNAO Expert Panel members are asked to forward the contact information of colleagues, coworkers, and clients to the RNAO Best Practice Guideline Development Team Lead, and they are invited to be stakeholders; individuals can register to become stakeholder reviewers via an online sign-up form on the RNAO website; in addition, this online form may be promoted through social media or at RNAO events to solicit reviewers. The RNAO website provides a short description of the BPG and invites reviewers to provide their contact information to receive the BPG when it is ready for stakeholder review. The names of all interested stakeholder reviewers are compiled into a database and accessed when the BPG is ready for review. The goal is to enlist a minimum of 50 reviewers representing a range of practice settings from local, provincial, national, and international jurisdictions.

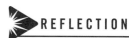

REFLECTION

How do stakeholder reviewers make an important contribution to the quality of BPGs and their uptake?

Timelines

Stakeholder reviewers have 2 weeks from the time they receive the guideline to respond. In general, stakeholder reviewers are asked to dedicate approximately 3 to 4 hours to review the guideline and to provide written feedback.

Stakeholder feedback

Feedback from external reviewers is collected by the RNAO Best Practice Guideline Development Team Lead using a brief questionnaire. Reviewers complete an online form; however, individuals also have the option to provide their feedback via mail or fax.

The questionnaire lists all the recommendations and asks the reviewer if the recommendation is clear (yes/no); if the reviewer agrees with the recommendation (yes/no); and if the evidence support is thorough (yes/no). A section for overall comments and general impressions is also provided by asking reviewers to consider the following three questions:

- Are there any significant gaps in the recommendations outlined that you believe should be addressed/included in this guideline? If so, please provide details of the gaps you have identified.

- Appendixes have been included in the draft guideline to support guideline implementation. Are they appropriate? Evidence-based? Are there any gaps in the content provided?

- Is there anything else you would like to comment on in order to strengthen this document? (e.g., Content: background context, research gaps, monitoring indicators. Format: flow, ease of readability, terminology/language, etc.); please feel free to comment in the space below.

The feedback from stakeholders is compiled by the RNAO Best Practice Guideline Development Team Lead and reviewed with the RNAO Expert Panel. Each point is addressed and discussed by the RNAO Expert Panel, and any changes to the guideline are noted. If no changes are made to the guideline as a result of the stakeholder review, the reason(s) are recorded. When all the comments have been addressed and the RNAO Expert Panel has come to consensus about the revisions, the document is ready for production through edit and design. Documentation of the stakeholder review process is maintained at the RNAO office for transparency and future reference.

PUBLICATION AND DISSEMINATION

Editing, design, and publication

Prior to publication, the guideline is professionally edited and then forwarded to a design company. Following final approval, the PDF document is posted to the RNAO website and printed. Hard copies are made available for purchase, and a free electronic version is made available for download from the RNAO website, www.RNAO.ca. Complimentary hard copies are distributed to all members of the Expert Panel and stakeholder reviewers, with a letter of appreciation and acknowledgement for their valuable contribution to the BPG development process. For dissemination of the guideline, it is sent to the NGC and GIN to be housed in their guideline databases. RNAO engages in a number of other dissemination and implementation activities that are discussed in other chapters.

Announcement of release of the new guideline

The announcement of a completed guideline is timed to coincide with other local, provincial, national, or international events of importance. Depending on the profile of the topic, RNAO considers the need to hold a stand-alone press conference, which at times is attended even by a minister of health or others (Di Costanzo, 2014). Other venues include a major conference where the BPG is introduced to live audiences. The announcement highlights the core elements of the guideline and directs the audience to the RNAO website: www.RNAO.ca. Expert Panel members are encouraged to share the new guideline within their organizations. Each new guideline enters RNAO's rich dissemination protocol, including: RNAO's *Registered Nurse Journal* and monthly *In the Loop*, the RNAO website, webinars, an app version of the guideline freely accessible online, health education fact sheets, and presentations at conferences to support uptake. All of these dissemination strategies are discussed in future chapters.

GUIDELINE UPDATING

RNAO has made a commitment to revise BPGs every 5 years following publication of the last edition as follows:

1. Each nursing BPG will be reviewed by a team of specialists (RNAO Expert Panel) in the topic area.

2. During the period between development and publication of a new edition, RNAO IABPG Centre staff will regularly monitor for new and relevant literature in the field.

3. Based on the results of this monitoring, RNAO IABPG Centre staff, in consultation with members of the original RNAO Expert Panel members and other specialists and experts in the field, may recommend the guideline be reviewed and revised earlier than the 5-year revision period.

4. Three months prior to the review milestone, the RNAO Best Practice Guideline Development Team Lead will commence the planning of the review process by developing a detailed work plan with target dates and deliverables for developing a new edition of the guideline.

GUIDELINE DEVELOPMENT ENHANCEMENTS

RNAO is continuing to improve its guideline development processes, making them as rigorous as possible. As discussed earlier this chapter, changes have been made in the systematic review processes, Expert Panel composition, and recommendation build. Refining of the recommendation build using a modified Delphi process and incorporation of recommendation grading are two new processes that have been introduced to strengthen the recommendations. The Delphi process has been discussed earlier in this chapter, and this section will focus on guideline grading.

GUIDELINE GRADING

Grading recommendations was a process used by organizations with a defined focus on the level and quality of evidence or type of study used to support that evidence. Many organizations use formal systems to grade evidence, including consideration of various contextual factors and recommendations and why this is important for clinicians. As organizations utilized different methods to denote high-grade or strong recommendations, it became confusing and inconsistent for clinicians and others to determine why one guideline called a particular recommendation strong, while others, based on the same evidence, did not. This sparked the need for a structured approach to identify, evaluate, and implement a grading methodology for recommendations.

A methodology of rating recommendations based solely on the level of evidence supporting that recommendation should be used with caution, because limitations exist on the availability of Type 1 (RCT) evidence. For example, there are extensive observational findings that support hand washing to reduce infection rates; however, there are no randomized controlled trials showing similar results. Alternatively, there are strong data from Randomized Control Trials (RCTs) showcasing that alcohol-based hand sanitizer solution is better at reducing infection rates than the use of latex gloves. As such, the recommendation to wash hands, of the utmost importance in infection control, is based on weaker evidence (observational findings) as compared to the cleansing method (RCT). Most would agree it is more important that hands are washed regardless of the method chosen.

GRADE

Globally, guideline developers inconsistently rate quality of evidence and grade strength of recommendations, thus creating challenges for guideline users when interpreting the grading system and related content. To understand the methods, the GRADE (the Grading of Recommendations, Assessment, Development and Evaluation) system, first reported in 2004, is advantageous for the following reasons (Atkins et al., 2004):

- Developed by a widely representative group of international guideline developers
- Clear separation between quality of evidence and strength of recommendations
- Explicit evaluation of the importance of outcomes of alternative management strategies
- Comprehensive criteria for downgrading and upgrading quality-of-evidence ratings
- Transparency in the process of moving from evidence to recommendations
- A discussion of benefits, harms, values, and preferences

- Pragmatic interpretation of strong versus weak recommendations for clinicians, patients, and policymakers
- Applicability to systematic reviews and health technology assessments

In 2006, the *BMJ* requested in its "Instructions to Authors" on bmj.com that authors preferably use the GRADE framework when submitting a clinical guideline article following its publication (Guyatt et al., 2008). This highlights the importance of evidence frameworks that move beyond level or quality of evidence to clearly state the strength of a recommendation.

The strength of recommendations is based on the quality of supporting evidence, the degree of uncertainty about the balance between desirable and undesirable effects, the degree of uncertainty or variability in values and preferences, and the degree of uncertainty about whether the intervention represents a wise use of resources.

Strong recommendations imply that most individuals will be best served by the recommended course of action, in which the panel is confident that:

- Desirable effects of an intervention outweigh its undesirable effects (strong recommendation for an intervention), or
- Undesirable effects of an intervention outweigh its desirable effects (strong recommendation against an intervention)

Weak recommendations are those for which the panel believes the:

- Desirable effects *probably* outweigh the undesirable effects (weak recommendation for an intervention), or
- Undesirable effects *probably* outweigh the desirable effects (weak recommendation against an intervention) but appreciable uncertainty exists

The quality of evidence is graded as high, moderate, low, or very low, based on likelihood that further research would change our confidence in the estimate of effect. The GRADE approach is based on a sequential assessment of the quality of evidence, followed by judgment about the balance between desirable and undesirable effects, and subsequent decision about the strength of a recommendation. Separating the judgments regarding the quality of evidence from judgments about the strength of recommendations is a critical and defining feature of the GRADE framework. GRADE stresses the necessity to acknowledge the values and preferences underlying the recommendations and postulates a systematic approach to grading the recommendations that can minimize bias and aid interpretation.

Unlike other appraisals, the GRADE framework emphasizes that weak recommendations in the face of high-quality evidence are common because of factors other than the quality of evidence that influence the strength of a recommendation. For the same reason, it supports strong recommendations based on evidence from observational studies. The emergence of "real world evidence" or observational data, including qualitative research, is required to support identification of interventions that are effective and not amendable to RCT methodology. SIGN (Scottish Intercollegiate Guidelines Network) released a policy statement in 2013 when moving from its previous system of assigning letter grades (ABCD) based mostly on the level of evidence (I–IV) to the GRADE methodology. Other guideline organizations, such as NICE (National Institute for Health and Care Excellence), have followed, and to date over 100 organizations from 19 countries have endorsed or use GRADE (GRADE working group, 2017). NICE is an independent public body that provides evidence-based national guidance and recommendations made by independent committees on a wide range of topics related to health and social care in England.

GRADE CERQual

The Confidence in the Evidence from Reviews of Qualitative Research (GRADE CERQual) is an approach developed in 2010 to facilitate a transparent and standard method for appraisal of qualitative literature. The World Health Organization (WHO) identified the need for the CERQual approach when attempting to develop a guideline that required qualitative evidence. Members of WHO and other international professionals formed a subcommittee of the GRADE working group to determine the components of the approach and conduct testing. CERQual requires review of qualitative evidence to determine confidence in *research findings*, defined as "data from primary studies that describe a phenomenon or aspect of a phenomenon" (Lewin et al., 2015, p. 3). The following four components are used to ascertain confidence in the research findings (Lewin et al., 2015):

1. **Methodological limitations**—Identify any issues in the design or conduct of the primary studies

2. **Relevance**—Assess the degree of consistency between the research findings for the body of evidence and the research question(s), specifically the population, phenomenon of interest, and setting

3. **Coherence**—Determine whether the patterns found in the data are adequately supported and explicated by the research findings

4. **Adequacy of data**—Evaluate the overall saturation, richness, and quantity of data available to corroborate the research findings

Confidence in the review findings, based on the four components, is ascribed one of four levels: high confidence, moderate confidence, low confidence, and very low confidence. Each of the levels represents varying degrees of confidence in the evidence ranging from "highly likely that review findings are a reasonable representation of the phenomenon of interest" to "not clear whether the review finding is a reasonable representation of the phenomenon of interest" (Lewin et al., 2015, p. 11). We anticipate that in the future, RNAO will incorporate the GRADE CERQual approach into the guideline development processes.

RNAO's application of GRADE

The alignment of GRADE and GRADE CERQual frameworks with RNAO guideline development methodology has resulted in changes to current processes that were previously outlined. Prior to the systematic review, the development team now conducts a gap analysis to ascertain specific areas of focus for the purpose, scope, research questions, and outcomes of the guideline. Based on the findings, the Expert Panel further informs these areas and finalizes the direction of the guideline. The panel votes on the PICO research questions and outcomes to ensure areas of highest priority are addressed in the guideline. The health science librarian continues to conduct the extensive literature search. When completed, two NRAs independently perform the title and abstract screening and relevance review.

The current evaluation of evidence, including the quality-appraisal tools (i.e., CASP, AMSTAR) is being replaced with the processes described in the GRADE and GRADE CERQual approaches. The data extraction tables are being transformed into the evidence profiles and summary of finding tables outlined by the GRADE and GRADE CERQual frameworks utilizing the GRADE pro software. The process of building recommendation statements has changed. The levels of evidence are eliminated. Instead, each new guideline as of 2018 and next editions of existing guidelines include GRADE and CERQual profiles and summaries, outlining the recommendations and strength of recommendations. The Expert Panel continues to reach consensus on the recommendations using the modified-Delphi technique. In 2017, RNAO pilot-tested this transition with two clinical and one healthy work environment guideline. This initial testing enabled the RNAO guideline development team to assess the processes and modify steps to ensure efficient integration of the GRADE and CERQual frameworks.

The topics relevant to nurse-led guidelines are diverse in subject matter, scope, population, and setting. This unique dynamic presents opportunities and challenges. We anticipate that systematic reviews will generate a multiplicity of study designs, including quantitative evidence amendable to meta-analysis, observational findings requiring narrative descriptions of GRADE criteria, and qualitative synthesis. Historically, when variability was found within one guideline topic area, future endeavours tend to generate similar results. As such, when quantitative and qualitative literature is used, the GRADE and CERQual evidence profiles are linked with the respective research question and its outcome to clearly and transparently demonstrate the basis for each recommendation statement.

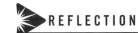 **REFLECTION**

What are the advantages of using the GRADE methodology in RNAO's BPG development process? Do you see any disadvantages, and if so how could they be overcome?

Appraisal of graded recommendations

AGREE researchers developed and validated the AGREE REX: AGREE Recommendation EXcellence tool (AGREE, no date). This instrument is a "useful, reliable, and valid knowledge resource to complement the AGREE II, on the clinical credibility and implementability of practice guideline recommendations" (AGREE, n.d.). The AGREE-REX is comprised of 1) an Assessment Instrument, 2) a User's Guide, and 3) a series of practical tools (Resource-Rex). Upon review of AGREE-REX and AGREE II, users may notice similarity with the NEATS tool created by NGC. The NEATS tool attempts to ascertain the clinical credibility, and feasibility of implementing recommendations with some of the other elements of guideline development methodology found in AGREE II.

RNAO'S EVOLUTION IN GUIDELINE DEVELOPMENT

This chapter has addressed all aspects of RNAO's rigorous BPG development process, along with the relevant background to guideline development in healthcare, as well as challenges and solutions. Included is our seven-step development process, use of emerging trends, new standards, and future directions. As a developer of quality guidelines for international uptake, RNAO uses all study types in systematic reviews, including quantitative and qualitative research. This is necessary to best respond to questions that affect day-to-day patient care and capture interventions that can improve patients' clinical and quality-of-life outcomes. In addition, RNAO has focused on three domains that are critical to achieve results: 1) evidence-based clinical practice recommendations, 2) educational recommendations regarding the knowledge clinicians need to have to implement best practices, and 3) what the organizations and/or health system needs to do to create work environments that optimize best practices uptake.

RNAO's culture is that of a learning organization constantly using quality improvement. As such, its guideline development processes are not static. They evolve as needed to align with international standards. For example, RNAO has moved from panels of all nurses to 50% nurses to ensure a multidisciplinary approach. RNAO was amongst the first guideline developers to include patients and people with lived experiences in both the planning and development of guidelines as Expert Panel members. Furthermore, RNAO launched its Patient and Public Engagement Council (PPEC) in 2016, and is the first nursing professional association to do so. Through the PPEC, the concept of equity has been prioritized and will now be reflected in the evidence framework that RNAO is creating to denote a strong recommendation.

"Having tragically lost my son to a drug overdose, being a member of the supervised injection services BPG gives great meaning and voice to his life."

–Cori Chapman, mother of Brad Chapman

RNAO guideline developers draft recommendations based upon the evidence from the systematic review and high-quality guidelines for the panel to examine, refine, and identify gaps. In addition, RNAO has implemented a robust consensus-building process, including the modified Delphi, to ensure all panel member voices are heard without undue influence from overbearing panel members. These last two processes provide a strong foundation for the implementation of GRADE. Over the course of 2017, RNAO has created its own nursing-led and -developed evidence framework to clarify and distinguish the level and quality of evidence with the strength of the recommendations. As of 2018, all new and next editions of existing guidelines include GRADE and CERQual profiles and summaries, outlining the recommendations and strength of recommendations.

In 1998, when RNAO embarked on the groundbreaking work of BPG development and shortly after implementation and evaluation, there were few other players in the field, and certainly no professional nursing organizations. Now nearly two decades later, RNAO is globally recognized for its leading-edge work in all aspects of evidence-based practice, and arguably is the "go to" organization when credible guidelines are necessary to address key clinical and healthy work environment issues that affect the practice of nurses and the public we serve.

RNAO has achieved these outcomes first and foremost by its dogged attention to guideline quality and capacity to continually improve its processes to be ever more rigorous and at the same time user-friendly. Guideline uptake and the differences these evidence-based tools make for patients as well as practitioners, organizations, and the system are the ultimate priorities.

KEY MESSAGES

- Quality guidelines that adhere to international development standards offer solutions to drive care quality, practice effectiveness, and improved health outcomes.

- RNAO's well-honed BPG development process is not static and continuously incorporates new international guideline standards.

- RNAO BPGs include top recommendations that influence practice, education, organizations, and the system. They also include evaluation indicators.

- RNAO BPG use and impact are facilitated by additional evidence-based resources including apps, quick summaries, online modules, and health education fact sheets.

- Guideline development processes continue to be advanced based on research and lived experiences.

REFERENCES

AGREE. (n.d.). *AGREE-REX: Recommendation EXcellence*. Retrieved from http://www.agreetrust.org/agree-research-projects/agree-rex-recommendation-excellence/

AGREE Collaboration. (2003). Development and validation of an international appraisal instrument for assessing the quality of clinical practice guidelines: The AGREE project. *Quality & Safety in Health Care, 12*(1), 18–23.

Almost, J., Wolff, A. C., Stewart-Pyne, A., McCormick, L. G., Strachan, D., & D'Souza, C. (2016). Managing and mitigating conflict in healthcare teams: An integrative review. *Journal of Advanced Nursing, 72*(7), 1490–1505. doi: 10.1111/jan.12903

Atkins, D., Eccles, M., Flottorp, S., Guyatt, G. H., Henry, D., Hill, S., . . . GRADE Working Group. (2004). Systems for grading the quality of evidence and the strength of recommendations I: Critical appraisal of existing approaches. *BMC Health Services Research, 4*(1), 38.

Brouwers, M. C., Kho, M. E., Browman, G. P., Burgers, J. S., Cluzeau, F., Feder, G., . . . AGREE Next Steps Consortium. (2010). AGREE II: Advancing guideline development, reporting and evaluation in health care. *CMAJ, 182*(18), E839–E842.

Cochrane Public Health (n.d.). *Unit Eight: Principles of Critical Appraisal*. Retrieved from http://ph.cochrane.org/sites/ph.cochrane.org/files/public/uploads/Unit_Eight.pdf

Dalkey, N., & Helmer, O. (1963). An experimental application of the DELPHI method to the use of experts. *Management Science, 9*(3), 458–467.

Di Costanzo, M. (2014, June 13). *Recommendations for first comprehensive nursing guideline on elder abuse released today.* Retrieved from http://rnao.ca/news/media-releases/2014/06/13/recommendations-first-comprehensive-nursing-guideline-elder-abuse-rel

Fineout-Overholt, E., & Johnston, L. (2005). Teaching EBP: Asking searchable, answerable clinical questions. *Worldviews on Evidence-Based Nursing, 2*(3), 157–160.

The GRADE working group. (2017). *Welcome to the GRADE working group.* Retrieved from http://gradeworkinggroup.org/

Grimshaw, J. M., Thomas, R. E., MacLennan, G., Fraser, C., Ramsay, C. R., Vale, L., . . . Donaldson, C. (2004). Effectiveness and efficiency of guideline dissemination and implementation strategies. *Health Technology Assessment, 8*(6), iii–iv, 1–72.

Grinspun, D., Melnyk, B. M., & Fineout-Overholt E. (2014). Advancing optimal care with rigorously developed clinical practice guidelines and evidence-based recommendations. In B. M. Melnyk & E. Fineout-Overholt (Eds.), *Evidence-Based Practice in Nursing & Healthcare. A Guide to Best Practice* (3rd ed.), (182–201). Philadelphia: Lippincott, Williams & Wilkins.

Guyatt, G. H., Oxman, A. D., Vist, G. E., Kunz, R., Falck-Ytter, Y., Alonso-Coello, P., . . . GRADE Working Group. (2008). GRADE: An emerging consensus on rating quality of evidence and strength of recommendations. *BMJ, 336*(7650), 924–926. doi: 10.1136/bmj.39489.470347.AD

Harripaul-Yhap, A., Dusek, B., Pearce, N., & Lloyd, M. (2015). Care transitions: A systematic review of best practices. *Journal of Nursing Care Quality, 30*(3), 233–239.

Hirst, S. P., Penney, T., McNeill, S., Boscart, V. M., Podnieks, E., & Sinha, S. K. (2016). Best-Practice Guideline on the prevention of abuse and neglect of older adults. *Canadian Journal on Aging, 35*(2), 242–260. doi: 10.1017/S0714980816000209

Institute of Medicine (IOM). (2011). *Clinical practice guidelines we can trust.* Washington, DC: The National Academies Press.

Institute of Medicine (IOM). (2011, March 23). *Press Release.* Retrieved from http://www.nationalacademies.org/hmd/Reports/2011/Clinical-Practice-Guidelines-We-Can-Trust/Press-Release.aspx

Legere, L. E., Wallace, K. Bowen, A., McQueen, K., Montgomery, P., & Evans, M. (2017). Approaches to health-care provider education and professional development in perinatal depression: A systematic review. *BMC Pregnancy and Childbirth, 17,* 239.

Lewin, S., Glenton, C., Munthe-Kaas, H., Carlsen, B., Colvin, C. J., Gülmezoglu, M., . . . Rashidian, A. (2015). Using qualitative evidence in decision making for health and social interventions: An approach to assess confidence in findings from qualitative evidence syntheses (GRADE-CERQual). *PLoS Med, 12*(10), e1001895. doi: 10.1371/journal.pmed.1001895

McHugh, M. (2012). Interrater reliability: The kappa statistic. *Biochem Medica, 22*(3), 276–282.

Melnyk, B. M., Grossman, D. C., Chou, R., Mabry-Hernandez, I., Nicholson, W., DeWitt, T. G., . . . Flores, G. (2012). USPSTF perspective on evidence-based preventive recommendations for children. *Pediatrics, 130*(2), 2011–2087.

National Guideline Clearinghouse. (n.d.). *National Guideline Clearinghouse Extent Adherence to Trustworthy Standards (NEATS) Instrument.* Retrieved from https://www.guideline.gov/documents/neats_instrument.pdf

Pati, D. (2011). A framework for evaluating evidence in evidence-based design. *Health Environments Research & Design Journal, 4*(3), 50–71.

Pluye, P., Robert, E., Cargo, M., Bartlett, G., O'Cathain, A., Griffiths, F., Boardman, F., Gagnon, M.P., & Rousseau, M.C. (2011). Proposal: A mixed methods appraisal tool for systematic mixed studies reviews. Retrieved from http://mixedmethodsappraisaltoolpublic.pbworks.com

Qaseem, A., Forland, F., Macbeth, F., Ollenschläger, G., Phillips, S., van der Wees, P., & Board of Trustees of the Guidelines International Network. (2012). Guidelines International Network: toward international standards for clinical practice guidelines. *Annals of Internal Medicine, 156*(7), 525–531.

Recalla, S., English, K., Nazarali, R., Mayo, S., Miller, D., & Gray, M. (2013). Ostomy care and management: A systematic review. *Journal of Wound, Ostomy and Continence Nursing, 40*(5), 489–500.

Schünemann, H. J., Hill, S. R., Kakad, M., Vist, G. E., Bellamy, R., Stockman, L., . . . Oxman, A. D. (2007). Transparent development of the WHO rapid advice guidelines. *PLoS Med, 4*(5), e119. https://doi.org/10.1371/journal.pmed.0040119

Schünemann, H. J., Wiercioch, W., Etxeandia, I., Falavigna, M., Santesso, N., Mustafa, R., . . . Akl, E. A. (2013). Guidelines 2.0: Systematic development of a comprehensive checklist for a successful guideline enterprise. *CMAJ, 186*(3), E123–E142.

Scottish Intercollegiate Guidelines Network (SIGN). (2013). *Policy statement on the grading of recommendations in SIGN guidelines.* Retrieved from http://www.sign.ac.uk/assets/sign_grading.pdf

Scottish Intercollegiate Guidelines Network (SIGN). (2017). SIGN 50: *A guideline developer's handbook.* Retrieved from http://www.sign.ac.uk/sign-50.html

Sharma, T., Bamford, M., & Dodman, D. (2016). Person-centred care: An overview of reviews. *Contemporary Nurse, 51*(2–3), 107–120.

Shekelle, P. G., Kravitz, R. L., Beart, J., Marger, M., Wang, M., & Lee, M. (2000). Are nonspecific practice guidelines potentially harmful? A randomized comparison of the effect of nonspecific versus specific guidelines on physician decision making. *Health Services Research, 34*(7), 1429–1448.

Suva, G., Sager, S., Mina, E. S., Sinclair, N., Lloyd, M., Bajnok, I., . . . Xiao, S. (2015). Systematic review: Bridging the gap in RPN to RN transitions. *Journal of Nursing Scholarship, 47*(4), 363–370. doi 10.1111/jnu.1214

Wennberg, J. & Gittelsohn, A. (1973). Small variations in health care delivery. *Science, 182*(4117), 1102–1108.

Wennberg, J. & Gittelsohn, A. (1982). Variations in medical care among small areas. *Science America, 246*(4), 120–134.

Wilding, R. & Wagner, B. (2012). Systematic review and the need for evidence. *Supply Chain Management: An International Journal, 17*(4). https://doi.org/10.1108/scm.2012.17717daa.001

Williams, P. L., & Webb, C. (1994). The Delphi technique: A methodological discussion. *Journal of Advanced Nursing, 19*(1), 180–186.

Woolf, S., Schünemann, H. J., Eccles, M. P., Grimshaw, J. M., & Shekelle, P. (2012). Developing clinical practice guidelines: Reviewing, reporting, and publishing guidelines; updating guidelines; and the emerging issues of enhancing guideline implementability and accounting for comorbid conditions in guideline development. *Implementation Science, 7*(61).

Ye, L., Goldie, C., Sharma, T., John, S., Bamford, M., Smith, P. M., . . . Schultz, A. S. (2017). Tobacco-nicotine education and training for health-care professional students and practitioners: A systematic review. *Nicotine & Tobacco Research.* https://doi.org/10.1093/ntr/ntx072

APPENDIX A: DETAILED TIMELINES FOR GUIDELINE DEVELOPMENT PROCESSES

Timeline Frame	Development Step	Development Phase	Activity
Month 1	Topic Selection	Identifying a topic	■ Decision for a new guideline or revision of existing guideline ■ Topics for possible guideline development are reviewed from multiple sources ■ Topics for guideline development are evaluated using a priority matrix ■ RNAO Best Practice Guideline Development Team Lead initiates planning process ■ Panel cochairs identified, one of whom is a PhD-prepared nurse
Month 1–3		Planning (as needed for new topics): Focus Groups Scoping review Refinement of purpose and scope	■ Recruitment of experts on topic for focus groups ■ Development of premeeting questions for focus-group participants to gather information on current practice, resources, research, and gaps in information on selected topic for guideline development ■ Information from focus groups gathered and transcribed into themes to assist RNAO Expert Panel in finalizing guideline purpose and scope
Month 1		Existing Guidelines Search	■ Search conducted for existing guidelines on topic selected for guideline development ■ Assessment of existing guidelines with AGREE II Instrument ■ High-quality existing guidelines identified for RNAO Expert Panel review at Panel Launch
Month 1	Expert Panel	Expert Panel Recruitment	■ Approximately 12–15 individuals are recruited to participate on the RNAO multidisciplinary Expert Panel ■ Panel matrix is used to support identification of roughly one-quarter each of direct-care clinicians, researchers, education/policy/system level, and patient/persons with lived experience. This includes 50% nurses, at least one physician, and other disciplines from relevant sectors of the health-care system ■ A terms of reference template (Appendix C) is developed for each guideline development Expert Panel and shared so each panel member understands his/her roles and the key deliverables and timelines for BPG development ■ Panel chair is identified ■ RNAO Expert Panel membership is finalized
Month 2	Expert Panel	RNAO Expert Panel Launch	■ Orientation to RNAO IABPG Centre guideline development program and methodology. ■ Refine the guideline purpose and scope based on identified themes from focus groups ■ Formulate Clinical Research Questions (CRQs) based on PICO ■ Identify search terms and databases with librarian to create the search strategy

Timeline Frame	Development Step	Development Phase	Activity
			■ Compile results of AGREE II assessments for Expert Panel to select guidelines that will inform guideline development
			■ RNAO Expert Panel members sign up for one of the following subgroups to work on: Evaluation & Monitoring Indicators (including NQuIRE®), Manuscript, Health Education Fact Sheets, and Mobile Device version of guideline
Months 3–8	Systematic Reviews	Systematic Literature Reviews: Identify and Select Evidence	■ A subgroup of the RNAO Expert Panel, panel chair, and RNAO IABPG Development Team Lead work with librarian on search strategy and systematic review processes
			■ NRAs conduct relevance reviews for each CRQ
			■ Two NRAs review article titles and abstracts independently to determine those for inclusion
			■ Where there are differences related to inclusion, the RNAO Best Practice Guideline Development Team Lead becomes the third-party decision-maker
Months 3–8		Systematic Literature Reviews: Quality Appraisal to Evaluate Evidence	■ Studies included accessed by two NRAs for quality
			■ Inter-rater reliability is checked between the NRAs prior to completion of quality appraisal of all articles
			■ Two NRAs critically appraise articles for quality using standardized tools
Months 3–8		Systematic Literature Review: Data Extraction and Final Report	■ The two NRAs review the appraised included studies and extract data into tables specific to each research question
			■ NRAs compile data extraction tables by research questions and compile a Narrative Summary of Themes report to present to Guideline Development Lead; this information is also made available to the Expert Panel as supplementary material
Month 8–9	Recommendation Development	Development of Draft Recommendations & Panel Consensus	■ Guideline development lead reviews data tables and narrative summary to draft recommendation statements and supporting evidence summaries. Research gaps and indicators for evaluation and monitoring practices associated with topic are also identified.
			■ Modified-Delphi technique utilized to build panel consensus on recommendations
			■ Draft recommendations and evidence summaries are shared with panel for review and anonymous vote
			■ Recommendations that reach consensus for inclusion are moved forward, for exclusion are removed
			■ Nonconsensus recommendations are discussed at in-person meeting, refined, and voted upon until consensus achieved
Month 3–10		Development of draft guideline	■ Sections of the draft guideline created by development lead include: purpose, scope, background information; guideline recommendations and supporting evidence; research gaps and future implications for research; implementation strategies; structure, process, and outcome indicators to support evaluation and monitoring of guideline implementation; and supporting tools for uptake in form of appendixes
			■ Guideline draft is reviewed and edited by the RNAO Expert Panel
			■ Permissions to reprint third-party content are requested and documented

continues

(Continued)

Timeline Frame	Development Step	Development Phase	Activity
Month 11	Stakeholder Review	External Stakeholder Review	▪ Reviewers (stakeholders, experts on topic of guideline) are identified through various methods—including open online application, social media recruitment, suggestions from the panel, and potential endorsers—to review guideline. Stakeholders represent individuals, organizations, and healthcare. Targeted recruitment is conducted to address any gaps, and a minimum of 50 stakeholders are invited to participate. ▪ Stakeholder questionnaire developed and posted online in a survey tool for stakeholder review of draft guideline. Feedback submissions required within 2 weeks from stakeholders. ▪ All feedback is compiled and reviewed by Guideline Development Lead and addressed and documented. ▪ Items for discussion are brought to RNAO Expert Panel to determine adjustments to guideline draft. Decisions are documented.
Month 12		Final Guideline Draft	▪ All internal and external comments are addressed and reviewed by the panel. ▪ Expert Panel reaches consensus on final version of the guideline.
Month 13	Guideline Publication	Final Draft production	▪ Final draft edited professionally ▪ Edited draft designed and published for online and print ▪ PDF version is posted on the RNAO website ▪ Hard copies are available through online purchase

Month 14–15		Publication: Dissemination and Uptake Activities
		
		Mobile Device Version of BPG
		
		Health Education Fact Sheet (HEFS)
		
		Manuscript for Publication
			▪ RNAO Expert Panel members who signed up for subgroup activities begin work on the following using templates:
			  ▪ Manuscript: to outline systematic review process on topic for guideline development
			  ▪ Health Education Fact Sheet: to outline key messages from guideline content to patients or healthcare providers
			  ▪ Mobile Device Version: key information required by clinicians for use on various mobile devices identified from design and proof for print draft version (following completion of final edit of guideline); RNAO BPG mobile app available for download
			▪ A draft summary of the content is completed according to the established templates
			▪ Manuscript submitted to journals until accepted
			▪ Health Education Fact Sheet put into HEF PDF template for upload to RNAO website after consensus reached on the content and health literacy review meets the Public Health Agency of Canada's recommendation for reading level
			▪ Guideline is submitted to NGC and GIN for inclusion into their databases

Month 15		Celebration – Release of the Guideline	▪ The release of the guideline is linked to a conference, event, or webinar session ▪ Guideline moves into dissemination and implementation through IABPG Centre's guideline implementation activities

APPENDIX B: EXAMPLE OF PRIORITY-IDENTIFICATION MATRIX

The intent of this matrix is to assist in identifying priority areas for guideline development, based on a systematic approach to reviewing the short list of identified topics. The outcome of the review is to have all reviewers consider the topics identified, the results of the initial searches, and select a maximum of three priority topics. The compiled results will be used to establish the topic for guideline development. The following criteria have been identified as key to topic selection:

- Topic is relevant to one or more key priority areas, identified by the Ministry of Health and Long-Term Care (MOHLTC): gerontology; home healthcare; mental healthcare; emergency care; primary healthcare

- Topic is within the scope of nursing practice and will impact both RNs and RPNs in a range of practice settings

- A multidisciplinary approach would be appropriate for development

- Topic builds on a previously developed guideline, or general topic area

- Potential for partnerships in development, external to MOHLTC

- Perceived need for the guideline, as identified by those submitting the topic for consideration

- Evidence to support guideline recommendations is available

- Consideration of other known guideline work on the topic area

Guideline topic	Key priority areas addressed* (identify all that may apply)	Topic will be applicable to a wide range of practice settings (Identify all that apply)	Multidisciplinary approach would be possible related to the topic	Topic builds on/supports other RNAO BPGs (Yes/No)	Potential for partnerships external to MHLTC	Rationale for BPG provided by the nurse identifying the topic is strong. (Yes/No) Comments	Evidence support is available to develop guideline (refer to summary of evidence template)	Guidelines have been developed on this topic previously	Recommen-dation	Suggested scope

APPENDIX C: TERMS OF REFERENCE TEMPLATE

RNAO BEST PRACTICE GUIDELINE PANEL

The Registered Nurses' Association of Ontario (RNAO) is the professional association representing registered nurses, nurse practitioners, and nursing students in Ontario. Since 1925, RNAO has advocated for healthy public policy, promoted excellence in nursing practice, increased nurses' contribution to shaping the healthcare system, and influenced decisions that affect nurses and the public they serve.

TERMS OF REFERENCE AND TIMELINE

The International Affairs and Best Practice Guidelines (IABPG) Centre houses the Best Practice Guidelines (BPG) Program, a signature program of RNAO. The program mandate is the development, dissemination, implementation, and evaluation of clinical and Healthy Work Environment Best Practice Guidelines. To date, the program has published 42 clinical BPGs, 12 System and Healthy Work Environment BPGs, and various implementation resources (e.g., two "Toolkits," one for implementing clinical practice guidelines and the other an Educator Resource; e-Learning Programs; mobile versions of guidelines; and Health Information Fact Sheets). The BPGs and other resources can be accessed online at www.RNAO.ca/bpg.

BPG PURPOSE

The proposed purpose of this guideline will be to identify evidence-based best practices for nurses (in collaboration with the interprofessional teams that they work with), on [insert topic]. The guideline will have relevance to all areas of clinical practice including public health, primary care, hospital care, home care, rehabilitation, complex care, and long-term care.

The guideline will provide recommendations in three main areas: 1) practice recommendations, including assessment, planning, intervention and evaluation; 2) education recommendations; and 3) organization/policy/system recommendations. All recommendations will be developed in accordance with the systematic review literature and expert opinion.

RNAO team members involved with this BPG:

- RNAO Program Manager/Guideline Development Lead
- RNAO Project Coordinator
- Nursing research associates (NRA)
- Associate Director of Guideline Development
- Director of RNAO's IABPG Centre

PANEL MEMBERS

The Expert Panel will be comprised of a broad representation of experts from nursing practice, administration, education, research, and policy, as well as other health professions and patient representatives.

PANEL RESPONSIBILITIES

The responsibilities of the panel members are as follows:

- Attend face-to-face meetings and virtual meetings.

- Read preparatory materials sent by the Guideline Team.

- Participate in a consensus development process to finalize recommendations (i.e., anonymous voting process). All panel members will be expected to vote prior to the recommendation build session and attend the session in person to deliberate on the day.

- Provide feedback on various drafts of the guideline throughout the development process.

- Participate in the development of other implementation and evaluation resources (e.g., health education fact sheet, nursing order sets, and outcome indicators).

- Identify appropriate stakeholders to review the draft guideline prior to publication.

- Support dissemination and implementation of the guideline.

In addition to the panel responsibilities above, the role of the panel cochairs is to:

- Support the Program Manager to guide the panel and ensure activities are being completed and timeline is being met.

- Assist with setting meeting agendas.

- Facilitate the BPG panel meetings with the Program Manager (as needed).

- Participate in cochair meetings with the Program Manager and Project Coordinator on a monthly basis (or as needed).

- Colead dissemination activities (e.g., BPG webinar launch) and assist with promoting and disseminating the completed guideline.

- Support panel group process including conflict resolution.

TERM

The guideline development panel will carry out its work over the estimated timeframe of approximately 15 months from [Start date].

MEETINGS/COMMITMENT

There will be up to three in-person meetings in Toronto and three to four virtual meetings over the guideline development period. In addition, the panel will be expected to work independently to review pre-reading materials (e.g., systematic review data tables, narrative summaries). They will also be required to participate in small-group work between face-to-face and virtual meetings. RNAO will provide access to a teleconference line and other support as needed. See the timeline that follows for more details about expected dates.

EXPENSES

RNAO will reimburse the costs of economy travel, accommodation, and meals for all in-person meetings (details outlining allowable expenses are found on RNAO's expense form). Toll-free numbers will also be provided for all calls to RNAO for the purpose of virtual meetings.

This process of guideline development involves seven stages (see the diagram in Figure C.1). The panel will be most actively involved in recommendation formulation and review.

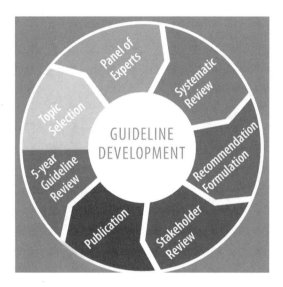

FIGURE C.1   Guideline development process diagram.

GUIDELINE DEVELOPMENT PLAN

Project Activities	June 2016	July 2016	Aug 2016	Sept 2016	Oct 2016	Nov 2016	Dec 2016	Jan 2017	Feb 2017	Mar 2017	Apr 2017	May 2017	June 2017	July 2017	Aug 2017	Sep 2017
Guideline Development Start	■															
1. One day in-person panel meeting: BPG launch	■															
2. Systematic review		■	■	■	■	■	■									
▪ Virtual panel meeting (teleconference/WebEx) for updates				■												
3. Recommendation formulation								■	■							
▪ Virtual panel meeting to prepare for recommendation build meeting								■	■							
▪ Two-day in-person panel meeting: recommendation build									■							
4. Developing draft of guideline												■	■			
▪ Virtual panel meeting to review draft guideline													■	■		
5. Stakeholder review															■	
▪ Panel Meeting (TBD: in-person or virtual) to review stakeholder feedback															■	
6. Guideline publication e															■	■
▪ Guideline dissemination (ongoing)																

APPENDIX D: RNAO HEALTH EDUCATION FACT SHEET

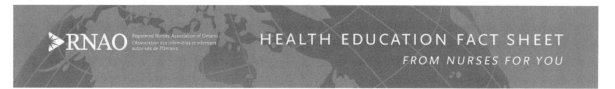

Delirium, dementia and depression: What is the difference?

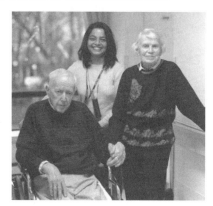

Many older adults are affected by delirium, dementia and/or depression. These conditions are not part of normal aging. Delirium, dementia and depression are different from one another, but it can be hard to distinguish between them because their signs and symptoms may be alike. Sometimes a person has more than one of these conditions at the same time. Alert health-care staff if you or someone you know shows any of these signs or symptoms.

Delirium is a condition that **comes on quickly** (within hours or days) and affects the brain. It is usually temporary, lasting one-to-seven days, but should be treated right away. Most times delirium is caused by a combination of factors.

Delirium may be caused by:

- having an illness
- staying in bed too long
- being in a noisy or confusing environment
- having pain

People at highest risk for delirium include:

- older adults
- people with depression or dementia
- people who have broken their hip
- people who have had major surgery (e.g. heart surgery)

Signs of delirium

- poor concentration
- difficulty remembering things
- confusion about time and place
- seeing or hearing things that are not there

- being sleepy or slow to respond
- problems eating or sleeping
- changes in personality
- not showing interest in things

These signs can come and go. Tell a health-care provider right away if you notice any of these signs. Delirium is a serious illness and needs to be **treated right away**.

Dementia is a disorder of the brain that can affect learning, memory, mood and behaviour. Dementia **develops slowly**, over several months or years. Dementia affects different people in different ways. Aging does not cause dementia but it is more common among older adults. One of the most common types of dementia is Alzheimer's disease.

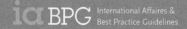

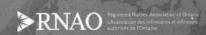

HEALTH EDUCATION FACT SHEET
FROM NURSES FOR YOU

Signs of dementia

- difficulty performing familiar tasks (e.g. banking, driving, brushing teeth)
- difficulties with thinking, problem solving, or learning new information or language
- memory loss that affects day-to-day activities
- not being able to find things (e.g. thinking someone took or moved something)
- confusion about time and place
- changes in personality, mood or behaviour
- loss of initiative (e.g. needing to be told what to do)
- poor or decreased judgment

Keep in mind that just because a person has dementia does not mean they cannot continue to live well and have meaning in their lives.

Depression is a medical illness. Having depression does not mean someone is weak. Many people have depression throughout their lives, while others suffer from depression as a result of a major change in their life, including:

- death of a loved one
- loss of independence (e.g. moving to a long-term care home)
- developing dementia or an illness

Signs of depression

- sleeping more or less than usual
- loss of interest in usual hobbies or activities
- low energy levels
- eating more or less than usual
- difficulty concentrating
- aches and pains
- constipation
- being agitated or irritable
- feely guilty, worthless, hopeless, full of regret
- thoughts of not wanting to live or of ending one's life

Depression should be taken seriously. Talk to a health-care provider if you or someone you know shows signs of depression. There are many treatment options available.

Getting help

Talk to a health-care provider right away if you or someone you know shows signs of delirium, dementia or depression. They can arrange for a proper assessment and connect you to the care or treatment you need. Also, ask them where you can get more information or support. You can learn more about delirium from RNAO's fact sheet, *Delirium: How you can help.*

This fact sheet was developed to go with the RNAO best practice guideline (BPG) *Delirium, dementia, and depression: Assessment and care, Second Edition* (2016). It is intended to increase your knowledge, and help you take part in decisions about your health or the health of a family member. RNAO's BPGs are available for public viewing and free download at RNAO.ca/bestpractices

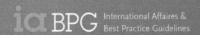

www.RNAO.ca/bestpractices

APPENDIX E: TOOLS FOR QUALITY APPRAISAL OF THE LITERATURE

Type of Study	Study Design	Quality-Appraisal Tool
Systematic Reviews	▪ Systematic Review ▪ Meta-Analysis ▪ Meta-Synthesis ▪ Literature Review	AMSTAR Appraisal Tool
Best Practice Guidelines	▪ Clinical Guideline	AGREE II Tool

Experimental	▪ Randomized Controlled Trials
	   –Double Blind
	   –Single Blind
	   –Non-Blind
		CASP RCT Appraisal Tool

Quasi-Experimental	Nonrandomized Trial Interrupted time series design Pre-Post Test with or without control group	(Pre-Post Test with no control group) Controlled Clinical Trial Tool adopted from National Institutes of Health (Quasi-experimental study with a control group) Cochrane Public Health Quasi-Experimental Appraisal Tool [Cochrane Public Health, n.d.]

Non-Experimental	▪ Cohort Studies
	   –Prospective Cohort
	   –Retrospective Cohort
	   –Time Series Study
		CASP Cohort Appraisal Tool

	▪ Case Control Studies –Nested Case Control	CASP Case Control Appraisal Tool

	▪ Descriptive Studies
	   –Cross Sectional Studies
	   –Prevalence Studies
		CASP Cross Sectional Appraisal Tool

Qualitative Studies	▪ Phenomenology ▪ Grounded Theory ▪ Ethnography ▪ Critical Social Theory	CASP Qualitative Appraisal Tool
Mixed Method Studies	▪ Mixed Method	Mixed Methods Appraisal Tool (Pluye et al., 2011)

APPENDIX F: RNAO STATEMENT ON LEVELS OF EVIDENCE USED IN SYSTEMATIC REVIEWS/GUIDELINES

The RNAO BPG development process uses the following Levels of Evidence:

Ia	Evidence obtained from *meta-analysis* of randomized controlled trials
Ib	Evidence obtained from at least one *randomized controlled trial*
IIa	Evidence obtained from at least one well-designed *controlled study without randomization*
IIb	Evidence obtained from at least one other type of well-designed *quasi- experimental study, without randomization*
III	Evidence obtained from *well-designed non-experimental descriptive studies, such as comparative studies, correlation studies, and case studies*
IV	Evidence obtained from expert committee reports or opinions and/or clinical experiences of respected authorities

Adapted from the Scottish Intercollegiate Guidelines Network (2017) and Pati (2011).

3

CREATING HEALTHY WORKPLACES: ENABLING CLINICAL EXCELLENCE

Irmajean Bajnok, PhD, MScN, BScN, RN
Althea Stewart-Pyne, MHSc, RN

LEARNING OBJECTIVES

After reading this chapter, you will be able to:

- Outline the origins of RNAO's healthy work environment evidence-based guidelines for nurses and other healthcare providers

- Understand the elements of a healthy work environment and how their synergy contributes to the multifaceted and complex nature of healthcare work settings

- Discuss key aspects of a healthy work environment embedded in RNAO's set of Healthy Work Environment (HWE) BPGs

- Describe how a healthy work environment influences outcomes for nurses, patients, organizations, and systems

INTRODUCTION

This chapter describes the strong links between work environments and the uptake of clinical Best Practice Guidelines (BPG) and the establishment of evidence-based practice cultures. The rationale for the development of Healthy Work Environment (HWE) BPGs is provided, alongside the model of a healthy work environment that guided the development process. The chapter also outlines the collaborative processes used to select the initial foundational HWE BPGs and how their impacts were evaluated in workplaces across health sectors. It explores the development of HWE BPGs in foundational areas and other themes. The chapter concludes with a review of the outcomes of HWE BPG implementation, including enhanced provider satisfaction and sustained uptake of clinical practice guidelines, which together have led to better client outcomes.

INITIATION OF HEALTHY WORK ENVIRONMENTS (HWE) BPGS

In Ontario in the early 2000s, the Ministry of Health and Long-Term Care (MOHLTC) began to explore the impact of the work environment in healthcare on providers, organizations, and clients, and approached the Registered Nurses' Association of Ontario (RNAO) to expand its successful evidence-based clinical Best Practice Guidelines Program (Grinspun, Virani, & Bajnok, 2002) to focus also on work environments. In 2003, RNAO took up the challenge to develop HWE BPGs with funding support from MOHLTC and from the Canadian government.

At the time of the request from the Ontario government, RNAO had begun to identify emerging evidence of the link between uptake of clinical best practices and characteristics of the work environment. We had noticed enthusiastic uptake in what we called healthy work environments (HWE). HWEs were also being discussed by others (Izzo, 2001; Lowe, 2002; Rycroft-Malone et al., 2002). Through its policy work, RNAO was also acutely aware of serious workplace issues as expressed by nurses and documented by scholars (Baumann et al., 2001; Cohen, Stuenkel, & Nguyen, 2009; Griffin et al., 2003; O'Brien-Pallas et al., 2005; RNAO, 2000).

Seminal work by Rycroft-Malone et al. (2002) concluded that evidence uptake in clinical practice is closely linked to healthcare work environments that support evidence-based practice and decision-making. The authors noted that within healthy work environments, the following components are generally present and they positively impact successful guideline implementation processes (Rycroft-Malone et al., 2002):

- Transformational leadership

- Effective structures/teamwork

- Rewards and recognition for work and years of service

- A learning culture that:

  - Values staff and clients

  - Promotes democratic decision-making

  - Utilizes multiple sources of information methods to provide feedback to staff

Other important research by Izzo (2001) and by Lowe (2002) emphasized characteristics that contribute to a healthy workplace. These include relationships with supervisors and coworkers, the presence of rewards and recognition, and a culture that:

- Is built on trust

- Values people

- Supports learning

- Provides opportunities for participation

- Provides timely, complete information

With its groundbreaking work in developing HWE BPGs, RNAO brought to the forefront a greater understanding that HWEs are not only critical for a vibrant workforce and high-performing organizations, but also imperative for clinical excellence and positive health outcomes for patients (Griffin et al., 2003).

DEFINITION OF A HEALTHY WORK ENVIRONMENT

RNAO defines *healthy work environments* as "practice settings that maximize the health and well-being of nurses [and all health care workers], quality patient outcomes and organizational and system performance and societal outcomes" (RNAO, 2013b, p. 8).

This definition reinforces that the work environment is integral to workers and what they do, and the impact of their work, as well as organization and system outcomes. Each of these areas, and the synergy between and amongst them, will be discussed in this chapter. When RNAO commenced this leading-edge work, there were few guides to direct the process. A decision was made at the outset to develop a comprehensive conceptual model for HWEs that reflected the multidimensional and complex nature of the healthcare workplace (RNAO, 2006b, 2006c, 2007a, 2007b, 2007c, 2008). The HWE Conceptual Model is used by each HWE BPG Expert Panel in its development work, and it is included as part of the introduction to each HWE BPG. Additionally, RNAO's rigorous clinical BPG development and related processes for uptake and impact assessment were used to guide the development, implementation, and evaluation of evidence-based tools to enhance the work environment.

THE HWE CONCEPTUAL MODEL

The development of the HWE Conceptual Model preceded the development of the HWE BPGs and built on relevant existing models (Baumann et al., 2001; DeJoy & Southern, 1993; Griffin et al., 2003; O'Brien-Pallas & Baumann, 1992). The RNAO model served to better explain the multiple levels, diverse factors, complex relationships, and synergistic impacts associated with HWEs for healthcare providers, patients, organizations, and the system (RNAO, 2006b, 2006c).

Figure 3.1 illustrates the factors and components, and the interactions among the key elements, that influence an HWE.

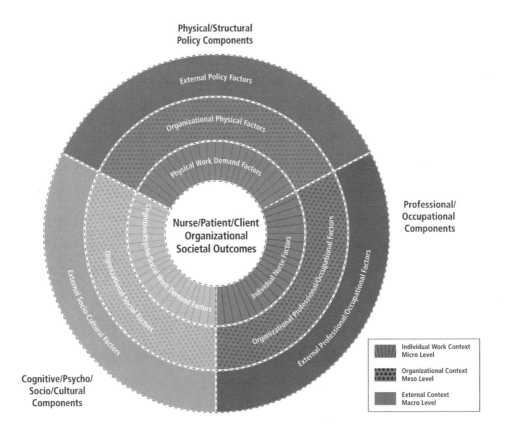

FIGURE 3.1 RNAO HWE Conceptual Model.

When you look at this, you may ask, "What is this model trying to tell me?"

This model presents the healthy workplace as a product of the interdependence amongst individual, organizational, and external system factors, and three different types of components: physical/ structural/policy, cognitive/psycho/socio/cultural, and professional/occupational components that are part of each of the factors. The factors are illustrated in three circles surrounding the central overall goal of HWEs—better outcomes for healthcare providers, patients, organizations, systems, and society as a whole, including healthier communities (Griffin et al., 2003). The components are illustrated in the three wedges that cut across each of the factors. The lines within the model are dotted to indicate the synergistic interactions amongst all levels and components of the model.

The model suggests that each individual practitioner's functioning is influenced by interactions between the individual and the individual's environment. Thus, interventions to promote HWEs must be aimed at multiple levels and components of the organization and the system. Similarly, interventions must influence not only the factors within the system and the interactions amongst these factors, but also the system itself (Green, Richard, & Potvin, 1996; Grinspun, 2000). The assumptions underlying the model are:

- Healthy work environments are essential for quality, safe patient care.

- The model is applicable to all practice settings and all domains of nursing.

- Individual, organizational, and external system-level factors are the determinants of healthy work environments for nurses.

■ Factors at all three levels impact the health and well-being of nurses, quality patient outcomes, organizational and system performance, and societal outcomes, either individually or through synergistic interactions.

■ At each level, there are physical/structural policy components, cognitive/psycho/social/cultural components, and professional/occupational components.

■ The professional/occupational components are unique to each profession, while the remaining components are generic for all professions/occupations.

Figure 3.2 highlights the physical/structural policy components at each level that influence an HWE.

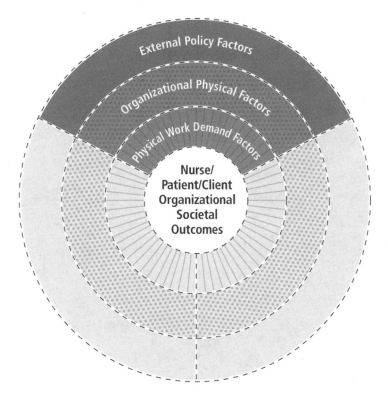

FIGURE 3.2 Physical/structural policy components.

The physical/structural policy components identified above in the top wedge of the circles are the physical characteristics and environment of the organization developed to respond to the physical work characteristics and work demands. They include the following:

■ Physical work demand factors (shown on the inner area of the wedge with striped lines) are those tasks that require effort and involve the physical capabilities of the nurse or care provider to deliver the care. An example of physical work demand factors could be the nature of the patient population that might require more physical lifting or rotating shifts.

■ Organizational physical factors (shown on the dotted area of the wedge) are both the existing characteristics and the structures and processes that the organization creates to provide a supportive work environment. An example of this might be the physical layout of the work setting and the design of multiple supply or equipment access points, such as computer terminals, to improve efficiency.

■ External policy factors (shown on the solid outer area of the wedge) include factors such as immigration policies; healthcare funding policies; legislative, trade, economic, and political influences external to the organization; and other agreements that have the potential to affect healthcare.

Figure 3.3 highlights the cognitive/psycho/socio/cultural components at each level that influence an HWE.

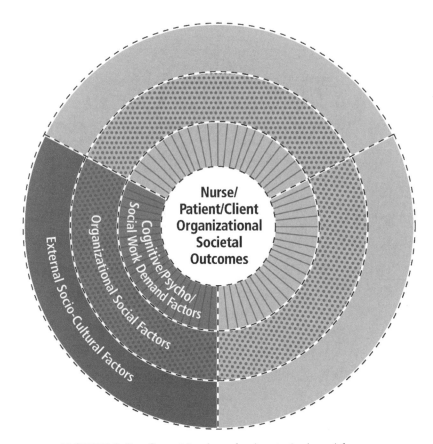

FIGURE 3.3 Cognitive/psycho/socio/cultural factors.

The cognitive/psycho/social/cultural components identified on the left lower wedge of the circles are the factors represented by the individual working in healthcare and as a member of society. They include the following:

■ Individual cognitive/psycho/social work demand factors (shown on the inner area of the wedge with striped lines) refer to those situations that require effective problem solving, coping, and communication by the individual. This kind of work demand requires cognitive, psychological, and social capabilities and effort (Grinspun, 2010). This applies to most nursing roles but could be more complex with specific patient populations.

■ Organizational social factors refer to factors such as the climate, culture, and values of the organization.

■ External socio-cultural factors: These are consumer trends, care preferences, family roles, diversity of the population and providers, and changing demographics. As an example, in the early 2000s we saw a relaxation of visiting policies with the trend to more patient-centeredness and inclusivity of families in care (Farmanova, Judd, Maika, & Wilkes, 2015). However, in 2004 with the advent of SARS (severe acute respiratory syndrome), there was an enormous move back to less open visiting policies (Rogers, 2004).

Figure 3.4 highlights the professional/occupational components at each level that influence an HWE.

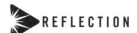

REFLECTION

When exploring these organizational factors in your own work setting, ask yourself the following questions: Does the organization value nursing? Are there visible supports for staff who work shift and opportunities for professional development?

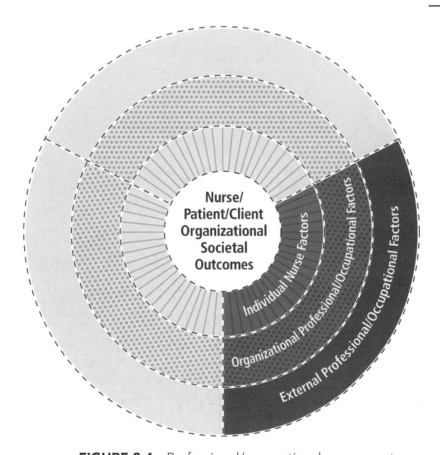

FIGURE 3.4   Professional/occupational components.

The details of this section of the model, shown on the right lower wedge of the circles, have been outlined here to be specific to nurses (and could be altered depending on the type of healthcare worker), whereas the other components of the model are applicable to all healthcare workers. They include the following:

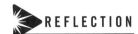
REFLECTION

Consider the following questions to assess this component in your organization: What level of autonomy for practice is supported? Is there a nursing committee that determines scope of practice for nurses in your organization?

- Individual nurse factors are the knowledge, skill, and personal attributes (such as age, education, and physical health and well-being) of the individual that determine response to the work demands.

- Organizational professional/occupation factors refer to the nature of the professional's role and supports within organization (e.g., level of autonomy, scope of practice).

- External professional/occupational factors refer to those factors outside of the organization that come as a result of policies and regulations, such as standards of practice and the regulated scope of practice from the regulatory body for nursing (e.g., standards of practice, certification, and ethical recruitment).

HWE BPG DEVELOPMENT METHODOLOGY

To meet our commitment to ensuring that every HWE BPG is based on the best available evidence, it was a given that RNAO would utilize the same rigorous Guideline Development process as for the clinical BPGs, and monitor and revise each guideline on a regular basis. The HWE BPG development process remains consistent with the clinical BPG process, and as the clinical BPG development methodology is refined and enhanced, the development processes for the HWE BPGs are modified to reflect the increased rigor. The HWE BPG development methodology includes the following steps:

- The topic is selected based on key issues/trends in healthcare, data from RNAO's Best Practice Spotlight Organizations (BPSO), input from nurse and other healthcare professionals, or recommendations from government and/or other healthcare task forces.

- A panel of nurses and inter-professionals is convened from a range of specialties, roles, and practices settings. Increasingly, the panels have national and international representation. We recruit nurses and inter-professionals who possess expertise in practice, research, policy, education, and administration related to the topic area. These individuals form the Expert Panel.

- The scope of the guideline is identified and defined through a process of discussion and consensus with internal RNAO partners and external subject-matter experts.

- The Expert Panel identifies key themes and concepts in the subject matter that direct the research questions for the systematic literature review search and provide an organizing framework for the guideline.

- Following retrieval of relevant literature by a qualified health sciences librarian, a systematic literature review is conducted by a team of qualified nurse researchers (part of RNAO's BPG development team). The findings are used to inform the development of recommendations from individual and team, organizational, and policy perspectives.

- Drafts of the guideline are developed through a consultative process with RNAO and the Expert Panel members. The drafts are reviewed and revised by the Expert Panel and members of RNAO's Guideline Development Team.

- The guideline is distributed for review, first to panel members and then to external stakeholders.

- All feedback from panel members and stakeholders is considered and changes are made as necessary by consensus and evidence.

- The recommendations and evidence are then finalized through an internal process and editorial review at RNAO.

- The Guideline Development Team reaches consensus on the final document.

- The HWE BPG is published and widely disseminated for use.

DEVELOPING HWE BPGS: WHERE TO START

As indicated, the initial goal of the Program was the development of foundational guidelines that would assist nurses and other clinicians with day-to-day workplace challenges, to facilitate their focus on clinical excellence. These foundational HWE BPGs were based on key topic areas identified using a grounded research approach in which, through a series of focus groups, nurses from across sectors and geographic areas in Canada were asked about key workplace issues they felt were critical to quality patient care. There was a high consistency in the results, which included six discrete topic areas that would become the foundational HWE BPGs.

These first six HWE BPGs were developed in partnership with the Joanna Briggs Institute (JBI), which carried out the systematic literature reviews related to each of the topic areas identified (Pearson et al., 2006a, 2006b, 2006c, 2007a, 2007b). At the time, JBI had just released its quality-appraisal and data-extraction tools for qualitative research, which were most appropriate in defining the evidence base for the HWE BPGs. Six foundational guidelines were published between 2006 and 2008, addressing: leadership; collaborative practice; workload and staffing; professionalism; diversity; and workplace health, safety, and well-being.

Recognizing the importance of leadership, collaboration, and capacity-building related to workplace issues, their impact, and resolution, the HWE BPGs were targeted to all levels of staff within organizations as well as a number of external stakeholders such as regulatory bodies, governments, and unions, thus supporting a team responsibility for workplace health. In keeping with this intent, the HWE BPGs included evidence-based individual- and team-oriented recommendations to support direct care clinicians in learning about HWEs and contributing to a healthy work environment. Also, evidence-based organizational and policy recommendations were designed to support health care organizations in creating and sustaining positive work environments. In addition, system-oriented recommendations were developed to garner the engagement of governments, unions, and regulatory and standard-setting bodies in addressing workplace issues. Figure 3.5 graphically displays and explains the types of recommendations included in RNAO's System and Healthy Work Environment BPGs.

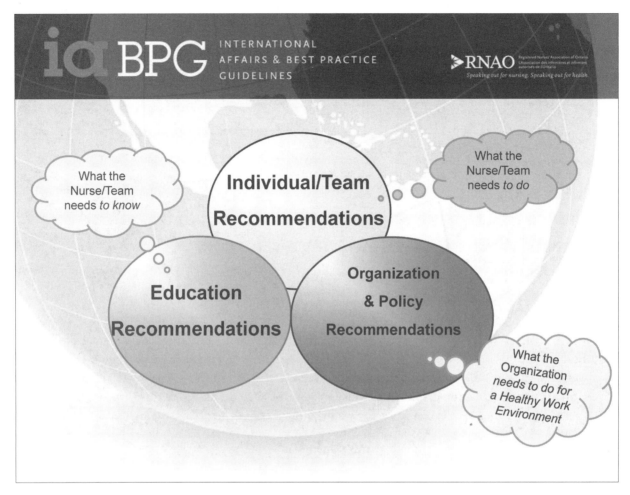

FIGURE 3.5 Types of recommendations included in RNAO's System and Healthy Work Environment BPGs.

THE FOUNDATIONAL HWE BPGS

The six foundational guidelines are:

- *Collaborative Practice Among Nursing Teams* (RNAO, 2006b)

- *Developing and Sustaining Effective Staffing and Workload Practices* (RNAO, 2007a)

- *Developing and Sustaining Nursing Leadership* (RNAO, 2006c)

- *Embracing Cultural Diversity in Health Care: Developing Cultural Competence* (RNAO, 2007b)

- *Professionalism in Nursing* (RNAO, 2007c)

- *Workplace Health, Safety and Well-Being of the Nurse* (RNAO, 2008)

The intent was to use these six guidelines as the initial focus for creating an HWE and then develop additional guidelines that stemmed from these foundational themes to enable further enhancement of the work environment. A short description of each foundational HWE BPG is provided in the following sections.

EFFECTIVE NURSING LEADERSHIP

Effective leadership is a pivotal aspect in all nursing roles whether the nurse practices directly with patients, in the field of education developing future leaders, as a researcher who mentors new researchers, or as an administrator or executive leader who provides support and guidance to staff (Cummings et al., 2010; Pearson et al., 2007a; RNAO, 2006c).

COLLABORATIVE PRACTICE

Strengthening team practice amongst all categories of nurses supports the practice setting for nurses. This guideline explores what fosters healthy work environments and effective teamwork amongst all categories of nurses in Ontario, Canada—the registered nurse, the registered practical nurse, and the nurse practitioner (Pearson et al., 2006c; RNAO, 2006c)

STAFFING, WORKLOAD, AND STRUCTURE

Staff mix for a specific practice setting is composed of various categories of nurses working intra-professionally and inter-professionally. Education, experience, skill mix, and leadership qualities have an enormous impact on the quality of nurse staffing. Nurse staffing is a complex process. An effective and formalized staffing plan requires an understanding of the complexity involved in patient care and in matching human resources (scope of practice, skills, number of staff, education, and experience) to patient needs (Pearson et al., 2006c; RNAO, 2007a).

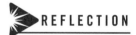

▶ REFLECTION

As you read these short descriptions of each HWE BPG, consider how decisions are made in your organizations, the workload patterns, and the physical facilities and resources available to support you in your role. What are the decision-making processes? Is there enough staff to support the complexity of patients and their care?

PROFESSIONALISM

This guideline recognizes eight qualities of a professional staff and, in addition, outlines how organizations and leaders support professional behaviours in nursing and other staff. Some questions in determining the degree of professionalism are (Pearson et al., 2006b; RNAO, 2007c): Does the staff have the necessary knowledge and skills? Does the nursing staff have a positive and professional attitude to support evidence-based practice? Does the organization have a positive view of the nursing profession? Have nurses been effectively supported through practice change in the past?

WORKPLACE CULTURE AND DIVERSITY

The degree to which the workplace culture supports and builds on diversity is a critical factor in HWEs, as well as in effective individual and team functioning.

This can be assessed by asking the following questions: What is the overall nature of the organization, in terms of how we think things should be done? What is seen as important? To what degree does the culture support change and evidence-based practice? Are the organizational values clear and evident in how and what decisions are made? Is there a culture of respect for all? Are all key stakeholder perspectives considered and incorporated? Are processes in place to evaluate decisions? (Pearson et al., 2007b; RNAO, 2007b)

WORKPLACE HEALTH, SAFETY, AND WELL-BEING OF THE NURSE

The health of nurses involves various complex components. These components are discussed in the guideline. They include the physical design of the organization, the work nurses do, working conditions, occupational hazards, injury and illness prevention, health promotion, organizational culture, and system supports (RNAO, 2008).

PILOT IMPLEMENTATION AND EVALUATION

Shortly after their release, the foundational HWE BPGs were evaluated through a 4-year, multisite study involving nine health care settings (acute care, mental health, and home care) in Ontario. A pre- and 3- and 6-month post- research study design was used. Units/teams in each setting were randomly assigned specific HWE BPGs to implement (RNAO, 2010). The results were extremely encouraging and demonstrated extensive engagement of nurses and other healthcare professionals in the HWE BPG implementation work. The findings also revealed the high value that was placed on this work and the perceived positive outcomes as expressed by staff in relation to: the effectiveness of teamwork, staff satisfaction, the quality of care, and patient outcomes (RNAO, 2010). In addition, it became clear that the HWE BPGs were useful across settings and sectors, and with a variety of nursing and other health professionals and staff.

These results fuelled widespread implementation, and the success of the foundational guidelines led to the development of other related HWE BPGs consistent with longstanding and emerging issues in healthcare work settings. The following list of HWE BPGs represents either a second edition of the foundational BPG or new themes:

- *Preventing and Managing Violence in the Workplace* (RNAO, 2009)

- *Preventing and Mitigating Nurse Fatigue in Health Care* (RNAO, 2011)

- *Managing and Mitigating Conflict in Health-Care Teams* (RNAO, 2012a)

- *Developing and Sustaining Interprofessional Health Care: Optimizing Patients/Clients, Organizational, and System Outcomes* (RNAO, 2013a)

- *Developing and Sustaining Nursing Leadership*, Second Edition (RNAO, 2013b)

- *Intra-Professional Collaborative Practice Among Nurses*, Second Edition (RNAO, 2016a)

- *Developing and Sustaining Safe, Effective Staffing and Workload Practices*, Second Edition (RNAO, 2017b)

As the Program has matured, the HWE BPG Program has expanded to focus on the health system, and the guidelines are now termed System and Healthy Work Environment BPGs. Examples of guidelines that reflect the health system include *Practice Education in Nursing* (RNAO, 2016c), and *Adopting eHealth Solutions: Implementation Strategies* (RNAO, 2017a).

A variety of resources has been developed, reflecting best practices in implementation science (RNAO, 2012c), that facilitate dissemination and uptake of the HWE BPGs. For example, *The Healthy Work Environments Quick Reference Guide* (RNAO, 2013c) includes summaries of all the HWE BPGs and was developed for managers to enable ease of use in the workplace. This resource was so popular that it was made available to all staff for online access. In addition, for a number of the BPGs, a summary of key guideline recommendations and assessment resources, called Tips and Tools, was developed and targeted to point-of-care nurses. The following Tips and Tools were developed for the following associated guidelines.

GUIDELINE	TIPS AND TOOLS RESOURCE
Preventing and Managing Violence in the Workplace (2009)	*Preventing and Managing Violence: Tips and Tools for Nurses* (2014e)
Preventing and Mitigating Nurse Fatigue in Health Care (2011)	*Managing and Mitigating Fatigue: Tips and Tools for Nurses* (2014c)
Managing and Mitigating Conflict in Health-Care Teams (2012a)	*Managing and Mitigating Conflict: Tips and Tools for Nurses* (2012b)
Developing and Sustaining Interprofessional Health Care: Optimizing Patients/Clients, Organizational, and System Outcomes (2013a)	*Developing and Sustaining Interprofessional Health Care: Tips and Tools for Health-Care Teams* (2014a)
Developing and Sustaining Nursing Leadership (2013b)	*Developing and Sustaining Nursing Leadership: Tips and Tools* (2014b) *Point-of-Care Leadership Tips and Tools for Nurses* (2014d)

For some of the BPGs—*Practice Education in Nursing* (2016c) and *Adopting eHealth Solutions: Implementation Strategies* (2017a)—a synopsis of the guideline was developed, incorporating evidence highlights and recommendations.

As noted earlier, the work environment needs to be healthy in order to support positive patient outcomes. By identifying and developing the foundational HWE BPGs, an awareness of the importance of the work environment was raised and has been sustained. In addition, it became clear that environmental readiness (reflecting issues in the workplace) was a critical factor in implementation science and incorporated in RNAO's clinical implementation resources (RNAO, 2012c).

CREATING HEALTHY WORKPLACES

Achieving HWEs for nurses requires that organizational leaders and individual practitioners commit to transformational change using interventions specific to the underlying workplace context and organizational factors (Lowe, 2004; RNAO, 2008). The HWE BPGs support this type of transformational change through the use of evidence-based recommendations that address unique nursing professional practice as well as common workplace issues. Evidence-based recommendations that address the individual provider, care teams, education for HWEs, and organizational and system policy incorporate a focus on the nurses' health and morale and ensuing ability to provide care, patient outcomes, and organizational and system performance (RNAO, 2006b, 2006c, 2007a, 2007b, 2007c, 2008).

Evidence about HWEs in healthcare settings and their broad impacts continues to mount. In a systematic review conducted by Lindberg and Vingard (2012), results strongly link the work environment and the ability to provide safe, quality care. In the review, the following nine (9) elements were identified as necessary to achieve a healthy workplace:

- Collaboration/teamwork
- Development of the individual
- Recognition
- Employee involvement
    - Positive, accessible, and fair leaders
    - Autonomy and empowerment
- Appropriate staffing
- Skilled communication
- Safe physical environment

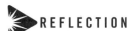

REFLECTION

Do you remember your first job? Maybe your first job was in nursing, or maybe another field. Chances are the first thing you will remember are the people. Staff relations and teamwork are critical aspects of the work environment.

All these areas are addressed in RNAO's 12 System and Healthy Work Environment BPGs.

HEALTHY WORK ENVIRONMENTS AND THE IMPACT ON HEALTHCARE SETTINGS

Organizations with HWEs recognize that people and their relationships are at the heart of their ability to achieve the mission within the context of the overall vision and strategic plan (Burgess & Purkis, 2010; RNAO, 2016a). The work environment and the multiple influences within the workplace (as delineated in the HWE Conceptual Model) have an impact on the mental and physical well-being of employees, including the cultural, social, and professional roles performed by nurses and other members of the inter-professional team.

WORK ENVIRONMENT AND NURSE OUTCOMES

It is important to examine the work environment as part of quality improvement to enhance nurse outcomes, and by extension patient outcomes (Baernholdt & Mark, 2009). Better support services, a smooth workflow, and a work environment that enables autonomous nursing practice and committed nurses contribute to strong nursing outcomes (Baernholdt & Mark, 2009).

Other factors from the work environment that impact nurse and ultimately patient outcomes are (Grinspun, 2002, 2003, 2007; Grinspun & Anyinam, 2014; O'Brien-Pallas & Hayes, 2010; Pearson, et al., 2007a; 2007b; RNAO, 2008):

1. Nursing workload

2. Casualization (or increasing numbers of temporary part-time staff) of the nursing workforce

3. The age demographic in many jurisdictions

4. Nursing leadership

5. Financial support

6. Respect

Chachula, Myrick, and Yonge (2015) examined the factors and basic psychosocial processes involved in the decision of newly graduated RNs in Western Canada to leave the profession on a permanent basis. The results of the study (Chachula et al., 2015) indicated that participants withdrew from their nursing identities in the absence of intrinsic and extrinsic rewards (e.g., support, validation, and legitimization of their roles).

Four interconnected categories were also reflected in the findings (Chachula et al., 2015):

1. Navigating the constraints of the healthcare system and workplace (e.g., strained, rigid, nonresponsive, bureaucratic, high patient loads, cutbacks, poor working conditions)

2. Negotiating social relationships, hierarchies, and troublesome behaviours (e.g., hierarchies, horizontal and lateral violence, bullying)

3. Facing fears, traumas, and challenges (e.g., sensitivity, patient deaths, critical feedback)

4. Weighing competing rewards and tensions (e.g., losing joy of nursing, weighing positives and negatives)

These findings relate directly to the work environment, and it has been suggested that the factors fuelling the ongoing shortage of nurses are the result of unhealthy work environments (Dunleavy, Shamian, & Thomson, 2003; Grinspun, 2010; RNAO, 2008, 2017b). This is compounded by funding models that make it challenging for workplaces to hire the most qualified staff to deliver and oversee the complex care required in today's health system. This has a definite impact on quality of care, as several studies have shown a link between positive patient outcomes and sufficient Registered Nurse staffing (Drach-Zahavy, 2004; Mattila et al., 2014; RNAO, 2016b).

Havaei, MacPhee, and Dahinten (2016) looked at skill mix in acute care settings and two nurse outcomes, namely emotional exhaustion and intention to leave. The findings identified that those with a higher level of emotional exhaustion, high workload, and exposure to lack of respect, and those seeking a change in their career were more likely to leave the profession altogether. Within the home care sector there were similar findings. That is, home care nurses who reported having an intention to leave desired to have: higher nurse-evaluated quality of care, greater variety of patients, more satisfaction with salary and benefits, greater income stability, greater continuity of patient care, greater meaningfulness in work, more positive relationships with supervisors, and higher work-life balance (Tourangeau, Patterson, Saari, Thomson, & Cranley, 2017).

WORK ENVIRONMENT AND PATIENT OUTCOMES

Patient outcomes associated with HWEs that reflect best practices related to staffing, staff mix, team-work, and leadership include:

- Decreased patient mortality and a higher value of care (Silber et al., 2016)
- Decreased adverse outcomes (McHugh et al., 2016)
- Better nurse staffing and work environments associated with increased survival of in-hospital cardiac arrest patients (McHugh et al., 2016)

Furthermore, many research studies and reviews have examined the positive patient outcomes that occur as a result of full-time nurse staffing (a critical component of a healthy work environment), many of which have cost-saving implications from a systems and organization-level perspective:

- Decreases in missed care (Zhu et al., 2012)
- Decreased unassisted falls (Staggs & Dunton, 2014)
- Decreased failures to rescue (Harless & Mark, 2010; Kane, Shamliyan, Mueller, Duval, & Wilt, 2007)
- Decreased cardiac arrest (Kane et al., 2007)
- Decreased hospital acquired pneumonia (Kane et al., 2007)
- Increased patient safety in ICU and surgical care (Kane et al., 2007)

WORK ENVIRONMENT AND ORGANIZATIONAL OUTCOMES

The nurses' work environment impacts the organizational outcomes; for example in the case of absenteeism, the cost to the organization and sector can be substantial (Aldana, 2001), and unless the root cause is addressed (e.g., leadership, workload, team dynamics, safety, not enough equipment and other resources), absenteeism due to illness, stress, and injury will continue to add costs to the bottom line, and by extension add risks to quality care (Aldana, 2001; Duffield et al., 2011; O'Brien-Pallas & Hayes, 2010; O'Brien-Pallas, Tomblin Murphy, & Shamian, 2008; RNAO, 2008, 2017b).

Organizations that adopt HWE principles and values—and take a comprehensive and collaborative approach to ensure workers can function in a safe and respectful atmosphere—are the most successful in BPG uptake, leading to better outcomes (Davies et al., 2006; Shamian & El-Jardali, 2007). Shamian and El-Jardali (2007) also acknowledged RNAO's HWE Program as having potential to create professional practice environments and ease the nursing recruitment and retention issues plaguing healthcare. HWEs promote nurse and employee well-being, engagement, retention, productivity, and patient safety, all of which affect the health system's costs (Cohen et al., 2009; O'Brien-Pallas et al., 2008). We need healthy nurses and other healthcare workers who are consistently present to affect good clinical outcomes for patients. Healthcare workers are one of the highest-risk groups for work-related injuries and illness in Ontario and across Canada. Statistics reveal that:

- The average number of days of work lost due to illness or disability was at least 1.5 times greater for workers in healthcare than the average for all workers (Canadian Institute for Health Information, 2005).

- The lost time injury rate in the healthcare sector in Ontario was 1.27 per 100 workers in 2015. Of this lost time, 12% was directly related to workplace violence (Ontario Ministry of Labour, 2017).

- Fifty-four percent (54%) of Ontario nurses have experienced physical abuse; 85% have experienced verbal abuse, and 19% have experienced sexual violence or abuse (Ontario Nurses Association, 2015).

Unhealthy work environments impact the ability to retain and recruit healthcare workers. Illnesses and injuries resulting from these unhealthy environments place additional pressure on coworkers, reduce providers' ability to meet their patients' needs, and, as discussed previously, may in some cases even cause people to consider leaving their profession (Chachula et al., 2015; Havaei et al., 2016; Public Services Health and Safety Association, 2011; Tourangeau et al., 2017).

Therefore, attention to work environments is critical to ensuring strong organizational outcomes, and managers and nurse administrators have a critical role in influencing the work environment through increasing nurse retention and preventing staff turnover, to ultimately improve patient care (Sellgren, Kajermo, Ekvall, & Tomson, 2009). Some factors that may help increase retention and decrease turnover include acknowledging the challenges faced by nurses (Sellgren et al., 2009); shared clinical decision-making and full-time employment (Grinspun, 2007); models of care delivery that promote continuity of caregiver (Grinspun, 2010; Meyer, Wang, Li, Thomson, & O'Brien-Pallas, 2009; RNAO, 2006a); promoting self-scheduling (Butler et al., 2011); work support programs (Luo, Lin, & Castle, 2013); appropriate working conditions (Nakamura et al., 2010); and staffing within budgeted levels (North et al., 2013). In 2015, the total days of work lost in healthcare occupations was reported to be 13.8 per worker (Statistics Canada, 2014). The financial benefits yielded from improvements in the work environment that lead to reduced absenteeism, improved productivity, and reduced healthcare costs for employees have been clearly documented (Aldana, 2001; RNAO, 2017b).

> **REFLECTION**
>
> *Reflecting on that first job again, do you recall if you worked alone or if other employees were an important part of your day-to-day experience? Did you feel supported? Did you feel part of a team? These are important considerations that influence the work environment and have a link to clinical outcomes for patients. Reflect on them also in relation to your current work position.*

WORK ENVIRONMENT AND HEALTH SYSTEM OUTCOMES

HWEs are also closely tied to the recruitment and retention of nurses who are critical in ensuring access to health services and sustaining the healthcare system (Laschinger, Wong, & Grau, 2012). An adequate supply of appropriately qualified registered nurses is central to a healthy work environment and to the provision of quality, evidence-based care (Frith, Anderson, Fan, & Fong, 2012; Trinkoff et al., 2011). In a spiralling down cycle, staff shortages impact retention, as nurses who are dissatisfied with the quality of care they can provide leave the workplace and may also leave the profession. Nursing shortages may in turn impact recruitment success at the organizational level (Berry & Curry, 2012; MacPhee, 2014; RNAO, 2000) because nurses do not want to work in unhealthy workplaces, and at the professional level, because potential nurses are looking for satisfying, meaningful work.

In Canada, data from the Canadian Institute for Health Information (CIHI) indicates there was a decline in the number of RNs, the first in almost two decades (CIHI, 2015). This emerging trend, at a time when patients and health issues across all sectors are becoming more complex (Lipsitz, 2012), does not bode well for healthy work environments or quality care. It behooves governments, professional bodies, unions, regulatory bodies, healthcare organizations, and individual managers and direct care nurses to work together to use the plethora of strong evidence available to shape healthy work environments.

IMPLEMENTING HWE BPGS

Implementing HWEs (see Chapter 4, *Forging the Way with Implementation Science*) and building a culture of safety for healthcare workers opens the door to developing a culture of evidence-based clinical practice. If the work environment issues are addressed, nurses and other clinicians and managers are freed to focus on delivering the highest-quality evidence-based care possible. Implementing HWE BPGs is not *instead of* implementing clinical BPGs, but in *support of* implementing clinical BPGs. The principles and practices of implementation science are as critical in implementing HWE BPGs as they are with clinical BPGs. The RNAO Implementation Toolkit (2012c) addresses principles of implementation science as they pertain to uptake of both clinical and System and Healthy Work Environment guidelines, and includes relevant exemplars specifically related to HWE BPGs to aid users. The case study on page 87 is one of many examples that demonstrate how attention to work environment issues enhanced the ability to advance evidence-based clinical practice.

HWE BPGS: EVALUATING IMPLEMENTATION PROCESSES AND OUTCOMES

Evaluation of approaches to creating healthy work environments using HWE BPGs is imperative and must be a factor at the outset of any initiatives to plan changes to improve the workplace. There are numerous tools for assessing and evaluating various components of the work environment, and within each of the RNAO HWE BPGs, there are evaluation guides and specific structure, process, and outcome indicators that can be used to measure the impact of implementing the BPG. The structural indicators refer to the supports needed to be available in the organization (e.g., people, physical entities, policies, accessible computers) that allow nurses and others to provide quality care in a workplace that supports staff health and well-being. The process indicators (e.g., education, team meetings, safety reviews) include the methods or the systems implemented and developed to achieve the outcomes. The outcomes measured examine the desired states for patients and providers resulting from the adoption of healthy work processes (Donabedian, 2005). Staff satisfaction and of course clinical excellence are also key indicators of the health of the work environment.

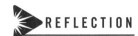

REFLECTION

When you are in a workplace, what are the indicators you usually use to determine the health of the work environment?

CASE STUDY

HWE BPGS AND CLINICAL EXCELLENCE: SCARBOROUGH AND ROUGE HOSPITAL'S EXPERIENCE

Representing the Birchmount and General sites of the Scarborough and Rouge Hospital (SRH) in Toronto, Canada, we began a focus on a healthy workplace as part of our Best Practice Spotlight Organization (BPSO) predesignation work. This decision followed a strong interest identified through focus groups, a review of incident reports, and leadership engagement. We knew that it was important for our work environment to be as healthy as possible, as we embarked on building trusting relationships amongst each other and working as a cohesive team to create clinical changes necessitated by clinical BPG implementation. This focus on a healthy workplace showed us that there were areas that required improvement.

We chose to implement the *Preventing and Managing Violence in the Workplace* (RNAO, 2009) HWE BPG, because workplace bullying was a worrisome factor that had preoccupied a number of our staff and leadership teams. We formed a working group, which included representatives from the inter-professional team, occupational health department, security, and the formal leadership. Using the individual, team, and organizational recommendations in the BPG, we identified and worked on a number of the evidence-based strategies presented. These strategies involved all staff and included: a hospital wide presurvey, a policy review, anti-bullying education, an improved response plan for incidents, as well as other training related to wellness and violence reduction. We also conducted regular monitoring of incident reports for trends and emerging issues, which were followed up by

leaders within the organization to ensure a timely response and contribute information to our committee for ongoing attention.

While all staff participated in the anti-bullying training and were impacted by the new policies and procedures, specific teams in identified areas carried out more targeted strategies such as creating anti-bullying charters for their units.

We conducted a post survey and as might be anticipated with more knowledge about what constituted bullying, greater attention to a respectful workplace, and clarity of the reporting processes, the post-implementation survey yielded a higher number of individuals reporting they had experienced violence in the workplace. These results helped us all to be more aware of the extent of the issue and work together to meet the higher expectations we were now setting.

The focus on this aspect of an HWE enabled staff to appreciate that their well being was important, and impacted staff morale and engagement. Our work on implementation of clinical Best Practice Guidelines was facilitated through this initial attention to a critical issue in the workplace and aided the staff to focus on evidence-based care for their patients knowing that the organization was supporting them. The successes of the clinical Best Practice Guidelines were in part due to the implementation of the HWE guidelines.

Permission to use by Scarborough and Rouge Hospital, Scarborough, Ontario, Canada.

Within NQuIRE (Nursing Quality Indicators for Reporting and Evaluation), RNAO's comprehensive international data system used to measure the impact of clinical BPG implementation, there are general human resource structural indicators, and process and outcome indicators related to each clinical BPG. The structural indicators are those factors and components that make up the work environment. To date in the NQuIRE data dictionaries, the structural indicators are reflective of the *Developing and Sustaining Safe, Effective Staffing and Workload Practices*, Second Edition (RNAO, 2017b), and the *Intra-professional Collaborative Practice Among Nurses*, Second Edition (RNAO, 2016a) HWE BPGs;

however, over time these indicators will expand to include aspects of other HWE BPGs. The value of measuring these indicators in relation to the process indicators (what the nurse does for the patient) and the outcome indicators (the patient's health status) is that it helps us better understand the impact of the healthcare work environment on practice (process indicators) and subsequently on patient outcomes. In a fiscally conscious environment, such knowledge is crucial to help us learn the best ways to maximize results and minimize costs.

INTO THE FUTURE

As we look forward to how the HWE BPGs can continue to support positive clinical outcomes for patients, as well as better provider and organizational outcomes, RNAO's focus is the ongoing up-dating of all HWE BPGs to reflect current evidence, incorporating the latest research in this area. In addition, RNAO will continue to take a lead role in promoting and supporting studies that explore the relationships between and amongst workplace structures and processes, and clinical, provider, and organizational outcomes.

RNAO's clinical BPGs will continue to include within the recommendations for organizations and health systems the top aspects of HWEs that enable sustained clinical practice change leading to better patient outcomes. In addition, as RNAO's NQuIRE matures, more of the HWE BPGs will be captured in the structural indictors, empowering a better understanding of the interconnection between evidence-based nursing practice and work environments. As pointed out in Chapter 1, quality patient care is both an individual and a collective responsibility.

CONCLUSION

This chapter showcases healthy work environments and their importance for clinical excellence and patient well-being through enhancing provider, organizational, and system outcomes. It highlights the urgent need for attention to work environments and why it is critical especially in healthcare. The chapter outlines the many resources developed by RNAO, including System and HWE BPGs, and how their use by practitioners and other stakeholders within and outside organizations can make a difference to the broad spectrum of outcomes they influence.

The work environment cannot be forgotten in any setting, as it is clear that those expected to carry out their roles need to have the right preparation and resources to do their work, as well as feel valued, respected, engaged, and acknowledged. This is vital in healthcare where the targets of care and service, our patients and families, are often the most vulnerable amongst us. What is good for nurses and other health workers—in terms of the work environment—is also good for patients.

KEY MESSAGES

■ Clinical excellence is fuelled by a number of factors, including the health of the work environment.

■ Uptake of evidence-based clinical guidelines is enhanced by attention to elements of the work environment that influence staff satisfaction, such as access to resources, trust, teamwork, rewards, and recognition.

■ Leadership in all roles and sectors is a critical work environment factor that impacts the ability of clinicians to uptake evidence and be able to deliver evidence-based practice every day and over time.

■ Measurement of clinical outcomes must go hand-in-hand with structural measurement of work environment indicators that help us determine the context for clinical excellence.

■ The RNAO System and HWE BPGs outline recommendations that help care providers (individuals and teams), organizations, and the system create healthy work environments for all, ultimately making a difference for patients.

REFERENCES

Aldana, S. (2001). Financial impact of health promotion programs: A comprehensive review of the literature. *American Journal of Health Promotion, 15*(5), 296–320.

Baernholdt, M., & Mark, B. A. (2009). The nurse work environment, job satisfaction and turnover rates in rural and urban nursing units. *Journal of Nursing Management, 17*(8), 994–1001.

Baumann, A., O'Brien-Pallas, L., Armstrong-Stassen, M., Blythe, J., Bourbonnais, R., Cameron, S., . . . Ryan, L. (2001, June). *Commitment and care: The benefits of a healthy workplace for nurses, their patients, and the system*. Ottawa, ON: Canadian Health Services Research Foundation and the Challenge Foundation.

Berry, L., & Curry, P. (2012). Nursing workload and patient care. Ottawa, ON: The Canadian Federation of Nurses Unions. Retrieved from https://nursesunions.ca/wp-content/uploads/2017/07/cfnu_workload_printed_version_pdf.pdf

Burgess, J., & Purkis, M. E. (2010). The power and politics of collaboration in nurse practitioner role development. *Nursing Inquiry, 17*(4), 297–308.

Butler, M., Collins, R., Drennan, J., Halligan, P., O'Mathuna, D. P., Schultz, T. J., . . . Vilis, E. (2011). Hospital nurse staffing models and patient and staff-related outcomes. Cochrane Database of Systematic Reviews, 7. doi:10.1002/14651858.CD007019.pub2

Canadian Institute for Health Information (CIHI). (2005). *Canada's health care providers: 2005 chartbook*. Retrieved from https://secure.cihi.ca/free_products/HCP_Chartbook05_e.pdf

Canadian Institute for Health Information (CIHI). (2015, June 23). *Regulated Nurses, 2014*. Ottawa, ON: CIHI.

Chachula, K. M., Myrick, F., & Yonge, O. (2015). Letting go: How newly graduated registered nurses in Western Canada decide to exit the nursing profession. *Nurse Education Today, 35*(7), 912–918.

Cohen, J., Stuenkel, D., & Nguyen, Q. (2009). Providing a Healthy Work Environment for Nurses: The Influence on Retention. *Journal of Nursing Care Quality, 24*(4), 308–315. doi: 10.1097/NCQ.0b013e3181a4699a

Cummings, G. G., MacGregor, T., Davey, M., Lee, H., Wong, C. A., Lo, E., . . . Stafford, E. (2010). Leadership styles and outcome patterns for the nursing workforce and work environment: A systematic review. *International Journal of Nursing Studies, 47*(3), 363–385. doi: 10.1016/j.ijnurstu.2009.08.006

Davies, B., Edwards, N., Ploeg, J., Virani, T., Skelly, J., & Dobbins, M. (2006). *Determinants of the sustained use of research evidence in nursing*. Retrieved from http://www.cfhi-fcass.ca/Migrated/PDF/ResearchReports/OGC/davies_final_e.pdf

DeJoy, D. M., & Southern, D. J. (1993). An integrative perspective on work-site health promotion. *Journal of Occupational Medicine, 35*(12), 1221–1230.

Donabedian, A. (2005). Evaluating the quality of medical care. *The Millbank Quarterly 83*(4), 691–729.

Drach-Zahavy, A. (2004). Primary nurses' performance: Role of supportive management. *Journal of Advanced Nursing, 45*(1), 7–16.

Duffield, C., Diers, D., O'Brien-Pallas, L., Aisbett, C., Roche, M., King, M., . . . Aisbett, K. (2011). Nursing staffing, nursing workload, the work environment and patient outcomes. *Applied Nursing Research, 24*(4), 244–255.

Dunleavy, J., Shamian, J., & Thomson D. (2003). Workplace pressures: Handcuffed by cutbacks. *Canadian Nurse, 99*(3), 23–26.

Farmanova, E., Judd, M., Maika, C., & Wilkes, G. (For Canadian Foundation for Healthcare Improvement). (2015, November). *Much more than just a visit: A review of visiting policies in select Canadian acute care hospitals*. Retrieved from http://www.cfhi-fcass.ca/sf-docs/default-source/patient-engagement/better-together-baseline-report.pdf?sfvrsn=10

Frith, K., Anderson, E. F., Fan, T., & Fong, E. (2012). Nurse staffing is an important strategy to prevent medication errors in community hospitals. *Nursing Economics, 30*(5), 288–294.

Green, L. W., Richard, L., & Potvin, L. (1996). Ecological foundation of health promotion. *American Journal of Health Promotion, 10*(4), 270–281.

Griffin, P., El-jardali, F., Tucker, D., Grinspun, D., Bajnok, I., & Shamian, J. (2003). What's the fuss about? Why do we need healthy work environments for nurses anyway? *Human Resources Database*. Retrieved from http://www.longwoods.com/content/18026

Grinspun, D. (2000). Taking care of the bottom line: Shifting paradigms in hospital management. In D. L. Gustafson (Ed.), *Care and consequence: Health care reform and its impact on Canadian women* (pp. 25–48). Halifax, NS: Fernwood Publishing.

Grinspun, D. (2002). A flexible nursing workforce: Realities and fallouts. *Hospital Quarterly, 6*(1), 79–84.

Grinspun, D. (2003). Part-time and casual nursing work: The perils of health-care restructuring. *The International Journal of Sociology and Social Policy, 23*(8/9), 54–70.

Grinspun, D. (2007). Healthy workplaces: The case for shared clinical decision making and increased full-time employment. *Healthcare Papers, 7*(Special Issue), 85–91.

Grinspun, D. (2010). *The social construction of nursing caring.* (Doctoral dissertation). Toronto, ON: York University.

Grinspun, D., & Anyinam, C. (2014). Leadership. In S. Coffey & C. Anyinam (Eds.), *Interprofessional health care practice* (1st ed.) (pp. 131–158). Toronto, ON: Pearson Canada Inc.

Grinspun, D., Virani, T., & Bajnok, I. (2002). Nursing Best Practice Guidelines: The RNAO (Registered Nurses' Association of Ontario) project. *Hospital Quarterly, 5*(2), 56–60.

Harless, D. W., & Mark, B. A. (2010). Nurse staffing and quality of care with direct measurement of inpatient staffing. *Medical Care, 48*(7), 659–663.

Havaei, F., MacPhee, M., & Dahinten, V. S. (2016). RNs and LPNs: Emotional exhaustion and intention to leave. *Journal of Nursing Management, 24*, 393–399.

Izzo, J. (2001). The shift in the work ethic and implications for employers. *Employment Relations Today, 28*(2), 53–61.

Kane, R. L., Shamliyan, T., Mueller, C., Duval, S., & Wilt, T. (2007). Nurse staffing and quality of patient care. Evidence Report/Technology Assessment, *151*, 1–115.

Laschinger, H., Wong, C., & Grau, A. (2012). The influence of authentic leadership on newly graduated nurses' experiences of workplace bullying, burnout and retention outcomes: A cross-sectional study. *International Journal of Nursing Studies, 49*(10), 1266–1276.

Lindberg, B., & Vingard, E. (2012). Indicators of healthy work environments—A systematic review. *Work, 41*(Supplement 1), 3032–3038.

Lipsitz, L. A. (2012). Understanding health care as a complex system: The foundation for unintended consequences. *JAMA : The Journal of the American Medical Association, 308*(3), 243–244. http://doi.org/10.1001/jama.2012.7551

Lowe, G. S. (2002). High-quality healthcare workplaces: A vision and action plan. *Hospital Quarterly, 5*(4), 49–56.

Lowe, G. S. (2004). *Thriving on healthy: Reaping the benefits in our workplaces.* [PDF document]. Retrieved from http://grahamlowe.ca/events/thriving-on-healthy-reaping-the-benefits-in-our-workplaces/

Luo, H., Lin, M., & Castle, N. G. (2013). The correlates of nursing staff turnover in home and hospice agencies: 2007 National Home and Hospice Care Survey. *Research on Aging, 35*(4), 375–392.

MacPhee, M. (2014). Valuing patient safety: Responsible workforce design. Ottawa, ON: Canadian Federation of Nurses Unions.

Mattila, E., Pitkanen, A., Alanen, S., Leino, K., Luojus, K., Rantanen, A., & Aalto, P. (2014). The effects of the primary nursing care model: A systematic review. *Journal of Nursing Care, 3*(6). http://dx.doi.org/10.4172/2167-1168.1000205

McHugh, M. D., Rochman, M. F., Sloane, D. M., Berg, R. A., Mancini, M. E., Nadkarni, V. M., . . . Aiken, L. H. (2016). Better nurse staffing and work environments associated with increased survival of in-hospital cardiac arrest patients. Medical Care, 54(1), 74–80.

Meyer, R. M., Wang, S., Li, X., Thomson, D., & O'Brien-Pallas, L. (2009). Evaluation of a patient care delivery model: Patient outcomes in acute cardiac care. *Journal of Nursing Scholarship, 41*(4), 399–410.

Nakamura, E., Tanabe, N., Sekii, A., Honda, A., Hoshino, E., Seki, N., . . . Suzuki, H. (2010). Staff nurses' intention to remain employed in small- and medium-sized hospitals, with a focus on their working conditions. *The Tohoku Journal of Experimental Medicine, 220*(3), 191–198.

North, N., Leung, W., Ashton, T., Rasmussen, E., Hughes, F., & Finlayson, M. (2013). Nurse turnover in New Zealand: Costs and relationships with staffing practises and patient outcomes. *Journal of Nursing Management, 21*(3), 419–428.

O'Brien-Pallas, L., & Baumann, A. (1992). Quality of nursing worklife issues: A unifying framework. *Canadian Journal of Nursing Administration, 5*(2), 12–16.

O'Brien-Pallas, L., & Hayes, L. (2010). Nursing workforce and health policy. In A. S. Hinshaw & P. Grady (Eds.), *Shaping health policy through nursing research* (pp. 231–249). New York, NY: Springer Publishing Co.

O'Brien-Pallas, L., Tomblin Murphy, G., & Shamian, J. (2008). *Final report: Understanding the costs and outcomes of nurses' turnover in Canadian hospitals (Nursing Turnover Study)*. University of Toronto: Nursing Health Services Research Unit.

O'Brien-Pallas, L., Tomblin Murphy, G., White S., Hayes, L., Baumann, A., Higgin, A., . . . Wang, S. (2005). *Building the future: An integrated strategy for nursing human resources in Canada—Research synthesis report of research findings*. Ottawa, ON: The Nursing Sector Study Corporation.

Ontario Ministry of Labour. (2017). *Health care sector injury statistics*. Retrieved from https://www.ontario.ca/document/health-care-sector-plan-2017-18/health-care-sector-injury-statistics

Ontario Nurses Association. (2015). *Violence should not be part of the job*. Retrieved from https://www.ona.org/wp-content/uploads/ona_flfeature_workplaceviolence_201505.pdf?x72008

Pearson, A., Pallas, L. O., Thomson, D., Doucette, E., Tucker, D., Wiechula, R., . . . Jordan, Z. (2006c). Systematic review of evidence on the impact of nursing workload and staffing on establishing healthy work environments. *International Journal of Evidence-Based Healthcare, 4*(4), 337–384.

Pearson, A., Porritt, K., Doran, D., Vincent, L., Craig, D., Tucker, D., . . . Long, L. (2006b). A systematic review of evidence on the professional practice of the nurse and developing and sustaining a healthy work environment in healthcare. *International Journal of Evidence-Based Healthcare, 4*(3), 221–261.

Pearson, A., Porritt, K. A., Doran, D., Vincent, L., Craig, D., Tucker, D., . . . Henstridge, V. (2006a). A comprehensive systematic review of evidence on the structure, process, characteristics and composition of a nursing team that fosters a healthy work environment. *International Journal of Evidence-Based Healthcare, 4*(2), 118–159. doi:10.1111/j.1479-6988.2006.00039.x

Pearson, A., Laschinger, H., Porritt, K., Jordan, Z., Tucker, D., & Long, L. (2007a). Comprehensive systematic review of evidence on developing and sustaining nursing leadership that fosters a healthy work environment in healthcare. *International Journal of Evidence-Based Healthcare, 5*(2), 208–253.

Pearson, A., Srivastava, R., Craig, D., Tucker, D., Grinspun, D., Bajnok, I., . . . Gi, A. A. (2007b). Systematic review on embracing cultural diversity for developing and sustaining a healthy work environment in healthcare. *International Journal of Evidence-Based Healthcare, 5*(1), 54–91.

Public Services Health and Safety Association. (2011). *What is a healthy work environment (HWE)?* Retrieved from http://www.healthyworkenvironments.ca/AboutUs.htm

Registered Nurses' Association of Ontario (RNAO). (2000) *Ensuring the care will be there: A report on recruitment and retention in Ontario*. Toronto, ON: Registered Nurses' Association of Ontario.

Registered Nurses' Association of Ontario (RNAO). (2006a). *Client centred care* (Revised Supplement). Toronto, ON: Registered Nurses' Association of Ontario.

Registered Nurses' Association of Ontario (RNAO). (2006b). *Collaborative practice among nursing teams*. Toronto, ON: Registered Nurses' Association of Ontario.

Registered Nurses' Association of Ontario (RNAO). (2006c). *Developing and sustaining nursing leadership*. Toronto, ON: Registered Nurses' Association of Ontario.

Registered Nurses' Association of Ontario (RNAO). (2007a). *Developing and sustaining effective staffing and workload practices*. Toronto, ON: Registered Nurses' Association of Ontario.

Registered Nurses' Association of Ontario (RNAO). (2007b). *Embracing cultural diversity in health care: Developing cultural competence*. Toronto, ON: Registered Nurses' Association of Ontario.

Registered Nurses' Association of Ontario (RNAO). (2007c). *Professionalism in nursing*. Toronto, ON: Registered Nurses' Association of Ontario.

Registered Nurses' Association of Ontario (RNAO). (2008). *Workplace health, safety and well-being of the nurse*. Toronto, ON: Registered Nurses' Association of Ontario.

Registered Nurses' Association of Ontario (RNAO). (2009). *Preventing and managing violence in the workplace*. Toronto, ON: Registered Nurses' Association of Ontario.

Registered Nurses' Association of Ontario (RNAO). (2010). *Pilot evaluation of implementation and update of healthy work environment Best Practice Guidelines: Final report*. Toronto, ON: Registered Nurses' Association of Ontario.

Registered Nurses' Association of Ontario (RNAO). (2011). *Preventing and mitigating nurse fatigue in health care*. Toronto, ON: Registered Nurses' Association of Ontario.

Registered Nurses' Association of Ontario (RNAO). (2012a). *Managing and mitigating conflict in health-care teams*. Toronto, ON: Registered Nurses' Association of Ontario.

Registered Nurses' Association of Ontario (RNAO). (2012b). *Managing and mitigating conflict: Tips and tools for nurses.* Toronto, ON: Registered Nurses' Association of Ontario. Retrieved from http://rnao.ca/sites/rnao-ca/files/CONFLICT_8.5_x_5.5_WEB.pdf

Registered Nurses' Association of Ontario (RNAO). (2012c). *Toolkit: Implementation of Best Practice Guidelines* (2nd ed.). Toronto, ON: Registered Nurses' Association of Ontario.

Registered Nurses' Association of Ontario (RNAO). (2013a). *Developing and sustaining interprofessional health care: Optimizing patients/clients, organizational, and system outcomes.* Toronto, ON: Registered Nurses' Association of Ontario.

Registered Nurses' Association of Ontario (RNAO). (2013b). *Developing and sustaining nursing leadership* (2nd ed.). Toronto, ON: Registered Nurses' Association of Ontario.

Registered Nurses' Association of Ontario (RNAO). (2013c). *The healthy work environments quick reference guide.* Toronto, ON: Registered Nurses' Association of Ontario. Retrieved from http://rnao.ca/sites/rnao-ca/files/HWE_PocketGuide2013.pdf

Registered Nurses' Association of Ontario (RNAO). (2014a). *Developing and sustaining interprofessional health care: Tips and tools for health-care teams.* Toronto, ON: Registered Nurses' Association of Ontario. Retrieved from: http://rnao.ca/sites/rnao-ca/files/IPC_TIPS_AND_TOOLS_0.pdf

Registered Nurses' Association of Ontario (RNAO). (2014b). *Developing and sustaining nursing leadership: Tips and tools.* Toronto, ON: Registered Nurses' Association of Ontario. Retrieved from http://rnao.ca/sites/rnao-ca/files/LEADERSHIP_16.5_x_8.5_WEB_0.pdf

Registered Nurses' Association of Ontario (RNAO). (2014c). *Managing and mitigating fatigue: Tips and tools for nurses.* Toronto, ON: Registered Nurses' Association of Ontario. Retrieved from http://rnao.ca/sites/rnao-ca/files/FATIGUE_8.5_x_5.5_WEB.PDF

Registered Nurses' Association of Ontario (RNAO). (2014d). *Point-of-care leadership tips and tools for nurses.* Toronto, ON: Registered Nurses' Association of Ontario. Retrieved from http://rnao.ca/sites/rnao-ca/files/POC_16.5_x_8.5_WEB_0.pdf

Registered Nurses' Association of Ontario (RNAO). (2014e). *Preventing and managing violence: Tips and tools for nurses.* Toronto, ON: Registered Nurses' Association of Ontario. Retrieved from http://rnao.ca/sites/rnao-ca/files/VIOLENCE_8.5_x_5.5_WEB.pdf

Registered Nurses' Association of Ontario (RNAO). (2016a). *Intra-professional collaborative practice among nurses* (2nd ed.). Toronto, ON: Registered Nurses' Association of Ontario.

Registered Nurses' Association of Ontario (RNAO). (2016b). *Mind the safety gap in healthy system transformation: Reclaiming the role of the RN.* Retrieved from http://rnao.ca/sites/rnao-ca/files/HR_REPORT_May11.pdf

Registered Nurses' Association of Ontario (RNAO). (2016c). *Practice education in nursing.* Toronto, ON: Registered Nurses' Association of Ontario.

Registered Nurses' Association of Ontario (RNAO). (2017a). *Adopting e-Health solutions: Implementation strategies.* Toronto, ON: Registered Nurses' Association of Ontario.

Registered Nurses' Association of Ontario (RNAO). (2017b). *Developing and sustaining safe, effective staffing and workload practices.* Toronto, ON: Registered Nurses' Association of Ontario.

Rogers, S. (2004). Why can't I visit? The ethics of visitation restrictions—Lessons learned from SARS. *Critical Care, 8*(5), 300–302. http://doi.org/10.1186/cc2930

Rycroft-Malone, J., Kitson, A., Harvey, G., McCormack, B., Seers, K., Titchen, A., . . . Estabrooks, C. (2002). Ingredients for change: Revisiting a conceptual framework. *Quality and Safety in Health Care, 11*(2), 174–180.

Sellgren, S. F., Kajermo, K. N., Ekvall, G., & Tomson, G. (2009). Nursing staff turnover at a Swedish university hospital: An exploratory study. *Journal of Clinical Nursing, 18*(22), 3181–3189.

Shamian, J., & El-Jardali, F. (2007). Healthy workplaces for health workers in Canada: Knowledge transfer and uptake in policy and practice. *HealthcarePapers, 7*(Sp), 6–25.

Silber, J. H., Rosenbaum, P. R., McHugh, M. D., Ludwig, J. M., Smith, H. L., Niknam, B. A., . . . Aiken, L. H. (2016). Comparison of the value of nursing work environments in hospitals across different levels of patient risk. *JAMA Surgery, 151,* 527–536.

Staggs, V. S., & Dunton, N. (2014). Associations between rates of unassisted inpatient falls and levels of registered and non-registered nurse staffing. *International Journal for Quality in Health Care, 26*(1), 87–92.

Statistics Canada. (2014). *Absence rates of full-time employees, 2013.* Retrieved from http://www.statcan.gc.ca/daily-quotidien/140424/dq140424g-eng.htm

Tourangeau, A. E., Patterson, E., Saari, M., Thomson, H., & Cranley, L. (2017). Work-related factors influencing home care nurse intent to remain employed. *Health Care Manage Rev, 42*(1), 87–97.

Trinkoff, A. M., Johantgen, M., Storr, C. L., Gurses, A. P., Liang, Y., & Han, K. (2011). Nurses' work schedule characteristics, nurse staffing, and patient mortality. *Nursing Research, 60*(1), 1–8.

Zhu, X. W., You, L. M., Zheng, J., Liu, K., Fang, J. B., Hou, S. X., . . . Zhang, L. F. (2012). Nurse staffing levels make a difference on patient outcomes: A multisite study in Chinese hospitals. *Journal of Nursing Scholarship, 44*(3), 266–273.

IMPLEMENTATION SCIENCE: SECOND PILLAR FOR SUCCESS

4

FORGING THE WAY WITH IMPLEMENTATION SCIENCE

Doris Grinspun, PhD, MSN, BScN, RN, LLD(hon), Dr(hc), O.ONT
Heather McConnell, MA(Ed), BScN, RN
Tazim Virani, PhD, RN
Janet E. Squires, PhD, RN

LEARNING OBJECTIVES

After reading this chapter, you will be able to:

- Recognize that transferring and ensuring uptake of Best Practice Guidelines (BPG) into day-to-day clinical work requires active and multilevel interventions

- Understand the multifaceted strategies that can be used to create sustained evidence-based practice (EBP) changes in clinical practice and in academia and how to deploy them

- Describe RNAO's evidence-based implementation resources that support BPG uptake in service and academia

- Discuss the latest trends in implementation science

INTRODUCTION

This chapter provides the foundation for the Registered Nurses' Association of Ontario's (RNAO) groundbreaking work on Best Practice Guideline (BPG) implementation at micro, meso, and macro levels of intervention. We discuss RNAO's signature implementation strategies and evidence-based implementation tools as they relate to individual healthcare providers, organizations, and the health system as a whole. We also share two key evidence-based implementation resources for service organizations and academia. We end the chapter with a discussion of the latest trends in implementation science including: integrated knowledge translation and patient engagement, technology enabled and arts-based knowledge translation, developmental evaluation, and the concept of deimplementation.

As discussed in Chapter 1, *Transforming Nursing Through Knowledge: The Conceptual and Programmatic Underpinnings of RNAO's BPG Program*, RNAO has nurtured the BPG Program to mature in an organic way informed by macro theories of social movements and whole-system change; meso frameworks of knowledge to action—in practice; theories of diffusion, innovation, and distributed knowledge; and continuous on-the-ground learnings from the field. Nowhere has this approach been more evident than in RNAO's implementation methodology. From the inception of the BPG Program, RNAO has had deliberate stakeholder engagement on a massive scale. RNAO's trademark as an "activist" professional association for policy matters is the cornerstone for all aspects of the BPG Program. Stakeholders embraced the collective opportunity to be engaged in the BPG Program and have generously contributed their unwavering commitment, expertise, and time. Their feedback is continuous and rich, always reinforcing that together we must ensure BPGs are truly implemented into practice and do not stay as books on the shelf. Thus, while rigorously developed BPGs are foundational to the BPG Program, robust and dynamic implementation is what gives it life in the day-to-day practice of clinicians, in organizations, and throughout the health system.

During the 1990s, when the Program began, the most common approach to support evidence-based practice in nursing was to conduct educational sessions (Forsetlund et al., 2009; Kitson, Harvey, & McCormack, 1998). RNAO quickly recognized that following such education, it was difficult for practitioners to implement what they had learned once they returned to their practice settings. Much depended on the support they had in their practice settings from colleagues and managers, as well as the availability of resources (Canadian Institutes of Health Research [CIHR], 2012b; Grinspun, Melnyk, & Fineout-Overholt, 2014; Kitson et al., 1998; RNAO, 2012). The same barriers or blockages exist as much today as they did when RNAO's BPG Program began. For example, are the necessary evidence-based tools available for guiding and documenting nursing interventions? How will other staff follow up on the interventions? Will they have the required supplies and equipment to support interventions? What the BPG Program has done through its implementation methodology is equip nurses with approaches and techniques to overcome challenges. These approaches and techniques are detailed next.

MULTILEVEL AND MULTIFACETED IMPLEMENTATION

From the outset of the BPG Program in 1999, it was clear to RNAO and its stakeholders that a multifaceted approach to implementing the BPGs was needed to achieve sustainable change in practice and positive health outcomes. The initial focus was on knowledge translation and transfer, and supporting practice changes by addressing enablers and barriers to making change happen (Grinspun, Virani, & Bajnok, 2002). The term "implementation science" was at the time just an emerging concept and not widely used or understood. Indeed, it was only in 2006 that the first journal dedicated to implementation science was launched. Its editors defined the concept as "the study of methods to promote the adoption and integration of evidence-based practices, interventions and policies into routine health care and public health settings" (Eccles & Mittman, 2006: p.1). RNAO's approach to support implementation of BPGs has evolved alongside the program. When the first guidelines were issued in 2001, RNAO's approach to supporting implementation was rudimentary. For the first year, we focused on three main approaches. First, we promoted the availability of the guidelines through a dissemination plan that included strategies such as an inaugural conference to introduce the guidelines to the nursing community, the publication of a series of articles related to various aspects of the BPG Program, distribution in hard copy to key stakeholders including schools of nursing, and ensuring the guidelines were accessible to the broader healthcare community and available for free download via the RNAO website. Second, we launched the Best Practice Champion Network with nurses from a variety of workplaces, trained by RNAO, to assist colleagues in implementing BPGs. Third, we identified service organizations to pilot the BPGs, and together we learned about effective implementation strategies. What follows are highlights of each level alongside the related implementation strategies, which are depicted in Figure 4.1 in the inner and outer circles of the implementation pillar of the BPG Program.

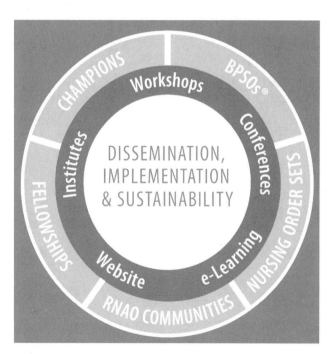

FIGURE 4.1   Implementation pillar of RNAO BPG Program.
© Registered Nurses' Association of Ontario. All rights reserved.

As Chapter 1 highlights, implementation has evolved from rudimentary to a sophisticated and comprehensive set of multilevel and multifaceted subprograms all aimed at optimizing evidence uptake, evidence sustainability, and Evidence Boosters. Indeed, the BPG Program works at three distinct and interrelated implementation levels: micro-level designed for individual nurses/health professionals, meso-level designed for organizations, and macro-level designed for health systems. What follows are highlights of each level alongside the related implementation strategies.

MICRO-LEVEL/INDIVIDUAL NURSE IMPLEMENTATION

The overall purpose of RNAO's intervention at the micro level is to work with nurses and other interested health professionals in developing their capacity as BPG leaders. Two key strategies are utilized: 1) the Best Practice Champion Network; and 2) the RNAO Learning Institutes.

BEST PRACTICE CHAMPION NETWORK

RNAO coined the term "Champion" in 2001 following a comprehensive literature review on change agents. The term "Champion" was chosen to describe individuals who promote, support, and defend evidence-based practice (EBP). They pave the way for developing EBP cultures, identifying resources and other sources of assistance. RNAO defined a *Champion* as someone who supports the use of BPGs and other evidence-based resources to inform clinical practice and decision-making. Champions come from a variety of clinical, educational, and management positions, and all work to enhance the use of the guidelines in a range of clinical and academic settings.

Champions are described by a variety of terms in the literature, including change agents, knowledge broker, sponsors, and internal entrepreneurs (Greenhalgh, Robert, Bate, MacFarlane, & Kyriakidou, 2005; Locock, Dopson, Chambers, & Gabbay, 2001). Rogers (2003), in his diffusion of innovation theory, refers to "change agents" who "influence clients' innovation-decisions in a direction deemed desirable by a change agency" (p. 366). Thompson, Estabrooks, and Degner (2006), as cited by Ploeg et al. (2010), conducted a concept analysis in this area and concluded that opinion leaders, facilitators, champions, linking agents, and change agents were basically all knowledge-transfer agents with different conceptual labels.

RNAO created a Best Practice Champions Network as a way to identify, support, and energize this group of change agents (Grinspun, Virani, & Bajnok, 2002). The Network, established in 2002, now consists of over 50,000 nurses, nursing students, other health professionals, support staff, and, more recently, members of the public who are knowledgeable and passionate about BPGs and actively motivate and guide their uptake in their organizations. Network members become Champions by participating in either a 1-day in-person workshop, a virtual learning series, or a self-directed eLearning program (RNAO, 2017b). The content of these orientation programs has been designed to provide Champions with numerous tools and strategies to promote and support the implementation of RNAO's BPGs in their organizations and to clarify and cement their role as a Champion. The basis of the curriculum for these educational offerings is the *Toolkit: Implementation of Best Practice Guidelines* (Bajnok, Grinspun, Lloyd, & McConnell, 2015; RNAO, 2012), discussed later in this chapter.

Once they have become Champions, members of the Network have access to various resources to advance their role, including newsletters, social networking, access to an online community of practice, workshops, seminars, and regular knowledge-exchange webinars at which Champions take the lead in presenting their work. RNAO Champions in Ontario also have access to funds that provide opportunities for networking and disseminating their work within their organization and scaling it out to their local community. The financial support for Champions across Canada and in other countries is dependent on local context and decisions. For example, in China, the Students' Association of Evidence-Based Nursing is supported and operated by graduate students of the Beijing University of Chinese Medicine (BUCM) School of Nursing. They are Best Practice Champions who train nursing undergraduate students from BUCM and other schools interested in evidence-based nursing. Supported by faculty, they also engage in translating BPGs and reviewing BPGs—an effective approach for spreading the BPSO knowledge and preparing more Champions. For details, see Chapter 14, *Overcoming Context and Language Differences: BPSO Trailblazers in China*.

A study of the RNAO Best Practice Champion Network conducted by Ploeg and colleagues (2010) found that RNAO Champions are change agents that take on multidimensional roles to support BPG implementation. These include educator, facilitator, mentor, leader, policy developer, and evaluator. They also found that Champions use many strategies targeted at various levels of the organization, attend to a range of stakeholders, and tailor their strategies to the organizational context. Three main categories and related subcategories associated with Champion diffusion strategies were identified in this study and are summarized in Table 4.1.

TABLE 4.1   DIFFUSION STRATEGIES OF RNAO CHAMPIONS

CATEGORY	RELATED SUBCATEGORIES
Dissemination of information about clinical practice guidelines	Providing education and creating awareness Acting as a resource to support and mentor nurses
Champions as persuasive practice leaders	Working through committees Participating in and leading interdisciplinary teams
Tailoring guideline implementation strategies to the organizational context	Exploring, auditing, and monitoring of best practices Making changes to documentation systems to incorporate best practice recommendations

Source: Ploeg et al., 2010

Champions are active knowledge disseminators of clinical information to nurses and other healthcare professionals. They are prepared facilitators who offer support and mentorship. Champions are persuasive practice leaders who work with various disciplines in all types and levels of positions to explain, convince, and help ensure that RNAO BPG implementation and recommendations permeate the organization. The Champions navigate complex webs of committees and working groups in their organizations and regions to move practice change forward. The relationships they build across interdisciplinary boundaries improve the uptake of behaviour change beyond the nursing profession. Finally, Champions are adapters who tailor implementation strategies to the organizational context. They accomplish this by exploring practices and auditing and monitoring implementation processes and patient outcomes. They make efforts to contextualize guidelines to make them accessible and applicable to staff and patients by developing policies and procedures to support practice change (Ploeg et al., 2010).

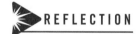

REFLECTION

Think about a recent practice change that took place within your workplace. Did "Champions" step forward to lead the implementation of the change? If so, what strategies did they use to support their peers in changing practice?

The findings of this study are consistent with the ongoing experience of RNAO's BPG implementation leads globally, who are working to implement and sustain evidence-based-practice cultures within their organizations. The following reflection on the role and impact of the Champions they work with mirror the views of others across the BPSOs:

> *"Having Best Practice Champions has had an impact on resident care. We are seeing better outcomes for residents. The Champions understand the evidence and the rationale for why things are done a certain way. Champions have brought our team together around the common goal of improving resident care."*
>
> —Sue Anderson, RN, Unit Manager and Michelle Varey, RPN, RAI Coordinator
> William George Extended Care—Meno Ya Win Health Centre
> Sioux Lookout, Ontario

RNAO BPG INSTITUTES

Capacity development of those responsible for leading guideline implementation didn't stop with the establishment of the Best Practice Champions Network in 2002. Feedback from those involved in the program at the time indicated that additional education and leadership development was necessary to support successful guideline implementation, evaluation, and sustainability. The format of an "Institute" was chosen to address this need, and the first annual Clinical BPG Institute was held in 2002 and was attended by nurses from a range of practice settings, all involved in the early days of RNAO's BPG implementation.

RNAO's BPG Institutes are now a signature professional development offering. The format remains as a multiday event (3–5 days) held in a learning environment, away from the day-to-day responsibilities of work and home. It includes evidence-based theory, input sessions, stories from the field engaging those who are actively implementing BPGs, networking, and the establishment of small working/reference groups known as Best Practice Knowledge Units (BKUs) that support individual and collective learning. A key outcome for participants is to utilize the knowledge and skill gained at the Institute to shape a plan related to guideline introduction, implementation, evaluation, and/or sustainability that they can mobilize within their workplace.

The original curriculum included elements of the RNAO (2002) *Toolkit: Implementation of Clinical Practice Guidelines* (Toolkit) and addressed: the basics of the types of evidence that inform practice, the link between research and practice, facilitation and clinical supervision, enabling evidence-based practice cultures, strategies to support clinical change, project management, stakeholder engagement, environmental readiness, action-plan development, and finally sustaining change and the change agent.

Over the years, feedback from participants indicated that a "booster" session would be helpful for those experienced in guideline implementation, and the curriculum was revised to include a "foundational" (5-day) and "advanced" (3-day) stream. The curriculum for the advanced stream assumes a strong understanding of the elements of the Toolkit and some guideline implementation experience. This program focuses on project management skills, quality improvement with an emphasis on spread and scaling up, strategic positioning, leadership in developing evidence-based practice cultures, and peer learning about successful implementation strategies to support clinical practice change. The curriculum for both the foundational and the advanced streams has been revised over the years to reflect the expanding knowledge of implementation science. The foundational stream in particular underwent a significant update with the publication of the second edition of the RNAO Toolkit in 2012. The pedagogical principles of adult education theory remain fundamental to these offerings.

For the past 8 years, the Institutes have been increasingly attracting members of the interprofessional team who are both engaged as faculty and/or attending for their own capacity development. This is paralleled with the move to increase the number of heath disciplines involved in RNAO's guideline development, as well as a recognition by organizational and health system leaders of the impact of nursing-led guidelines on the interprofessional team and the need for all stakeholders to be involved in establishing evidence-based-practice cultures.

The following comment about the June 2017 *Clinical BPG Institute* reflects the overall views of the participants about this learning event:

> *"The RNAO Best Practice Clinical Institute was an absolute pleasure to attend. I attended the Clinical Institute with high expectations of professional growth and it exceeded them in every way! The knowledge, networking opportunities, and awareness of the BPGs that I was able to bring back to my facility has been a great help!"*
>
> —Matthew Léveillé, BScN, RN, RAI-C
> Staff Education Coordinator
> Muskoka Landing Long-Term Care
> Huntsville, ON

What began as a modest offering in 2002 has evolved into a "must attend" professional development opportunity always booked to capacity. Moreover, today, in addition to the foundational BPG Institute (RNAO, 2017a), RNAO offers topic-specific Institutes including a focus on enhancing nursing executive leadership and clinical programs based on its BPGs in the area of wound care (clinical and program planning streams), chronic disease management, and mental health and addiction. Many of the institutes have been tailored to different contexts, such as those produced in partnership with First Nations in Canada. The quote below demonstrates the high value placed on the collaborative approaches used in the development of these programs to ensure context relevance, as well as the impact on knowledge, skills, and empowerment they have had on participants:

> *"The First Nations and Inuit Health Branch (FNIHB), Ontario Region has worked with RNAO over the past 7 years as they have planned, delivered and evaluated a number of learning events for the front line nurses. Basing these events on the RNAO Best Practice Guidelines has been a stellar opportunity. With the help of a comprehensive planning committee, the week-long events modeled after the RNAO Learning Institutes have been tailored to the First Nations context, and focused on areas such as mental health and addiction, chronic disease management,*

and wound care. Each of the institutes has had a broad reach targeting nurses in a variety of locations, and has reflected critical best practice guidelines such as diabetic foot ulcer, managing chronic conditions, pressure injury, and substance use. In addition, these capacity building events have helped us create a network of nurses working with the First Nations population to help champion evidence-based practice, healthy work environments, and culturally competent care."

–Vanessa L. Follon, RN, BScN
Assistant Director of Nursing
Regional Coordinator—Home and Community Care Program
Ontario Region/First Nations and Inuit Health Branch

MESO-LEVEL/ORGANIZATIONAL LEVEL IMPLEMENTATION

The overall purpose of RNAO's intervention at the meso level is to support service and academic organizations in optimizing evidence uptake, evidence sustainability, and Evidence Boosters. Three key strategies are utilized: 1) *Toolkit: Implementation of Best Practice Guidelines* (for service organizations), 2) *Educator's Resource: Integration of Best Practice Guidelines* (for academia), and 3) *Best Practice Spotlight Organizations*. Each is discussed in the following sections.

IMPLEMENTING BEST PRACTICE GUIDELINES INTO CLINICAL PRACTICE: TOOLKIT

When the RNAO published its first guidelines in 2001, the guidelines were pilot tested in a range of practice settings across the continuum of care. Champions, then called clinical resource nurses (CRNs), led the implementation and were a critical enabler for effective practice change. During this evaluation phase, these CRNs identified the need for a consistent approach to the planning and implementation of practice changes that were based on the RNAO BPG recommendations, and they asked RNAO to develop a "guideline on how to implement guidelines." This was the impetus for the development of the *Toolkit: Implementation of Clinical Practice Guidelines* (RNAO, 2002). An interprofessional panel of researchers and practitioners, including some of the CRNs, worked to identify evidence to support the development of the Toolkit through the synthesis of systematic reviews, primary studies, and the expert opinion of panel members. The Toolkit was designed to be a user-friendly, evidence-based tool to facilitate guideline implementation within healthcare organizations. The goals of the Toolkit included a focus on helping those responsible for guideline implementation:

- Identify important factors in their organization that influence the adoption process

- Gain the support of Champions and key stakeholders

- Assess organizational support and readiness to adopt the guidelines

A case study approach was utilized, with sample templates and blank templates provided for ease of use. As such, it provided sound direction to organizations and their leaders about how best to ready a setting for change and how to plan, resource, and implement a carefully crafted set of strategies to achieve success (DiCenso et al., 2002).

An evaluation of the Toolkit conducted by Dobbins and colleagues concludes that this evidence-based resource showed promise as a useful guide for those responsible for guideline implementation (Dobbins, Davies, Danseco, Edwards, & Virani, 2005). They also recommended periodic updates to ensure it continues to reflect the current evidence in implementation science. Based on these findings, feedback from those using the Toolkit, and an updated review of the state of implementation science globally, the Toolkit was revised, and its second edition was published in 2012 (RNAO, 2012). The second edition addresses comments from users that indicated more attention was needed to the important issue of maintaining change in the clinical setting and strategies to promote long-term sustainability. The panel that was convened to develop the second edition reviewed various models and frameworks that considered sustainability as an element of the implementation process. They chose the Knowledge-to-Action (KTA) framework, which is the foundation of the current edition of this resource. It was also renamed to *Toolkit: Implementation of Best Practice Guidelines* to recognize its utility in implementing both clinical and healthy work environment guidelines.

The KTA framework was developed through a concept analysis of 31 action theories to make sense of what happens during the knowledge translation/implementation process by considering both knowledge creation and action. This framework takes a systems perspective and recognizes that implementation is a social process and that adaptation of research evidence is necessary in order to take both local context and culture into account. The KTA process identifies the ideal phases or categories of action that are believed to be important when attempting to implement change (Graham & Tetroe, 2010).

The KTA model (as depicted in the Toolkit, 2012, in Figure 4.2) is composed of two phases: 1) the Knowledge Creation process, which is presented as a triangle; and 2) the Action Cycle, which circles around the model and represents the activities or processes required to move the knowledge (evidence) into practice. It should be noted that there are bidirectional arrows between elements of the action cycle, as it is not a linear process, and aspects of the cycle will need to be revisited at various phases of implementation.

The Knowledge-to-Action framework provides the foundation for the Toolkit, with its chapters representing the various steps in the Action Cycle. Table 4.2 provides a high-level summary of the content of the Toolkit and the focus of each chapter.

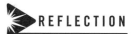

REFLECTION

What implementation models or change theories are you familiar with? What are the similarities/differences between those models/ theories and the KTA framework?

REVISED KNOWLEDGE-TO-ACTION FRAMEWORK

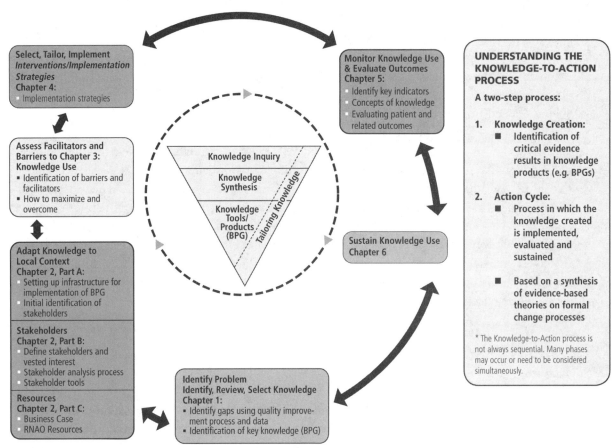

Adapted from "Knowledge Translation in Health Care: Moving From Evidence to Practice."
S. Straus, J. Tetroe, and I. Graham. Copyright 2009 by Blackwell Publishing Ltd. Adapted with permission.

FIGURE 4.2   Knowledge-to-Action framework as depicted in *Toolkit: Implementation of Best Practice Guidelines* (RNAO, 2012).

TABLE 4.2   CHAPTERS OF THE TOOLKIT: IMPLEMENTATION OF BEST PRACTICE GUIDELINES (RNAO, 2012)

CHAPTER	CONTENT
Introduction: Setting the Stage	▪ Overview of the Toolkit
Chapter 1: Identify Problem: Identify, Review, Select Knowledge	▪ A problem is defined and best practices that may be helpful to resolve the problem are identified. ▪ Identify a BPG to determine if current practice is consistent with the best practice, or whether a change in practice is needed (gap analysis).

CHAPTER	CONTENT
Chapter 2A: Adapt Knowledge to Local Context	▪ Choose a knowledge product (BPG) that reflects best evidence to address the identified problem.
	▪ Recommendations can be adapted to suit the organizational context.
Chapter 2B: Stakeholders	▪ Involve staff and stakeholders to ensure that the chosen knowledge product will meet the needs and best fit the organizational culture.
Chapter 2C: Resources	
Chapter 3: Assess Facilitators and Barriers to Knowledge Use	▪ Incorporate an assessment of the environment and the relevant stakeholders to maximize outcomes.
	▪ Identify key facilitators such as group interactions, positive staff attitudes, leadership support, interdisciplinary Champions, as well as inter-organizational collaboration.
	▪ Determine critical barriers including lack of knowledge, negative attitudes, and resistance to change.
Chapter 4: Select and Tailor Implementation Interventions and Strategies	▪ Incorporate an implementation plan that considers stakeholder assessment and engagement, the local context, as well as the evidence on effective implementation strategies.
Chapter 5: Monitor Knowledge Use & Evaluate Outcomes	▪ Measure knowledge product use by adherence to the recommendation or changes in knowledge, behaviours, and/or attitudes.
	▪ Evaluate the impact of implementing knowledge products.
	▪ This phase is central to effective implementation and should be considered throughout all of the earlier phases.
Chapter 6: Sustain Knowledge Use	▪ Plan for long-term improvement of care outcomes based on effective implementation of knowledge products.
	▪ Dependent on supportive leadership, facilitative human resources, and ongoing staff education
	▪ Requires adaptability and integration of new knowledge into dynamic and evolving practice environments

The Toolkit has been utilized extensively in Ontario, across Canada, and internationally to direct a structured, systematic approach to the implementation process. It has been translated into multiple languages, which has supported its global reach. The following quotes from those who have used the Toolkit to lead practice change highlight its effectiveness in both local and international contexts:

". . . [T]he gap analysis tools located in the Toolkit easily helped identify where our long-term care home was excelling and where there was room for improvements. The Toolkit assisted our home in creating an annual strategic plan to evaluate our required programs, formulate home specific education plans, monitor changes, and guide our nurses to provide the most current, evidence-based care."

—Sara Le, RN
Director of Resident Care
Tilbury Manor Nursing Home

"The Toolkit has been used to support our staff to implement the RNAO guidelines. We were introduced to the Toolkit early in our BPSO work, and it has made a significant difference in how we approach practice change, by providing a methodology that all staff are able to understand and utilize."

—Maribel Esparza-Bohórquez, RN, MSc
Chief of Nursing Division, Clinica FOSCAL, Bucaramanga, Colombia

INTEGRATING BEST PRACTICE GUIDELINES INTO CURRICULA: EDUCATOR'S RESOURCE

The engagement of stakeholders in the academic sector is critical to support integration of BPGs in the undergraduate nursing curriculum. A Request for Proposals issued in 2003 resulted in the selection of eleven academic institutions that proposed projects to integrate BPGs into various undergraduate nursing courses. These projects resulted in significant innovations, with faculty and students collaborating on project conceptualization and execution. As these projects were being completed, RNAO and the academic organizations involved in this work recognized the need for a resource that would capture key learnings and inform nurse educators in both academic and practice settings about successful approaches to integrating evidence-based practice into curriculum. The outcomes from these educational projects were shared with the nursing community via RNAO's multidimensional dissemination strategy, and ultimately informed the development of the *Educator's Resource: Integration of Best Practice Guidelines* (RNAO, 2005a).

RNAO's Educator's Resource was developed by a team of experts from academia and those responsible for staff development in practice settings from across the continuum of care. The development process included a review of the relevant literature and the creation of a guiding framework to organize the key components. The draft Educator's Resource was reviewed by over 70 external stakeholders representing academic and service organizations, including the Canadian Association of Schools of Nursing and the College of Nurses of Ontario (the provincial nursing regulatory body). Their feedback was compiled, discussed by the panel, and based on consensus, incorporated into the final document (RNAO, 2005a).

RNAO's Educator's Resource is designed to help educators in academic or practice settings to plan, implement, and evaluate learning events for nurses and the interprofessional team, whether staff or students, to promote integration of BPGs into practice. We recommend that this resource be utilized in conjunction with the *Toolkit: Implementation of Best Practice Guidelines* (RNAO, 2012) and the guidelines themselves.

The Educator's Resource has been structured to provide "need to know" and "nice to know" content. Chapters are organized utilizing the framework for Integration of Best Practice Guidelines into learning events (Figure 4.3) as its foundation.

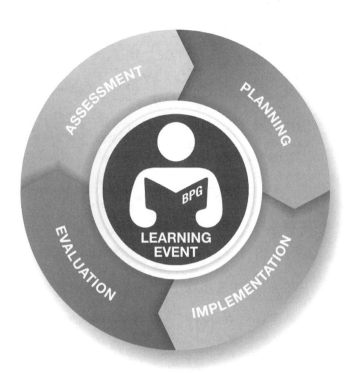

FIGURE 4.3 Framework for Integration of Best Practice Guidelines into learning events (adapted from RNAO, 2005a, p. 9).

The Framework in Figure 4.3 represents nursing as a knowledge-based profession, integrating both the art and science of nursing. These elements are enhanced through the integration of BPGs into practice. The intended outcome is enhanced quality of nursing practice and clinical outcomes. This four-step framework incorporates the student, the guideline(s), the learning event, and the educator. At the center of the framework is the learner and the learner's interaction with the BPG. Surrounding the learner/BPGs are the activities the educator should consider in order to deliver a successful learning event. These activities include the elements of the nursing process: Assessment, Planning, Implementation, and Evaluation. These elements are depicted in a circular manner because the interaction of teaching and learning is cyclical, and aspects of the framework may occur simultaneously (RNAO, 2005a, p. 9).

The Educator's Resource is divided into six chapters to guide readers through the elements of the framework as they design a learning event. Each chapter is structured in a similar way and includes (RNAO, 2005a, p. 10):

- What is this chapter about? (outlines the steps of the framework element)
- Steps (description of the steps and specific discussion of content relevant to the chapter)
- Scenarios (two case studies that apply information from the chapter)
- Key points (summary of the chapter)
- References
- Tips, Tools and Templates (ready-to-use materials)

Table 4.3 provides a summary of the chapters of the Educator's Resource, representing the various elements of the guiding framework and the key content addressed.

TABLE 4.3   CHAPTERS OF THE EDUCATOR'S RESOURCE: INTEGRATING BEST PRACTICE GUIDELINES (RNAO, 2005A)

CHAPTER	CONTENT
Chapter 1—Setting the Stage	■ What is the Nursing Best Practice Guidelines Program? ■ What is the purpose of the Educator's Resource? ■ Who can benefit from the Educator's Resource? ■ How was the Educator's Resource developed? ■ Roadmap to using the Educator's Resource ■ Scenarios, References ■ Tips, Tools and Templates
Chapter 2—Assessment for the Learning Event	■ Step 1: Assess the Environment ■ Step 2: Assess the Educator ■ Step 3: Assess the Learner ■ Step 4: Conduct a Learning Needs Assessment ■ Step 5: Assess the Group ■ Key Points, Scenarios, References ■ Tips, Tools and Templates
Chapter 3—Planning the Learning Event	■ Step 1: Integrate BPG content into the curricula of an academic or practice setting ■ Step 2: Identify facilitators and driving forces for integration of BPG content ■ Step 3: Identify barriers to integrating BPG content, and strategies to overcome them ■ Step 4: Identify partnerships for BPG education ■ Step 5: Facilitate the integration of BPG content into learning events ■ Step 6: Identify and allocate resources ■ Step 7: Plan for content ■ Step 8: Develop a learning plan ■ Step 9: Plan for contingencies ■ Key points, scenarios, references ■ Tips, Tools and Templates
Chapter 4—Implementing Teaching/Learning Strategies	■ Step 1: Choose teaching/learning strategies ■ Step 2: Implement teaching/learning plan ■ Key points, scenarios, references ■ Tips, Tools and Templates
Chapter 5—Evaluation	■ Step 1: Review your endpoint ■ Step 2: Evaluate the learning event ■ Step 3: Evaluate the learner ■ Step 4: Review and implementation of evaluation ■ Key points, scenario, references ■ Tips, Tools and Templates

CHAPTER	CONTENT
Chapter 6—Enrichment Materials	▪ Nursing Best Practice Guidelines Program ▪ Assessing your learners ▪ Planning the learning event ▪ Implementing the learning plan ▪ Evaluation ▪ References

The Educator's Resource is a unique tool that has been widely utilized to support the integration of BPGs into curricula within Ontario, across Canada, and internationally. It is available for free download from the RNAO website (RNAO, 2005a). As a result of the international interest in this resource, it has been translated into Spanish, and this version can also be assessed on the RNAO website (RNAO, 2005b).

BEST PRACTICE SPOTLIGHT ORGANIZATIONS

A key organizational strategy to support meso-level implementation is the Best Practice Spotlight Organization (BPSO) Designation. Launched in 2003, the Designation has proven to be the most successful implementation tool to foster evidence-based organizations through BPG implementation and sustainment, as well as to measure sustained implementation impact on patients, organizational, and health system outcomes. As described in Chapter 1, *Transforming Nursing Through Knowledge: The Conceptual and Programmatic Underpinnings of RNAO's BPG Program*, the BPSO Designation is an opportunity for health and academic organizations to formally partner with RNAO over a 3-year period. Following this period, if successful, the organization becomes a Designated BPSO, with renewal biennially, pending achievement of deliverables. The goal of the partnership is to create EBP cultures through systematic implementation of multiple RNAO BPGs.

Chapter 6, *Best Practice Spotlight Organization: Implementation Science at Its Best*, details the BPSO objectives, types of BPSOs, as well as RNAO's requirements for, and supports to, BPSOs. Chapters 7, 8, 9, 10, 13, 14, 15, and 17 each bring to the reader the lived experiences of BPSOs in various health sectors and academia—from the founding BPSOs to more recent ones, in all sectors, and in various places around the globe. Thus, what follows is a high-level analysis of what has made them so successful from an implementation science perspective.

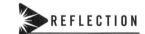 **REFLECTION**

Thinking about practice change initiatives within your workplace that have not been successfully sustained, how do you think the outcome may have been different with committed support from all levels of the organization?

The BPSO Designation enables organizations to commit to a focus on patient care and clinical excellence, using the latest evidence to inform practice and optimize outcomes. The systematic implementation of BPGs has helped advance government priorities within organizations, as well as enhance clinical, provider, and organizational outcomes. Through the BPSO Designation, healthcare and academic organizations have made progress in positively influencing provincial, national, and international health systems.

Since the inception of the program, BPSOs have effectively used and contributed to implementation science in developing creative strategies for successfully implementing BPGs, as well as by sustaining and spreading their uptake. BPSOs have also enhanced their understanding of evaluation and the importance of data quality, increased their capacity to effectively monitor and evaluate guideline impact, and developed mechanisms to share results with the staff implementing practice changes to support sustainment (RNAO, 2015).

The following testimony highlights the impact of the BPSO Program on BPG uptake resulting in better patient *outcomes:*

> *"[In our organization as a BPSO] RNAO Best Practice Guidelines provide guidance and enhanced patient care supporting evidence-based practice. The guidelines have provided rigor and enhanced clarity to all healthcare professionals. The impact of the best practice guidelines ensures favourable patient outcomes and experience while advancing the nursing profession."*

> —Suzanne Robichaud
> Vice-President of Clinical Programs and Chief Nursing Officer
> Hôpital Montfort—RNAO BPSO
> Ottawa, Ontario

MACRO-LEVEL/HEALTH SYSTEM IMPLEMENTATION

The third level of implementation for the BPGs is the macro level, targeted at health system implementation. The goal here is to scale out the implementation efforts across the health system in Ontario, across Canada, and internationally. Five years from the outset of the BPG Program, system levers were identified to enable long-term sustainability of the guidelines and the impact the guidelines have on the health of people. Several key initiatives were instituted:

- In 2004, with funding from Health Canada, a Pan-Canadian tour was delivered involving 24 full-day, free workshops and numerous webinars focused on evidence-based practice and the uptake of BPGs. The engagement was phenomenal, with over 2,000 nurses participating from across the country. This high level of interest resulted in requests for workshops from organizations in various parts of Canada that were interested in expanding their utilization of evidence-based practice.

- Several impactful, system-level initiatives have been launched throughout the years to advance the uptake of evidence, and in particular RNAO's BPGs, across specific sectors or in focused areas of practice. For example, in the long-term care sector, funding was secured by RNAO to hire Long-Term Care Best Practice Coordinators whose role is to support practice advancement in LTC homes based on guideline recommendations. Chapter 11, *Evidence-Based Practice in Long-Term Care*, expands on this important initiative. Similarly, a specific multifaceted strategy was developed for smoking cessation, including an interactive website (www.TobaccoFreeRNAO.ca), Champions dedicated to smoking cessation, and collaboration with a range of provincial and national government stakeholders working to reduce tobacco use. Chapter 10, *Scaling Up and Out: System-Wide Implementation Initiatives*, highlights this and two additional RNAO-led provincial and national implementation initiatives in the areas of mental health and addiction and falls prevention.

■ In 2017, RNAO launched an *Implementation Research Collaboratory*—a partnership between RNAO, BPSOs, and researchers from around the world to identify, develop, and test indicators for successful and sustained guideline implementation. The inaugural activity of the Collaboratory, as part of a larger program of research, is a commissioned study to refine, validate, and operationalize the RNAO *Indicators and Sub-Indicators of the Best Practice Guideline Implementation Framework*. The study will result in a comprehensive framework of indicators of BPG implementation, identifying specific implementation strategies and processes that will be incorporated into the Nursing Quality Indicators for Reporting and Evaluation (NQuIRE) for routine collection by BPSOs (Squires, Gifford, Grinspun, Grdisa, & McConnell, 2017). The intent is to expand implementation science knowledge through studying actual experiences of our global BPSO network.

LATEST PERSPECTIVES ON IMPLEMENTATION SCIENCE

As we have seen throughout this chapter, transferring knowledge and ensuring uptake of evidence-based practices (EBPs) into our day-to-day clinical work does not automatically happen. It requires the purposeful interventions described and studied in the field of implementation science (Grinspun, Virani, & Bajnok, 2002; Grinspun, Melnyk,& Fineout-Overholt., 2014). RNAO is at the forefront of this relatively young field, which will continue to evolve based on lived experiences and research. What follows are emerging implementation science approaches that are impacting knowledge uptake in nursing and healthcare.

INTEGRATED KNOWLEDGE TRANSLATION AND PATIENT ENGAGEMENT

There is increasing acceptance in implementation science of the importance of adopting an integrated knowledge translation (iKT) approach to both producing and translating knowledge into practice. *iKT* refers to a collaborative, participatory, action-oriented, community-based approach to research that results in the co-production of knowledge (CIHR, 2012a). The cornerstone of iKT is that it involves engaging and integrating stakeholders (also known as knowledge users) into the full research process from conceptualization through to interpretation and dissemination of findings. The stakeholders can and should vary greatly depending on the project. They can range from policy- and decision-makers from the community up to the federal level, researchers, members of the public including patients and families, members of industry, healthcare providers of all levels, and the media (CIHR, 2012a). Knowledge, when produced in this unique paradigm, is then already in part "owned" by the participants, who are in a much better position and willing to act on the knowledge than if they are simply informed about it. Hence, an iKT approach naturally facilitates implementation of knowledge. RNAO was ahead of most in following this approach since the inception of the BPG Program.

Patient engagement is a special case of iKT that is increasingly receiving attention in Canada and internationally. *Patient engagement* occurs when "patients meaningfully and actively collaborate in the governance, priority setting, and conduct of research, as well as in summarizing, distributing, sharing, and applying its resulting knowledge" (CIHR, 2014, p. 1). Given that this is a relatively new way of doing research for many, scientific evaluations of experiences with patient engagement in research studies are limited. However, existing evaluations are promising, revealing that engaging the public early in the design of studies, ideally at the planning stage, not only ensures that the research is relevant to their concerns but also leads to better results and improved translation of the knowledge produced into practice (Nass, Levine, & Yancy, 2012). The inclusion of the public at the micro level in the RNAO's Best Practice Champion Network, and at the meso level in organizational specific BPSO implementation activities, demonstrates the application of the principles inherent in iKT and patient engagement.

TECHNOLOGY-ENABLED KNOWLEDGE TRANSLATION

The digital age has revolutionized the way people access information, communicate, and collaborate. Technology-enabled knowledge translation refers to the use of digital information and communication technologies to accelerate knowledge translation efforts. With the universality of the Internet, the proliferation of approaches in communication and social networking, and the continuous improvements in technologies from electronic notebooks to smartphones, there are now rich opportunities for technology-enabled knowledge translation in most healthcare settings.

The use of social media is one example of technology that is increasingly used as a tool for knowledge translation in healthcare. *Social media* is defined as the set of tools and networking platforms allowing people to connect, communicate, and collaborate via web-based technology (Jue, Marr, & Kassotakis, 2009). Examples of social media include: e-communities; hosted image and video services; social networking sites such as Facebook and Twitter; blogs; and wikis (Oakley & Spallek, 2012). While social media is still a relatively new tool for knowledge translation and has not yet received extensive scientific evaluation, there are, in theory, several reasons to consider its use. For example, because billions of people use social media, it provides a venue for quick dissemination of health information to large numbers and diverse stakeholders. It also stimulates conversation between stakeholders, which can include how the knowledge can be used to advance practice (Ndumbe-Eyoh & Mazzucco, 2016). Additionally, it creates "communities of practice" around specific topics of interest; it provides flexibility in when and how to deliver knowledge; and it has built-in metrics for evaluation of knowledge dissemination such as numbers of shares (a means of publicizing a post further to one's contacts) and likes (a symbolic way of letting others know that one values or appreciates the post) (Hemsley & Mason, 2013). RNAO, as a professional association, is extremely active in social media and utilizes a variety of platforms including Twitter, Facebook, Instagram, Pinterest, Periscope, and YouTube, amongst others, for knowledge mobilization related to both policy matters and the BPG Program.

ARTS-BASED KNOWLEDGE TRANSLATION

Arts-based knowledge translation has emerged recently as a novel, nontraditional approach to moving knowledge into practice. Although arts-based methods are relatively new to nursing and healthcare generally, they are very well established in other fields, predominantly education and the social sciences. Arts methods such as storytelling, visual arts, and drama offer alternative ways of communicating knowledge about healthcare. Arts-based knowledge translation holds immense potential for providing new and unique ways of engaging diverse stakeholders, especially patients and families, on important healthcare issues. The approach uses experiential and interactive aspects of health and is boundary-crossing, as it requires collaboration between individuals from very diverse professional backgrounds (e.g., physicians, nurses, storytellers, artists, and filmmakers). Arts-based knowledge translation represents an exciting paradigm shift, whereby knowledge translation is viewed as a creative, dynamic process rather than a passive linear process as originally thought (Parsons & Boydell, 2012). The RNAO utilized arts-based knowledge translation as a strategy in a limited way at a BPG conference held in the early 2000s, where a small theatre company was engaged to bring to life key recommendations of several foundational Best Practice Guidelines and highlight the impact of quality nursing care on patients and their families. Several BPSOs have incorporated the art of storytelling in their Champion development workshops as an innovative strategy to facilitate engagement, influence value shifts, and share outcomes.

DEVELOPMENTAL EVALUATION

Although not conventionally thought of as an approach to knowledge translation in healthcare, developmental evaluation holds great potential for facilitating meaningful practice change due to the importance it places on context. With developmental evaluation, assessments are made of where things are and how things are unfolding in an organization with respect to the implementation of specific knowledge. This helps determine which knowledge-translation strategies hold promise, which ones currently used ought to be abandoned, and what new efforts should be tried (Patton, 2010). What is most novel and promising about this approach for knowledge translation is that instead of trying to "control" for context, it recognizes the crucial importance of context and adapting to the context to make knowledge translation happen.

DEIMPLEMENTATION

Much of the emphasis in knowledge translation is rightfully placed on implementation of knowledge—getting best practice knowledge used in practice. But equally important, and a currently rising trend, is *deimplementation*—getting ineffective or potentially harmful knowledge out of practice. Deimplementation is merely the opposite of implementation; therefore, it is likely to require different approaches and thoughtful ways to: 1) identify practices that should be deimplemented and then 2) to design strategies to deimplement these practices. This newly emerging field of deimplementation, also known as deinvestment, is still in its infancy but has sparked a lot of interest, with much ongoing investigation by knowledge-translation researchers in Canada and internationally. It is argued that "deimplementing practices reflects a recommitment to evidence-based healthcare" (Prasad & Ioannidis, 2014, p. 4).

CONCLUSION

Making significant practice changes requires intervention and ongoing attention at multiple levels—micro, meso, and macro. At the micro level, RNAO's Best Practice Champions demonstrate their value daily, serving as motivators, problem solvers, and mentors for evidence-based practices. They identify barriers that block and enablers that support practice change, and they funnel this knowledge in appropriate ways at the practice and organizational levels. At the meso level, BPSOs have transformed the organizational culture of service organizations to one where evidence-based practice is the norm. BPSOs leverage the capacity of their Champions and utilize a range of approaches to successfully implement Best Practice Guidelines.

These approaches have been founded in implementation science and the systematic approach to practice change outlined in the *Toolkit: Implementation of Best Practice Guidelines* (RNAO, 2012), resulting in positive impacts on client, practitioner, and organizational outcomes. By linking evidence-based practice to evidence-based policy, scaling up implementation, and engaging key stakeholders and the public, practice and policy changes at the macro level are achieved as described throughout this book. Looking to the future, RNAO's cutting-edge *Implementation Research Collaboratory* will contribute new knowledge on the most effective implementation strategies and tools to ensure optimal uptake of evidence to continuously enhance nursing practice and improve outcomes for patients, organizations, and health systems everywhere.

KEY MESSAGES

- Successful implementation programs require attention at the micro level of individual practitioners, meso level of organizations, and macro level of regions and health systems.

- Champions at all levels of the organization have been shown to effectively facilitate the uptake of evidence in practice.

- Implementation frameworks have been successfully utilized to support the integration of BPGs in clinical practice and educational curriculum.

- Organization-level strategies to focus BPG implementation have proven successful across a range of settings and contexts.

- Wide stakeholder engagement—involving stakeholders in a variety of roles and in all sectors—supports the uptake of evidence-based practices in service and academic organizations.

REFERENCES

Bajnok, I., Grinspun, D., Lloyd, M., & McConnell, H. (2015). Leading quality improvement through Best Practice Guideline development, implementation, and measurement science. *Med UNAB, 17*(3), 155–162.

Canadian Institutes of Health Research (CIHR). (2012a). *Guide to knowledge translation planning at CIHR: Integrated and end-of-grant approaches.* Retrieved from http://cihr-irsc.gc.ca/e/documents/kt_lm_ktplan-en.pdf

Canadian Institutes of Health Research (CIHR). (2012b). *Moving into action: We know what practices we want to change, now what? An implementation guide for health care practitioners.* Retrieved from http://www.cihr-irsc.gc.ca/e/documents/lm_moving_into_action-en.pdf

Canadian Institutes of Health Research (CIHR). (2014). *Patient engagement.* Retrieved from http://www.cihr-irsc.gc.ca/e/45851.html

DiCenso, A., Virani, T., Bajnok, I., Borycki, E., Davies, B., Graham, I., Harrison, M., . . . Scott, J. (2002). A toolkit to facilitate the implementation of clinical practice guidelines in healthcare settings. *Hospital Quarterly, Spring,* 55–60.

Dobbins, M., Davies, B., Danseco, E., Edwards, N., & Virani, T. (2005). Changing nursing practice: Evaluating the usefulness of a Best Practice Guideline implementation toolkit. *Canadian Journal of Nursing Leadership, 18*(1), 34–45.

Eccles, MP & BS, Mittman. (2006). Welcome to Implementation Science. *Implementation Science,* 1:1 doi:10.1186/1748-5908-1-1

Forsetlund, L., Bjørndal, A., Rashidian, A., Jamtvedt, G., O'Brien, M. A., Wolf, F., . . . Oxman, A. D. (2009). Continuing education meetings and workshops: Effects on professional practice and health care outcomes. Cochrane Database of Systematic Reviews, 2, CD003030. doi: 10.1002/14651858.CD003030.pub2

Graham, I., & Tetroe, J. (2010). The knowledge to action framework. In J. Rycroft-Malone & T. Bucknell (Eds.). *Models and frameworks for implementing evidence-based practice: Linking evidence to action* (pp. 207–222). Oxford, UK: Wiley-Blackwell, Sigma Theta Tau International Honor Society of Nursing.

Greenhalgh, T., Robert, G., Bate, P., MacFarlane, F., & Kyriakidou, O. (2005). *Diffusion of innovations in health service organizations: A systematic literature review.* Maldne, MA: Blackwell.

Grinspun, D., Melnyk, B. M., & Finout-Overholt, E. (2014). Advancing optimal care with rigorously developed clinical practice guidelines and evidence-based recommendations. In B. M. Melnyk & E. Fineout-Overholt (Eds.). *Evidence-based practice in nursing and health care: A guide to best practice* (3rd ed.) (pp. 182–201). Philadelphia, PA: Wolters Kluwer.

Grinspun, D., Virani, T., & Bajnok, I. (2002). Nursing Best Practice Guidelines: The Registered Nurses' Association of Ontario project. *Hospital Quarterly, 5*(2), 56–60.

Hemsley, R., & Mason, R. M. (2013). Knowledge and knowledge management in the social media age. *Journal of Organizational Computing and Electronic Commerce, 23*(1–2), 138–167.

Jue, A. L., Marr, J. A., & Kassotakis, M.E. (2009). *Social media at work: How networking tools propel organizational performance.* San Francisco, CA: Jossey-Bass.

Kitson, A., Harvey, G., & McCormack, B. (1998). Enabling the implementation of evidence based practice: A conceptual framework. *Quality in Health Care,* 7, 149–158.

Locock, L., Dopson, S., Chambers, D., & Gabbay, J. (2001). Understanding the role of opinion leaders in improving clinical effectiveness. *Social Science & Medicine, 53*(6), 745–757.

Nass, P., Levine, S., & Yancy, C. (2012). *Methods for involving patients in topic generation for patient-centered comparative effectiveness research: An international perspective.* (Research Priorities White Paper for the Patient-Centered Outcomes Research Institute [PCORI]). Retrieved from http://www.pcori.org/assets/Methods-for-Involving-Patients-in-Topic-Generation-for-Patient-Centered-Comparative-Effectiveness-Research-%e2%80%93-An-International-Perspective.pdf

Ndumbe-Eyoh, S., & Mazzucco, A. (2016). Social media, knowledge translation, and action on the social determinants of health and health equity: A survey of public health practices. *Journal of Public Health Policy, 37*(S2), S249–S259.

Oakley, M., & Spallek, H. (2012). Social media in dental education: A call for research and action. *Journal of Dental Education, 76*(3), 279–287.

Parsons, J., & Boydell, K. (2012). Arts-based research and knowledge translation: Some key concerns for health-care professionals. *Journal of Interprofessional Care, 26*(3), 170–172.

Patton, M. Q. (2010). *Developmental evaluation: Applying complexity concepts to enhance innovation and use.* New York, NY: Guilford Publications.

Ploeg, J., Skelly, J., Rowan, M., Edwards, N., Davies, B., Grinspun, D., . . . Downey, A. (2010). The role of nursing best practice champions in diffusing practice guidelines: A mixed methods study. *Worldviews on Evidence-Based Nursing, 7*(4), 238–251. doi: 10.1111/j.1741-6787.2010.00202.x.

Prasad, V., & Ioannidis, J. (2014). Evidence-based de-implementation for contradicted, unproven, and aspiring healthcare practices. *Implementation Science, 9*(1). https://doi.org/10.1186/1748-5908-9-1

Registered Nurses' Association of Ontario (RNAO). (2002). *Toolkit: Implementation of clinical practice guidelines*. Toronto, ON: Registered Nurses' Association of Ontario.

Registered Nurses' Association of Ontario (RNAO). (2005a). *Educator's resource: Integration of best practice guidelines*. Retrieved from http://rnao.ca/bpg/guidelines/resources/educators-resource-integration-best-practice-guidelines

Registered Nurses' Association of Ontario (RNAO). (2005b). *Recursos para el docente*. Retrieved from http://rnao.ca/bpg/resources/recursos-para-el-docents

Registered Nurses' Association of Ontario (RNAO). (2012). *Toolkit: Implementation of Best Practice Guidelines* (2nd ed.). Toronto, ON: Registered Nurses' Association of Ontario.

Registered Nurses' Association of Ontario (RNAO). (2015). *2014–2015 Best Practice Spotlight Organization impact survey: Summary of survey results*. Retrieved from http://rnao.ca/sites/rnao-ca/files/FINAL_RNAO-BPSO_Impact_Survey_from_Printer.pdf

Registered Nurses' Association of Ontario (RNAO). (2017a). *Best Practice Guidelines clinical institute: Program overview*. Retrieved from http://rnao.ca/sites/rnao-ca/files/2017_Institute_Foundational_Agenda.pdf

Registered Nurses' Association of Ontario (RNAO). (2017b). *RNAO best practice champion eLearning course*. Retrieved from http://elearning.rnao.ca

Rogers, E. M. (2003). *Diffusion of innovations* (5th ed.). New York, NY: Free Press.

Squires, J., Gifford, W., Grinspun, D., Grdisa, V., & McConnell, H. (2017). Identifying, refining, validating and operationalizing indicators and sub-indicators of Best Practice Guideline implementation and sustainability: A framework to drive measurement. *Research Proposal–RNAO Commissioned Study*. Toronto, ON: Registered Nurses' Association of Ontario.

Thompson, G., Estabrooks, C., & Degner, L. (2006). Clarifying the concepts in knowledge transfer: A literature review. *Journal of Advanced Nursing, 53*(6), 691–701.

5

TECHNOLOGY AS AN ENABLER OF EVIDENCE-BASED PRACTICE

Rita Wilson, MEd, MN, RN
Irmajean Bajnok, PhD, MScN, BScN, RN

LEARNING OBJECTIVES

After reading this chapter, you will be able to:

- Understand the importance of technology as an enabler of evidence-based practice

- Outline RNAO's technology-related resources that support evidence-based practice

- Describe nursing order sets and their benefits

- Determine strategies to integrate the nursing order sets as clinical decision supports in evidence-based practice

- Define the concept of International Classification for Nursing Practice (ICNP) as a standardized nursing language and explain its benefits

- Delineate key recommendations from RNAO's eHealth-related BPG, *Adopting eHealth Solutions: Implementation Strategies*

INTRODUCTION

The paradigm shift in healthcare in recent years has resulted in a new focus on the use of technology to increase efficiency, enhance patient safety, and optimize health outcomes. With this paradigm shift came a solution to the dilemma of the widely reported 17-year lag between the production of research evidence and its integration into practice (Kumar, 2012). This recognition of technology as an enabler of evidence-based practice was the catalyst for RNAO to develop implementation resources to more effectively facilitate ease of access to its Best Practice Guidelines (BPG) at the point of care.

This chapter describes RNAO's advancement into the world of technology where its current focus is the development of innovative eHealth resources to promote evidence-based practice. Key resources discussed in this chapter include: 1) an app that enables clinicians to access the RNAO guidelines on mobile devices such as smartphones and tablet computers; 2) nursing order sets that simplify the process of integrating BPGs into electronic health information systems; and 3) a BPG to enhance the involvement of healthcare leaders, nurses, and other clinicians in all phases of an eHealth implementation.

EHEALTH

eHealth is defined by the World Health Organization (WHO) as "the use of information and communication technologies (ICT) for health" (WHO & International Telecommunication Union [ITU], 2012, p. 1). Its primary goal is to enhance the flow of information, using technological means, to more effectively support healthcare delivery and the management of health systems (WHO & ITU, 2012). eHealth supports a variety of needs in the health sector.

In hospitals, eHealth encompasses (but is not limited to) the use of information and communications technologies to support administrative systems, patient care services (e.g., telemedicine, diagnostic services, medication management, healthcare delivery), and consumer health services (e.g., patient portals) (Health Canada, 2010). In the home care and public health sectors, eHealth facilitates remote patient monitoring and clinicians' access to information through the use of mobile technology (e.g., smartphones and tablet computers) (Health Canada, 2010). Further, in the long-term care sector, eHealth is evident in the use of computer systems by nurses and other care providers for electronic documentation, order entry, and electronic prescribing (Health Canada, 2010).

Since the introduction of eHealth as a national and provincial strategy to revolutionize and modernize healthcare delivery, RNAO has been actively advocating for nurses to be fully engaged throughout the process. The added value of registered nurses and nurse practitioners at the decision-making tables ensures their perspectives are adequately reflected in the eHealth infrastructure. Moreover, their contributions during the planning stages positively influence the design of electronic health information systems that are user-friendly and clinically relevant for nurses and other clinicians (RNAO, 2017a).

Beginning in 2005, RNAO has kept pace with the trends in hospitals and other health organizations to leverage technology to support care delivery. In that year, RNAO launched its nursing and eHealth program (with funding from the Ontario Ministry of Health and Long-Term Care) to empower nurses to adopt and effectively utilize eHealth innovations and evidence-based eResources (RNAO, 2006, 2009, 2013b). Over several years of working in partnership with the Ontario Government, RNAO developed evidence-based eLearning and educational resources to inform nurses and other clinicians about eHealth and its benefits and applicability to nursing and the entire healthcare sector. RNAO also built a cadre of approximately 1,500 eHealth Champions to lead and support the adoption of eHealth amongst nurses and other clinicians.

In 2009, following the outstanding successes of the eHealth Champions, RNAO was funded to head the Nurse Peer Leader Project through Canada Health Infoway's (Infoway) Clinician Support Network Program. Infoway is Canada's national body that aims to optimize the use of eHealth to increase value for individuals and the health system.

Within its broad mandate, Infoway extends tremendous effort to increase clinician engagement in eHealth through regional clinician support network projects that target nurses, pharmacists, and physicians across the country. The RNAO Nurse Peer Leader Project resulted in a network of 14 nurses throughout the province of Ontario, Canada, who worked within all sectors (including academia), to raise awareness of eHealth and its value in nursing. In addition to this "unfreezing" role, peer leaders also provided nursing input to eHealth decision-making locally and regionally, often role modeling effective use of eHealth in nursing. These peer leaders were part of a network that was supported through education and professional development in eHealth and change management, and they spread an active virtual community of practice and interactive coaching. Their roles paved the way for greater involvement of nursing in eHealth decision-making and led to a further successful Infoway-funded Ontario Peer Leader Project with RNAO in partnership with the Ontario Medical Association. This initiative, which extended from 2012 to 2014, focused on advancing the adoption of eHealth in primary care.

The eHealth champions and peer leaders were both creating and noting the trend for a greater readiness amongst nurses to adopt eHealth in day-to-day practice activities. This trend was a catalyst for the launch of RNAO's first eHealth innovation in 2011—the *RNAO Nursing Best Practice Guidelines* app, designed for use on mobile devices such as smartphones and tablet computers (Wilson, Bajnok, & Costa, 2015).

RNAO NURSING BEST PRACTICE GUIDELINES APP

The *RNAO Nursing Best Practice Guidelines* app (see Figure 5.1) was developed to facilitate access to condensed versions of over 50 clinical and healthy work environment guidelines at the point of care (Bajnok, Burkoski, & Doran, 2012; Doran et al., 2010, 2012; RNAO, 2016a). With this new electronic resource, nurses have access to the practice recommendations, related evidence, and teaching tools at their fingertips. The app has quickly become a popular resource used by nurses and other clinicians around the world (RNAO, 2016a). For many nurses, it became a critical professional practice aid to prepare for patient care, answer questions during care delivery, conduct health teaching with patients, access clinical resources, and serve as a reference to support practice decisions (Doran et al., 2010, 2012).

Just prior to the 5-year anniversary of its launch, in an effort to refine and expand the app's utility, RNAO conducted a survey of end users in 2015. The survey results prompted an upgrade of the app to provide an even more user-friendly resource with advanced functionality aimed at enhancing the practice of nurses and other clinicians, globally.

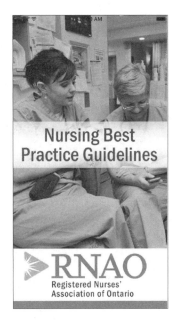

"Glad to have the BPGs in a portable, fast, well-organized format. A great tool to utilize to ensure delivery of quality care!"

"Thank you—this is incredible! For nurses working in home care and other areas where computers and Internet aren't available, this is the perfect resource for the most up-to-date evidence-based practices."

"Amazing!! Quick evidence-based information at your finger tips! A must for students and nurses in any setting."

FIGURE 5.1 *RNAO Nursing Best Practice Guidelines* app with quotes from users.
Reprinted from RNAO, 2016a. ©Registered Nurses' Association of Ontario. All rights reserved.

The upgraded app incorporates the following design features and functionality:

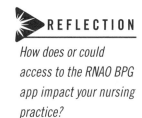

- Concise, clinically relevant, evidence-based guidelines to assist with the assessment, decision-making, and management of patients with a variety of health conditions (e.g., stroke, ostomy, pain, and pressure injury)

- Guidelines categorized by subject/topic (i.e., chronic disease management, addiction and mental health, care of older persons, etc.) with the option to display the guidelines in alphabetical order

- Enhanced search functionality for quick reference

REFLECTION

How does or could access to the RNAO BPG app impact your nursing practice?

The app's usability was an important consideration during the redesign. The International Organization for Standardization (ISO) defines usability as the "extent to which a system, product or service can be used by specified users to achieve specified goals with effectiveness, efficiency and satisfaction in a specified context of use" (ISO 9241-11, 2016, para. 2). Multiple usability sessions involving nurses and other health professionals were conducted prior to the release of the revised app. The usability of the the final product was ranked very high by the end users. A contributing factor to the app's usability is the inclusion of consistent headings to organize the content of the condensed clinical and healthy work environment guidelines (shown in Figure 5.2).

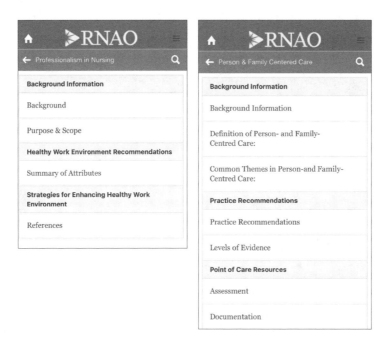

FIGURE 5.2 *RNAO Nursing Best Practice Guidelines* app—Standardized headings used for clinical and healthy work environment guidelines.

The app is available for free download for Apple and Android mobile devices from the App Store and Google Play Store, respectively. Since its relaunch in 2015, the app has been downloaded by hundreds of users in over 70 countries across the globe, affirming the value of the app in assisting clinicians with point-of-care decision-making and in promoting evidence-based practice. Through such tools as the app, clinicians' point-of-care access to evidence-based resources translates into appropriate and timely healthcare interventions for their patients, leading to optimal health outcomes.

Mobile devices represent one of two groundbreaking ways that RNAO is leveraging technology to enable evidence-based practice; the other is nursing order sets.

NURSING ORDER SETS

As originally designed, beginning in 1999, the RNAO BPGs were intended to be used in environments with paper-based communications tools, health records, and clinical resources. With the increasing use of electronic health information systems, RNAO devised a novel implementation strategy to seamlessly integrate the BPGs within these systems. In 2011, RNAO began developing, disseminating, and actively supporting the adoption and evaluation of nursing order sets.

The term *order set* is used to describe a list of orders or interventions that are recommended for specific patient diagnoses, conditions, and treatment (Idemoto, Williams, & Blackmore, 2016; Slavik Cowen & Moorhead, 2014). An order set may support clinical decision-making at the point of care as a paper-based resource or as a resource embedded within an electronic health information system (Wilson et al., 2015).

Order sets were originally associated with physician orders, but more recently, the term has been increasingly used in reference to interventions that fall within the domain of nursing (Canadian Association of Schools of Nursing, 2012; RNAO, 2012). A case in point is the study by Drake and colleagues (Drake, Redfern, Sherburne, Nugent, & Simpson, 2012), which referred to a standardized pressure ulcer nursing order set that existed in the hospital where they conducted their research. The order set was introduced to help nurses conduct pressure ulcer risk assessments and implement preventive measures for at-risk patients. Similarly, Kruse and Rigotti (2014) examined the effectiveness of adding a screening question for second-hand smoke exposure to an existing nursing admission order set.

RNAO's nursing order sets complement the specific clinical Best Practice Guideline from which they are derived by distilling the practice recommendations into evidence-based, actionable intervention statements that can be used to formulate a person's plan of care (Wilson, 2013). Table 5.1 shows two practice recommendations from the RNAO (2013a) guideline *Assessment and Management of Foot Ulcers for People with Diabetes*, Second Edition, and the corresponding action-oriented interventions in the nursing order set.

TABLE 5.1 BPG PRACTICE RECOMMENDATIONS AND CORRESPONDING ACTION-ORIENTED INTERVENTIONS IN NURSING ORDER SET

PRACTICE RECOMMENDATIONS ASSESSMENT AND MANAGEMENT OF FOOT ULCERS GUIDELINE	ACTION-ORIENTED INTERVENTIONS ASSESSMENT AND MANAGEMENT OF FOOT ULCERS NURSING ORDER SET
1.1 Identify the location and classification of foot ulcer(s) and measure length, width, and depth of wound bed.	❑ Assess foot ulcer(s) using a validated tool on admission or initial contact ▪ Identify the location and classification of the foot ulcer(s). ▪ Measure the length, width, and depth of the wound bed using a consistent tool.
4.0 Monitor the progress of wound healing on an ongoing basis using a consistent tool, and evaluate the percentage of wound closure at 4 weeks.	❑ Observe and measure pressure ulcers on an ongoing basis using the PUSH Tool ▪ Evaluate the percentage of wound healing at 4 weeks. ▪ If a 50% reduction in surface area is not achieved in 4 weeks, a comprehensive reassessment of the client and treatment plan should be conducted before advanced healing technologies are considered.

As can be seen, the nursing order sets are tools to translate evidence into practice and reduce variation in care by outlining the specific interventions required and when and how they should be carried out. Furthermore, the integration of these order sets into electronic health information systems increases clinicians' access to evidence-based interventions to inform their practice, whenever and wherever they need them (Wilson, 2013).

An added feature of RNAO's nursing order sets is their flexibility. They can be readily incorporated into any electronic health information system or clinical context (e.g., acute care, primary care, long-term care, home care, or community care) (Wilson, 2013). This flexibility was a significant consideration during the development process.

DEVELOPMENT PROCESS

In their evidence-based analysis, Healthcare Human Factors (HHF) (2009) noted variability in the order set development process related to the type of methodology and the type of developers used. In some instances, the methodology was consensus of opinion. In others, the order set development process was informed by evidence. The HHF report also identified two types of order set developers: in-house clinicians, and working groups composed of clinicians from different organizations. In the latter case, the order sets are often made available to other healthcare organizations either as part of a library or embedded in a computerized provider order entry system.

RNAO uses a hybrid methodology when developing its order sets, beginning with a detailed analysis of the evidence-based practice recommendations and the corresponding evidence published in the Best Practice Guideline (see Figure 5.3). This step ensures that pertinent nursing intervention statements and clinical decision support resources are included in the nursing order set.

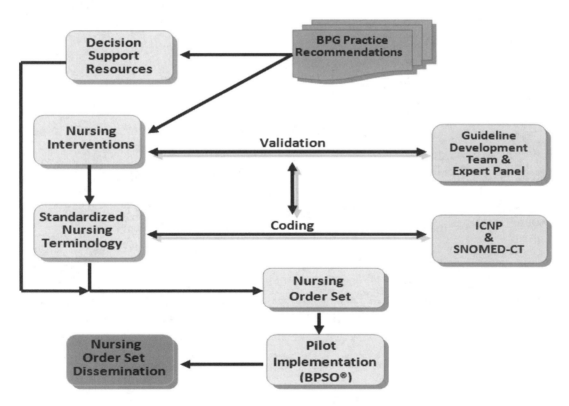

FIGURE 5.3   Nursing order set development process.
Reprinted from Wilson et al., 2015. Used with permission.

Individual nursing intervention statements are drafted in accordance with two international nursing-specific standards: 1) Health informatics: Categorical structures for representation of nursing diagnoses and nursing actions in terminological systems (ISO 18104:2014) (ISO, 2014); and 2) International Classification for Nursing Practice (ICNP) 7-Axis Model (International Council of Nurses [ICN], 2009). The ICN developed ICNP as the international standardized terminology language to describe the work that nurses do (Coenen & Kim, 2010).

Upon completion, the draft intervention statements are validated using a collaborative approach involving RNAO's guideline development team of registered nurses and members of the expert panels who developed the BPG. Once validated, a working group composed of a nursing informatician from the RNAO and expert terminologists from the ICN map the interventions to ICNP. *Mapping* is the process by which similar or related concepts or terms are formally interrelated using a standardized terminology language such as the ICNP numerical coding system (Wieteck, 2008). By assigning the same numerical code to each of these terms or concepts (e.g., pressure injury, pressure ulcer, and decubitus ulcer), the electronic health information system is able to recognize them as synonyms (Wieteck, 2008). Therefore, using a standardized terminology language facilitates the extraction of more accurate data for quality-improvement initiatives, policy development, and research (Wilson, 2013).

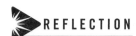

REFLECTION

Consider the importance of embedding specific nursing interventions in the electronic health record as part of the plan of care.

The ICN has mapped their ICNP codes to the Systematized Nomenclature of Medicine-Clinical Terms (SNOMED CT) as part of their Harmonization Agreement with the International Health Terminology Standards Development Organization (IHTSDO) (Kim, Hardiker, & Coenen, 2014). Globally, SNOMED CT is considered the most comprehensive terminology language used to facilitate the exchange of health information (National Library of Medicine [NLM], 2016). Through this collaboration, it is also now possible to map the RNAO nursing order sets to SNOMED CT. This is the recommended approach if the order sets are being embedded in an electronic health information system that has SNOMED CT built in.

A large academic and research hospital in Ontario, Canada recently embedded RNAO's nursing order sets in Epic. This electronic health information system uses SNOMED CT as a terminology language (IHTSDO, 2017). The staff involved in the implementation were required to cross reference the ICNP codes in the nursing order set to the SNOMED CT codes embedded in Epic (see Table 5.2).

By linking these terminology languages behind the scenes in Epic—for example, when clinicians add a diagnosis to the problem list by selecting an existing term—the corresponding SNOMED CT concept is automatically selected. This cross-referencing enhances the organization's ability to use the technology to provide evidence-based clinical decision support and increase its reporting capabilities (IHTSDO, 2017).

TABLE 5.2   MAPPING ICNP CODES IN NURSING ORDER SETS TO SNOMED CT CODES IN EPIC

NURSING ORDER SET INTERVENTION STATEMENT	ICNP CODE IN THE ORDER SET	ICNP PREFERRED TERM (2015 RELEASE)	SNOMED CT CODE IN EPIC	SNOMED CT FULLY SPECIFIED NAME (2016–01–31 RELEASE)
Assess for infection using clinical assessment techniques	10002821	Assessing susceptibility to infection	370782005	Assessment of susceptibility for infection (procedure)
Obtain a comprehensive health history on admission or initial contact	10030687	Admission Assessment	406152008	Admission assessment (procedure)
Implement diabetic foot ulcer care protocol	10031117	Diabetic Ulcer Care	711027007	Diabetic ulcer care (regime/therapy)
Perform physical examination of affected limb(s) on admission	10032258	Physical Examination	5880005	Physical examination procedure (procedure)

KEY FEATURES AND POTENTIAL BENEFITS

Several key features in the design of RNAO's nursing order sets make them valuable for nurses. First, the order sets are composed of evidence-based, actionable nursing intervention statements. By embedding the nursing order sets within electronic health information systems, nurses will immediately have access to the best available evidence at their fingertips, reducing the research-to-practice gap.

Second, the interventions within the order sets are aligned with each component of the nursing process: assessment, planning, implementation, and evaluation. The American Nurses Association (ANA) describes the *nursing process* as "the common thread uniting different types of nurses who work in varied areas" (ANA, 2013, para. 1). Therefore, using the nursing process as the organizing framework for the nursing order sets ensures their congruence with the typical nursing workflow (Yildirim & Özkahraman, 2011). It is important to note that although the order sets are intended to support nurses' workflow, none of the intervention statements are preselected. This approach ensures that the nurses use the order sets as a clinical decision support resource rather than a substitute for their own clinical decision-making.

Third, each intervention statement in the order set is linked to the practice recommendations from which they were derived. To illustrate this point, consider the subset of the *Reducing Foot Complications for People with Diabetes Nursing Order Set* (RNAO, 2015) shown in Figure 5.4.

The numbers shown in the column with the heading "PR#" reflect the practice recommendations from which the interventions displayed to the left of the column were derived. For example, the intervention statement "assess risk for foot ulceration/amputation at least annually in all clients with diabetes 15 years or older and more frequently for those at higher risk" was derived from practice recommendations "1.0-2.0."

The actual practice recommendations published in the BPG (RNAO, 2007) are:

1.0   "Physical examination of the feet to assess risk factors for foot ulceration/amputation should be performed by a healthcare professional;

1.1   This examination should be performed at least annually in all people with diabetes over the age of 15 and at more frequent intervals for those at higher risk; and,

2.0   Nurses should conduct a foot risk assessment for clients with known diabetes. This risk assessment includes the following: history of previous foot ulcers; sensation; structural and biomechanical abnormalities; circulation; and self-care behaviour and knowledge."

In addition to linking the practice recommendations to the intervention statements, the order sets provide a summary of the supporting evidence that is also accessible at the point of care.

Fourth, intervention statements in the order set that are supported by the strongest evidence (e.g., meta-analyses, systematic reviews of randomized controlled trials, or randomized controlled trials) are displayed in bold font. One example of this feature is evident in the intervention "Teach about basic foot care" in Figure 5.4, which appears in bold font indicating strong evidence for this intervention.

Reducing Foot Complications for People with Diabetes Nursing Order Set	PR#
See Associated Document for Practice Recommendations (PR). Interventions printed in **bold font** are supported by the strongest evidence.	
Assessment	
❑ **Assess risk for foot ulceration/amputation at least annually in all clients with Diabetes 15 years or older and more frequently for those at higher risk (10042678)** • Obtain history and perform physical examination • The foot risk assessment includes: history of previous foot ulcers; sensation; structural and biomechanical abnormalities; circulation; and self-care behaviour and knowledge Associated Documents: Risk Assessment Algorithm; Diabetes Foot Assessment/Risk Screening Guide; Use Of The Semmes-Weinstein Monofilament and Structural and Biomechanical Abnormalities	1.0-2.0
❑ Classify and document risk for foot ulceration/amputation • Based on assessment of risk factors, clients should be classified as "lower" or "higher" risk for foot ulceration/amputation • Inform client of his/her foot risk status	6.0 3.0
Planning	
❑ Refer clients at higher risk for foot ulceration/amputation to their primary care provider/ specialized (10032567) • Diabetes or foot care treatment/education teams as appropriate	6.0
Implementation	
❑ **Teach about basic foot care (10042825)** • All people with Diabetes should receive basic foot care education; reinforce at least annually Associated Document: Basic Foot Care Education For People With Diabetes	4.0-5.2

FIGURE 5.4   Subset of *Reducing Foot Complications for People with Diabetes Nursing Order Set.*
Reprinted from RNAO, 2015.

Fifth, the nursing order sets include associated documents that are clinical decision support resources derived from the guidelines. Associated documents include resources such as decision trees, algorithms, risk factors, signs and symptoms of adverse conditions, and educational material. Below is an example of an associated document contained in the nursing order set *Working with Families to Promote Safe Sleep for Infants 0–12 Months of Age* (RNAO, 2016d). Associated documents can be integrated into electronic health information systems as reference documents and made available to clinicians whenever and wherever they are needed.

ASSOCIATED DOCUMENT USED AS AN EDUCATIONAL RESOURCE

Strategies to create safe sleep environments for infants:

- Place the infant in a crib, cradle, or bassinet that meets the Canadian safety regulations.

- Keep out any extra items in the sleep environment other than the mattress and a fitted sheet.

- Do not place loose blankets, quilts, or comforters near the infant, between the mattress and the sheet, or under the infant.

- Use caution regarding swaddling of infants.

- Avoid overheating of the infant by placing them in fitted one-piece sleepwear that is comfortable at room temperature and avoid the use of additional blankets.

Reprinted from RNAO, 2016d. ©Registered Nurses' Association of Ontario. All rights reserved.

The sixth feature, ALERTS, promotes the use of technology as an enabler of evidence-based practice. In each order set, ALERTS are displayed in red font to draw attention to specific practices or factors that might jeopardize patient safety. One example from the nursing order set *Assessment of Stroke Patients Receiving Acute Thrombolytic (r-tPA)* (RNAO, 2016c) is: "Monitoring vital signs is important to reduce the risk of secondary brain injury and improve outcomes" (see Figure 5.5). This feature will be particularly useful for nurses using electronic health information systems with more advanced functionality such as triggers and reminders that can be preprogrammed to generate alerts.

A seventh feature is the cross-referencing of the intervention statements in the nursing order sets to the international nursing standardized terminology language (i.e., ICNP). A key advantage of adopting ICNP is the ability to identify synonymous terms and concepts that are used to represent nursing data in electronic health information systems by assigning the same numerical codes to these terms and concepts. ICNP codes are stored in tables built into the technology behind the scenes and referenced as needed when data are extracted for analysis, research, or interoperability—the exchange of information amongst healthcare facilities.

One example of a use case for ICNP codes is the researcher who needs to extract data from different healthcare agencies to perform comparative analyses to establish benchmarks. Another potential use case is the nurse manager who needs to extract and analyze data to evaluate the adoption of a particular evidence-based practice.

Assessment of Stroke Patients Receiving Acute Thrombolytic Therapy (r-tPA) Nursing Order Set	PR#
See Associated Document for Practice Recommendations (PR) The interventions displayed in bold font are supported by the strongest evidence	
ALERT: Nurses should recognize the sudden/new onset of the signs and symptoms of stroke as a medical emergency to expedite access to time dependent stroke therapy; "time is brain"	2.0
Assessment	
☐ Perform neurological assessment on admission (10036772) Associated Document: Neurological Assessment Tools	3.0
☐ Assess vital signs (T, BP, RR, HR, SpO₂) on admission (10032113) *ALERT: Monitoring vital signs is important to reduce the risk of secondary brain injury and improve outcomes*	3.0
☐ Screen for dysphagia risk within 24 hours of the client regaining consciousness post stroke (10050155) **NOTE:** Nurses with the appropriate training should screen for dysphagia using a validated tool, in all practice settings	6.0-6.1
☐ Maintain NPO (including oral medication) until dysphagia risk assessment completed (10044793)	
☐ Assess client's/caregiver's learning needs/readiness (10002781)	13.0
Planning	
☐ Collaborate with interprofessional team, and client/family regarding client-centered plan of care that incorporates advanced, palliative and end of life care planning (10035915)	4.1

FIGURE 5.5 ALERTS in a stroke nursing order set.

RNAO's nursing order sets simplify the evaluation of guideline implementations by seamlessly capturing data on key process and outcome measures for further analysis using data analytics software. RNAO's Nursing Quality Indicators for Reporting and Evaluation (NQuIRE) is one example of a data analytics system. It is used by Best Practice Spotlight Organizations (BPSO), which are healthcare organizations or academic institutions from around the world that have entered into a formal agreement with RNAO to implement BPGs (three in international sites and five in Canadian sites) over a 3-year period and evaluate the impact. NQuIRE collects organization-level data on human resource structural indicators as well as nursing-sensitive process and outcome indicators designed to systematically monitor adoption of the practice changes recommended in the guidelines and evaluate their impact on patient outcomes.

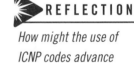

REFLECTION

How might the use of ICNP codes advance nursing practice?

NURSING ORDER SETS IN ACTION

This section showcases nursing order sets in action through an RNAO Canada Health Infoway partnership. RNAO's nursing order sets are vendor neutral. They may be embedded within any electronic health information system, irrespective of the vendor. Since their introduction in 2012, nursing order sets have been implemented by more than 30 healthcare organizations across the spectrum of care including primary care, acute care, home care, and long-term care.

Given RNAO's past successes with Infoway's Peer Leader Model, discussed earlier in this chapter, in 2015 Infoway awarded RNAO funding that allowed them to demonstrate the impact of embedding ICNP-encoded nursing order sets within multiple electronic health information systems to enable automatic data capture and retrieval to support outcome evaluation (Punch, 2017). The main objectives of the project were to train nurse peer leaders across selected project sites to:

1. Promote clinician engagement and adoption of the following advanced clinical e-functions:

    a) e-Clinical decision support: Nursing order sets (embedded in electronic health information systems) that were derived from the following RNAO Best Practice Guidelines:

    ■ *Assessment and Management of Foot Ulcers in People with Diabetes*

    ■ *Assessment and Management of Pressure Injuries for the Interprofessional Team*

    ■ *Strategies to Support Self-Management in Chronic Conditions: Collaboration with Clients*

    b) e-Performance measurement: Technology-enabled data collection and extraction using the ICNP terminology language.

    c) e-Clinical analytics: RNAO's NQuIRE data system to measure the impact of implementing the guidelines.

2. Enhance clinicians' capacity to effectively use patient e-services (i.e., viewing electronic resources) to promote self-management of existing foot ulcers and pressure injuries and prevent the formation of new ones.

Four project sites were selected through a Request for Proposal process, representing home care, long-term care, and two hospital settings. Three of the sites were Designated BPSOs (see Chapter 6).

The project was a resounding success, as depicted in the Infographic on the RNAO Nurse Peer Leader Network Project, displayed in Figure in 5.6. The image shows project details and outcomes from provider, organization, and patient perspectives. As demonstrated, provider and organizational outcomes included integrating nursing order sets in four different types of electronic health information systems; enhancing provider knowledge and expertise; and strengthening evidence-based practice—in assessment, planning, sustained practice change, and evaluation—through technology support. In addition, for patients, results showed improvements in wound healing time and reduced risks and complications, all leading to higher quality of life.

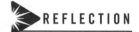 **REFLECTION**

In what ways do nursing order sets embedded in the electronic health record support consistent use of evidence-based practice?

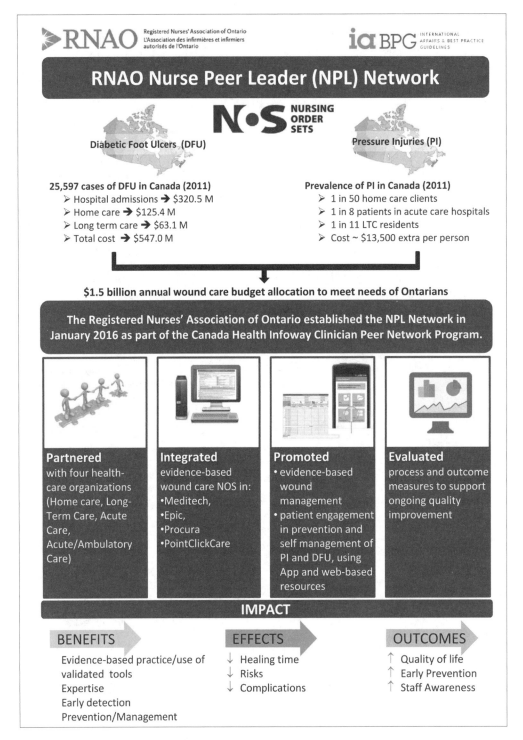

FIGURE 5.6 Infographic on RNAO Nurse Peer Leader Network Project.

NURSING ORDER SET CASE STUDIES

The following case studies provide examples from three healthcare organizations that were part of the RNAO Nurse Peer Leader Network Project. Each case highlights a different focus the organizations took in bringing the project to life in their context. Case 1, a home care setting, used the evidence-based nursing order set to design an app to promote self-management of foot ulcers in patients with diabetes. Case 2 features an acute care setting in which evidence-based practice is facilitated by embedding the nursing order sets for three BPGs into Meditech, their electronic health information system. In Case 3, a long-term care facility used an innovative nursing order set design that enabled providers to see the assessments and interventions together as a unified care plan, enhancing the nursing process.

CASE STUDY

NURSING ORDER SETS IN HOME CARE

In 2015, RNAO awarded a Canadian home-care agency the BPSO Designation after they met the rigorous requirements of the 3-year candidacy program. To date, the agency has implemented seven BPGs across their organization. Four of these guidelines were implemented with the support of nursing order sets embedded within Procura, their electronic documentation system. By embedding RNAO's ICNP-encoded nursing order sets within Procura, direct-care clinicians use the evidence-based intervention statements to generate care plans and inform their practice. In addition, the nursing order sets provide increased ability to collect and monitor data for key process and outcome indicators to support continuous quality improvement (RNAO, 2017b).

Recently, the home care agency utilized an innovative approach to implement the nursing order set *Strategies to Support Self-Management in Chronic Conditions: Collaboration with Clients* (RNAO, 2016b). They designed, developed, and implemented a self-management app and a self-management health coach portal based on the content of the nursing order set. Their goal was to use technology as an enabler of evidence-based wound management for clients with diabetes-related foot ulcers.

The app was piloted in one branch of the home care agency for 5 months. Prior to the implementation of the app, no clients were engaged in the self-monitoring of their foot ulcers.

After the deployment of this resource in the pilot site, there was a consistent upward trend from 10 clients in the first month to 18 clients engaged in this activity when the project ended. Through the use of this innovative approach, clients had direct access to a health coach who provided self-management support and monitored their progress (RNAO, 2017b).

Clients used the self-management app to (RNAO, 2017b):

- Complete a self-management readiness assessment questionnaire that includes a depression screening tool and questions to assess their knowledge of diabetes and foot care

- Identify goals with their health coach

- Self-monitor their symptoms

- Access relevant educational resources

- Enter and track their appointments

- Speak or send a message directly to their health coach

CASE   STUDY

NURSING ORDER SETS IN ACUTE CARE

A Canadian acute care hospital that was also awarded the BPSO Designation in 2015 has implemented nine of RNAO's BPGs to bridge its research-to-practice gap, ensuring that the most current available knowledge is being applied to the care provided to patients and families (RNAO, 2017b). The implementation of three of these guidelines was facilitated by embedding the corresponding nursing order sets within Meditech, the hospital's electronic health information system.

Embedding the intervention statements into the Meditech system made it easy for clinicians to use RNAO's evidence-based guideline and order sets to prevent and manage pressure injuries. Furthermore, the ICNP codes that were built into the back end of the system enabled the organization to collect data for key process and outcome indicators as clinicians completed their electronic

documentation. This implementation strategy also simplified the process of extracting meaningful data to evaluate the impact of the guideline on practice and health outcomes (RNAO, 2017b).

The data obtained from the system to evaluate the process and outcome measures revealed that patients with pre-existing pressure injuries had their wounds assessed on admission 100% of the time. There was also evidence that the monthly average of patients with pressure injuries who received pressure reduction management ranged from 83% to 100% over an 8-month period. The average rate of healing pressure injuries ranged from 25% to 100% monthly. These results provide clear data about which interventions are effective and should be reinforced, and which should be reviewed, revised, and/or refined.

CASE   STUDY

NURSING ORDER SETS IN LONG-TERM CARE

A large Canadian for-profit organization implemented nursing order sets in two of its long-term care homes in Ontario (RNAO, 2017b). The order sets were embedded in PointClickCare, the organization's electronic health information system. The organization is not a BPSO.

The nursing order sets were embedded within the care planning methodology as user-defined assessments. This design enabled direct-care staff to view the complete order sets as distinct entities within the system. This design was markedly different compared to other software applications where components of the order sets are typically built as separate entities in the system. For example, assessments are built separately from the related interventions. Therefore, clinicians are seldom aware that these components are part of a nursing order

set. In contrast, by building the nursing order sets as user-defined assessments, care providers were able to see the assessments and interventions together in one document. This design also allowed the organization to use an innovative approach to incorporate the ICNP codes into the system on the front end, which increased the staff's awareness of this standardized terminology and provided the added value of using the codes to extract data for ongoing monitoring, evaluation, and continuous quality improvement (RNAO, 2017b).

Care providers readily adopted the nursing order sets, which they affectionately termed "my new best friend." By completing and then checking off the interventions in the nursing order sets, the care providers were assured that the residents were receiving evidence-based care.

RNAO's evidence-based nursing order sets are expediting knowledge translation across sectors, as can be seen through the experiences of these three organizations, which represent three different sectors. Each of these organizations demonstrated that technology-enabled guideline implementation, using nursing order sets as clinical decision support resources, reinforce and sustain evidence-based practice. The innovative use of the order sets in the app in one organization also highlighted the potential for technology-enabled patients' self-management informed by the best evidence. Lastly, ICNP-encoded nursing order sets seamlessy facilitated technology-enabled data collection and retrieval for quality monitoring and evaluation.

EHEALTH BPG: ADOPTING EHEALTH SOLUTIONS

While many of the health resources described herein have been developed with extensive nursing and clinician input and user feedback, this is not always the case. When more attention is paid to "getting it done" rather than to "getting it done right" in relation to eHealth, the system experiences loss of time, money, and opportunities for high-quality healthcare. The next section highlights RNAO's development of a System and Healthy Work Environment BPG to reinforce the importance of nursing and other clinician involvement in eHealth adoption in healthcare.

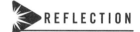

REFLECTION

In your workplace, how is technology used to support evidence-based practice? Consider how engaged in eHealth you are or could be in your nursing role.

The eHealth BPG, *Adopting eHealth Solutions: Implementation Strategies*, was incubated early in 2016, during discussions between RNAO and Canada Health Infoway (RNAO, 2017a). The decision was made to partner and produce a BPG to help executive nurses and other key healthcare stakeholders, including clinicians, effectively lead and support the implementation and adoption of digital health solutions across Canada. Infoway's Chief Nursing Executive cochaired the BPG development panel along with a nurse informatics expert and administrative lead in a large urban acute care setting.

The evidence-based guideline published by RNAO in February 2017 was specifically designed to enhance the eHealth capacity of (RNAO, 2017a):

- Healthcare leaders, nurses, and other health professionals in practice, education, administration, and informatics to optimize their involvement in the procurement, design, implementation, adoption, and optimization of an eHealth solution

- Healthcare executives and clinical/nonclinical leaders, educators, and administrators at the organization and system levels to effectively identify and address the eHealth education needs of the healthcare workforce

- Government agencies, administrators, and policymakers to identify and implement relevant evidence-based policies that support health system transformation and nationwide health information exchange by addressing known barriers to eHealth adoption at the national and jurisdictional levels

"We believe this guideline is a key resource for healthcare executives, frontline nurses and other healthcare providers, and helps us achieve Infoway's vzision of healthier Canadians through innovative digital health solutions."

—Michael Green
President and CEO
Canada Health Infoway

The guideline was developed by an international and interprofessional panel of experts using RNAO's rigorous and systematic guideline development process. Panel members included patient partners, healthcare executives, nurses, and other health professionals from a range of settings (including informatics, practice, education, research, and policy) (RNAO, 2017a).

All panel members, with the exception of the patient partners, had considerable expertise in eHealth implementations. Furthermore, several had previously been actively involved in implementations that resulted in their organizations attaining Stage 6 or higher on the Healthcare Information and Management Systems Society (HIMSS) Electronic Medical Record Adoption Model (EMRAM). The EMRAM provides an eight-point (0–7) scale to measure the extent to which a healthcare organization uses technology to support care delivery (HIMSS Analytics, 2017). The higher the score on the EMRAM, the closer the organization is to achieving a paperless environment.

The patient partners were chosen because of their personal experiences with the healthcare system and the impacts of receiving care in environments without access to electronic health information. They all supported the use of technology as an enabler to increase clinicians' knowledge and decision-making capacity.

The guideline development process included a systematic review of the peer-reviewed literature and a targeted review of the grey literature to identify the best available evidence to answer the following research questions:

1. What individual- and organizational-level factors contribute to high-quality electronic health information systems and their successful adoption?

2. What education and training do individuals/organizations need to lead and support high-quality electronic health information system implementations and adoption?

3. What system-level factors contribute to high-quality, technology-enabled health service delivery and successful health systems transformation?

Relevant articles and resources published in English from January 2006 to March 2016 were included. A total of 178 peer-reviewed articles and 56 grey literature resources were deemed relevant. Draft guideline recommendations were formulated using the evidence obtained from the literature review. A modified-Delphi technique was employed to obtain panel consensus (i.e., the identity of the panel members was not concealed, but their individual responses to the draft recommendations were concealed from the other members of the group).

The Expert Panel identified 26 evidence-based recommendations that address known micro-level, meso-level, and macro-level barriers to the successful implementation of eHealth solutions. In the BPG, these recommendations are categorized as individual/organization, education, and system/policy.

KEY INDIVIDUAL/ORGANIZATION RECOMMENDATIONS

There are fifteen (15) individual/organization recommendations focusing on micro- and meso-level factors that contribute to the implementation, adoption, and optimal utilization of high-quality eHealth solutions to realize the intended return on investment. These are summarized in the following five bulleted statements (RNAO, 2017a):

- Garner visible executive sponsorship throughout all phases of the Hospital Information System (HIS) implementation.

- Create a specialized chief nursing information officer (CNIO) role as a critical element to advance clinical adoption in healthcare organizations.

- Use formal change and project management methodologies to fully engage relevant stakeholder groups throughout all phases of the implementation for optimal implementation and adoption.

- Incorporate usability processes throughout to enhance individual and organizational efficiencies, effectiveness, and user satisfaction.

- Develop an ongoing post-implementation operational plan that includes data governance structures and processes that support sustainability.

KEY EDUCATION RECOMMENDATIONS

There are four education recommendations that focus on the eHealth education infrastructure required to facilitate the acquisition of informatics competencies by healthcare executives and health professionals. They include (RNAO, 2017a):

- Health organizations and academic institutions will develop an education and training infrastructure that provides opportunities for key stakeholders to develop role-specific informatics competencies.

- Healthcare organizations will facilitate integration of role-specific informatics competencies within executive and professional practice leadership roles using a shared accountability model.

- Nurses and other health professionals will take responsibility for being up-to-date with role-specific eHealth competencies.

- Healthcare organizations will facilitate access to health information, empowering individuals to assume greater responsibility for self-management of their health and to engage in informed dialogue with their health professionals.

KEY SYSTEM/POLICY RECOMMENDATIONS

There are seven system/policy recommendations that address the structure, process, and policy requirements at the macro level to realize the long-term goals of nationwide electronic health information exchange and health systems transformation. They include that national and jurisdictional agencies responsible for eHealth work with key relevant stakeholders and (RNAO, 2017a):

- Develop a comprehensive strategy to achieve nationwide interoperability

- Collaborate to establish an effective governance structure that provides strong, coordinated leadership and works in conjunction with regulatory bodies and professional associations to achieve its eHealth goals

- Provide incentives to foster development of innovative next-generation eHealth solutions

- Develop strategies to mitigate the initial costs for health organizations to adopt eHealth solutions and ongoing financial barriers

- Develop and strategically implement education and training policies to build eHealth capacity in the workforce

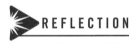

REFLECTION

How could the eHealth BPG be used in your workplace to enhance eHealth adoption?

- Collaborate with regulatory bodies and professional associations to accelerate the adoption of eHealth solutions

- Ensure that the necessary telecommunications infrastructure is in place in remote communities to support the implementation of eHealth solutions

The guideline provides structure, process, and outcome indicators to monitor and evaluate the impact and effectiveness of its implementation as well as links to a variety of related tools. Table 5.3 depicts a sample of such indicators for selected recommendations.

TABLE 5.3 STRUCTURE, PROCESS, AND OUTCOME INDICATORS FOR MONITORING AND EVALUATING THE EHEALTH GUIDELINE

STRUCTURE	PROCESS	OUTCOME	TOOLS
RECOMMENDATIONS 1.1-1.2			
▪ Executive leadership established a formalized governance structure with roles, responsibilities, and sponsorship to guide and support all phases of the implementation of the eHealth solution.	▪ Governance structure established with diverse representation (e.g., interprofessional and cross-functional) and clearly delineated roles and responsibilities.	▪ Governance structure supports successful implementation of the eHealth solution.	▪ Sample governance structures (see pages 31–32 and Appendix E).
RECOMMENDATIONS 1.3			
▪ Organization implemented policies and procedures to support a comprehensive organizational readiness assessment in the early planning phase.	▪ Organization completed a readiness assessment that included individual, organizational, and technical dimensions. ▪ Organization addressed all gaps identified.	▪ Organization demonstrated individual, organizational, and technical readiness.	▪ Standardized organizational readiness assessment tool (see page 34 and Appendix F).

CONCLUSION

Healthcare has scaled a new paradigm since the introduction of eHealth. Globally, eHealth is recognized for its potential to add efficiency to the system as a whole. However, for the system to realize this ideal and engender person-centered care and evidence-based clinical practice, clinicians and patients have to be fully engaged in the design, development, and testing of the resources and tools developed.

This chapter has outlined the work of a professional association in advocating for and enabling clinician and patient engagement in eHealth. The key resources developed by RNAO for clinicians to support technology-enabled evidence-based practice have been described. It is through continued design, development, and use of such resources, and engagement in ongoing research, that we will harness the full power of technology to promote safe, high-quality, evidence-based practice. Finally, co-creating resources that empower patients and all users of the health system with knowledge and self-care capacity will truly lead us to a person-centered healthcare system.

KEY MESSAGES

▪ The RNAO BPG app enables nurses to access the practice recommendations, related evidence, and teaching tools at their fingertips.

▪ Nursing Order Sets expedite knowledge translation.

▪ ICNP codes simplify the evaluation of guideline implementations by seamlessly capturing data on key process and outcome measures.

▪ There is strong evidence to support the value add of using a systematic, participatory approach to eHealth adoption in healthcare.

REFERENCES

American Nurses Association (ANA). (2013). *The nursing process*. Silver Spring, MD: American Nurses Association. Retrieved from http://www.nursingworld.org/EspeciallyForYou/What-is-Nursing/Tools-You-Need/Thenursingprocess.html

Bajnok, I., Burkoski, V., & Doran, D. (2012, October). Enhancing evidence-based nursing practice and quality patient care through information technology [Presentation]. RNAO Conference, *Knowledge, the power of nursing: Celebrating Best Practice Guidelines and clinical leadership*. Conference conducted in Toronto, ON.

Canadian Association of Schools of Nursing. (2012). *Nursing informatics entry-to-practice competencies for registered nurses*. Ottawa, ON: Canadian Association of Schools of Nursing. Retrieved from http://www.casn.ca/2014/12/nursing-informatics-entry-practice-competencies-registered-nurses-2/

Coenen, A., & Kim, T.Y. (2010). Development of terminology subsets using ICNP. *International Journal of Medical Informatics*, 79(7), 530–538.

Doran, D., Haynes, B. R., Estabrooks, C. A., Kushniruk, A., Dubrowski, A., Bajnok, I., . . . Bai, Y. Q. C. (2012). The role of organizational context and individual nurse characteristics in explaining variation in use of information technologies in evidence based practice. *Implementation Science*, 7(1), 122. Retrieved from https://implementationscience.biomedcentral.com/articles/10.1186/1748-5908-7-122

Doran, D., Paterson, J., Clark, C., Srivastava, R., Goering, P. N., Kushniruk, A. W., . . . Jedras, D. (2010). Supporting evidence-based practice for nurses through information technologies. *Worldviews on Evidence-Based Nursing 2010*, 7(1), 4–15. Retrieved from https://inf-fusion.ca/~/media/nurseone/page-content/pdf-en/supporting_evidence-based_practice_for_nurses_through_information_technologies.pdf

Drake, J., Redfern, W., Sherburne, E., Nugent, M., & Simpson, P. (2012). Pediatric skin care: What do nurses really know? *Journal for Specialists in Pediatric Nursing*, 17, 329–338.

Health Canada. (2010). *eHealth*. Retrieved from https://www.canada.ca/en/health-canada/services/health-care-system/ehealth.html

Healthcare Human Factors. (2009). *Order sets in healthcare: An evidence-based analysis*. Retrieved from https://www.colleaga.org/sites/default/files/attachments/Patient-Order-Sets_Report_OHTAC_UHNHHF_Feb_10_Final.pdf

HIMSS Analytics. (2017). *Electronic medical record adoption model*. Retrieved from http://www.himssanalytics.org/emram

Idemoto, L., Williams, B., & Blackmore, C. (2016). Using lean methodology to improve efficiency of electronic order set maintenance in the hospital. *BMJ Quality Improvement Reports*, 5(1), u211725.w4724. doi:10.1136/bmjquality.u211725.w4724

International Council of Nurses (ICN). (2009). *ICNP version 2*. Geneva, CH: International Council of Nurses.

International Health Terminology Standards Development Organization. (2017). *12.2 Appendix B-Vendor case studies: 12.2.10 Epic*. Retrieved from https://confluence.ihtsdotools.org/display/DOCANLYT/12.2.10+Epic

International Organization for Standardization. ISO 18104:2014. (2014). *Health informatics: Categorical structures for representation of nursing diagnoses and nursing actions in terminological systems*. Retrieved from https://www.iso.org/standard/59431.html

International Organization for Standardization. ISO 9241-11.2 (en). (2016). *Ergonomics on human-system interaction—Part 11: Usability: Definitions and concepts*. [ISO online browsing platform]. Retrieved from https:// www.iso.org/obp/ui/#iso:std:iso:9241:-11:dis:ed-2:v2:en:sec:A.7

Kim, T. Y., Hardiker, N., & Coenen, A. (2014). Inter-terminology mapping of nursing problems. *Journal of Biomedical Informatics, 49,* 213–220.

Kruse, G. R., & Rigotti, N. A. (2014). Routine screening of hospital patients for secondhand tobacco smoke exposure: A feasibility study. *Preventive Medicine, 69,* 141–145.

Kumar, S. (2012). Using technology to close the evidence-practice gap: A south Australian experience. *The Internet Journal of Allied Health Sciences and Practice, 10*(4), Article 3. Retrieved from http://nsuworks.nova.edu/ijahsp/vol10/iss4/3/

National Library of Medicine (NLM). (2016). *Supporting interoperability: Terminology, subsets and other resources.* Retrieved from https://www.nlm.nih.gov/hit_interoperability.html

Punch, D. (2017). Bold strategies: Put the work in during the early stages. *Registered Nurse Journal, 29*(3), 26–29.

Registered Nurses' Association of Ontario (RNAO). (2006). *Nursing's involvement in Ontario's eHealth strategy: Project report prepared for the Ministry of eHealth and Long Term Care.* Toronto, ON: RNAO.

Registered Nurses' Association of Ontario (RNAO). (2007). *Reducing foot complications for people with diabetes.* Toronto, ON: RNAO.

Registered Nurses' Association of Ontario (RNAO). (2009). *Nursing's involvement in Ontario's eHealth strategy: Project report prepared for the Ministry of eHealth and Long Term Care.* Toronto, ON: RNAO.

Registered Nurses' Association of Ontario (RNAO). (2012). *Nurses educator eHealth resource: Integrating eHealth into the undergraduate nursing curriculum.* Toronto, ON: RNAO.

Registered Nurses' Association of Ontario (RNAO). (2013a). *Assessment and management of foot ulcers for people with diabetes* (2nd ed.). Toronto, ON: RNAO.

Registered Nurses' Association of Ontario (RNAO). (2013b). *Nursing's involvement in Ontario's eHealth strategy: Project report prepared for eHealth Ontario.* Toronto, ON: RNAO.

Registered Nurses' Association of Ontario. (2015). *Reducing foot complications for people with diabetes* [Nursing order set]. Toronto, ON: RNAO.

Registered Nurses' Association of Ontario (RNAO). (2016a). *RNAO Nursing Best Practice Guidelines* (App). Retrieved from https://itunes.apple.com/us/app/rnao-nursing-best-practice/id386783615?mt=8

Registered Nurses' Association of Ontario (RNAO). (2016b). *Strategies to support self-management in chronic conditions: Collaboration with clients nursing order set.* Toronto, ON: RNAO.

Registered Nurses' Association of Ontario (RNAO). (2016c). *Stroke assessment across the continuum of care nursing order set.* Toronto, ON: RNAO.

Registered Nurses' Association of Ontario (RNAO). (2016d). *Working with families to promote safe sleep for infants 0–12 months of age nursing order set.* Toronto, ON: RNAO.

Registered Nurses' Association of Ontario (RNAO). (2017a). *Adopting eHealth Solutions: Implementation strategies.* Toronto, ON: RNAO.

Registered Nurses' Association of Ontario (RNAO). (2017b). *RNAO nurse peer leader network: Final evaluation report.* Toronto, ON: RNAO.

Slavik Cowen, P., & Moorhead, S. (2014). *Current issues in nursing* (8th ed.). St. Louis, MO: Mosby.

Wieteck, P. (2008). Furthering the development of standardized nursing terminology through an ENP-ICNP cross-mapping. *International Nursing Review, 55,* 296–304.

Wilson, R. (2013, July). Nursing order sets standardize care across sectors, geographical areas. *Hospital News.* Retrieved from: http://www.hospitalnews.com/nursing-order-sets-standardize-care-across-sectors-geographical-areas/

Wilson, R., Bajnok, I., & Costa, T. (2015). Promoting evidence-based care through nursing order sets. *MedUNAB, 17*(3), 176–181.

World Health Organization (WHO) and International Telecommunication Union (ITU). (2012). *National eHealth strategy toolkit: Overview.* Geneva, CH: WHO & ITU. Retrieved from http://www.who.int/ehealth/publications/overview.pdf?ua=1

Yildirim, B., & Özkahraman, S. (2011). Critical thinking in nursing process and education. *International Journal of Humanities and Social Science, 1*(13), 257–262.

BEST PRACTICE SPOTLIGHT ORGANIZATION: IMPLEMENTATION SCIENCE AT ITS BEST

Irmajean Bajnok, PhD, MScN, BScN, RN
Doris Grinspun, PhD, MSN, BScN, RN, LLD(hon), Dr(hc), O.ONT
Heather McConnell, MA(Ed), BScN, RN
Barb Davies, PhD, RN, FCAHS

LEARNING OBJECTIVES

After reading this chapter, you will be able to:

- Describe the RNAO Best Practice Spotlight Organization (BPSO) Designation as a global meso- and macro-level knowledge translation (KT) strategy

- Identify key requirements of the BPSO Designation and how they are informed by implementation science

- Understand how the Knowledge-to-Action framework guides the work of the BPSOs and RNAO's consultation and approaches for support

- Discuss the importance of using a change management approach in BPG implementation activities and how that is addressed in the BPSO Designation

- Outline how the types and models of BPSO contribute to widespread Best Practice Guideline (BPG) uptake and sustained use

- Determine factors that contribute to the success of BPSOs in implementing and sustaining BPGs

- Gain an appreciation of collective identity and how it is cultivated amongst BPSOs globally

INTRODUCTION

In 2003, RNAO launched a highly successful organizational knowledge-transfer strategy: the Best Practice Spotlight Organization (BPSO) Designation. Through this strategy, service and academic organizations formally partner with RNAO to systematically implement RNAO's clinical Best Practice Guidelines (BPG)—augmented with System and Healthy Work Environment guidelines; sustain and spread the use of BPGs; and create a culture of evidence-based practice (Bajnok, Grinspun, Lloyd, & McConnell, 2015). Academic BPSOs integrate RNAO's evidence-based guidelines throughout the curriculum. In the ensuing years, the BPSO Designation has:

- Been awarded to health service organizations in all sectors and in academic institutions

- Involved nurses, faculty, students, and other healthcare professionals (including physicians, social workers, occupational therapists, physiotherapists, speech therapists, dieticians, and nonregulated staff)

- Spread to 12 countries around the world

- Been the impetus for implementation of all of RNAO's 41 clinical and 12 System and Healthy Work Environment BPGs

- Resulted in changes in practice and the work environment the world over

- Improved health and clinical outcomes and quality of life for clients

- Enhanced organizational performance

- Contributed to healthcare cost savings

This chapter discusses key aspects of the BPSO Designation, including its initial vision almost 15 years ago (Di Costanzo, 2013; Grinspun, 2011), its key objectives, current requirements, and place in the global healthcare community today. The chapter concludes with a look at the future in relation to sustaining BPSO and BPSO Host Designates and maintaining quality.

WHY BPSOS

In 2002, following the preparation of numerous BPG Champions (Grinspun, Virani, & Bajnok, 2002), to help implement the first published RNAO BPGs, it became clear that Champions, while necessary to evidence use, were not sufficient to create a sustained organizational culture of evidence-based practice. Nor could they alone make new practices and the use of new knowledge "stick" within their practice area and across the organization. It was obvious that enduring practice change took a team and consideration at multiple levels in an organization. In addition, it took concerted effort, organizational commitment, leadership, and knowledge about both best clinical evidence and best evidence in implementation science (Grinspun, 2011; Grinspun, Melnyk, & Fineout-Overholt, 2014; Higuchi, Davies & Ploeg, 2017; Melnyk & Fineout-Overholt, 2015; Melnyk et al., 2016; Ploeg, Davies, Edwards, Gifford, & Miller, 2007).

RNAO's vision was to foster evidence-based organizations so that BPGs could be readily implemented using the Champions and other members of the team with the goal of achieving better client, provider, organizational, and system outcomes. Central to the vision was the rigorous BPG development process that RNAO had honed over the previous 5 years (Bajnok et al., 2015; Grinspun, 2011; Grinspun et al., 2014; Grinspun et al., 2002); the early attention RNAO paid to moving the best evidence into daily practice by building individual capacity; and the wide dissemination of guidelines through its broad network of nurses, healthcare professionals, and health system and policy stakeholders (Grinspun, Lloyd, Xiao, & Bajnok, 2015).

Through feedback from Champions and specially trained Clinical Resource Nurses, RNAO began to cultivate opportunities to engage with entire organizations to support them in key activities to implement Best Practice Guidelines throughout their institutions. As a result of these early activities, the BPSO Designation was conceived and inaugurated in 2003 (Bajnok et al., 2015; Di Costanzo, 2013; Grinspun, 2011) as an opportunity for healthcare organizations to formally partner with RNAO to systematically implement and sustain BPGs in practice and evaluate their impact. The BPSO Model is a practice model that incorporates structures, processes, and evaluation methods to support sustained use of Best Practice Guidelines and deliver improved outcomes for patients, providers, and the organization.

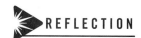

REFLECTION

Have you ever tried to initiate practice change based on a clinical practice guideline in your organization? What were the challenges? How would it have been more effective if the entire organization was on board with what you were attempting to achieve?

BPSO OBJECTIVES

The specific objectives of this innovative BPG uptake endeavour are to:

- Establish dynamic, long-term partnerships that focus on making an impact on patient care through supporting knowledge-based nursing practice

- Demonstrate creative strategies for successfully implementing nursing Best Practice Guidelines at the individual and organizational levels

- Establish and deploy effective approaches to evaluate implementation activities, utilizing structure, process, and outcome indicators

- Identify effective strategies for system-wide dissemination of guideline implementation and outcomes

SELECTING THE BPSOS

Beginning in 2003, the first BPSOs were selected through a competitive request-for-proposal application process. This resulted in nine BPSOs representing sectors including home healthcare, acute care, and rehabilitation care in the Canadian provinces of Ontario and Quebec. These pioneer BPSOs paved the way for the now-coveted BPSO Designation. From the outset there were very specific supports offered by RNAO and clear deliverables expected of the BPSOs.

Today, as in previous years, through the formal application process, applicants are required to demonstrate their commitment to engaging in the BPSO Designation at all levels in the organization, their short- and long-term objectives for BPSO, as well as their experiences and characteristics that will ensure success. Organizations also identify which BPGs they have selected to implement and how they were chosen. Over the ensuing years, the process has become more refined and rigorous; however, the key elements of organizational commitment and intent to sustain this work have been consistent, as has been the provision of RNAO coaching and consultation support and attention to principles of knowledge translation (KT).

Due to the high interest in the BPSO Designation in Canada and around the world, a number of information resources have been designed for potential BPSOs such as webinars, question-and-answer sessions, in person presentations, the BPSO website, and the "Steps to Becoming a BPSO" flyer (see Appendix A to view a copy of the flyer). They inform and support the application process for organizations that see the high value of the BPSO Designation, as expressed in the quote below by a chief nursing executive at a large hospital.

> *"If you want to propel nursing professional practice forward and succeed at achieving highly reliable, safe care in your organization, become a BPSO."*

—Vanessa Burkoski, RN, BScN, MScN, DHA
Chief Nursing Executive
Humber River Hospital

In their evaluation, Ploeg et al. (2007) found that factors at the individual, organizational, and environmental (systems) level influenced BPG implementation, many of which are foundational to the BPSO Designation. These include leadership support, Champions, teamwork and collaboration, professional association support, and inter-organizational collaboration and networks.

THE BPSO DESIGNATION

Fifteen years later, the BPSO Designation is well recognized around the world and acknowledged as an award-winning innovation (Health Council of Canada, 2012; Kirschling & Erikson, 2010; WHO, 2015) that is closing the gap between the knowledge we have and how we use it in our practice (Melnyk, 2017).

As BPSOs, organizations agree to engage in a 3-year qualifying experience that is formalized as a partnership and delineated in a signed BPSO Agreement between the organization and the RNAO (RNAO, 2017a). The elements of the agreement include what the organization (BPSO) commits to and what supports the RNAO will provide. The mutual mandate is that the organization develops a supportive and sustainable infrastructure; builds capacity; implements multiple BPGs; disseminates the processes and outcomes of their BPSO activities; and evaluates the impacts on practice, clients, and the organization as a whole. These are recommended organizational strategies based in implementation science that contribute to building environments for evidence-based practice to flourish and health outcomes to improve (Grinspun et al., 2014; Melnyk, 2014).

Following the 3-year qualifying period, pending achievement of all required deliverables, the organization becomes a Designated BPSO. This recognition acknowledges the organization's achievements in the systematic implementation and evaluation of evidence-based practices while demonstrating an evidence-based culture. As a BPSO Designate, the engagement is ongoing as BPSOs focus on sustaining the practice changes they implemented, spreading their work, and implementing new BPGs. They also continue contributing data to NQuIRE, RNAO's robust international data system for measuring BPG impacts on clients and providers (Grinspun et al., 2015), and myBPSO, RNAO's electronic reporting system for BPSOs. In addition, BPSO Designates become mentors for new BPSO organizations locally, nationally, and internationally—a much-needed resource for those organizations starting to implement best practices (Bajnok et al., 2015; Melnyk, 2014). The BPSO Designation is renewed every 2 years based on achievement of the requirements.

THE BPSO HOST MODEL

The RNAO BPSO Designation has experienced a very rapid spread globally, which precipitated RNAO to redesign the BPSO Designation in 2012 to include opportunities for broad global support and spread through the BPSO Host Model—a type of BPSO satellite (Albornos-Munoz, González-María, & Moreno-Casbas, 2015; Bajnok et al., 2015; Grinspun, 2011). The BPSO Hosts support organizations in their jurisdiction to become BPSOs and work directly with them. BPSO Direct organizations focus on evidence-based practice in their own institutions; they receive support from and report to a BPSO Host.

The BPSO Hosts currently established represent government agencies, academic conglomerates, regulatory bodies, and labour unions. The requirements for success as a BPSO Host are that they must:

- Demonstrate capacity to engage organizations in their jurisdiction to become BPSO Directs with them

- Request and review applications through a request-for-proposal process

- Formalize relationships with selected organizations through a BPSO Agreement

- Provide support to their BPSO Directs to achieve outcomes

- Monitor the outcomes achieved

- Report to RNAO through myBPSO, as a BPSO Host and on behalf of all its BPSO Direct organizations

- Measure and report on outcomes

BPSO Hosts enter into a BPSO Host Agreement with RNAO (RNAO, 2017b), committing to use RNAO's methodologies and materials and RNAO's approaches to coaching, monitoring, and evaluation.

BPSO Hosts meet regularly with RNAO to share successes and challenges and gain support for their Host activities. To date, Spain (through the Nursing and Healthcare Research Unit [Investén-iscci] Institute of Health Carlos III), Australia (through the Australian Nursing and Midwifery Federation [ANMF]—SA Branch), and Italy (through the Collegio IPASVI Milano—Lodi—Monza e Brianza), amongst others, have been involved in the BPSO Designation through the BPSO Host Model. These BPSO Hosts, with RNAO's support, lead the BPSO Designation in their jurisdictions and have successfully initiated and sustained this innovative and highly effective organizational KT strategy. Below is a quote from the BPSO Host Sponsor and the BPSO Host Lead in Italy reinforcing pride in being a BPSO Host and the impact of their work with outcomes apparent in their BPSO Directs.

"As the first BPSO Host in Italy we are very proud to be working in partnership with RNAO to bring Italy the BPGs through the BPSO model to improve nursing care and education. We are excited to begin as a Host with two BPSOs—a service BPSO and an academic BPSO—that are partner organizations. Already we have experienced great benefits in the practice of nursing, our relationships with doctors, and nursing morale. In the university it is strengthening the curriculum specifically in the areas of BPG implementation."

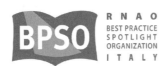

—Giovanni Muttillo, RN, MsN
President of the Collegio IPASVI Milano-Lodi Monza-Brianza
Director of Health Professions at the Local Health Agency of Teramo
Scientific Director of BPSO Host, Italy

—Loris Bonetti, PhD, RN, MsN
Councilor of the Collegio IPASVI Milano-Lodi Monza-Brianza
Expert in clinical nursing research at the Oncology Institute of Southern Switzerland,
IOSI, Bellinzona(Ch)
Nurse Leader of the BPSO Host, Italy

New BPSO Hosts are currently being developed in Chile, Nova Scotia (Canada), and Peru. Table 6.1 summarizes the various types and models of BPSOs within the BPSO Designation.

TABLE 6.1 TYPES AND MODELS OF BPSO DESIGNATION

TYPES OF BPSOS	DESCRIPTION
Service	Focus on evidence-based practice to impact client and organizational outcomes by integrating BPGs in service organizations at the point of care. ■ Any health sector (i.e., public health, primary care, hospital, home care, long-term care)
Academic	Focus on evidence-based nursing education to impact student learning, and ultimately client outcomes, by integrating BPGs in academic curricula.

MODELS OF BPSOS	DESCRIPTION
BPSO Direct	The organization develops a relationship with a BPSO Host and meets deliverables over a 3-year qualifying period to become a BPSO Designate. In countries where RNAO has a BPSO Host, BPSO Directs in that country receive support from that BPSO Host and report to that BPSO Host. In countries where RNAO has not established a BPSO Host, BPSO Directs receive support from RNAO and report to RNAO.
BPSO Host	The organization develops a relationship with RNAO to oversee the BPSO Designation in their jurisdiction and support their BPSO Directs. All BPSO Hosts receive support from RNAO and report to RNAO.

BPSO IMPLEMENTATION STRATEGIES

The implementation consultation and coaching strategies used by RNAO and the specific BPSO Agreement requirements are grounded in implementation science (Gallagher-Ford, 2014; Grinspun et al., 2014; RNAO, 2012; Stetler, Richie, Rycroft-Malone, & Charns, 2014; Straus, Tetroe, & Graham, 2013). The following seven implementation strategies are embedded in the formal agreements organizations sign with RNAO once selected to be a BPSO (Bajnok et al., 2015):

1. Use a systematic, planned approach to implementation (RNAO, 2012)

2. Incorporate change principles in the guideline implementation process (Grol, Wensing, Eccles, & Davis, 2013; Haines, 2005; Heath & Heath, 2010; Kotter, 2012)

3. Engage leaders in all roles, both formal and informal (including BPSO Sponsors, BPSO Leads, Champion Leaders, Champions, BPG Leaders, and BPSO Steering Committee members), in all stages of BPG implementation (Aarons et al., 2016; Gifford, Davies, Tourangeau, & Lefebre, 2011; Higuchi et al., 2017; Stetler et al., 2014; Straus et al., 2013)

4. Align BPG implementation to the organization's priorities to include the vision, mission, and strategic plan; quality-improvement initiatives; and government directives (Higuchi, Downey, Davies, Bajnok, & Waggott, 2013; Melnyk, 2014; Ploeg et al., 2007)

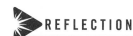

REFLECTION

Think about past experiences you have had in attempting to make practice change based on clinical practice guidelines. How would attention to these seven elements assist in BPG implementation?

5. Select approaches to implementation informed by assessments of facilitators and barriers to knowledge uptake, and level of knowledge of the practice change (RNAO, 2012; Straus et al., 2013)

6. Integrate BPG recommendations into organizational processes, structures, and roles to enable dynamic sustainment (Chambers, Glasgow, & Stange, 2013; Maher, Gustafson, & Evans, 2010)

7. Interact with a broader network of organizations striving for similar goals related to creating evidence-based cultures and implementing evidence-based guidelines (Melnyk, 2014; Straus et al., 2013)

RNAO COACHING AND CONSULTATION

The BPSO Host Coaches, including the RNAO Coaches working with their BPSO Directs, use the RNAO (2012) *Toolkit: Implementation of Best Practice Guidelines* and the Knowledge-to-Action framework (Straus et al., 2013) to guide their regular consultative sessions with BPSOs. This assists the BPSO Directs in making progress to achieve the BPSO requirements and deliverables over the 3-year period prior to designation. These deliverables are monitored by the BPSO Hosts and by RNAO for their BPSO Directs.

The monitoring process occurs in a variety of ways as established by BPSO Hosts to mirror the processes used by RNAO. These include regular meetings with Coaches, scheduled presentations to the BPSO knowledge exchange networks required in each BPSO Host jurisdiction, and semi-annual written reports to the BPSO Host (or to RNAO in cases where there is not a jurisdictional Host).

All BPSOs submit their reports through myBPSO, the online reporting system launched by RNAO in October 2015 to capture the specific deliverables related to guideline implementation, capacity development, dissemination, sustainability, and evaluation. The report auto-populates with previously inputted data, so BPSO Leads need to populate reports with new information only. The frequency of reporting is either biannually, or in the case of Designated BPSOs, annually. The evaluation data and other relevant contextual information from myBPSO are critical complements to NQuIRE's indicator data. During the 3-year predesignation period, the formal BPSO Agreement is renewed annually pending performance reviews. Following designation, agreements are renewed every 2 years, again based on achievement of deliverables. These processes are the same for service and academic BPSOs.

A SYSTEMATIC IMPLEMENTATION PROCESS

Elements of the Toolkit (RNAO, 2012) that are part of the BPSO performance expectations and used as indicators of success are outlined below. These are described in detail in Chapter 4, *Forging the Way with Implementation Science*. The Toolkit (RNAO, 2012), a handbook of implementation science for BPG uptake, informs the curriculum for the RNAO BPG Champion program and the RNAO Clinical BPG Institute, both of which inform the BPSO Orientation Program. The elements are derived from the Knowledge-to-Action Model (Graham et al., 2006; Straus et al., 2013) and include:

- Leaders at all levels make a commitment to support facilitation of guideline implementation.

- Guidelines are selected for implementation through a systematic, participatory process.

- Specific guideline recommendations are tailored to the local context.

- Stakeholders that will be impacted by the implementation of the guidelines are identified and engaged in the implementation process.

- Environmental readiness assessment for implementation is conducted for its impact on guideline uptake.

- Barriers and facilitators to use of the guideline are assessed and addressed on an ongoing basis.

- Interventions are selected that consider barriers and facilitators within the organization.

- Guideline use is systematically monitored and sustained.

- Action plans for sustainability of practice changes are developed, reviewed, and updated on a regular basis.

- Evaluation of the impacts of guideline use is embedded into the process.

- Adequate resources to complete the activities related to all aspects of guideline implementation are made available.

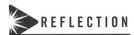 **REFLECTION**

After reviewing the RNAO (2012) Implementation Toolkit, think about how you may have used it in the past, or might use it in the future, to create practice change.

These elements ensure a systematic implementation process and are used by senior administration BPSO sponsors, BPSO Leads, Champion Leaders, BPG Champions, and BPG Leaders.

ENSURING BPSO SUCCESS

There are a number of features delineated as expectations that make the BPSO Designation a most effective knowledge translation (KT) strategy to bring evidence to sustained daily use in practice. These are recognized as strategies "that work" and continue to be espoused in the literature (Melnyk, 2014). They have been honed over the last 15 years of the BPSO Designation based on implementation science research and experiential knowledge and are included in the BPSO Agreement. They represent the following elements: development of an infrastructure, capacity building, implementation, dissemination, monitoring and reporting progress, evaluation, as well as audit and feedback. Each is discussed next.

INFRASTRUCTURE

The BPSO Agreement reinforces that it is important to create an infrastructure. It involves individuals in key roles; defined reporting relationships; linkages to committees that oversee and make strategic decisions about BPG implementation and resource allocation, and to existing structures that make and implement operational decisions to support guideline implementation (RNAO, 2017b). Many of these elements are supported by Grol et al. (2013).

The BPSO infrastructure must not be separate from the ongoing business of the organization and must be tightly connected to existing groups focused on professional practice and quality/risk management, such that the BPSO and guideline implementation are part of the organization's mainstream operations. Moreover, and as indicated previously, organizations are advised to leverage their mission, vision, strategic directions, and quality-improvement activities to align with the BPSO goals (Bajnok et al., 2015). These are also characteristics recommended by Melnyk (2014).

In exploring the roles of system and organizational leadership in evidence-based intervention, Aarons et al. (2016) demonstrated strong relationships between transformational leadership and visible support, and success in evidence-based intervention. In addition, the authors noted the importance of alignment, in support for evidence-based practice (EBP), amongst leadership at the clinical, middle management, and executive levels. This important point is supported by many who have studied success factors in EBP implementation (Aarons et al., 2016; Bajnok et al., 2015; Chambers et al., 2013; Gifford et al., 2011; Higuchi et al., 2017; Melnyk, 2014; Rogers, 2003; Stetler et al., 2014). The BPSO Host and Direct Models creates clear expectations for strong links between the support and mentoring of leadership at the executive nurse level—and indeed all levels in the organization—in order to fuel success in initiating and sustaining EBP.

Key deliverables in relation to the infrastructure expectations of a BPSO Direct include:

- Formation of a steering committee consisting of key stakeholders fully engaged with the BPSO work, including the BPSO Sponsor, BPSO Lead, Champion Leaders, BPG Leaders and Champions, and other stakeholders who will be impacted by, or who can influence, its success

- Identification of a BPSO Sponsor, who is usually the Chief Nurse Executive or equivalent role, who champions the BPSO Designation within the senior team and organization and supports the BPSO Lead

- Appointment of a BPSO Lead who is able to devote at least half of her work time to lead the BPSO, manage deliverables, carry out related activities, and be the organization's link to RNAO (in some cases, depending on the organizational context, the BPSO Sponsor may also act as the BPSO Lead)

- Creation of BPG implementation teams and BPG Leaders who lead the implementation team; become experts on the topic and the BPG; and work with the BPSO Lead to develop and monitor implementation strategies from practice change, to policy reviews and revision, to education activities for direct-care nurses and others

- Development of Champions in all roles who work directly with their peers in knowledge broker, ambassador, teaching, mentoring, and role-modeling activities

- Establishment of key reporting and decision-making processes, as depicted in a model describing their BPSO infrastructure

Years of working with BPSOs have demonstrated that when these structures are in place, the BPSO Designation is valued, visible, integrated, and aligned with organizational priorities, achieved in a timely manner, and sustained for the long term.

CAPACITY BUILDING

It is critical that education be provided to staff in all roles so they can lead and support the practice changes resulting from the BPG implementation (Melnyk, 2017). The RNAO BPSO Direct Agreement stipulates several capacity-building requirements that must be undertaken by staff.

Capacity-building activities generally begin with the BPSO Orientation Program, to which each BPSO must send representatives as stipulated in the BPSO Agreement, including the Chief Nurse as the BPSO sponsor, BPSO Lead, and Champion Leaders. Other and ongoing capacity-building activities include: development and maintenance of a cohort of Best Practice Champions; attendance at RNAO's Clinical BPG Institute; involvement in monthly virtual knowledge-exchanges sessions for qualifying BPSOs and quarterly sessions for Designate BPSOs; and attendance at the annual in-person BPSO Knowledge Exchange Symposium. The attention to ensuring key leaders in the BPSO have a strong EBP knowledge base, an understanding of RNAO's BPGs and the BPSO, is well founded in the literature. Implementation science experts have reached a strong consensus that an understanding of evidence-based practice (Bajnok et al., 2015; Grinspun et al., 2014; Melnyk, 2017; Melnyk et al., 2014; Stetler et al., 2014), and in particular of the science of creating and sustaining practice (Gallagher-Ford, Buck, & Melnyk, 2014; Grol et al., 2013; Higuchi et al., 2017) change, is imperative if BPGs are to be implemented by nursing and other staff.

BPSO ORIENTATION

The BPSO Orientation is a 2-day program scheduled for BPSOs in Ontario, or a 5-day program scheduled for sites outside Ontario. For Ontario sites, the 2-day session is scheduled as a launch, with engagement of Ontario's Chief Nurse, other members of the government, the RNAO CEO, and the

RNAO BPG Team, including the BPSO Coaches. The agenda includes details of the RNAO BPG Program and the BPSO Designation, as well as the steps to get started as a BPSO. It also provides for interaction amongst BPSOs and an opportunity for each BPSO to showcase its site, the BPGs selected, and its overall plans.

This helps to build a foundation for the peer networks all BPSOs become a part of and begins to cultivate the collective identity of the new BPSO cohort as a member of the global BPSO community (see Chapter 1 for an introduction and discussion of the concept of collective identity). Following this, the BPG Institute (outlined in detail in Chapter 4) serves as an orientation for the BPSOs who send representatives to the Institute according to their organization size as stipulated in the BPSO Agreement. This 5-day program provides specific knowledge and application sessions based on implementation science to help in BPG implementation and related deliverables expected of BPSOs.

For international BPSOs, there are some differences that arise because of distance and the travel and scheduling requirements for RNAO International BPSO Coaches, who lead the orientation sessions in international jurisdictions. International BPSOs must send representatives to the initial BPSO Orientation Program, which is a 5-day BPSO launch and education session hosted by the BPSO site. Since the orientation is on site and scheduled for one or two new BPSOs at a time, the organizations send substantial numbers of staff to this session, generating much energy and imparting new knowledge and skills on a large scale that fuel a successful start-up. In some cases, like in the Latin-American BPSO consortium described in Chapter 15, two countries—Chile and Colombia—joined together for their BPSO Orientation Program, creating a strong and unique bonding that has characterized that region since.

The BPSO launch portion of this orientation serves as an introduction of the program to key government, nursing, and other health professional stakeholders in the country or jurisdiction, and showcases the organization and its goals in becoming a BPSO. In addition, it begins to create a strong sense of collective identity amongst all attendees about their profile as a BPSO and membership in the global BPSO network. This identity is demonstrated, for example, in proud displays of the BPSO logo on nursing units, on written documents (including organizational letterhead), Champion buttons, and uniforms. The logo is country-specific, and in Figure 6.1 the logos for China, Colombia, and Qatar are displayed as examples.

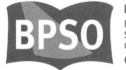 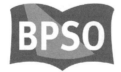 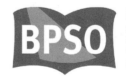

FIGURE 6.1 Logos for China, Colombia, and Qatar.
© Registered Nurses' Association of Ontario. All rights reserved.

The BPSO Orientation Program and the BPG Learning Institutes are identified as training programs in RNAO's Training of Trainers (TOT) Model in which the RNAO BPSO International Coaches, as Master Trainers, train the BPSO Sponsors, BPSO Leads, and Champion Leaders, who in turn train Champions and BPG Leaders in 1- to 2-day workshops in their jurisdictions.

A key factor in BPG uptake in the BPSOs is the focus on the process of change or adoption of the innovation (Grol et al., 2013) and the transition process (Bridges, 1991) or becoming an evidence-based culture. BPSO Sponsors, BPSO Leads, and Champion Leaders learn how to use the change process throughout all aspects of the adoption cycle (Rogers, 2003). Different theories of change are incorporated in their education, including:

- Rogers' (2003) insights on the rate of adoption of change and the categories of adopters

- Conner (2006), who recognizes eight stages of change beginning with first contact and awareness and ending with institutionalization and internalization to secure the new practices

- Kotter's (2012) eight-step change process starting with the burning platform, which helps change agents align the change to organizational realities and create the motivation for change

- The ADKAR model (Hiatt, 2006) which highlights the role of education in change

- Heath & Heath (2010), who focus on practical ways of initiating and sustaining change

In addition, the RNAO Toolkit, reinforcing Lewin's change theory, recognizes the importance of psychological safety (Schein, 1996) as clinicians try out new evidence-based practices.

The BPSO Orientation Program and BPG Learning Institute portray change using Haines's (2005) work, which depicts the ups and downs of change as akin to a rollercoaster ride, and indeed multiple rollercoasters and waves of change, in the nonlinear process of adoption of best practices through transition (Bridges, 1991). The rollercoaster of change shown in Figure 6.2 becomes very symbolic for BPSO Leaders around the world both as they measure their own reactions to change compared to their colleagues, and as they gain knowledge about the predictable responses to change and the need for perseverance (Haines, 2005). This content and the related methodology used in discussion and application, like much of the common content in these orientation sessions, begin to shape the collective identity of BPSOs as members of a global EBP movement.

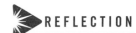

REFLECTION

Think about a situation you have been in where a new approach was introduced. How was change theory used? How could it have been used to enhance the success of the change? Why do you think collective identity is important in large system change?

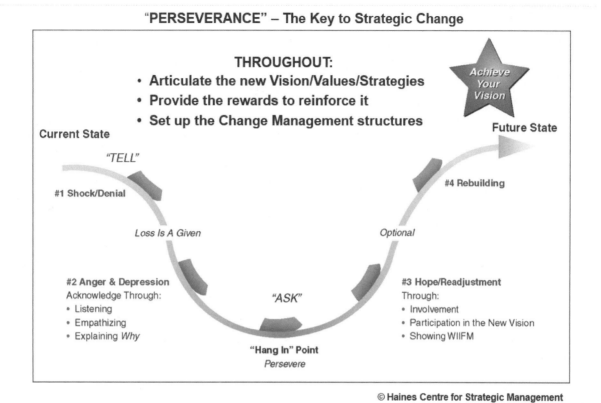

FIGURE 6.2 The Rollercoaster of Change™.
© 2007 Stephen Haines—Haines Centre for Strategic Management. Used with Permission.

CHAMPIONS

RNAO requires in its BPSO Direct and BPSO Host Agreements that BPSOs develop 15% of their nursing staff as Best Practice Champions, who will provide the inspiration and motivation for the change (RNAO, 2017b). This is consistent with diffusion theory that defines *critical mass* as the degree of momentum or energy needed to initiate and sustain a change (Rogers, 2003). The recommended number required to reach critical mass according to Rogers (2003) is 10% to 30% of the target group. RNAO's selection of 15% reflects the combined estimations of innovators (2.5%) and early adopters (13.5%) when adopters are plotted on the adoption curve. Our experience throughout 15 years has been that this number, when maintained and in most cases exceeded, does sustain the momentum for BPG uptake.

The Champion development process begins with staff members being selected by their unit team lead/manager or volunteering to take on this role. They become Champions by participating in a 1-day, in-person workshop; a virtual learning series; or via a self-directed eLearning program. By becoming a Champion, those involved commit to facilitating and leading BPG implementation amongst their peers. Other healthcare professionals are encouraged to become Champions, and hundreds have been prepared through the RNAO Champion program. In addition, there are now thousands of nurses, nursing students, support staff, and more recently members of the public, who have become part of the RNAO Best Practice Champion Network.

BPG CLINICAL LEARNING INSTITUTE

RNAO's Clinical BPG Institute, now in its 16th year, provides an opportunity for nurses and other healthcare professionals to gain knowledge, understanding, and opportunities to apply elements of the Toolkit (RNAO, 2012) to an action plan for guideline implementation. Use of a multifaceted action plan was a key recommendation of Higuchi et al. (2017), based on a study of eight pioneer BPSOs. Participants come to the BPG Institute with an idea of an evidence-based clinical innovation they want to implement and leave with a clear plan of how to bring knowledge to action. Both the Champion's workshop and the BPG Learning Institute are based on the RNAO Implementation Toolkit (2012).

BPSO KNOWLEDGE EXCHANGE SESSIONS

Knowledge exchange sessions with peer BPSOs provide an opportunity to learn from each other's successes and challenges. BPSOs are required to present regular, comprehensive updates to their peers for information, feedback, and problem-solving. The annual BPSO Knowledge Exchange Symposium is hosted by RNAO for all BPSOs, including those who have been designated and those in the pre-designation period. The goals of the Symposium are knowledge exchange, collaboration, celebration, and networking. BPSOs share lessons learned, Designated BPSOs mentor new BPSOs, and implementation science experts bring new knowledge to the group. Leaders from all BPSOs are expected to attend and present their progress during networking sessions that are a highlight of the event.

COACHING AND SUPPORT

Engagement with a BPSO Coach is another key strategy that is embedded in the BPSO Designation. Harvey et al. (2002) emphasized the role of facilitation while leading practice change and introduced the role of external facilitators who utilize an outreach model to work with organizations, providing advice, networking, and support to help them establish the required practice changes. Pre-Designation BPSOs have an assigned experienced implementation expert from RNAO (BPSO Coach) whom they must meet within the first 3 months of becoming a BPSO and maintain regular contact with over the 3-year period. The role of the Coach has recently expanded to include a site visit for the purposes of observing "on the ground" implementation and evaluation. Coaches provide consultation, role modeling, referral to key resources, and early identification of challenges to achieving BPSO Designation.

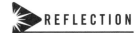

REFLECTION

How do staff with knowledge about implementation science influence BPG uptake and development of an evidence-based practice culture in an organization? Are the principles transferable to other aspects of nursing and patient care?

SUSTAINED IMPLEMENTATION

During the 3-year pre-designation period, Canadian BPSOs are required to implement a minimum of five clinical BPGs (three across the entire organization), and international BPSOs are required to implement a minimum of three (one across the entire organization). This difference in requirement acknowledges the fact that Canadian nurses have had ready access to the RNAO BPG Program and its resources since its inception; it also recognizes that there may be differences in context in international settings related to EBP. BPSOs must determine where (units, programs, teams) the implementation will take place and utilize the practice recommendations to direct the clinical interventions. The education recommendations are used to ensure staff have the knowledge and skill to carry out the clinical interventions, and the organization/policy recommendations to support sustainment of the practice change. These requirements ensure that the practice changes "stick" because of knowledge-able and committed staff, and that the necessary structures and processes are in place to embed the new practices.

All BPSOs are required to develop a sustainability plan focused on organizational structures, processes, and roles and to keep the plan updated to share with RNAO through the required reporting. These elements are strongly supported by Chambers et al. (2013) and Maher et al. (2010) in their discussions of sustainability as part of implementation of EBP. The partnership amongst BPSOs and RNAO provides many opportunities for organizations to receive and give feedback. This enables RNAO and the BPSOs to adapt and modify their approaches based on outcomes, changes in evidence, and changes in context both at the organizational and the system levels. As reinforced by Chambers et al. (2013) in "The Dynamic Sustainability Framework," sustained practice is not a static concept, and there is high recognition for sustainment that evolves over time based on current best evidence.

DISSEMINATION

Given the value of reflection and regular progress reviews, BPSOs are required in their formal agreement to consolidate their work and share it in a public way. This is achieved through professional presentations at local, provincial, national, and/or international conferences; sharing the resources they develop on the RNAO website; or by participating as faculty for RNAO professional development offerings. RNAO also expects that the BPSO will feature its BPSO activities on its organization's website, and more recently it has become a requirement to establish a social media presence through which BPSO work can be disseminated. Finally, development and submission of manuscripts related to the BPSO Designation process and outcomes for publication in peer-reviewed journals is an expectation during the predesignation period and continues post-BPSO Designation. This deliverable contributes to capacity building within BPSOs; positions the BPSO and its leaders locally and beyond, thus strengthening their status in their organizations and communities; facilitates emerging clinical and nursing knowledge for wide consumption; and demonstrates the ever-expanding knowledge base of the nursing profession. BPSOs share their progress on this deliverable in the semi annual or annual report to RNAO.

MONITORING AND REPORTING PROGRESS

As a way of monitoring that all deliverables are met—aside from the opportunities afforded through the regular knowledge exchange meetings, in-person Symposiums, and interaction with the BPSO Coaches—predesignate BPSO Directs and Hosts submit a formal written report to RNAO on a semi-annual basis. As previously mentioned, the reporting format is available online through myBPSO and requires an update on all deliverables. For Designated BPSOs, the reporting requirement is an annual submission, with designation renewal every 2 years. For Canadian BPSO Directs, the IABPG Director and Associate Director of Guideline Implementation and Knowledge Transfer, as well as the BPSO Coach, conduct a virtual meeting with the BPSO Lead, Sponsor, and other members of the BPSO team to discuss the report. For international BPSOs and BPSO Hosts, these meetings are led by either the RNAO CEO or the Director of the International Affairs and Best Practice Guidelines Centre, as their identified Coach.

The ARCH Model (Baker, Turner, & Bush, 2015)—which includes Self **A**ssessment, **R**einforcement, **C**orrection, and **H**elp with an action plan—is used to guide and focus the discussion, ensure two-way communication, identify and reinforce strengths, and outline plans to address any challenges. Follow-up notes are communicated to the BPSO, including areas to address immediately, and areas to be addressed in the next report. At year end, decisions are made to determine if the BPSO has met the annual deliverables in order to move to the next year. At the end of the 3-year period, a review is conducted to determine whether the deliverables have been met sufficiently to enable designation. There have been situations in which, due to competing priorities, staffing changes, or major organizational restructuring, BPSOs require an extension of 6 months to a year in order to achieve the deliverables required for designation. In all cases, these BPSOs have been successful within the extended qualifying timeframe.

EVALUATION

With the establishment of NQuIRE, the evaluation and monitoring deliverable has become robust and consistent across BPSOs (Grinspun et al., 2015). From the outset, BPSOs are expected to collect baseline data for key human resource structure indicators and for process and outcome indicators related to the BPGs they are implementing. Service BPSOs submit monthly data on a quarterly basis to NQuIRE and share their results in their regular written reports to RNAO (Grinspun et al., 2015). Academic BPSOs do not yet submit data to NQuIRE. However, they identify, measure, and report on key indicators such as: BPGs' influence on the overall curriculum, course objectives and content; teaching methodology; student knowledge; and student practice skills.

BPSO HOSTS

BPSO Host organizations have specific deliverables they must meet as part of the signed Agreement with the RNAO Host Organization (RNAO, 2017b). These deliverables focus on actions and accomplishments necessary in their role of recruiting, initiating, and overseeing a cadre of BPSO Directs in their jurisdiction, all of whom must have a signed BPSO Direct Agreement with the Host. BPSO Hosts are supported and monitored by RNAO and are divided between RNAO's CEO and the IABPG Director. The Latin America BPSO Consortium (composed of BPSO Directs in Chile, Colombia, and Portugal, as well as BPSO Hosts in Chile, Peru, and Spain.) also report to RNAO's CEO, who is fluent in Spanish. RNAO's focus in coaching and monitoring is on the BPSO Host itself and its role in the oversight of its BPSO Directs. RNAO's focus extends to those BPSO Directs only to determine the BPSO Host's progress and its ability to meet the deliverables.

AUDIT AND FEEDBACK

In addition to the numerous monitoring strategies used, and based on the views that observing BPSOs in their own context and providing direct feedback on their performance as assessed against the standards (Ivers et al., 2012) is conducive to enhanced behaviours, RNAO conducts a formal, annual, onsite audit of its BPSO Directs and the BPSO Hosts. The value of audit and feedback is reinforced by Ivers et al. (2014), based on the results of an in-depth analysis of a systematic review of 140 studies in which they examined effects on professional practice when audit and feedback were included as a critical aspect of the care processes. Ivers and colleagues (2014) concluded that while there was variation in impact on professionals and patients, audit and feedback were effective in situations in which there was a high learning curve involved in uptake of the new practices and when the feedback was provided by a supervisor or colleague, verbally and in writing, with intention to follow up and an action plan. Audit and feedback were also more effective when targeted to nonphysicians.

Our audit and feedback process meets the above criteria and has become an effective way for us to determine the fidelity of the BPSOs in relation to the program requirements outlined in the BPSO Agreements. The intent is to help BPSO Directs and BPSO Hosts not only to modify their behaviours when they are not meeting expectations, but also to learn what they are doing well in order to sustain these actions. Consistent with the findings of Ivers et al. (2014), the BPSO Coaches are involved in the audit, and they provide verbal and written feedback to the BPSO about their progress. Specific audit tools, aligned with the relevant requirements, have been developed for BPSO Hosts, and academic and service BPSO Directs, and serve as guides to the auditors and as teaching tools during feedback sessions. These sessions also include a focus on specific action plans to be addressed and the timeframe. The audit and feedback processes are outlined in more detail in Chapter 12, *RNAO's Global Spread of BPGs: The BPSO Designation Sustainability and Fidelity*.

SUMMARY OF BPSO REQUIREMENTS

These key deliverables required of qualifying and Designated BPSOs are evidence-based, achievable, and, over a 3-year period and beyond, create the momentum and the milieu needed for sustainment and expansion of evidence-based practice changes. They are summarized here:

- Develop a BPSO infrastructure with structures, people, and processes:
  - Build capacity throughout the organization related to the clinical practice change and an enhanced understanding of knowledge-translation methodologies
  - Participate in regular knowledge exchange sessions with other BPSOs as part of a peer network
  - Act as a mentor or be mentored by others
  - Establish and maintain an informed and engaged cadre of Champions

- Utilize a systematic approach to implementation focused on practice change, education of clinicians and support staff, and embedding the new practices in organizational structures and processes:
  - Consult with the RNAO BPSO Coach to assist with challenges and strategies
  - Develop clear plans for evaluation, including submission of data to NQuIRE, with a focus on structure, process, and outcome indicators and how the results of this data will be shared with staff
  - Disseminate results through professional presentations and scholarly publications
  - Provide regular reports through myBPSO to RNAO focused on key deliverables

The BPSOs consistently identify these requirements and deliverables, in particular the formal partnership and resources and supports from RNAO, as key to their success (RNAO, 2015).

They are all elements of implementation science, and each has been used in some program of evidence-based practice development. The BPSO Designation has bundled this entire set of implementation science practices and principles into one comprehensive knowledge-translation initiative that has achieved proven results and created a collective identity the world over.

As discussed in Chapter 1, *Transforming Nursing Through Knowledge: The Conceptual and Programmatic Underpinnings of RNAO's BPG Program*, BPSOs have an interactive and shared journey, with a clear orientation of their action as well as the opportunities and constraints in which their action takes place. They find motivation amongst themselves and in one another. They recognize that they share certain orientations in common and on that basis decide to act together. BPSOs have active relationships amongst themselves and are intellectually and emotionally invested in their individual and collective success.

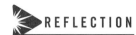
REFLECTION

For each of the major deliverables discussed above, identify why you think they are necessary in creating sustained practice change based on implementation of Best Practice Guidelines.

RNAO'S COMMITMENTS

The BPSO Designation is a partnership between RNAO and the BPSO, mobilized by the collective identity and goals of better outcomes for patients, nurses, other providers, organizations, and the health system as a whole. The partnership reinforces full engagement of BPSOs around the world in all aspects of the designation and espouses the philosophy of sustained capacity building. RNAO's commitments to the BPSO Directs and BPSO Hosts are seen as critical to their ability to meet the deliverables, establish a culture of evidence-based practice, and contribute to sustained capacity building. They include:

- Rigorously developed evidence-based guidelines and implementation resources, all freely available for download on the RNAO website

- Access to technology-enabled implementation resources such as the RNAO BPG app and the evidence-based Nursing Order Sets

- NQuIRE, RNAO's comprehensive indicator database system to measure BPG impact

- Support for opportunities to become a BPSO and be part of a formal BPSO network

- BPSO consultation and coaching from knowledge transfer, guideline development, and evaluation experts

- Provision of comprehensive and relevant capacity-building, networking, and information-sharing resources, and professional development opportunities

- Facilitation of knowledge-transfer forums such as the virtual BPSO Community of Practice, annual BPSO Knowledge Exchange Symposium, and regular BPSO Knowledge Exchange meetings

- RNAO's technology-enabled reporting system, myBPSO

- Review of required BPSO reports submitted through myBPSO, and provision of timely interactive feedback

- Promotion of BPSOs and their work through media features, opportunities for publication, and local and international mentoring connections

- Opportunities to mentor other BPSOs and to be part of the Certified BPSO Orientation Trainer network and the Certified Trained BPSO Auditor network (see details in Chapter 12)

BPSO SUCCESS FACTORS

The BPSO Designation is internationally renowned and has been a resounding success in demonstrating the uptake and sustained use of Best Practice Guidelines. The BPSO Designation's strategic approach has served to trigger the development of evidence-based cultures, improve patient care, and enrich the professional practice of nurses and other healthcare providers. At the time of writing, there were 7 BPSO Hosts composed of 125 BPSOs Direct that represent over 550 healthcare organizations and academic institutions in 12 countries and 5 continents.

CONCLUSION AND FUTURE CONSIDERATIONS

While this initiative has incubated, RNAO and all the BPSOs and BPSO Hosts remain vigilant in ensuring nothing interferes with gains made. They work continuously in partnership to reduce the knowledge-to-practice gap and to extend the BPSO Designation in current jurisdictions and scale out to new ones. The future will see more formalized approaches to sustained capacity building, including more Champion Leaders, BPG Leaders, Mentors, and Coaches identified from BPSO Hosts and BPSO Directs around the world. Plans are in place to support the rapid growth of BPSO Directs in Canada, China, and Eastern Europe; as well as to launch and develop BPSO Hosts in Canada, Chile, China, Peru, and several European countries.

RNAO's infrastructure; credibility as a professional association that speaks out for health and for nursing; and its broad practice, education, administration, research, and policy networks fuel its ability to sustain and grow the BPSO Designation. This crucial global initiative of KT is making it possible for healthcare organizations to establish evidence-based cultures; for nurses passionate about evidence-based care to thrive and lead knowledge-based change; and for clients to take comfort in knowing that the best evidence is being used to inform their care. The BPSO Direct and BPSO Host Models have been tested over 15 and 6 years respectively and have demonstrated that the BPSO Designation model fits a variety of global contexts.

As outlined in this chapter, RNAO's groundbreaking meso- and macro-level KT strategy, the BPSO Designation, is successful largely because of a set of requirements embodied in a signed formal agreement between the BPSO and RNAO. The Agreement ensures that organizations are clear about the expectations they must achieve and what supports and resources RNAO commits to provide. The explicit understanding is that with this type of partnership, organizations will be assured of achieving a culture of evidence-based practice and uptake of multiple BPGs. The RNAO BPSO Designation provides a proven model that brings knowledge to action through multiple interrelated strategies and evidence-based resources. This leads to more rapid practice change based on best evidence, and results in better patient and organizational outcomes. The world's patients deserve nothing less.

KEY MESSAGES

- A combination of principles and practices derived from implementation science literature, when applied at the organizational level, provides success in closing the knowledge-to-practice gap in healthcare.

- Leadership in all roles is critical to initiate and sustain development of an evidence-based practice culture.

- Understanding and applying change theory is a critical aspect of initiating and fostering sustained BPG uptake.

- Attention to all aspects of evidence-based practice—from rigorous guideline development to capacity building focused on both clinical knowledge and implementation science principles, evaluation, and sustainment—is necessary to achieve results.

- Organizations aiming to create an evidence-based culture benefit from working closely with both experts and peers striving for similar goals.

- There is a greater likelihood of success when the goal to achieve an evidence-based culture is aligned with the organizational vision, mission, and strategic priorities.

- Global uptake of evidence-based practice in nursing enables consistent approaches to care, facilitates intra- and inter-professional communication and collaboration, enhances opportunities for research, and ultimately strengthens the profession and its impact on clients.

REFERENCES

Aarons, G., Green, A., Trott, E., Willging, C., Torres, E., Ehrhart, M., . . . Roesch, S. (2016). The roles of system and organizational leadership in system-wide evidence-based intervention sustainment: A mixed-methods study. *Administration and Policy in Mental Health, 43*, 991–1008.

Albornos-Munoz, L., González-María, E., & Moreno-Casbas, T. (2015). Best Practice Guidelines implementation in Spain: Best practice spotlight organizations. *MedUNAB, 17*(3), 163–169.

Bajnok, I., Grinspun, D., Lloyd, M., & McConnell, H. (2015). Leading quality improvement through Best Practice Guideline development, implementation, and measurement science. *Med UNAB, 17*(3), 155–162.

Baker, S. D., Turner, G., & Bush, S. C. (2015, November). ARCH: A guidance model for providing effective feedback to learners [Education column]. *Society of Teachers of Family Medicine*. Retrieved from http://www.stfm.org/NewsJournals/EducationColumns/November2015EducationColumn

Bridges, W. (1991). *Managing transitions: Making the most of change*. Reading, MA: Addison-Wesley.

Chambers, D. A., Glasgow, R. E., & Stange, K. C. (2013). The dynamic sustainability framework: Addressing the paradox of sustainment amid ongoing change. *Implementation Science, 8*, 117. doi: 10.1186/1748-5908-8-117

Conner, D. (2006). *Managing at the speed of change: How resilient managers succeed and prosper where others fail*. New York, NY: Random House Publishing Group.

Di Costanzo, M. (2013). Becoming a BPSO. *Registered Nurse Journal, 25*(2), 12–26.

Gallagher-Ford, L. (2014). Implementing and sustaining EBP in real world healthcare settings: A leader's role in creating a strong context for EBP. *Worldviews in Evidence-Based Nursing, 11*(1), 72–74.

Gallagher-Ford, L., Buck, J., & Melnyk, B. M. (2014). Leadership strategies and evidence-based practice competencies to sustain a culture and environment that supports best practice. In B. M. Melnyk & E. Fineout-Overholt (Eds.), *Evidence-based practice in nursing & healthcare: A guide to best practice* (3rd ed.) (pp. 235–247). Philadelphia, PA: Wolters Kluwer.

Gifford, W., Davies, B., Tourangeau, A., & Lefebre, N. (2011). Developing team leadership to facilitate guideline utilization: Planning and evaluating a three-month intervention strategy. *Journal of Nursing Management, 19*, 121–132.

Graham, I. D., Logan, J., Harrison, M. B., Straus, S. E., Tetroe, J., Caswell, W., . . . Robinson, N. (2006). Lost in knowledge translation: Time for a map? *Journal of Continuing Education in the Health Professions, 26*(1), 13–24.

Grinspun, D. (2011). Guias de practica clinica y entorno laboral basados en la evidencia elaboradas por la Registered Nurses' Association of Ontario (RNAO) (Evidence based clinical practice and work environment guidelines prepared by the Registered Nurses' Association of Ontario). *Enfermeria Clinica* (Clinical Nursing), *21*(1), 1–2.

Grinspun, D., Lloyd, M., Xiao, S., & Bajnok, I. (2015). Measuring quality of evidence-based care: NQuIRE-Nursing Quality Indicators for Reporting and Evaluation data-system. *MedUNAB*, *17*(3), 170–175.

Grinspun, D., Melnyk, B. M., & Fineout-Overholt, E. (2014). Advancing optimal care with rigorously developed clinical practice guidelines and evidence-based recommendations. In B. M. Melnyk & E. Fineout-Overholt (Eds.), *Evidence-based practice in nursing & healthcare: A guide to best practice* (3rd ed.) (pp. 182–201). Philadelphia, PA: Wolters Kluwer.

Grinspun, D., Virani, T., & Bajnok, I. (2002). Nursing Best Practice Guidelines: The Registered Nurses' Association of Ontario project. *Hospital Quarterly*, *5*(2), 56–60.

Grol, R., Wensing, M., Eccles, M., & Davis, D. (2013). *Improving patient care: The implementation of change in health care* (2nd ed.). London, UK: John Wiley & Sons.

Haines, S. (2005). *Leading strategic change.* San Diego, CA: Systems Thinking Press.

Haines, S. (2007). *The natural cycles of life and change.* Retrieved from http://hainescentre.com/rollercoaster/

Harvey, G., Loftus-Hills, A., Rycroft-Malone, J., Titchen, A. I., Kitson, A., McCormack, B., . . . Seers, K. (2002). Getting evidence into practice: The role and function of facilitation. *Journal of Advanced Nursing*, *37*(6), 577–588.

Health Council of Canada. (2012). *Understanding clinical practice guidelines: A video series primer.* Retrieved from http://healthcouncilcanada.ca/tree/CPG_Backgrounder_EN.pdf.pdf

Heath, C., & Heath, D. (2010). *Switch: How to change things when change is hard.* New York, NY: Random House.

Hiatt, J. M. (2006). *ADKAR: A model for change in business, government and our community.* Loveland, CO, U.S. Prosci Research.

Higuchi, K., Davies, B., & Ploeg, J. (2017). Sustaining guideline implementation: A multisite perspective on activities, challenges and supports. *Journal of Clinical Nursing*, 1–12. doi: 10.1111/jocn.13770

Higuchi, K., Downey, A., Davies, B., Bajnok, I., & Waggott, M. (2013). Using the NHS sustainability framework to understand the activities and resource implications of Canadian nursing guideline early adopters. *Journal of Clinical Nursing*, *22*(11–12), 1706–1716.

Ivers, N., Jamtvedt, G., Flottorp, S., Young, J. M., Odgaard-Jensen, J., French, S. D., . . . Oxman A. D. (2012). Audit and feedback: Effects on professional practice and healthcare outcomes. *Cochrane Database of Systematic Reviews*, *6*, CD000259. doi: 10.1002/14651858.CD000259.pub3

Ivers, N., Sales, A., Colquhoun, H., Michie, S., Foy, R., Francis, J. J., . . . Grimshaw, J. M. (2014). No more 'business as usual' with audit and feedback interventions: Towards an agenda for a reinvigorated intervention. *Implementation Science*, *9*, 14. doi: 10.1186/1748-5908-9-14

Kirschling, J., & Erickson, J. (2010). The STTI practice academe collaborative partnership award: Honoring innovation, partnership and excellence. *Journal of Nursing Scholarship*, *42*(3), 286–294.

Kotter, J. P. (2012). *Leading change.* Boston, MA: Harvard Business Review Press.

Maher, L., Gustafson, D., & Evans, A. (2010). *NHS Sustainability Model.* Retrieved from http://www.institute.nhs.uk/sustainability

Melnyk, B. M. (2014). Building cultures and environments that facilitate clinician behaviour change to evidence-based practice: What works? *Worldviews in Evidence-Based Nursing*, *11*(2), 79–80.

Melnyk, B. M. (2017). The difference between what is known and what is done is lethal: Evidence-based practice is a key solution urgently needed. *Worldviews in Evidence-Based Nursing*, *14*(1), 3–4.

Melnyk, B. M., & Fineout-Overholt, E. (2015). *Evidence-based practice in nursing & healthcare: A guide to best practice* (3rd ed). Philadelphia, PA: Wolters Kluwer.

Melnyk, B. M., Gallagher-Ford, L., Koshy, B. K., Troseth, M., Wygarden, E., & Szalacha, L. (2016). A study of chief nurse executives indicates low prioritization of evidence-based practice and shortcomings in hospital performance metrics across the United States. *Worldviews in Evidence-Based Nursing*, *13*(1), 6–14.

Ploeg, J., Davies, B., Edwards, N., Gifford, W., & Miller, E. P. (2007). Factors influencing BPG implementation: Lessons learned from administrators, nursing staff and project leaders. *Worldviews in Evidence-Based Nursing*, *4*(4), 210–219.

Registered Nurses' Association of Ontario (RNAO). (2012). *Toolkit: Implementation of Best Practice Guidelines* (2nd ed.). Toronto, ON: Registered Nurses' Association of Ontario.

Registered Nurses' Association of Ontario (RNAO). (2015). *2014–2015 Best Practice Spotlight Organization impact survey: Summary of survey results.* Retrieved from http://rnao.ca/sites/rnao-ca/files/FINAL_RNAO-BPSO_Impact_Survey.pdf

Registered Nurses' Association of Ontario (RNAO). (2017a). *Best Practice Spotlight Organizations (BPSO).* Retrieved from http://rnao.ca/bpg/bpso

Registered Nurses' Association of Ontario (2017b). *RNAO Best Practice Spotlight Organization (BPSO).* Retrieved from http://rnao.ca/sites/rnao-ca/files/RNAOBPSOFactSheetApril2017.pdf

Rogers, E. (2003). *Diffusion of innovations* (5th ed.). New York, NY: Free Press.

Schein, E. H. (1996). Kurt Lewin's change theory in the field and in the classroom: Notes toward a model of managed learning. *Systems Practice and Action Research*, *9*(1), 27–47.

Stetler, C. B., Richie, J. A., Rycroft-Malone, J., & Charns, M. P. (2014). Leadership for evidence-based practice: Strategic and functional behaviour for institutionalizing EBP. *Worldviews in Evidence-Based Nursing*, *11*(4), 219–226.

Straus, S., Tetroe, J., & Graham, I. D. (Eds). (2013). *Knowledge translation in health care: Moving from evidence to practice* (2nd ed.) Oxford, UK: Wiley-Blackwell.

World Health Organization (WHO). (2015). *Nurses and midwifes: A vital resource for health. European compendium of good practices in nursing and midwifery towards Health 2020 goals*. Copenhagen, Denmark: WHO Regional Office for Europe. Retrieved from http://www.euro.who.int/en/health-topics/Health-systems/nursing-and-midwifery/publications/2015/nurses-and-midwives-a-vital-resource-for-health.-european-compendium-of-good-practices-in-nursing-and-midwifery-towards-health-2020-goals

APPENDIX A: STEPS TO BECOMING A BEST PRACTICE SPOTLIGHT ORGANIZATION (BPSO)

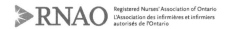 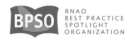

RNAO Best Practice Spotlight Organization® (BPSO)

The Registered Nurses' Association of Ontario

RNAO is the professional body representing registered nurses, nurse practitioners and nursing students in Ontario, Canada. We advocate for healthy public policy, promote excellence in nursing practice, and empower nurses to actively influence and shape decisions that affect the profession and the public they serve.

The RNAO Best Practice Guidelines Program

The RNAO's Nursing Best Practice Guideline (BPG) program was launched in November of 1999[1] and has, to date, produced 53 clinical and system and healthy work environments guidelines; a toolkit[2] to aid in the implementation of RNAO guidelines in practice settings; an educator's resource[3] to facilitate guideline implementation in the nursing curriculum and a range of educational programs offered across Canada and internationally. The uptake of the published guidelines is supported using a multi-pronged approach that includes a focus on individual capacity development, through the Best Practice Champion Network®[4] and RNAO institutes; organizational implementation through the Best Practice Spotlight Organization (BPSO) program; and health-system wide implementation. The guidelines, related tools, and implementation resources are available on RNAO's website at RNAO.ca/bestpractices

BPSO® Program Overview

The BPSO program supports BPG implementation at the organizational level. It was established in 2003, is internationally renowned, and has been successful in demonstrating the uptake and utilization of best practice guidelines.[56] The program's strategic approach has served to promote the development of evidence-based cultures, improve patient care and enrich the professional practice of nurses and other health-care providers. The end goal is to optimize nursing care, patient and organizational outcomes through the use of RNAO BPGs by promoting a culture of evidence-based nursing practice and management decision-making. There are two models of the BPSO Designation, one is the BPSO Direct and the other is the BPSO Host. More specific information related to the BPSO Host Model is included later in this document.

---

[1] Grinspun, D., Virani, T., & Bajnok, I. (2002). Nursing best practice guidelines: The RNAO (Registered Nurses' Association of Ontario) project. *Hospital Quarterly, 5*(2), 56-60.
[2] Registered Nurses' Association of Ontario. (2002). *Toolkit: Implementation of clinical practice guidelines.* Toronto, Canada: Registered Nurses' Association of Ontario.
[3] Registered Nurses' Association of Ontario, (2005) *Educator's Resource: Integration of Best Practice Guidelines.* Toronto, Canada: Registered Nurses' Association of Ontario.
[4] Ploeg, J., Skelly, J., Rowan, M., Edwards, N, Davies, B , Grinspun, D., Bajnok, I. Downey, A. (2010) The Role of Nursing Best Practice Champions in Diffusing Practice Guidelines: A Mixed Methods Study. Worldviews on Evidence-Based Nursing http://onlinelibrary.wiley.com/journal/10.1111/(ISSN)1741-6787/earlyview
[5] Kirschling, J. & Erickson, J. (2010). The STTI Practice Academe Collaborative Partnership Award: Honoring Innovation, Partnership and Excellence. Journal of Nursing Scholarship, 42(3), 285-204.
[6] Registered Nurses' Association of Ontario. (March-April 2013). *Registered Nurse Journal.*

The objectives of the BPSO program are to:

1. Establish dynamic, long-term partnerships that focus on making an impact on patient care through supporting knowledge-based nursing practice;
2. Demonstrate creative strategies for successfully implementing nursing BPGs at the individual and organizational level;
3. Establish and utilize effective approaches to evaluate implementation activities utilizing structure, process and outcome indicators; and
4. Identify effective strategies for system-wide dissemination of BPG implementation and outcomes.

BPSOs commit to a three-year BPSO qualifying experience, through which a formal partnership is established that defines the role of RNAO and the expected deliverables of the BPSO. During the three-year period, BPSO organizations focus on enhancing their evidence-based nursing practice and decision making cultures, with the mandate to implement and evaluate multiple clinical practice guidelines.

At the end of the three-year period, and assuming all deliverables are met, the BPSO organizations become "Designated BPSOs." As designated BPSOs, organizations focus on sustainability, and are committed to continue the implementation and evaluation of best practice guidelines in their organization and within the system. The BPSO designation is renewable every two years.

Steps to Becoming a BPSO

1. Submit evidence of readiness and commitment to implementing and evaluating at least five clinical BPGs (Canada) or three clinical BPGs (international) as a BPSO pre-designate in a proposal according to the BPSO Request-for-Proposal format. This proposal should include information for each BPG identifying why they were selected, strategies that will be utilized for implementation, expected outcomes for patients, providers and the organization, and means of evaluating these outcomes.
2. Sign a letter of agreement committing to a three-year partnership to become a BPSO Designate.

Responsibilities of the BPSO Direct

1. Identify a BPSO lead from your organization.
2. Develop a Steering Committee and program structure.
3. Identify a cadre of Champions (15 per cent of nursing staff) who will participate in a Champions orientation and support the uptake of evidence-based practices.
4. Send two or three staff/faculty to RNAO BPG related institutes each year, or alternately RNAO could deliver the institute in your organization.
5. Meet with other BPSO leads each month in Knowledge Exchange Teleconferences.
6. Commit to sending up to two staff to in-person Knowledge Exchange Symposiums each year* (optional for international BPSOs).
7. Enter data for structure, process and outcome indicators tailored to BPGs implemented through NQuIRE.
8. Submit an online report every six months and meet with the RNAO BPSO team via teleconference/virtual to review.
9. Disseminate outcomes from the BPSO qualifying experience, including tools and resources
10. Following achievement of the BPSO Designation, which is contingent on meeting all deliverables in the letter of agreement, commit to sustaining, expanding and spreading BPG implementation, and providing support to other BPSO pre-designates in a mentor role.

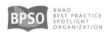

The RNAO Responsibilities in relation to the BPSO Direct

1. Provide access to published and electronic RNAO BPGs to the BPSO.
2. Provide the BPSO with an orientation to the RNAO International Affairs and Best Practice Guidelines Centre, the BPSO program and to specific guidelines, as appropriate.
3. Support the BPSO to develop and deliver an orientation to the best practice guideline and BPSO programs.
4. Provide training to the BPSO in the implementation of nursing BPGs using a train-the-trainer approach.
5. Provide support for implementation, through access to resources such as the Best Practice Champions Network including the Champion Workshops/eLearning program, the Implementation Toolkit, and Educator's Resource, BPG APPs and other implementation resources.
6. Provide expert consultation on guideline dissemination, implementation, uptake, evaluation and sustainability, on an ongoing basis and more formally through a regular BPSO teleconference involving other BPSOs at a similar BPG implementation stage.
7. Facilitate the establishment of a network of BPSO project leaders, for the purposes of knowledge transfer and exchange, and lead this network in regular knowledge exchange sessions to facilitate effective BPG implementation and evaluation.
8. Meet virtually (through web-based technology or telephone meetings) on a twice yearly basis, and as mutually agreed and/or as necessary, with the BPSO to review reports, monitor progress and provide recommendations.
9. Provide a coach for the BPSO for the three-year BPSO qualifying period. The BPSO coach serves as a point of contact for the BPSO organization, and their role will include consultation, coaching, linking with resources, referrals and site visits as necessary.
10. Identify and direct appropriate research opportunities to the BPSO.
11. Acknowledge the participation of the BPSO and its key individuals, teams, and units (as determined by the BPSO) in implementing and evaluating the selected best practices guidelines.

BPSO Host Model

The RNAO BPSO Host Model is a feature of the national/international BPSO program. A BPSO Host Organization enters into a formal agreement with RNAO to oversee the RNAO BPSO program in the country or region where it is located. The BPSO Host is responsible for all aspects of the BPSO program from selecting the BPSO organizations interested in becoming BPSOs to reporting progress back to RNAO. Generally the BPSO Host acts as the liaison between RNAO and the BPSOs in the specific country or region.

As the service and/or academic organizations become BPSOs, to implement, disseminate and evaluate RNAO best practice guidelines, the BPSO Host provides support by monitoring through regular meetings and reporting processes. The BPSO Host then reports to the RNAO with updates from the BPSOs as well as an overview of successes, challenges, questions and issues of the BPSO program in that country or region.

BPSO Host Organization Responsibilities

1. Selecting BPSOs within the region jurisdiction using RNAO Request-for-Proposal methodology.
2. Establishing a contract with the BPSO organizations as per the RNAO BPSO agreement prototype, outlining the expected deliverables and requirements to be adhered to over the three year period.
3. Launching the BPSO program in the region using an orientation session of all selected BPSOs involving nursing staff/faculty in all roles, and other stakeholders.

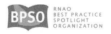

4. Committing resources to training in the implementation of RNAO's nursing BPGs using a train-the-trainer approach and RNAO's materials and approach.

5. Organizing and coordinating Institutes, based on the RNAO Implementation Toolkit, Champion Workshop curriculum and supporting materials developed in partnership with RNAO for local training and advancement of the implementation of nursing best practice guidelines.

6. Supporting the development of a network of Best Practice Champions, and BPG Institute attendees, within the country to build capacity and share implementation/evaluation experiences.

7. Hosting monthly knowledge exchange sessions of the BPSO leads from each BPSO organization to review, support and monitor progress as well to facilitate exchange of challenges, successes and lessons learned among the regional BPSOs.

8. Hosting an annual regional BPSO knowledge exchange event (symposium) to bring together representatives from all BPSO organizations to share progress, identify strengths and key outcomes, address challenges and make plans to enhance and spread and sustain this activity.

9. Requesting progress reports from each BPSO every six months during the pre-designate period and following review, holding meetings with each BPSO to discuss the report identifying overall progress, strengths, recommendations for change and further support needed.

10. Identifying a liaison person from the Host Organization for each BPSO to provide specific supports as necessary to the BPSO organization.

11. Monitor the deliverables/requirements that each BPSO must adhere to during the BPSO experience.

12. Facilitate the research and evaluation of the BPSO Program within the country, particularly through the RNAO Nursing Quality Indicators for Reporting and Evaluation® (NQuIRE®) data system. NQuIRE is comprised of quality indicators related to nursing practice, client clinical outcomes and organizational structure relevant to the guidelines selected for implementation.

13. Facilitate the dissemination activities of the BPSOs within the region.

14. Engaging in regular knowledge exchange, monitoring, planning and evaluation sessions with RNAO and other Host Organizations, at the initiation of and throughout the BPSO Program implementation.

The RNAO Responsibilities in relation to the BPSO Host

RNAO provides support for implementation, through training, as well as access to all available resources such as the draft contract agreement for BPSOs, reporting prototypes, Best Practice Champions Network including the Champion Workshops, the Implementation Toolkit, and Educator's Resource, BPG APPs and other implementation resources. RNAO also engages with the BPSO Host in regular meetings, and offers expert mentorship and consultation on guideline dissemination, implementation, uptake, sustainability and evaluation. Furthermore, the BPSO Host and BPSOs in the country or region are paired with mentor organizations, who have experienced the BPSO program.

For More Information

Contact us at BPSO@RNAO.ca.

Visit the Best Practice Spotlight Organization program website at www.RNAO.ca/bpg/bpso.

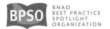

THE BPSO PIONEERS: CREATING, SUSTAINING, AND EXPANDING EVIDENCE-BASED CULTURES THROUGH THE BPSO DESIGNATION

Shirlee M. Sharkey, CHE, MHSc, BScN, BA
Nancy Lefebre, FCCHL, Extra Fellow, CHE, MScN, BScN
Karen L. Ray, MSc, RN
Anne-Marie Malek, CHE, MHSA, BN, RN
Barbara Bell, CHE, MN, BScN, RN
Ru Taggar, MN, RN
Beth O'Leary, PMP
Tracey DasGupta, MN, RN

LEARNING OBJECTIVES

After reading this chapter, you will be able to:

■ Describe roles of innovators and early adopters in implementation of Best Practice Guidelines (BPG) and creation of evidence-based practice cultures

■ Identify how to utilize successes and challenges in implementing large-scale change

■ Outline strategies for sustainment of BPGs

■ Understand the contribution of leadership at the executive level in creating an evidence-based practice culture

■ Determine lessons learned through the Best Practice Spotlight Organization (BPSO) Designation experience

INTRODUCTION

Quality patient, provider, and organizational outcomes are the primary aim of today's healthcare system (Canadian Institute of Health Information [CIHI], 2013). Care must be based on current evidence to ensure results are achieved in the best and most effective way possible (DiCenso, 2003). This has led to the original mandate of the Registered Nurses' Association of Ontario (RNAO): to create clinical Best Practice Guidelines and embrace implementation science processes to change practice (Grinspun, Virani, & Bajnok, 2002). This chapter describes the experience of three organizations, from different healthcare sectors in Ontario, that each achieved the RNAO Best Practice Spotlight Organization (BPSO) Designation. They are: 1) Saint Elizabeth, a home healthcare organization; 2) West Park Healthcare Centre, a rehabilitative care organization; and 3) Sunnybrook Health Sciences Centre, an acute care organization. In sharing our journeys, we outline the decision to engage in evidence-based practice (EBP); our successes and challenges in implementing Best Practice Guidelines (BPG) over an 18-year period; sustainability strategies; and finally, how each organization will take its BPSO work into the future.

The profound link between nursing work environments and healthy outcomes is one that all three organizations were quick to discover (Duffield et al., 2011; Purdy et al., 2010). The culture of an organization needs to be safe and supportive, leading to effective recruitment and retention as well as job satisfaction. In the beginning, early adopter organizations used to guide leadership strategies intuitively to create a culture of inquiry and respect for nurses and the care they provided. Today, we are fortunate to have RNAO's Healthy Work Environment (HWE) BPGs (see Chapter 3, *Creating Healthy Workplaces: Enabling Clinical Excellence*)—including the *Developing and Sustaining Nursing Leadership* BPG (RNAO, 2013c) and the RNAO Implementation Toolkit (2012)—that articulate useful leadership practices and implementation strategies.

The *Developing and Sustaining Nursing Leadership* BPG provides an organizing framework to guide leadership behaviours to result in "a healthy work environment and healthy outcomes for the patient/client, nurse, team, organization and the system" (RNAO, 2013c, p. 16) (see Figure 7.1). This framework addresses the context for leadership capabilities, at the organizational and personal levels, transformational leadership practices, and relevant outcomes to be considered. The guideline is supported by significant empirical evidence and is both helpful and relevant to nurse leaders in a variety of roles. Further, it describes:

- Leadership practices that result in healthy outcomes for patients/clients, organizations, and systems

- Anticipated outcomes of effective nursing practices

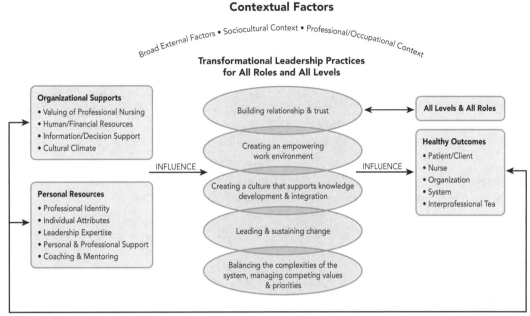

Contextual Factors

Broad External Factors • Sociocultural Context • Professional/Occupational Context

**Transformational Leadership Practices
for All Roles and All Levels**

Organizational Supports
• Valuing of Professional Nursing
• Human/Financial Resources
• Information/Decision Support
• Cultural Climate

Personal Resources
• Professional Identity
• Individual Attributes
• Leadership Expertise
• Personal & Professional Support
• Coaching & Mentoring

INFLUENCE

Building relationship & trust

Creating an empowering
work environment

Creating a culture that supports knowledge
development & integration

Leading & sustaining change

Balancing the complexities of the
system, managing competing values
& priorities

INFLUENCE

All Levels & All Roles

Healthy Outcomes
• Patient/Client
• Nurse
• Organization
• System
• Interprofessional Tea

Conceptual Model for Developing and Sustaining Leadership: RNAO Healthy Workplace BPG

FIGURE 7.1 Conceptual model for developing and sustaining leadership.
Reprinted with permission of the Registered Nurses' Association of Ontario (2013c).

Following is a series of case studies reflecting the successful work of the three organizations using the BPSO Designation strategy and related supports to develop an evidence-based culture in their organizations.

C A S E   S T U D Y

SAINT ELIZABETH

Saint Elizabeth is a Canadian social enterprise that provides home care, health solutions, and education to people where they are and when they need it. With more than 100 years of community health expertise, the not-for-profit charitable organization has provided 50 million care exchanges in the past decade alone and currently employs a team of 9,000 nurses, rehabilitation therapists, and personal support workers. Saint Elizabeth staff is highly mobile, geographically dispersed, and anchored in local neighbourhoods. Care is delivered in home and community settings across Canada to children, adults, and seniors, with services ranging from prevention and wellness to post-op care and the management of chronic conditions such as diabetes, wounds, and hospice palliative care.

GETTING STARTED

In the early days, before the advent of the BPSO Designation, Saint Elizabeth took a leadership role in pilot testing two RNAO guidelines: *Assessment and Management of Venous Leg Ulcers* (2004a) and *Establishing Therapeutic Relationships* (2006b). At that time, there was a paucity of published literature to guide the process of integrating evidence into clinical practice.

Accordingly, we used Rogers' Diffusion of Innovations Theory (Rogers, 1995) to explore how, why, and the rate at which new ideas spread. During the pilot, the guidelines were implemented at Saint Elizabeth as well as two other partner organizations. As a BPG implementation pioneer, this experience informed our early learnings related to infrastructure requirements, the role of organizational culture, and the need for tailored education strategies. The pilots allowed us to learn on a small scale before implementing guidelines across the organization to achieve the BPSO Designation.

MOVING TOWARD EVIDENCE-BASED PRACTICE

In 2003, Saint Elizabeth's vision was to be a "knowledge and care exchange company"—one that created, managed, utilized, and shared knowledge for the advancement of patient care and health outcomes, with a strong evidence base underpinning both decision-making (i.e., evidence-informed decision making [EIDM] [DiCenso, Ciliska, & Guyatt, 2005]) and healthcare practice. Working with the EIDM model (see Figure 7.2) and in partnership with our staff, we set forth to create a climate of critical inquiry and a culture that supported the use of evidence from the bedside to the boardroom. The opportunity to broadly implement and evaluate BPGs in partnership with RNAO provided the resources, focus, and a strategic catalyst for advancing our vision.

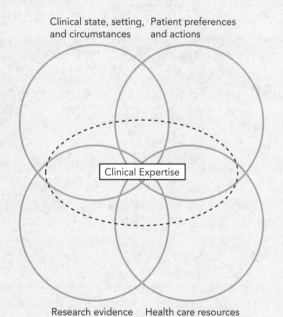

FIGURE 7.2   A model for evidence-based clinical decisions.
DiCenso et al., 2005. Used with permission.

To advance our knowledge and support a rigorous approach, a site visit was made to the University of Iowa Hospital (UIH), a well-known innovator and leader in the field of evidence-based practice. During discussions with staff at many levels—from direct care to executive leadership—we explored the role of organizational culture, leadership, infrastructure, processes, data collection, analysis, and reporting. An appreciative inquiry (AI) (Stavros, Godwin, & Cooperrider, 2015) approach was then used to document and categorize successful strategies into key themes such as education, reward and recognition, performance expectations, infrastructure supports, info-structure, culture, and external environment. Stavros et al. (2015) suggest that AI is a fundamental shift in perspective that focuses on the best in the organization and its people, leading to recognition of strengths and inspiring hope about new possibilities. This approach impacted our individual (micro), organization (meso), and system (macro) level strategies, which were tailored and aligned to our organizational environment and formed the basis of our implementation road map.

To ensure success moving forward, Saint Elizabeth put several structures in place that were consistent with the BPSO requirements (RNAO, 2017). First, a Project Leader was designated to ensure strategic alignment with the organization's vision of knowledge leadership. Second, internal structures were created to achieve integration and alignment with other activities and priorities throughout the organization. At the outset, we established a BPSO Steering Committee that included senior and local leaders as well as representation from professional practice, service delivery, research, and communications. Implementation was further supported by a dedicated project management team. Once the committee structures were in place, an Environmental and Stakeholder Assessment as outlined in the *RNAO Toolkit: Implementation of Best Practice Guidelines* (2012) was conducted in all implementation sites.

SUCCESSES

As a Designated BPSO, Saint Elizabeth has been involved in testing, developing, and implementing over 30 RNAO Best Practice Guidelines. Initially, we decided to implement one guideline at a time across 24 local sites, in order to promote staff engagement and full integration of the BPG. The project management team worked closely with each site to creatively solve problems, identify collective strategies, and meet overall timelines. This kept us on track and promoted collaboration and recognition between corporate and local teams. The clinical network was complemented by a strong working relationship with the local site manager, who helped ensure adequate staffing to deliver high-quality care, data collection, and evidence-based decision-making based on clinical outcomes.

The BPG initiative helped us to improve clinical outcomes, knowledge transfer, and professional relationships across the organization. Knowledge flowed from our advanced practice consultants at the corporate level, to the local clinical resource network, and out into community practice. In some specialty areas such as hospice palliative care, local clinical resource nurses played an active role as guideline Champions, providing consultation and mentoring to their peers (Ploeg et al., 2010). The BPG initiative provided the Champion preparation workshops and connection to a broad BPG Champion Network, and helped us identify the clinical and geographic areas where our Champion network was strongest, as well as the areas that needed further support and development. Since the initial implementation of the BPG related to wound care, excellent outcomes have been maintained:

- 100% wound reduction occurs at 30 days, exceeding our target every quarter year over year

- 100% of wounds healed at 12 weeks or less

In addition, in palliative care, related to pain and intensity we have:

- Successfully maintained threshold for pain and distress intensity for palliative patients, exceeding best practice targets (≤4/10) recommended by Cancer Care Ontario (Cancer Quality Council of Ontario, 2017)

To meet the BPSO requirements and implement and sustain BPGs, strategies for knowledge transfer included educational packages, documentation, and policies and procedures based on BPG evidence. Education was provided through a "train-the-trainer" approach that was flexible to local needs and designed to actively involve direct-care nurses based on their work schedule and practice reality. While we initially planned to deliver education during weekly team meetings, we quickly recognized that

a more creative approach was required. Accordingly, an eLearning program and virtual resource center was created that could be accessed from anywhere, 24/7. Nurses were further supported by virtual Communities of Practice that provided a forum for peer and expert support, as well as access to literature.

Through our work with indigenous communities across Canada, Saint Elizabeth saw an opportunity to further spread BPGs and support healthy outcomes beyond our own organization when we incorporated the guidelines into our First Nations, Inuit and Métis Program. For example, diabetes and diabetic foot ulcers are a significant challenge in First Nation communities (Martens, Martin, O'Neil, & MacKinnon, 2007), and education and skills in treating diabetic foot ulcers was a key focus of our BPG work. In Manitoba, we partnered with the Assembly of Manitoba Chiefs (AMC) on a Health Canada–funded project that focused on the prevention, treatment, and care of diabetic foot ulcers within a wait-times framework. As part of this project, we incorporated the *RNAO Assessment and Management of Foot Ulcers for People with Diabetes BPG* (2013a) into the education for community nurses and health workers and provided skills training, resources, and equipment to help with ulcer care (Saint Elizabeth Health Care and Assembly of Manitoba Chiefs, 2011). This initiative demonstrates creativity, commitment, and success in spreading and sustaining evidence-based practice to other locations and cultures. AMC went on to obtain federal funding to assist several Manitoba communities with technology to track patients and ensure treatment and follow-up.

Ensuring adequate treatment for people with diabetes also helped Saint Elizabeth strengthen external relationships in Ontario. For example, while implementing the BPG for *Subcutaneous Administration of Insulin for People with Type 2 Diabetes* (RNAO, 2009), it became evident that we were seeing a large population of patients that required more holistic care for diabetes. This led us to implement the guideline for *Reducing Foot Complications for People with Diabetes* (RNAO, 2004b, 2007b). Additionally, it highlighted the need for wound-dressing products and offloading devices for this population, and as a result, we improved communication with our funding partners and strengthened our alliance with local hospital clinics and physicians specializing in wound care.

"When nurses adhered to and advocated for use of recommendations in the RNAO's BPGs, patients' care has improved, in some cases, dramatically. The BPGs now help nurses structure client care and 'articulate what we're trying to do and why.' They also boost nurses' confidence when talking to patients and other practitioners."

—Kay McGarvey, Saint Elizabeth CRN, Toronto SDC

CHALLENGES

The nature of home care and our multisite environment presented some unique challenges related to BPG implementation. Community health nurses are knowledge workers who are highly autonomous, mobile, and geographically dispersed. Therefore, our implementation strategies had to be flexible and adaptable to this unique practice reality. At the time, our organization was growing rapidly, and many changes were taking place in the external environment that resulted in the need for ongoing recruitment and onboarding of new staff. Our orientation was revised to incorporate the BPSO initiative, and the ongoing engagement of preceptors and Champions in transferring knowledge was critical (Ploeg et al., 2010).

Another area of challenge was evaluation. Although we had a strong Continuous Quality Improvement program, much of the data we were collecting was related to the service delivery process, rather than specific clinical indicators and outcomes. The BPSO Designation helped us to improve our data-collection tools and processes to provide timely feedback on care outcomes. Moreover, as most visiting nurses were already using mobile phones, we were able to collect clinical data more easily at the point of care and follow it across visits with this technology, empowering nurses in the home to take more leadership in making decisions and changing the care plan as needed based on outcomes.

SUSTAINABILITY

Sustainability is a critical component of the BPSO Designation, and perhaps the most important factor to consider when implementing Best Practice Guidelines. If guidelines are not integrated within an organization, practice will quickly return to its previous state. To prevent this, it is important to embed the guidelines in every aspect of care delivery so that best practice becomes part of "usual care." At Saint Elizabeth, the day-to-day BPG implementation and sustainability were integrated into our Clinical Program structure. The advanced practice nurse for each specific area takes a leadership role in monitoring clinical outcomes and updating education, documentation, policies, and procedures with emerging evidence. They work with regional directors, clinical resource nurses, clinical networks, and local Champions to support ongoing education and improvements. The advanced practice nurse also supports the integration of the guidelines across the care continuum by adapting them for use in all of our healthcare services, including personal support and rehabilitation.

To foster ongoing strategic alignment, Saint Elizabeth kept the BPSO initiative within the permanent leadership role of the Manager of Knowledge Translation, under the direction of the Vice President of Knowledge, Practice and Clinical Services. This allowed us to continue to work with external partners to ensure evidence was created and used across the healthcare system. As an example, we partnered with other BPSO organizations such as West Park Healthcare Centre (see Case Study) to implement the RNAO Healthy Workplace BPG for *Developing and Sustaining Nursing Leadership* (2013c). We are also continuously involved with RNAO in creating new guidelines and resources, educating and mentoring new BPSO member organizations, and working with the collaborative RNAO/University of Ottawa Nursing Best Practice Research Centre (NBPRC). Table 7.1 outlines the BPSO requirements and opportunities through RNAO that have been and continue to be effectively used by Saint Elizabeth to support initial and sustained use of BPGs. Our ongoing relationship with RNAO has played a key role in supporting and sustaining the shift to an evidence-based culture and fostering leadership, empowerment, and professionalism amongst staff at Saint Elizabeth.

TABLE 7.1 BPSO REQUIREMENTS AND OPPORTUNITIES ENABLING IMPLEMENTATION AND SUSTAINABILITY

BPSO REQUIREMENTS SUPPORTING BPG IMPLEMENTATION	BPSO REQUIREMENTS AND OPPORTUNITIES THAT SUPPORT SUSTAINMENT
Formal BPSO Status and BPSO Designation	Membership on RNAO BPG panels
Ongoing access to BPSO Leadership team at RNAO	Member of panel to review other BPSO Proposals
Scheduled follow-up knowledge exchange sessions with RNAO and other BPSOs	Member of panel to review applications to RNAO fellowship opportunities
RNAO Toolkit (2012) and systematic approach to BPG implementation	Contributing to knowledge dissemination activities such as learning events or BPG-related conferences
Champion Workshops	Manuscript submission requirements of the BPSO Designation
Semi-Annual Status Reports required to be submitted to RNAO	Contributing data to NQuIRE and utilizing real-time reports on process and outcome indicators
Research/BPSO Liaison position required	Ongoing evaluation and research support from the RNAO/University of Ottawa Nursing Best Practices Research Centre
Practice Fellowships to support development of advanced clinical skill offered through RNAO	Mentorship work with new BPSOs to provide education and support

Perhaps the most important factors in sustaining the BPGs have been RNAO's enhanced focus on BPG evaluation through establishment of NQuIRE (Nursing Quality Indicators for Reporting and Evaluation), an international BPG-related data base system of indicators (see Chapter 16, *Evaluating BPG Impact: The Development and Refinement of NQuIRE*), and Saint Elizabeth's data collection and submission to this system through our Continuous Quality Improvement program. This process has been augmented by electronic collection of information, which is now part of our audit and feedback process. An evaluation of Saint Elizabeth's process was recently undertaken by Gifford et al. (2016), which showed that operational and clinical leaders are using the data to inform planning. Our next step is to expand information sharing with direct-care nurses to further improve practice.

"To see the evolution of our organization as one that uses evidence from the bedside to the boardroom to give the best care possible to get the best care outcomes for our clients and to engage our staff in that process . . . that's why we continue to be a BPSO."

—Nancy Lefebre
Saint Elizabeth Chief Clinical Executive and Senior Vice-President of Knowledge and Practice

THE FUTURE

Over time, organizations evolve around emerging themes that influence their future direction. In 2003, the theme of "knowledge" was informing Saint Elizabeth's evolution as a company and BPSO. Today, themes such as digitization and the consumer experience (Advisory Panel on Healthcare Innovation, 2015) are at the forefront, and as a result, BPGs and knowledge are being integrated into a digital framework that is anchored in person- and family-centered care, utilizing aspects of RNAO's *Person and Family Centred Care* BPG (2015). In this work, reflecting the approach in the BPG, our patients and their families are central in the care process as empowered, respected partners (RNAO, 2002, 2006a, 2006b, 2010,

2014). In the future, evidence-informed decision making (EIDM) will continue to evolve with more emphasis on management decision-making in addition to clinical care. This is already happening within and outside of our organization based on the rapid growth of big data and predictive analytics (Canada Health Infoway, 2013). In response to growing consumer engagement in health, outcome measures will eventually include more patient reported outcomes and a larger focus on the patient and family experience. The ongoing integration and sustained used of Best Practice Guidelines will be based on innovative knowledge-transfer strategies as we create and deliver new models of care, automate our processes, and design the practice environment of tomorrow.

CASE STUDY

WEST PARK HEALTHCARE CENTRE

West Park Healthcare Centre (the Centre) is located in Toronto, Ontario, Canada, and provides a range of post-acute and tertiary rehabilitation services aimed at assisting people to "get their life back" following life-altering illness or injuries. Rehabilitation and complex continuing care are core to the Centre's hospital-based programs and include inpatient, outpatient, outreach, and day services. Subspecialization is the hallmark of the Centre's program offerings, which are focused on helping individuals with difficult health challenges (such as advanced lung disease, tuberculosis, long-term ventilation, strokes, acquired brain injuries, amputation, and traumatic injuries) reclaim their lives and realize their potential.

GETTING STARTED

Over the years, the Centre's programs and services have evolved to meet the changing needs of our patient populations as well as various health system changes. Recruitment and retention challenges, along with significant financial pressures, led the Centre on a path to transforming its care delivery model in the late 1990s. In concert with changes to the care delivery model, the professional practice portfolio was realigned to ensure the

successful implementation of the new care delivery model and concomitant evolution of the practice setting. A centralized professional practice structure was established, led by a director of professional practice, and supported by new roles that included advanced practice nurses and nurse practitioners who were focused on advancing professional practice and improving the quality of patient care.

Our early experience with the RNAO BPGs began prior to our BPSO candidacy, with quality-improvement work in the area of pressure (wound) injury prevention and management. At the time, one of our advanced practice nurses (APNs) was involved in the first RNAO BPG development panel on pressure (wound) injuries and led the Centre's improvement work in this area. Advanced Practice Nurses at the Centre are registered nurses prepared at the graduate level with in-depth nursing knowledge and clinical expertise to meet the needs of the patients. Post-implementation results demonstrated a 55% improvement in the incidence of pressure injuries and provided a compelling case for the ongoing commitment to a comprehensive and sustained approach to BPG uptake.

MOVING FORWARD WITH EVIDENCE-BASED PRACTICE

The changes in our professional practice structure provided clear, senior accountability for professional practice and enhanced the qualifications for practice leaders, thereby positioning the Centre to move forward with the creation of an evidenced-based practice setting. The Centre's core values of respect, innovation, excellence, and accountability anchored our commitment to developing an evidence-informed culture.

Recognizing the cultural shift that would be required to move in this direction, the Lawler's Star Model (1996)—a conceptual framework for cultural alignment—was utilized to guide our implementation efforts (Galbraith, 2001; Lawler, 1996), making sure that all our organizational structures and processes were aligned with and could support an evidence-based culture. See Figure 7.3.

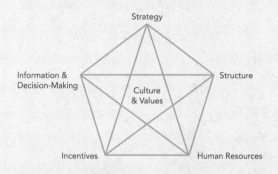

FIGURE 7.3 The Star Model.
Galbraith, J. R. Retrieved from http://www.jaygalbraith.com/services/star-model. Used with permission.

By the time we received our BPSO Designation in 2006, the Centre was in the process of implementing three additional BPGs: *Assessment and Management of Pain* (RNAO, 2013b); *Client Centered Care* (RNAO, 2002); and *Prevention of Falls and Fall Injuries in the Older Adult* (RNAO, 2011b).

Similar to the Saint Elizabeth case study, a systematic approach to the implementation and evaluation of the BPGs was put in place, using project management methodology and drawing on strategies from the RNAO BPSO consultation and coaching support and the RNAO Implementation Toolkit (2012). Our Advanced Practice Nurses led the majority of implementation teams. Implementation-

focused education and approaches were developed, both internally and with external assistance, and reflected creative strategies such as puzzles, role-playing, and various experiential learning processes to engage staff. A key difference in the Centre's approach was the creation of an interprofessional working group to build linkages across disciplines and programs to promote collaborative practice.

SUCCESSES

The nurse leaders who navigated this journey brought clear vision and foresight to the work, along with proven implementation experience, content expertise, and passion. In addition to personal resources, these nursing leaders influenced practice and outcomes through relationship building, creating an empowering work environment, and leading change (RNAO, 2013c). Although we experienced turnover in some leadership positions (discussed later in "Challenges"), consistent executive leadership enabled a continued focus and commitment to the BPSO mandate.

The linchpin of our success, then, was the pivotal role of our nursing leaders: resource nurses, advanced practice nurses, chief nursing officers, and chief nursing executives. Each contributed to our success through a deep understanding of:

- The fundamental benefits of the BPGs in advancing patient care and clinical practice

- The alignment of the BPSO mandate with the organization's vision and values

- The changing needs of our patients

- The imperative for quality improvement, innovation, and sustainable care delivery solutions

Shifting the culture of health organizations toward evidence-based practice is a big undertaking, and many stakeholders played a key role. Senior leaders were committed and engaged throughout the process, providing critical consideration in our implementation approach and thoughtful decisions on how and where to launch new BPGs. This helped to create a compelling "Call to Action" throughout the organization, successful co-created approaches, and an effective multimodal communication strategy.

Also key to the Centre's success was an interprofessional project team that ensured a collaborative approach to guideline implementation, clinical evaluation, and research. Interprofessional team members included APNs in gerontology and rehabilitation, clinical informatics, psychology, clinical pharmacy, and medicine. This approach encouraged expression of diverse perspectives and led to guideline adaptations that were specific to our patient populations, as well as implementation and evaluation strategies specific to our practice setting context. We also drew on the Community of Practice that was available to us through RNAO, which provided access to clinical experts, education, mentorship, and knowledge exchange opportunities for our staff.

Today, we continue to realize the benefits of sustained BPG use as evidenced in a number of human resource and clinical outcome indicators. Indicators reflecting job satisfaction consistently outperform the benchmark, as demonstrated in the results of our 2013 employee engagement survey results (see Figure 7.4).

"The scholarship domain of my CNS practice has been supported through the BPSO work in enabling me to make contributions to the development of nursing knowledge and evidence-based practice."

—Barbara Anderson (Cowie), CNS/Nurse Continence Advisor

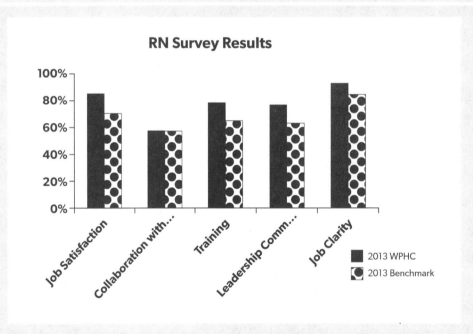

FIGURE 7.4   NRC, Employee Experience Survey, 2013.
Used with permission.

Clinical outcomes also continue to improve, as demonstrated by the implementation of the pain BPG resulting in a reduction of more than 50% of patients reporting pain over several years, and improving our performance well beyond provincial average. See Figure 7.5, which is based on data compiled by West Park Healthcare Centre from the Canadian Institute of Health Information Complex Continuing Care Reporting System Facility Level Reports for West Park Healthcare Centre, 2006–07, 2009–10, 2012–13, 2015–16, and 2016–17 Q1–3.

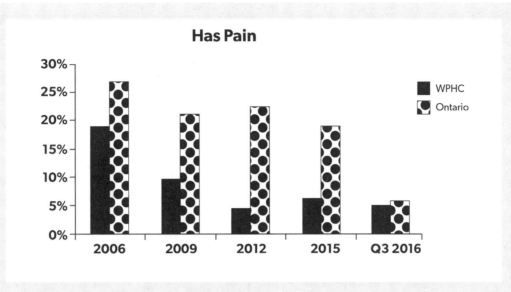

FIGURE 7.5   Reported Pain, West Park Healthcare Centre versus Ontario Scores.
Used with permission.

"Critical to our success were the nurse leaders who navigated the Centre on this journey and provided clear vision, determination and foresight to the work. As a BPSO, West Park's BPG implementation journey has encouraged a spirit of inquiry, enabled interprofessional collaboration and inspired the practice of our staff."

–Anne-Marie Malek, President and CEO

CHALLENGES

One of the biggest challenges in being an early adopter was that we were the only rehabilitation and complex continuing care hospital designated as a BPSO in the beginning. We did not have the benefit of being able to consult with a peer hospital through the process or while developing implementation resources. Implementation and sustainability require a long-term view of the allocation of resources, including the ongoing engagement and development of staff, the redesign of care processes, and the development of various clinical tools such as the incorporation of BPGs into the electronic patient record.

Environmental factors such as competing practice and corporate initiatives, clinical events such as the outbreak of severe acute respiratory syndrome (SARS) in Ontario, Canada in 2003, as well as senior nursing and clinical leader turnover presented further challenges to our implementation of the BPGs. Turnover of nursing leaders had a profound impact as it resulted in a loss of expertise and created a "stop/start" effect on relationships and engagement with staff.

However, adversity helped us reaffirm our commitment to the BPSO Designation mandate, engage new leaders, and become more flexible and creative in our implementation approaches. In fact, many of these challenges were made easier through our partnership with RNAO and the exchange of ideas and shared learning, which provided support to the APNs leading the implementation. Today one of our greatest challenges continues to be the enduring effort toward practice development, an enabling methodology that supports the ongoing implementation and sustainability of BPGs.

SUSTAINABILITY

More than a decade after our BPSO Designation, we have realized the value of this work time and time again and remain committed to our BPSO mandate. Committed leadership and an empowered practice environment are essential to sustaining the work. Our sustainability strategies have included the use of technology to embed BPGs in nursing documentation, access to clinical data to measure outcomes, and continued engagement in the RNAO activities outlined in Table 7.1. We have been steadfast in our vision to create an evidenced-based practice setting, and the value of that commitment has been pivotal to improving patient care and advancing professional practice at the Centre.

To facilitate and sustain practice change, the Centre adopted the practice development methodology (Manely, McCormack, & Wilson, 2008) to guide systematic change and enable nurses to transform culture and the context of care. According to Manely et al. (2008), practice development is based on a person-centered philosophy and supported by facilitators who help staff reflect on their practice identifying the nature of the experience and its impact on patients and on them personally and professionally. This methodology aligned well with RNAO's healthy workplace BPGs (see Chapter 3, *Creating Healthy Workplaces: Enabling Clinical Excellence*) and the knowledge-translation literature as reflected in RNAO's Implementation Toolkit (2012) and has guided our communications, knowledge building, behaviour change, recognition, and integration of BPGs into the fabric of

the Centre. Through a facilitative strategy, teams are empowered to focus on excellence through continuous improvement by setting and monitoring standards and targets.

At the same time, increased access to clinical information and decision support have further advanced clinical and administrative decision-making. Quality indicators and the balanced scorecard approach highlighted performance successes and opportunities. In addition to existing quality indicators, RNAO's NQuIRE provides a comprehensive data system to systematically monitor human resource structure, process, and outcome indicators, increasing our ability to evaluate the outcomes of BPG implementation. The inventory of available BPGs is reviewed on an ongoing basis as we identify gaps and plans for the future. For example, our focus on palliative care led to using the *End of Life Care During the Last Days and Hours BPG* (RNAO, 2011a), to develop and implement comfort interviews. In fulfilling a BPSO Designate requirement, and in keeping with the professional practice goals of the staff, a manuscript detailing the process and outcomes was then written and accepted for publication in a journal as a means to disseminate our learnings and findings (Konietzny & Anderson, 2018).

"BPGs provide an evidence informed foundation from which practice can be developed. That foundation is critical to the advancement of nursing care and improved patient outcomes."

—Barbara Bell, former Chief Nursing Executive

THE FUTURE

With the increasing complexity of patient populations, BPG implementation and sustainability will continue to be essential to the pursuit of excellence in clinical practice and patient care. As a BPSO, we have seen just how fundamental the implementation of BPGs has been to improving patient care and advancing professional practice at the Centre. BPGs have and will continue to

encourage a spirit of inquiry, enable interprofessional dialogue, and inspire the practice of nurses at various stages of their careers (RNAO, 2007a). As our programs and services evolve to meet the changing needs of the patients we serve, so must practice and care delivery. RNAO's rigorously developed BPGs, and their attention to knowledge transfer and evaluation, are effective tools for accomplishing this.

SUNNYBROOK HEALTH SCIENCES CENTRE

Sunnybrook is a large academic health sciences center that is fully affiliated with the University of Toronto, located in Toronto, Ontario, Canada. With 1.2 million patient visits each year, Sunnybrook has established itself across three campuses and is home to Canada's largest trauma center. Sunnybrook has nine clinical programs and 10,000 staff who support our vision: "To invent the future of healthcare."

GETTING STARTED

Sunnybrook Health Sciences Centre (SHSC) began its BPSO journey in 2012 with the primary purpose of selecting and implementing RNAO BPGs that would have the greatest impact on the health outcomes and well-being of our patients. The BPSO initiative was aimed at establishing ways to integrate new learning and evidence into practice and at increasing communication about patient outcomes and care delivery. We also recognized that the initiative aligned well with our Interprofessional Collaboration Strategy to foster collaborative relationships. Consequently, at the onset of our BPSO candidacy, we were deliberate in leveraging the talent and experience of *all* our staff with a vision "to achieve a collaborative interprofessional practice environment that focuses on what matters and what is important to patients." To date, we have been successful in meeting our objectives and the BPSO deliverables, and as a result we have realized significant impacts to practice, education, research, and leadership.

As part of achieving these results, we invested significant time and energy in developing a comprehensive plan in which we:

- Used the RNAO Implementation Toolkit (2012) as a map

- Connected with leaders at organizations with prior BPSO experience

- Built our own knowledge and expertise through formal learning programs such as the RNAO BPG Institute

- Adopted frameworks for implementation and sustainability

- Created an Interprofessional Best Practice Steering Committee and supporting infrastructure

- Engaged programs to identify opportunities for focus

- Developed an implementation plan, staging best practice work across the years of BPSO candidacy

In addition, in a large and complex organization, we understood the necessity of giving this work distinct recognition. Together with our Communications and Media Leaders, we created a tagline—"Best Practice Matters"—and visuals (Figure 7.6) that were and continue to be used to highlight best practice through communication and awareness-raising strategies.

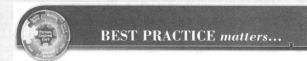

FIGURE 7.6 Sunnybrook Health Science Centre's "Best Practice Matters" logo.
Used with permission.

SUCCESSES

At the beginning of our BPSO candidacy, one of our key successes was the significant alignment created with our Nursing Council, a body that has nursing representation from units across the hospital. From the first year of candidacy to today, Nursing Council members have been engaged as key stakeholders: informing, advising, being involved in implementation, and serving as the conduit for best practice with other health professions. The Best Practice Steering Committee helped to ensure the inclusion of BPSO work in nonclinical areas such as human resource hiring practices, staff orientation, performance reviews, and the 2017–2020 Quality Strategic Plan.

Aligning BPGs within our Quality Improvement Plans has been a focus since the beginning, and we have continued to add indicators for person-centered care, falls risk reduction, patient mobilization, and delirium accuracy over the last few years. This provided additional visibility of these interventions both internal and external to the organization. As well, a BPG Dashboard (Figure 7.7) was created to align with our corporate Quality Improvement Portal and profile quarterly metrics for each best practice. Over time and with support, teams are growing in their ability to review performance, discuss improvement, and create local Action Plans to enhance patient outcomes. They use three guiding questions to assist them in reviewing their data:

1. What is our current status?

2. How are we moving toward the target?

3. What do we need to do to continue to improve?

"Clinicians will make things happen, when they understand why change is necessary."

—Sonia Dyal

APN of the Mental Health Department & Elaine Avila, Clinical Educator of inpatient oncology units

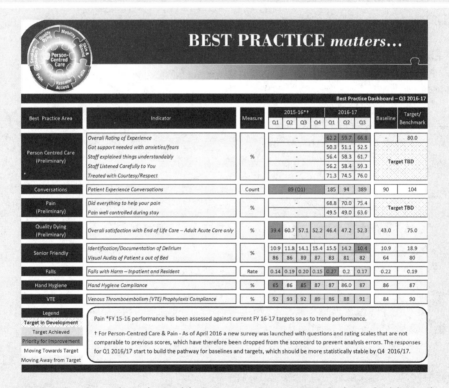

FIGURE 7.7   Sunnybrook Health Sciences Centre's BPG data dashboard.
Used with permission.

As a result of these quality initiatives, we have seen patient outcome improvements including the following:

- Pressure ulcer incidence reduction from 6.4% (2011) to 4.7% (2016)

- Quality Dying percent positive satisfaction scores, rising from 43% Q4, 2012/13 to 68% Q4, 2016/17

- Positive trends in both our patient experience and pain results on the new Canadian Patient Experience Survey tool

- Falls with harm/1,000 patient days meeting target in 8 of 12 quarters

- Mobilizing 80% of patients three times daily across 31 patient care units, for over 3 years

- Delirium accuracy, prevention, and management enhancements

- 2,395 Advanced Care Planning conversations documented since 2015

Other work is ongoing where future organization-wide impact is anticipated, including in areas related to violence management and prevention and managing high-risk behaviours.

SHSC began entering data within the RNAO's NQuIRE comprehensive data system in 2016. Data are being submitted for three RNAO Best Practices Guidelines—*Assessment and Management of Pain* (2013b), *Prevention of Falls and Fall Injuries in Older Adults* (2011b), and *Assessment and Management of Pressure Injuries for the Interprofessional Team* (2016)—from units in our Oncology, Rehab, Trauma, and Musculosketal Programs. We are in the relatively early stages of submission, anticipating the data will provide greater understanding of our process and outcome measures and the interplay with our human resources structural indicators (e.g., staffing, skill mix, absenteeism, and agency use).

In addition to being part of the Quality Improvement Program, staff at Sunnybrook is also encouraged to participate in Practice Based Research & Innovation (PBRI) activities. A very interesting part of our story has been the increasing interest and alignment between the two initiatives. As testament to this, of the 26 PBRI applications submitted for work in 2017/18, 11 are directly linked to best practice priorities. For each of these submissions, a Best Practice Lead serves as mentor, facilitating connectivity of the work and sustainability post-fellowship. Previous fellowship opportunities have achieved significant results, such as a 40% rise in patient mobilization, a 34% rise both in pain assessment every 4 hours and in pain reassessment post analgesic administration, change in dressing-change frequency, and adoption of a care-bundling tool.

A tremendous success has been the development of over 550 interprofessional direct-care staff as Champions, exceeding the 15% BPSO requirement. Champions are individuals who bring passion to patient care improvement and actively promote, educate, and inspire others to implement change and to adopt evidence into everyday care. Each Champion participates in an introductory Quality Improvement workshop endorsed by the RNAO as consistent with the RNAO BPG Champion Network Curriculum and led by our Quality and Patient Safety Department. The workshop provides Champions with the fundamental knowledge and tools to lead and sustain change. Then they work with their local teams to lead quality-improvement work based on BPG implementation and showcase their results in hospital-wide events.

To support the Champions, we created a new and innovative role of "Best Practice Change Coordinator." Change Coordinators are clinicians who know how things work, have connections with colleagues, and can translate theory into practice. In each of our candidacy years, we hired three interprofessional direct-care staff to mentor Champions approximately 2 days per month. Due to the success of this strategy, this important role has been sustained. As a result of this development opportunity, many Champions have gone on to post-graduate studies, while each of our Change Coordinators has moved on to formal leadership roles.

"As a Best Practice Change Coordinator I am learning and growing through experiences with Champions and leaders across the hospital. I am most proud to feel that together we are improving care for our patients."

—Marcia Fisher, Best Practice Change Coordinator

CHALLENGES

At Sunnybrook, we are thrilled to see the many accomplishments that have been achieved through our BPSO journey. As with any journey, there have been bumps in the road, and twists and turns that have caused us to reflect and challenge ourselves to ask, "Could it be even better if . . . ?" Limited time, competing demands, and advancing significant change in a large, multisite organization are amongst our greatest challenges. Despite their best intentions, staff often struggle to take on additional work and are challenged to find time to focus on initiatives, plan interventions, attend meetings, and engage colleagues to foster ideas for change.

We feel the solutions lie in the challenges themselves, and we continuously ask ourselves to think innovatively to:

- Bundle and integrate best practices so they are not viewed as additive

- Influence leaders' perspectives to help them recognize that modeling BPGs is one of the greatest ways to influence change

- Build technology that captures data and facilitates access to what we need to know

- Engage the organization to focus and collaborate on key priorities and solutions, recognizing that some will carry greater priority at different times

We believe that when the organization is engaged in ongoing dialogue about what "even better" looks like, we can co-create a future that makes sense, is meaningful, and has great impact.

SUSTAINABILITY

We began our BPSO journey explicitly intending to establish a process that would support all our work going forward. We have developed and continued to refine aspects of our program, building on what works and evolving what does not. We have a large Champion delegation, engaged local leaders, true credibility for best practice throughout the organization, and reporting mechanisms that have been ingrained and are aligned with key organizational priorities. Best Practice has had the support of Operations Directors who have made this work a priority within their programs. Reporting occurs on a regular basis to our Interprofessional Quality Committee, which provides additional advice and support. We also continue to take advantage of all the RNAO activities as outlined in Table 7.1. While we still have much to do, the structures clearly are in place to sustain Best Practices into the future.

THE FUTURE

At Sunnybrook, we are working very hard to continuously develop mechanisms to support Champions and enable them to know easily where focus is required to optimize patient outcomes and improve the patient experience. A formidable practice change that has resulted from this work is the identification and implementation of a system-wide approach to patient engagement. In 2012, prior to the development of the related RNAO BPG, *Person and Family Centred Care* (2015), 158 patient and family partners and 238 staff were asked to identify the recommendations needed to move forward with a person-centered approach to care. As a result of ongoing stakeholder engagement, and with the support of RNAO's BPGs, Sunnybrook is integrating consistent processes to standardize engagement and promote a seamless system of care for our patients.

We are also very excited about the recent launch of Sunnybrook's new Quality and Strategic Plan that not only articulates the key work that is needed across the organization but also engages staff in action-oriented improvement through quality conversations. We continue to share stories at our hospital—stories of connection and of inspiration, of care experiences and leadership. We are learning and growing together, endeavouring to ensure optimum patient outcomes are an obsession for all.

REFLECTIVE QUESTIONS

Thinking about the three case studies presented in this chapter:

1. What is the context for BPGs in your organization?

2. How might you leverage communication technology such as RNAO's BPSO Community of Practice (which connects all BPSOs around the world through a secure, technology-enabled sharing and discussion platform) in your implementation of BPGs?

3. Which of the leadership practices outlined in RNAO's Leadership BPG (2013c) would be most beneficial in beginning to implement BPGs within your organization?

4. Which leadership practices would be most beneficial in sustaining BPGs within your organization?

CONCLUSION

In conclusion, implementing and sustaining evidence-based practice is an important step in realizing improved care delivery and quality outcomes. Leadership is required at all levels of a BPSO, along with strategies that change and evolve over time. Leaders in the first BPSO pioneer cohort (first two case studies) took a brave step into the unknown, using many new educational techniques and electronic platforms, emerging evidence on implementation science, and tools and resources that were being developed "on the run." Fortunately, the BPSOs that followed (the Sunnybrook Health Sciences Centre case study) were able to learn from these experiences and "leap frog" forward in developing new approaches to engagement, implementation methods, and reporting systems. Our hope is that the discussion of our experience will provide some insight for others on or considering this journey. Although it is not for the faint of heart, the effort is very worthwhile as the use of BPGs ultimately improves outcomes for patients, nurses and other providers, health organizations, and the health system as a whole.

KEY MESSAGES

This chapter has outlined the experience of three BPSOs that implemented and sustained numerous RNAO BPGs over the past 18 years. Although each organization has had a unique experience, we found several common key messages across the organizations. Many of our insights build on the five transformation leadership practices found in the *Developing and Sustaining Nursing Leadership* BPG (RNAO, 2013c).

BUILD RELATIONSHIPS AND TRUST

Implementing and sustaining BPGs really comes down to listening to staff through appreciative inquiry mechanisms (Stavros et al., 2015) and working with them in order to provide the best knowledge possible and build teams and partnerships. Therefore, communication with stakeholder groups throughout the implementation stage is paramount to keeping everyone engaged. Understanding the organization's vision and strategic alignment of evidence-based practice is imperative. A key lesson learned was that although it is important to have a solid communication plan during implementation, it is equally as important to sustain internal communication and have a strategy that will continue to profile, celebrate, and recognize BPSO initiatives.

CREATE AN EMPOWERING WORK ENVIRONMENT

The work environment has a significant impact on care delivery and is an important aspect of implementation and sustainability. Staff must feel that they are respected and have the professional knowledge and skills they need to perform their roles. It is important that the staff feels part of a shared vision and understand that best practice achievements are the result of coordinated efforts from all staff. Time, planning, focus, leadership, structure, and resources are all critical inputs to evidence-based practice. While the initial implementation was focused on nursing, care today is delivered by interprofessional teams, which means organizations need an approach that promotes interprofessional collaboration in order to empower all workers and sustain momentum across disciplines. As well, it is imperative to have Champions at all levels of the organization to raise awareness about the use of evidence and to celebrate those using the guidelines to achieve quality care.

CREATE A CULTURE THAT SUPPORTS KNOWLEDGE DEVELOPMENT AND INTEGRATION

Part of an empowering work environment also includes a culture that supports knowledge development and integration. This vision needs to trickle down from senior management to the program level, where experts in clinical care help select appropriate guidelines for the setting, adapt them to suit the organization, and translate them into standardized or customized recommendations. Education needs to be available to all staff, and knowledge needs to be integrated into documentation systems for point-of-care data collection into the Continuous Quality Improvement system. These outcomes need to be reviewed through data dashboards in order to help identify areas of focus and improvement.

LEAD AND SUSTAIN CHANGE

Change can be difficult! It is a process that takes time and requires multiple strategies to achieve in practice, as identified in Chapter 4 of the RNAO Implementation Toolkit (2012). Challenges can be exacerbated by high staff growth, turnover, and the need to provide staff with time out of the work environment to receive BPG and implementation science education. Project Leaders need to be nimble, resilient, committed to the initiative, and flexible in their approach. The staff needs to be coached to talk with their colleagues, support the collective to realize change, and celebrate patient outcome improvements. Leaders should also look outside their organization to other BPSOs for tools, resources, and support; to RNAO coaches and experts; and the many capacity-building opportunities provided through RNAO such as the BPSO Knowledge Exchange Symposiums.

BALANCE COMPLEX ENVIRONMENTS AND MANAGE COMPETING VALUES AND PRIORITIES

Lastly, do not expect implementation to be a linear process; there will be a lot of ups and downs along the way given the complexity of organizations and health systems. It is vitally important you advocate for the proper resources, link BPG work to other strategic initiatives, and embed BPG implementation into the day-to-day operations through various processes such as patient safety initiatives, quality assurance programs, and accreditation. When faced with multiple demands and competing priorities, take a step back, review how you can dovetail projects together, and adjust your approach. And never give up; perseverance and creativity pay off by delivering results that are good for patients, and all involved will feel proud.

REFERENCES

Advisory Panel on Healthcare Innovation. (2015). *Unleashing innovation: Excellent healthcare for Canada—Executive summary*. Retrieved from http://www.healthycanadians.gc.ca/publications/health-system-systeme-sante/summary-innovation-sommaire/alt/summary-innovation-sommaire-eng.pdf

Canada Health Infoway. (2013, May 6). *Emerging technology series: Big data analytics in health* [White paper]. Retrieved from https://www.infoway-inforoute.ca/en/component/edocman/resources/technical-documents/emerging-technology/1246-big-data-analytics-in-health-white-paper-full-report

Canadian Institute of Health Information (CIHI). (2013). *A performance measurement framework for the Canadian health system*. Retrieved from https://secure.cihi.ca/free_products/HSP_Framework_Technical_Report_EN.pdf

Cancer Quality Council of Ontario. (2017). *Cancer System Quality Index (CSQI) 2017*. Retrieved from http://www.csqi.on.ca/

DiCenso, A. (2003). Research: Evidence-based nursing practice: How to get there from here. *Nursing Leadership, 16*(4), 20–26. Retrieved from http://www.electronichealthcare.net/content/16257

DiCenso, A., Ciliska, D., & Guyatt, G. (2005). Introduction to evidence-based nursing. In A. DiCenso, G. Guyatt, & D. Ciliska (Eds.), *Evidence-based nursing: A guide to clinical practice* (pp. 3–19). St. Louis, MO: Elsevier Mosby.

Duffield, C., Diers, D., O'Brien-Pallas, L., Aisbett, C., Roche, M., King, M., . . . Aisbett, K. (2011). Nursing staffing, nursing workload, the work environment and patient outcomes. *Applied Nursing Research, 24*, 244–255.

Galbraith, J. R. (2001). *Designing organizations: An executive guide to strategy, structure, and process*. San Francisco, CA: Jossey-Bass Publishing.

Gailbraith, J. R. The Star Model. Retrieved from http://www.jaygalbraith.com/services/star-model

Gifford, W., Davies, B., Rowan, M., Egan, M., Lefebre, N., & Brehaut, J. (2016). Understand audit and feedback to support falls prevention and pain management in home health care. *Home Health Care Management & Practice, 28*(2), 79–85.

Grinspun, D., Virani, T., & Bajnok, I. (2002). Nursing Best Practice Guidelines: The Registered Nurses' Association of Ontario Project. *Hospital Quarterly, 5*(2), 56–60.

Konietzny, C. & Anderson, B. (2018). Comfort Conversations in Complex Continuing Care: Assessing Patients' and Families' Palliative Care Needs. *Perspectives, 39, 4. (pending release of Journal)*

Lawler, E. E. (1996). *From the ground up: Six principles for building the new logic corporation*. San Francisco, CA: Jossey-Bass Publishing.

Manely, K., McCormack, B., Wilson, V. (Eds.). (2008). *International practice development in nursing and healthcare*. Oxford, UK: Blackwell Publishing Ltd.

Martens, P., Martin, B., O'Neil, J., & MacKinnon, M. (2007). Diabetes and adverse outcomes in a First Nations population: Associations with healthcare access and socio-economic and geographical factors. *Canadian Journal of Diabetes, 31*(3), 223–232.

Ploeg, J., Skelly, J., Rowan, M., Edwards, N., Davies, B., Grinspun, D., . . . Downey, A. (2010). The role of nursing best practice champions in diffusing practice guidelines: A mixed methods study. *Worldviews on Evidence-Based Nursing, 7*(4), 238–251.

Purdy, N., Spence Laschinger, H., Finegan, J., Kerr, M., & Olivera, F. (2010). Effects of work environments on nurse and patient outcomes. *Journal of Nursing Management, 18*(8), 901–913.

Registered Nurses' Association of Ontario (RNAO). (2002). *Client centered care*. Toronto, ON: Registered Nurses' Association of Ontario.

Registered Nurses' Association of Ontario (RNAO). (2004a). *Assessment and management of venous leg ulcers*. Toronto, ON: Registered Nurses' Association of Ontario.

Registered Nurses' Association of Ontario (RNAO). (2004b). *Reducing foot complications for people with diabetes*. Toronto, ON: Registered Nurses' Association of Ontario.

Registered Nurses' Association of Ontario (RNAO). (2006a). *Client centred care* (Supplement). Toronto, ON: Registered Nurses' Association of Ontario.

Registered Nurses' Association of Ontario (RNAO). (2006b). *Establishing therapeutic relationships*. Toronto, ON: Registered Nurses' Association of Ontario.

Registered Nurses' Association of Ontario (RNAO). (2007a). *Professionalism in nursing*. Toronto, ON: Registered Nurses' Association of Ontario.

Registered Nurses' Association of Ontario (RNAO). (2007b). *Reducing foot complications for people with diabetes* (Supplement). Toronto, ON: Registered Nurses' Association of Ontario.

Registered Nurses' Association of Ontario (RNAO). (2009). *BPG for subcutaneous administration of insulin in adults with type 2 diabetes*. Toronto, ON: Registered Nurses' Association of Ontario.

Registered Nurses' Association of Ontario (RNAO). (2010). *Strategies to support self-management in chronic conditions: Collaboration with clients*. Toronto, ON: Registered Nurses' Association of Ontario.

Registered Nurses' Association of Ontario (RNAO). (2011a). *End-of-life care during the last days and hours*. Toronto, ON: Registered Nurses' Association of Ontario.

Registered Nurses' Association of Ontario (RNAO). (2011b). *Prevention of falls and fall injuries in the older adult*. Toronto, ON: Registered Nurses' Association of Ontario.

Registered Nurses' Association of Ontario (RNAO). (2012). *Toolkit: Implementation of Best Practice Guidelines* (2nd ed.). Toronto, ON: Registered Nurses' Association of Ontario.

Registered Nurses' Association of Ontario (RNAO). (2013a). *Assessment and management of foot ulcers for people with diabetes* (2nd ed.). Toronto, ON: Registered Nurses' Association of Ontario.

Registered Nurses' Association of Ontario (RNAO). (2013b). *Assessment and management of pain* (3rd ed.). Toronto, ON: Registered Nurses' Association of Ontario.

Registered Nurses' Association of Ontario (RNAO). (2013c). *Developing and sustaining nursing leadership* (2nd ed.). Toronto, ON: Registered Nurses' Association of Ontario.

Registered Nurses' Association of Ontario (RNAO). (2014). *Care transitions*. Toronto, ON: Registered Nurses' Association of Ontario.

Registered Nurses' Association of Ontario (RNAO). (2015). *Person and family centred care*. Toronto, ON: Registered Nurses' Association of Ontario.

Registered Nurses' Association of Ontario (RNAO). (2016). *Assessment and management of pressure injuries for the interprofessional team* (3rd ed.). Toronto, ON: Registered Nurses' Association of Ontario.

Registered Nurses' Association of Ontario (RNAO). (2017). *Best Practice Spotlight Organization (BPSO) requirements*. Retrieved from http://rnao.ca/bpg/bpso/become

Rogers, E. (1995). *Diffusion of innovations* (4th ed.). New York, NY: Free Press.

Saint Elizabeth Health Care and Assembly of Manitoba Chiefs. (2011). *Patient wait time guarantee pilot project for the prevention, care and treatment of foot ulcers of people living with diabetes in Manitoba First Nations*. Retrieved from https://www.saintelizabeth.com/FNIM/About-Us/Initiatives/Manitoba-First-Nations-Patient-Wait-Times-Guarante.aspx

Stavros, J., Godwin, L., & Cooperrider, D. (2015). Appreciative inquiry: Organization development and the strengths revolution. In W. J. Rothwell, J. M. Stavros & R. L. Sullivan (Eds.), Practicing organization development: A guide to leading change and transformation (4th ed.) (pp. 96–116). Toronto, ON: Wiley.

West Park Healthcare Centre Compilation of Reports. (2016). Based on Canadian Institute of Health Information (CIHI) Complex Continuing Care Reporting System, Facility Level Reports for West Park Healthcare Centre. (2006–07, 2009–10, 2012–13, 2015–16, and 2016–17 Q1–3).

8

CREATING EVIDENCE-BASED CULTURES ACROSS THE HEALTH CONTINUUM

Carol Timmings, MEd (Admin), BNSc, RN
Barbara Heatley O'Neil, MAdEd, BScN
Leeann Whitney, MAEd, BScN, RN
Holly Quinn, MHS, BScN, RN
Sonya Canzian, MHSc, RN, CNN(C)

LEARNING OBJECTIVES

After reading this chapter, you will be able to:

- Describe the BPSO experience of four different health sector organizations: public health, hospital, primary care, and home care

- Give examples of how different organizations achieved, sustained, and continue to expand an evidence-based culture across the four health sectors

- Demonstrate the common and unique organizational implementation strategies in creating and sustaining a BPSO evidence-based culture

- Analyze which methods could be applied in other health settings to achieve BPSO Designation and an evidence-based culture

ACKNOWLEDGMENTS

The authors want to acknowledge the following contributors to this chapter:

- Toronto Public Health:

    - May Tao: RN, BScN, MSN, CCHN(C) Health Promotion Specialist
    - Katie Dilworth: RN, BScN, MHSc-HP, CCHN(C) Supervisor Nursing Quality Practice

- North Bay Nurse Practitioner-Led Clinic:

    - Terri MacDougall: NP-PHC, MScN IBCLC
    - Johanna Fonteine: RN

- Bayshore Home Health:

    - Janet Daglish: CMC, PMP, National Director, Business Development & Government Relations
    - Anna Cooper: RN, BScN, MN, Clinical Practice Leader/BPSO Lead
    - Tanya Baker: RN, BScN, Clinical Practice Manger/BPSO Lead

- St. Michael's Hospital:

    - Ella Ferris: RN, MBA, Former Executive Vice President, Programs and Chief Nursing and Health Disciplines Executive
    - Lianne Jeffs: RN PhD, FAAN, St. Michael's Hospital Volunteer Chair in Nursing Research, Scientist, Keenan Research Centre, Li Ka Shing Knowledge Institute
    - Murray Krock: RN, BScN, MN, Director, Nursing Practice and Education Professional Practice
    - Ashley Skiffington: RN, BScN, Med, Evidence-Based Practice Nursing Manager

INTRODUCTION

Healthcare today demands the understanding and implementation of evidence-based practices across the care-continuum. Patients/clients and their families should not be required to expend more time and energy thinking about the quality of the care they will receive than they do to stay healthy or to manage a specific disease. Patients/clients and their families require care at various times from a variety of providers. Transitions across the continuum of care should ideally be based on the same high-quality and evidence-based practices regardless of clinical specialty, location, day of the week, or time of day.

As the leaders of five organizations in Ontario individually grasped these concepts on a day-to-day basis, they each began their quest to seek out the best sources of evidence and to implement them in a sustainable way. Each of them turned to the Registered Nurses' Association of Ontario (RNAO) to acquire Best Practice Guidelines (BPG) to understand how to implement and sustain them, and finally to position their organizations to become Best Practice Spotlight Organizations (BPSO). Each undertook a unique approach related to: their motivation to become a BPSO, getting started, successes, challenges, and overall organizational impact. In this chapter, each leader discusses this unique approach, what BPSO looks like in their organization today, and their perspectives on the future.

TORONTO PUBLIC HEALTH BPSO EXPERIENCE

Toronto Public Health (TPH) serves 2.8 million residents and employs 1,800 staff, including 750 nurses. TPH's mission is to reduce health inequities and improve the health of the whole population. Innovative programs, direct services, partnerships, health communication, health monitoring, and advocacy for healthy public policies help to prevent sickness and disease, promote health, and improve the quality of people's lives.

Population health aims to improve the health of the entire population and is the primary approach in public health work. Its programs, services, and health policies focus on responding to the needs of vulnerable populations and advocating for attention to social determinants of health (Public Health Agency of Canada [PHAC], 2012).

LEARNING FROM THE PAST

In late 2002, a previously unknown disease emerged from China called severe acute respiratory syndrome, or SARS, spreading across the globe over the course of several weeks (Health Canada, 2003). About 8,500 persons worldwide were diagnosed with probable SARS during the epidemic, and there were over 900 deaths (Health Canada, 2003). Toronto was the epicenter for the SARS epidemic, which placed unprecedented demands on the public health system, challenging capacity for outbreak containment, surveillance, information management, and infection control. In the years following, the response was analyzed revealing systemic deficiencies in the public health system in Canada. We learned that Canada's ability to fight an outbreak such as SARS was tied more closely to the specific strengths of the public health system than to the general capacity of our publicly-funded healthcare system (Health Canada, 2003). A strong national call to improve public health services resulted.

System change included a new *Ontario Agency for Health Protection and Promotion* and revised *Ontario Public Health Standards* (Ministry of Health and Long-Term Care[MOHLTC], 2008), which established minimum requirements for fundamental public health programs and services. Both the new agency and standards would build an evidence-based culture for public health practice

in Ontario. Instead of planning programs and services in response to public demand or spotty use of evidence, all public health programs and services would be based on evidence. Further, a "capacity review" of the public health system called for increased public accountability including evidence-based programming and performance monitoring and reporting (Capacity Review Committee, 2006).

Key to the recommendations following SARS was a plan to rebuild the public health workforce with a range of activities from defining competencies through introduction of master's programs and professional development for staff (Joint Task Group on Public Health Human Resources, 2005). Advancing practice would require integration of evidence.

BPSO AND TPH: PERFECT ALIGNMENT

This increased focus on evidence, accountability requirements, and human resource recommendations post-SARS was aligned with internal directions at Toronto Public Health (TPH). With a strategic orientation toward innovative and outstanding service, a new professional practice model was being developed to enable the highest quality of professional practice. This mechanism would enhance the development of professional nursing leadership in the organization, facilitating the creation of mechanisms to support excellence in nursing practice, a catalyst toward TPH becoming part of the RNAO BPSO initiative. BPGs, with practice recommendations based on current and quality research, ensured the evidence was available. BPSO made integration of the evidence possible.

TPH staff had been involved in the development and integration of many RNAO Best Practice Guidelines (BPG) in the past, paving the way toward exploration of the merits of becoming a BPSO. A readiness assessment by nursing leaders found willingness and opportunity to improve evidence-based service and determined TPH was ideally situated to become a BPSO to positively impact evidence-based practice. An initial gap analysis (RNAO, 2012c) identified four BPGs to implement throughout the organization.

Fostering the development of others and building teams to encourage collaboration and cooperation are recognized as key to achieving results (Community Health Nurses of Canada, 2015). The initiative would need the buy-in of the senior management and practice support networks. A TPH BPSO structure was established to enable collaboration and support. The structure was designed to consist of a central steering committee as well as BPG implementation teams, each supported by Champions.

The steering committee is composed of one member from each of the BPG teams (currently 12) and is connected to the chief nursing officer and medical officer of health as well as professional practice supports (see Figure 8.1).

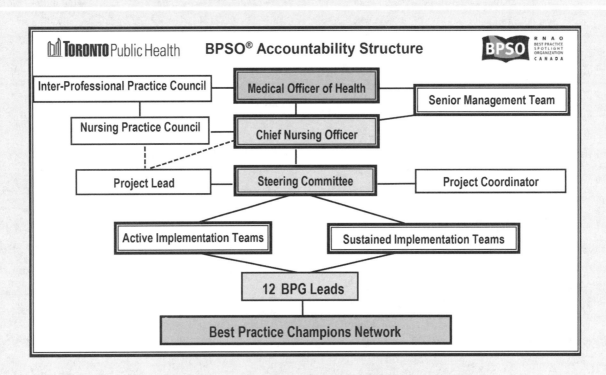

FIGURE 8.1 TPH BPSO accountability structure.
Used with permission.

Each BPG team works to initiate, implement, and evaluate recommendations from its guideline and has a cadre of Champions to work with from across the organization.

The Champion model is well established in the literature as an effective method of knowledge transfer (Flodgren et al., 2011; Kitson, 2009; Ploeg et al., 2010). An enthusiastic and committed group of over 260 BPG Champions has been recruited from several program areas and disciplines to assist with implementation. Champions are assigned to specific BPG implementation and evaluation activities based on skill sets and relevance to programs. An orientation webinar, tailored to public health practice, is provided to new Champions, enabling them to understand the overall BPSO initiative and the role and significance of being a Champion. The primary responsibility of Champions is to be a resource for their colleagues as an "expert" about their BPG. Champions post signage at their workstations, so colleagues are aware they are Champions and can seek them out as necessary (see Figure 8.2).

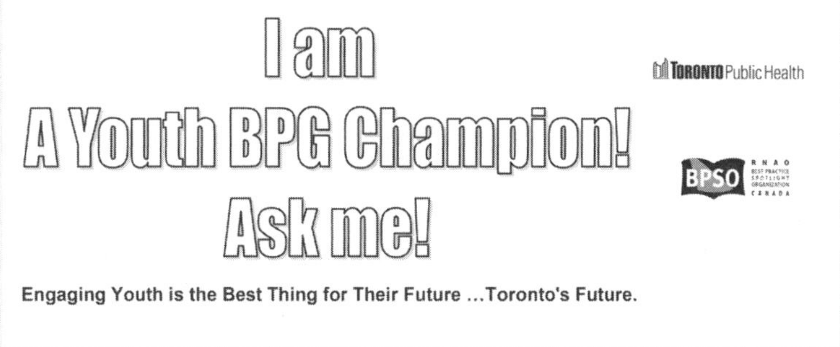

FIGURE 8.2 Champion desk sign.
Used with permission.

Champions are provided with ongoing professional development and support and, in turn, they provide training and support to their colleagues. One innovative strategy was training Champions in storytelling as an additional knowledge-transfer tool. Champions proved to be competent and knowledgeable public health practitioners who quickly shifted to evidence-based practice, contributing to excellence in public health. The Champion role is an excellent opportunity to develop leadership capacity.

COLLABORATION FOR SUCCESS

Although BPSO was initiated by nursing at TPH, its implementation is interdisciplinary and across the organization. Collaboration between professionals in a variety of program areas and with external partners has enhanced a systematic integration of evidence. Examples include the *Primary Prevention of Childhood Obesity* BPG team and the *Integrating Smoking Cessation into Daily Practice* BPG team.

The *Primary Prevention of Childhood Obesity* (RNAO, 2014c) BPG team has over 100 Champions who implement and evaluate the guideline. Public Health Nurses (PHNs) and Registered Dieticians collaborate to build capacity with schools in addressing strategies to reduce childhood obesity in 18 (and counting) Toronto schools. Nurses from the *Integrating Smoking Cessation into Daily Practice* (RNAO, 2003c) BPG team work with staff from across the organization to provide cessation counselling and nicotine replacement therapy to Toronto residents who would not otherwise have access to this evidence-based cessation tool. Partnership with other smoking cessation stakeholders has enabled sustained support for clients starting a quit attempt.

CUSTOMIZED SOLUTIONS TO FIT THE PRACTICE CONTEXT

The BPSO Initiative is part of a bigger picture to systematically integrate evidence into practice. TPH's unique role in health promotion in a population health context sometimes requires adaptation of BPG content to fit the public health context. The *Woman Abuse: Screening, Identification and Initial Response* BPG (RNAO, 2005f), for example, suggests universal screening "each time the health history is updated" (p.23), which is not appropriate for TPH group programs where clients attend multiple sessions. Occasionally at the adaptation stage, there is a need to conduct further research or literature reviews to ensure a fit with the strong prevention and health promotion philosophy in public health. The *Preventing and Addressing Abuse and Neglect of Older Adults* (RNAO, 2014b) BPG team completed a literature review to further define elder abuse prevention and to adapt strategies to fit the public health practice context.

START SMALL, THINK BIG

Best Practice Guideline recommendations are piloted in a small program team first and then evaluated (start small). Once the intervention's effectiveness is demonstrated, the intervention is scaled up to other programs and teams in the organization. Results are often disseminated internally at knowledge translation events and externally through publications and conferences (think and act BIG), contributing to systematic integration of evidence into practice. All levels of the organization are involved, from the Board of Health to the direct-care staff, to enhance practice and sustain the change.

CHALLENGES

During TPH's first year of BPSO candidacy, the organization experienced infrastructure challenges, taxing the staff and senior management (a 6-week labour disruption, and a level 5 H1N1 pandemic). These unforeseen challenges delayed the rollout of the BPSO events, necessitating compression of candidacy activities the following year. Managing the BPSO Designation required orienting new staff to assist and keeping a sharp focus on the work plan. TPH successfully moved forward and achieved designation in the required 3-year timeframe.

Evaluation of BPG implementation in public health practice can be a challenge. Measuring the success of implementation depends on the identification of measurable outcome indicators. Health outcomes for clients receiving public health intervention will often not be measurable until years after the intervention (e.g., increased rates of smoking cessation resulting in decreased rates of lung cancer). BPG teams have acknowledged this and are evaluating intermediate outcomes such as changes in client behaviour or awareness as well as outcomes related to staff learning and behaviour.

A TRANSFORMATIVE EXPERIENCE

The BPSO experience at Toronto Public Health has been transformative. It has increased our commitment to evidence-based practice and increased our staff competence, as well as their confidence that they are using the very best evidence available and making a measurable difference in the quality of service our clients receive.

A comprehensive evaluation conducted by TPH demonstrated that the experience of being a BPSO Designate has had positive benefits, including an increase in the use of evidence and knowledge sharing and increased collaboration amongst programs and interdisciplinary staff. Staff engagement in BPSO at all levels has contributed to organizational success in BPG implementation and sustainability (Toronto Public Health, 2011).

Toronto Public Health, the largest health unit in Canada, plays a leadership role for other public health organizations. As a BPSO, TPH soundly demonstrates the impact of creating and sustaining an evidence-based culture. Through full engagement and mobilization of the interprofessional team, sustained use of evidence-informed practice has made a difference in the health of the population in the City of Toronto.

CASE STUDY

BLUEWATER HEALTH BPSO EXPERIENCE

Bluewater Health—with locations in Sarnia and Petrolia, Ontario, Canada—is a fully accredited, 326-bed community hospital. With close to 2,500 staff, professional staff, and volunteers, Bluewater Health provides an array of specialized acute care, complex continuing care, allied health, and ambulatory care services. State-of-the-art facilities contribute to Bluewater Health's Mission: We create exemplary healthcare experiences with patients and families every time.

BLUEWATER'S MOTIVATION TO BECOME A BPSO

In 2009 and 2010, clinical practice professionals at Bluewater Health (BWH) were reviewing processes and procedures, seeking the evidence and rationale behind them in preparation for the move to a new hospital site in Sarnia. We recognized that some were based on habit and the practicality of locations of equipment, departments, and sites. The evidence required to ensure we were using current best practices and maximizing the opportunity to work collaboratively in the new environment was found in the RNAO's Best Practice Guidelines (BPG).

In October 2011, we submitted our proposal to RNAO to become a candidate to achieve BPSO Designation. Our quest began when the various professions engaged in focus groups to choose 7 BPGs for implementation, out of the possible 31 RNAO BPGs, that applied to our setting. Our selections were:

■ *Client Centred Care* (RNAO, 2002a)

■ *Supporting and Strengthening Families through Expected and Unexpected Life Events* (RNAO, 2002f)

■ *Establishing Therapeutic Relationships* (RNAO, 2002c)

■ *Strategies to Support Self-Management in Chronic Conditions: Collaboration with Clients* (RNAO, 2010e)

■ *Integrating Smoking Cessation into Daily Nursing Practice* (RNAO, 2003c)

■ *Assessment and Management of Pain* (RNAO, 2009a)

■ *Prevention of Falls and Fall Injuries in the Older Adult* (RNAO, 2002d)

GETTING STARTED

We launched our BPSO journey in April 2012. Year one focused on the recruitment of 98 Best Practice Champions to lead the work. We developed structures and processes to support implementation and evaluation of recommendations, and our Interprofessional Champion Model promoted a collaborative approach to both practice and patient- and family-centered care (RNAO, 2002a, 2009b).

Our intention was to begin with the *Client Centred Care* BPG (RNAO, 2002a). It was immediately evident that the work associated with the implementation of the *Client Centred Car*e (RNAO, 2002a), *Supporting and Strengthening Families through Expected and Unexpected Life Events* (RNAO, 2002f), and *Establishing Therapeutic Relationships* (RNAO, 2002c) guidelines was so aligned and integrated that we moved forward with all three together. They became known as the "big three." Best Practice Champions led the spread of the "big three" on

each of their units, with peer-to-peer learning, leadership support, and engagement (RNAO, 2007, 2013b, 2016b).

TWO NOTEWORTHY SUCCESSES

The BPSO journey was hard-wired into the Mission Statement, Strategic Plan, and Performance Goals. During Strategic Planning (fall 2012), there was a desire to "hardwire" our care philosophy into quality and safety initiatives. Dialogue began with Standing Committees of the Board to articulate themes and goals. The process was inclusive, innovative, and warm. We brought ideas through our stories. There was energy from the bedside to the boardroom about what authentic patient- and family-centered care (PFCC) would mean to care providers and to the way we partner with patients and families in care. This resulted in the 2013–2015 Strategic Goal, "Embed Patient & Family-Centred Care," and the creation of supporting "We will" statements:

We will:

■ Create a patient- and family-centered care strategy and action plan

■ Establish a Patient Experience Partner Council and a PFCC Advisory Council

■ Engage Patient Experience Partners (PEPs) in quality-improvement initiatives

■ Develop a plan to educate our people on PFCC principles and care strategies

■ Implement the RNAO BPGs—*Client Centred Care* (RNAO, 2002a), *Establishing Therapeutic Relationships* (RNAO, 2002c), and *Supporting and Strengthening Families in Expected and Unexpected Life Events* (RNAO 2002f)

We introduced Emily. Following broad consultation and site visits to exemplars in client-centered care, we began to explore the notion of naming *our patient,* as a way to really embrace client- and family-centered care (Toussaint, Gerard, & Adams, 2010). After much discussion of our findings and full engagement of staff through storytelling, we made the decision to name our patient. The name Emily was chosen, and each of us had an influence on Emily's experience of care, regardless of role. Emily came to represent every patient and family we had cared for in the past, were currently caring for, and would care for in the future (Jennings, O'Neil, Bossy, Dodman, & Campbell, 2016)

Emily debuted at the 2013 launch of our Strategic Plan as a collage of images of all of us—patients and families, care providers, physicians, support service staff, students, volunteers—engaged in giving and receiving care. Emily represented every face amongst us. Staff, physicians, and volunteers can find themselves in the Emily image (see Figure 8.3). The picture was present for events including BPG launches and knowledge exchange events. A newsletter was developed, and direct-care leaders named it "Dear Emily."

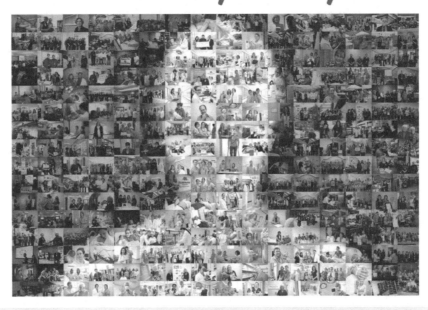

FIGURE 8.3 Emily image.
Used with permission.

Our Patient Advocate engaged patients and family members to create the Patient Advisory Council. A new volunteer role, the Patient Experience Partner (PEP), was launched. One of our PEPs shared her reaction to the Strategic Plan: "Emily's symbolic presence is our inspiration. She is the reason we do what we do."

TWO NOTEWORTHY CHALLENGES

Implementation barrier: We do that already. The implementation of the "big three" required us to reflect on every activity surrounding care. In early discussions with providers, we heard, "We do that already." Movement forward required imagining what inclusivity in care could look like when we intentionally asked ourselves about opportunities to invite patients and families into care as equal partners at point of care, on our units, and on our committees, including the Quality Committee of the Board for discussion about adverse events. We encountered scepticism, reluctance, and eventually a willingness to begin.

Courage required. It took courage to unveil the image of Emily and to explain this abstract notion. There was anxiety that the idea could be seen as "fluff," with the risk that the initiatives surrounding it, including the Strategic Plan and the journey to become a BPSO, could be tainted and our initiatives derailed. The courage and energy came from knowing that, regardless of role, whether in clinical, support, or administrative services, each of us could relate to Emily when we opened our hearts to the idea. We, or someone in our family, may have *been* Emily. If any one of us could be Emily, then how we deliver care becomes personal. Emily has brought focus to our conversations, our initiatives, our attitudes, our environment, and our culture.

OVERALL ORGANIZATIONAL IMPACT OF BPSO AND THE EMILY EFFECT

Over the course of our BPSO journey, we saw positive results in employee engagement scores and patient satisfaction scores. Comparing 2011 engagement scores with 2013, we achieved a 16% improvement in Quality Care; 19% improvement in Involvement in Decisions; and a 20% improvement in Positive Work Environment. Our overall employee-engagement score was 6% higher than other hospitals in Ontario.

When 2,500 staff, physicians, and volunteers began to think differently about Emily and to see the benefits of the "big three" BPGs on our culture, they experienced, in varying degrees, the meaningfulness of what we can do collectively. Emily has given the BPGs a face, a voice, and a realization that quality care based in evidence really does matter. As Champions made the alignment with all of the BPGs, they made the connections to Emily. Conversations and stories about Emily are increasingly shared across the organization. BPSO Initiatives implemented have taken on a higher relevance as Emily has provided us with a shared vision of what the patient experience and our culture can be. We received our Best Practice Spotlight Organization Designation in June 2015.

Also in 2015, the National Research Corporation, Picker Institute confirmed that our performance indicators on the Canadian Patient Satisfaction survey documents in several areas were above average and that they "were coming to visit BWH to see what we were doing." The Picker Institute was mapping patient-centered-care best practices, processes, and cultural attributes of the 99th percentile performers from publicly reported standardized patient experience data sets in Canada, Europe, and the U.S. BWH had achieved top performance in multiple dimensions of patient-centered care in comparison to other hospitals reporting in Ontario, with improvement in Access to Care, Physical Comfort, Respect for Patient Preference, Continuity and Transition, Coordination of Care, and Overall Rating scores. They wrote a case study profiling Bluewater Health as a high performer in delivering client-centered care based on exemplary performance on the acute care dimension of Access to Care (National Research Corporation, 2015).

SUSTAINING AND EXPANDING

Nearing the conclusion of the 2013–2015 Strategic Plan and with the achievement of our stated goals, there was a desire to take the "We will" commitments and refine them into statements that held specific and measurable relevance for each of us. Fourteen focus groups were held with 100 individuals from diverse roles including nurses, physicians, allied health professionals, management, support staff, patients, volunteers, PEPs, and family members. They were asked to recall moments of exemplary care. Together they drafted the "I will" statements that are called "My Promise to Emily" (Ontario Hospital Association, n.d.).

I promise you and your family I will:

- Respect you as an individual on a unique healthcare journey

- Take time to address your concerns and calm your fears

- Involve you whenever decisions are being made about you

- Be your advocate

Bluewater Health wrote the Mission Statement: "We create exemplary healthcare experiences *for* patients and families every time," about 8 years ago. It guided us beautifully for many years. As we introduced Emily, we began to question the appropriateness of the word *for*. We wondered if we had moved so far as to change the word to *with*. After receiving our BPSO Designation, we began the work of the Strategic Plan 2016–2021. The new plan is called "Kaleidoscope of Care." The image of Emily is at the center. At the board retreat, spring 2016, it was decided that the Mission Statement would officially be changed to, "We create exemplary healthcare experiences *with* patients and families every time."

Becoming a BPSO has given us renewed energy. Creating a culture where this kind of caring can occur is perhaps the greatest effect of Emily to date. Many of our staff spoke about BPSO and Emily at events in Canada and the United States in order to share our successes and challenges and be a mentor and role model for others. The philosophy of evidence-based patient- and family-centered care that we desired 8 years ago is now hard-wired into our mission statement and our culture, where we have re-engaged with the human experience of caring.

CASE STUDY

NORTH BAY NURSE PRACTITIONER-LED CLINIC BPSO EXPERIENCE

The North Bay Nurse Practitioner-Led Clinic (NBNPLC) is one of 25 Nurse Practitioner-Led Clinics in Ontario, Canada. Nurse Practitioner-Led Clinics are an innovative model for delivery of comprehensive primary healthcare in Ontario, Canada, that are "led" by nurse practitioners at a governance and administrative level. The NBNPLC opened its doors in the Nipissing District in northern Ontario in 2011 to help meet the demand of people seeking primary care. Clinic staff, including nurse practitioners, registered nurses, and social workers, work to their full scope of practice as defined by the regulatory colleges.

IN THE BEGINNING

In 2011, as a new organization with healthcare providers coming together from all areas of the health system, the NBNPLC was challenged to incorporate evidence-based procedures into the process of providing primary care. The team set a goal to define what processes could be performed similarly by all members of the healthcare team, based on the best available evidence, while maintaining the priority of patient-centeredness in a relationship-based model of healthcare.

The team developed the following goals to guide all care and service provided at the clinic.

- Provide safe, ethical care with prevention as a key outcome for patient care

- Base delivery of care on the best available scientific knowledge to all those who could benefit, and refrain from providing interventions when evidence suggests otherwise (Choosing Wisely Canada, n.d.)

- Avoid waste and find ways to improve processes based on Lean implementation (Toussaint et al., 2010)

- Intake patients who are underserved and need primary care, while at the same time implementing same-day access to appointments

- Provide equitable care that does not vary in quality based on gender, ethnicity, income, sexual orientation, or religion

- Provide care that is respectful and responsive to patient needs, values, and preferences

In order to help ourselves achieve these goals, we applied to RNAO to become a BPSO, with the successful outcome of achieving BPSO Designate status. Central to its success, the whole clinic (14 staff) became involved in implementation of five clinical BPGs, namely: *Integrating Smoking Cessation into Daily Practice* (RNAO, 2003c), *Assessment and Management of Pain* (RNAO, 2009a), *Interventions for Postpartum Depression* (RNAO, 2005c), *Woman Abuse: Screening, Identification and Initial*

Response (RNAO, 2005f), *Strategies to Support Self-Management of Chronic Conditions* (RNAO, 2010e); and one HWE BPG—*Collaborative Practice Among Nursing Teams* (RNAO, 2006). When working with the RNAO BPGs, because this was an interprofessional initiative, the NBN-PLC team made an intentional decision to use terms that were inclusive of all healthcare professionals. Over the 3 years of BPSO candidacy, six workgroups were formed, with a lead who organized and facilitated meetings with those who self-identified as wanting to work on BPG implementation in the clinic. In 2015–2016, as a BPSO Designate, the clinic implemented two more clinical BPGs, namely *Breastfeeding Best Practice Guidelines for Nurses* (RNAO, 2003a) and *Nursing Management of Hypertension* (RNAO, 2005d).

System-wide implementation meant that all staff working at the clinic were involved in all aspects of BPG uptake, including prioritizing which BPGs to implement first and using the RNAO BPG Toolkit (RNAO, 2012c) to ensure a systematic methodology. For example, many staff were familiar with the *Integration of Smoking Cessation into Daily Practice* BPG (RNAO, 2003c), and one of the nurse practitioners was already a smoking cessation BPG Champion, so that BPG was identified as our first priority.

All BPGs were chosen based on the issues identified in the patient population we serve, as well as available practice Champions and available local resources. Because of the targeted support from RNAO that was provided over the 3 years pre-Designation, all staff became BPG Champions, and each took on various lead positions for one of the six BPG workgroups.

Results of work by the individual groups were shared with the clinic team at bimonthly BPG meetings. Process maps, standardized documentation procedures, and coding in the Electronic Health Record (called Nightingale) helped communicate and sustain practice changes. Various reporting formats were created along the way, including a BPG Dashboard (see Figure 8.4). The segment of the dashboard included in the figure demonstrates, in the graph on the left side, the number of patients screened preimplementation of the RNAO Pain BPG (RNAO, 2009a), and, in the graph on the right side, the number of patients screened post-implementation. The differences are striking, and they have consistently grown and been sustained. NQuIRE was also utilized to track structural, process, and outcome measures, in relation to this and other guidelines.

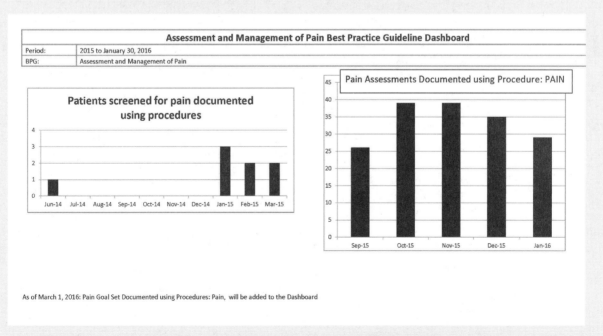

FIGURE 8.4 Dashboard showing patients screened for pain documented using procedures, before and after implementation of the *Assessment and Management of Pain* BPG (2009a). Used with permission.

STAKEHOLDER INVOLVEMENT IS KEY

Stakeholders were involved throughout our BPG journey and continue to be utilized based on their mandates, interest, time availability, and influence. The model for stakeholder participation that guided us suggests at least four different ways people and agencies can support a cause (Ontario Agency for Health Protection and Promotion [Public Health Ontario], 2015). These include:

1. As part of the "Core"

2. "Involved" in the work

3. "Supportive" of the cause

4. "Informed"

Using this model, it was identified that stakeholder support did not always require attending meetings or being part of the "core" group.

Attention to stakeholder involvement desired by the "core" group ensured a good match between stakeholders and the goals for the project, such that they could be involved in ways that were consistent with what they could contribute. This also enabled new stakeholders to emerge over time. An example was our partnership with the North Bay-Parry Sound District Health Unit, which was engaged as a "supportive" stakeholder for many of the BPGs implemented and continues to support us when there is a "fit."

As our work progressed and became more public and our stakeholder circle expanded, not only were we called on locally as leaders of best practices, but provincially as well. Our processes were distributed to the Ontario Nurse Practitioner-Led Clinic Network for use by others. An example of this was with the *Assessment and Management of Pain* BPG (RNAO, 2009a), which was adapted to be

consistent with the change to scope of practice for nurse practitioners in the spring of 2017 (College of Nurses of Ontario, 2017). Process maps and tools were distributed upon request to other Nurse Practitioner-Led Clinics (see Figure 8.5).

Another successful strategy for implementation was the engagement of BScN students from Nipissing University. Nursing students participated over a semester with clinic staff and patients on the *Strategies to Support Self-Management of Chronic Conditions: Collaboration with Clients* BPG (RNAO, 2010e) to create educational resources for patients. These students collaborated with patients to establish goals and develop action plans as directed through the BPG recommendations. The client-driven action plans were actively utilized in guiding self-care and were monitored by students, patients, and staff throughout the semester, with documentation of progress.

A key lesson from our BPSO journey was that the implementation of innovations can radically affect professionals' daily work processes and requires considerable time and willingness to learn. The adoption of new ways of practice implies an interruption of past-learned behaviours on the part of practitioners. Also, the BPSO journey has created a paradigm shift in control and power out of the hands of providers and into the hands of those who receive care. In 2018, we cannot regard patients as passive, but rather as equal, participatory partners who contribute to their own healthcare. The guidelines are congruent with this change and encourage the use of motivational interviewing and mutual goal setting. Combine this with scope-of-practice changes (such as the ability of nurse practitioners to prescribe narcotics and benzodiazepines in 2018), and the environment is both exhilarating and challenging. This quote by one of our nurse practitioners reinforces the feelings of our staff, fully engaged in our BPSO adventure:

"Through the BPSO Designation work at NBNPLC, I gained new knowledge and clarified my role as a nurse practitioner and a knowledge professional. It reinforced that I want to belong to and contribute to a culture of best practice. Know better, do better."

—Terri MacDougall, Nurse Practitioner (NP)

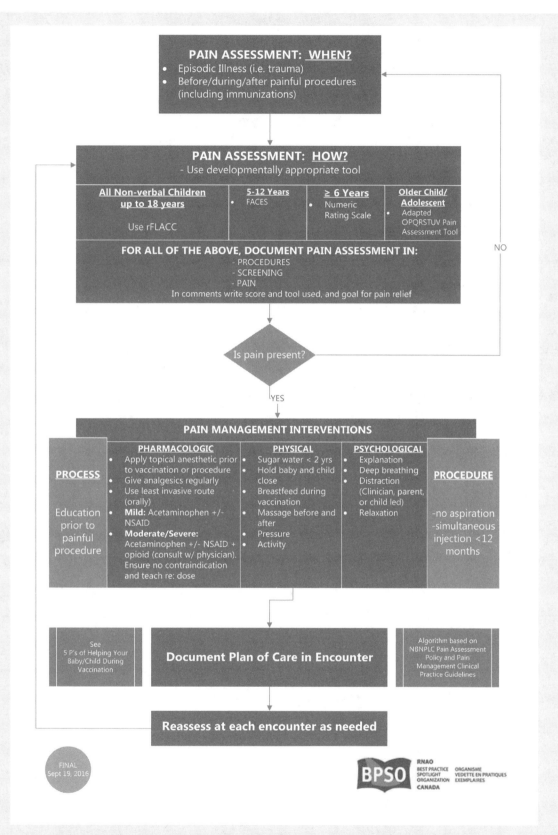

FIGURE 8.5   Protocol for pain assessment and management of the child.
Used with permission.

The challenges of taking the time to truly ascertain patients' concerns and needs—as well as pay attention to documentation and data collection requirements—are real issues (Young, Roberts, & Holden, 2017). These are issues we have to be mindful about as we maintain a client- and family-centered approach within our context of evidence-based practice and a focus on quality care and outcomes.

LEADERSHIP AS KEY TO SUCCESS

Managerial leadership by both the executive director, as a registered nurse, and the clinical director, as a nurse practitioner, provided encouragement and allowed time for staff to work on implementation tools and report back at meetings. Both leaders role-modeled a creative, adaptive, and supportive approach, and implementation of BPGs became part of the culture of evidence-based practice at the NBNPLC.

GREATEST CHALLENGE

One of the greatest challenges along the way was of staffing changes. However, with RNAO's support we focused on development of Champions, learned from our work at regular BPG update meetings, and developed and used BPG-related clinical decision supports for assessment, intervention, and documentation. All of these activities helped us keep up the momentum and continually improve.

SUSTAINABILITY FOR A SMALL TEAM

Early in our implementation phase, members of the NBNPLC team used the National Health System (NHS) Institute for Innovation and Improvement Sustainability Model (Maher, Gustafson, & Evans, 2010) to determine how best to sustain the work and current and future achievements. The Sustainability Model is a diagnostic tool that is used to predict the likelihood of sustainability for an improvement initiative. Areas of strength to support the BPSO work and outcomes identified by our team included: fit with organization's strategic aims and culture; clinical leadership engagement; staff behaviours toward sustaining the change; staff involvement and training to sustain the process; effectiveness of the system to monitor progress; and credibility of the evidence. The areas of improvement included: infrastructure for sustainability; senior leadership engagement; adaptability of improved processes; and benefits beyond helping our patients. An action plan was created that included sustaining our journey forward as we continue with implementation in the years to come.

Our journey as an RNAO BPSO and our continuous reflection on our efforts has enabled us to systematically implement and sustain new best practices and measure their impact. Providing timely data to the BPG-focused NQuIRE database system to assess progress has prompted an outcomes orientation and created a culture of enduring evidence-based practice, leading to better health outcomes for our clients.

BAYSHORE HEALTHCARE LTD. BPSO EXPERIENCE

Bayshore HealthCare is one of the country's leading providers of home and community healthcare services and a Canadian-owned company. Its services are purchased by government care programs, insurance companies, workers' compensation boards, healthcare organizations, the corporate sector, and the public. We serve Canadians coast to coast through over 60 branch offices and over 100 community clinics, and we employ approximately 12,000 full-time or part-time staff, including over 4,000 registered nurses as well as occupational health and safety specialists, occupational therapists, physiotherapists, speech and language rehab, social workers, dieticians, pharmacists, pharmacy technicians, physicians, dentists, personal support workers, and other unregulated care providers.

MOTIVATION TO BECOME A BPSO

Creating an evidence-based culture at Bayshore and subsequent application to be a BPSO was initiated by our clinical leaders, who identified the need to refocus the way we made organizational choices. The vision involved moving from task-based work to achieving clinical outcomes and would infiltrate through all levels of decision-making including strategic planning processes, informing evidence-based care planning, and ensuring the delivery of the best-quality home healthcare. Operational leadership agreed. That led to participation in the rigorous RNAO BPSO application process, following which, in 2012, Bayshore was selected to become a national Best Practice Spotlight Organization.

Our goal was to provide sustainable, superior, and trusted service to our clients and customers, and our objectives were to support ongoing improvement in our programs, clinical leadership capacity, and research opportunities. This fit well with our organizational objectives to create a great employee experience throughout the career journey and a care experience at Bayshore that ensures an enduring relationship with the client and family during the care processes.

One of the initial steps was creating a strong clinical quality accountability framework, followed by building an infrastructure and identifying necessary resources to support it. A specialized team of prepared clinicians would be instrumental in driving change in clinical and operational policies, processes, and systems. These team members were educated to be experts in promoting change at the clinician level through knowledge translation and guided workflows to drive informed decision-making at the front line.

HOW WE STARTED

Foundational to supporting system changes and creating robust electronic clinical management and learning systems was changing the culture at the front line to one of an evidence-based approach. Bayshore's vision statement embodies our commitment to client-centered care: "to enhance the quality of life, independence and dignity of Canadians in their homes," and our values capture our commitment to improvement in clinical capacity and nursing practice excellence. Our vision helped drive the cultural change needed.

At Bayshore, we knew that the best way to realize our vision was to provide the decision support tools, education, and coaching to our direct-care staff so that they could be prepared with the most relevant and up-to-date nursing knowledge, be secure in their work environment, and feel safe and supported by the organization.

The BPSO work has helped us to further reinforce our values in a demonstrable way and to further our mission to make a difference in our clients' lives. We understood that this would require commitment to embracing the culture of best practices in nursing; supporting and engaging nurses throughout our organization; and allocating resources to national, branch, and direct-care levels.

The BPSO Agreement outlined the scope for the project, and a steering committee was established to support leadership and decision-making. There were subcommittees developed at a working group level to take on specific aspects of work such as policy development. Capacity building was critical to create a long-term plan through an identified cohort of nurses. We engaged a critical mass of nurses as BPG Champions to support guideline implementation and evaluation, and we created a network of BPG Champions across the entire organization in Canada. We worked with the RNAO BPSO Coach and other designated mentor organizations to develop guideline implementation capacity; we felt greatly supported in this work.

Cultural change was initiated through a core team of six RNAO eHealth Best Practice Champions who worked on our first BPG implementation back in 2006. They introduced the Healthy Work Environment BPGs, which guided us in the review and revision of many of our policies, including human resource, clinical, and operational policies, to set the stage for implementing clinical BPGs.

Data would drive our learning and our care. Metrics to track implementation and evaluation were included under the domains of nursing practice, clinical outcomes, and organizational structure. We were well positioned to participate in research projects, with our data being uploaded into the NQuIRE database. We created a bridge for data interface between our electronic clinical management systems and the RNAO NQuIRE system to support evidence to inform revisions to processes based on outcomes and BPG content.

BUILDING A CULTURE OF EVIDENCE-BASED PRACTICE

One of the greatest challenges in providing home care clinical services is the remote nature of work. Our nurses often have limited clinical history and background information about the clients and their current health status upon initiating care. Initially, with client consent, our home care nurse conducts a risk and hazard assessment that creates an understanding of each client's environmental context and identifies potential risks for each client as well as the care team. Examples of potential risks may include presence of scatter-mats that could be a fall hazard for the client, or dogs or guns that could be a hazard for the care team visiting the home.

Care at Bayshore has evolved significantly over the years since BPSO implementation, in transitioning from general assessment and care plan templates to algorithmic care pathways that guide clinicians to prepare evidence-based care plans. These pathways were based on RNAO's BPGs. The pathway-based approach was foundational

to moving toward the eventual implementation of RNAO nursing order sets (NOS) for specific population-based care, which required a robust electronic clinical management information system.

Subsequently, during our BPSO candidacy period from 2012 to 2015, Bayshore was able to implement BPGs that were aligned with our strategic direction, including *Person-and Family-Centred Care* (RNAO, 2015); *Supporting and Strengthening Families Through Expected and Unexpected Events* (RNAO, 2002f); *Prevention of Falls and Fall Injuries in the Older Adult* (RNAO, 2002d); *Oral Health: Nursing Assessment and Interventio*n (RNAO, 2008a); and *Assessment and Management of Pain* (RNAO, 2009a). These BPGs were considered vital in providing client-focused care that was inclusive of family and caregivers. Our organization purposefully wanted to enhance support for unregulated care providers through the transfer of authority process, and for our clinicians providing care to our client population across all types of community care, and programs across Canada. We also chose BPGs to implement within clinical domains to strengthen our signature programs: Wound Care; Hospice Palliative Care; Paediatrics; and Frail Elderly. Following our BPSO Designation, we added BPGs including *Facilitating Client Centred Learning* (RNAO, 2012a) and *Strategies to Support Self-Management in Chronic Conditions: Collaboration with Clients* (RNAO, 2010e).

SUSTAINING THE CHANGES

Sustainability requires vigilance and continued investment as a BPSO, communicating what it stands for and keeping it at the front of Bayshore's thinking and philosophy. There has been a steady buy-in from clinicians across the organization. The challenge is keeping the focus on driving evidence-based care and more importantly keeping it relevant to what is impacting Bayshore and the home care sector. As our clinical practice leaders have recognized, all guidelines have to be considered in relation to the home care context, and the better we do this, the better the fit and potential for sustained use.

The development and deployment of Bayshore's Clinical Accountability Model has supported sustainability of BPG implementation. This approach is fundamental to achieving outcomes, working within integrated or bundled funding models (see Figure 8.6).

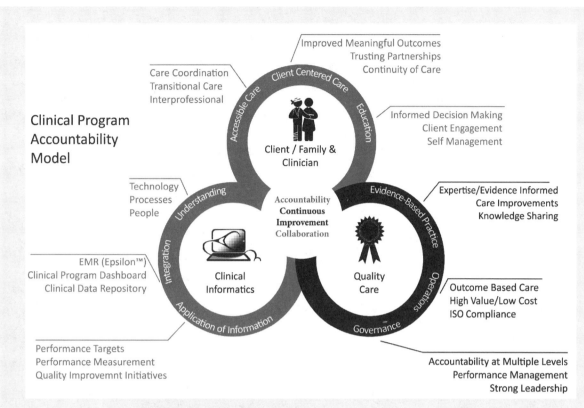

Clinical Program Accountability Model

Client Centered Care

Accessible Care

Education

Care Coordination
Transitional Care
Interprofessional

Improved Meaningful Outcomes
Trusting Partnerships
Continuity of Care

Informed Decision Making
Client Engagement
Self Management

Client / Family & Clinician

Accountability
Continuous Improvement
Collaboration

Understanding

Technology
Processes
People

Integration

Evidence-Based Practice

Expertise/Evidence Informed
Care Improvements
Knowledge Sharing

Clinical Informatics

Quality Care

Operations

EMR (Epsilon™)
Clinical Program Dashboard
Clinical Data Repository

Outcome Based Care
High Value/Low Cost
ISO Compliance

Application of Information

Governance

Performance Targets
Performance Measurement
Quality Improvemnt Initiatives

Accountability at Multiple Levels
Performance Management
Strong Leadership

FIGURE 8.6 Bayshore's Clinical Accountability Model.
Used with permission.

SUCCESSES AND CHALLENGES AS A BPSO

As a BPSO, Bayshore was able to grow clinical leadership, and evidence-based clinical and management decision-making, through the candidacy and designation maintenance BPSO phases. Our structures and span of control were modified to create more effective and efficient service models based upon evidence. The successes from our investment in evidence-based practice through the BPSO Designation are that we:

- Influenced system changes to support evidence-based practice (e.g., funders' use of evidence in reporting requirements that are aligned with RNAO nursing order sets)

- Supported discussions with government funders to move from measuring only operational process indicators to clinical outcome indicators

- Increased our ability to build capacity as an organization through the implementation of the Healthy Work Environment BPGs, which addressed the challenge of managing change and transformation to sustain an evidence-based practice culture (*Developing and Sustaining Nursing Leadership* [RNAO, 2013c]; *Managing and Mitigating Conflict in Health-Care Teams* [RNAO, 2013d]; and *Intra-Professional Collaborative Practice Among Nurses* [RNAO, 2016b])

- Were able to deploy across all groups of care providers including registered nurses, unregulated caregivers, pharmacists, therapists, and nonclinical operational and business employees

- Successfully spread RNAO BPGs across the country

- Maximized impact as a knowledge organization through evidence-based practice, nursing order set use, and evaluation of data over time

We knew there were going to be possible barriers to implementing and sustaining our work. Risks were identified and quantified, and strategies were developed to respond. Some of the earliest challenges that were identified and mitigated included:

- Ongoing senior management support, not just commitment at start-up

- Lack of commitment to dedicated resources over time

- Failing to include all staff, including direct-care clinicians

- Not having systems in place to monitor outcomes

- Not having local clinical leaders and Champions at the point-of-client-care delivery

THE IMPACT ON BAYSHORE

We have worked with the RNAO BPSO Coaches, mentors, and BPSO Designates to implement BPGs to access existing expertise and to assist in quality-improvement outcome monitoring. This has been a strong partnership with over 5 years of investment in clinical leadership, systems development, and learning and knowledge frameworks that have transformed the organization to reflect a culture of evidence-based care.

Bayshore has been on a significant journey from implementing initial BPGs to leading the entire organization toward accountable, evidence-based care. Our clinical leadership and Champion network was foundational in our ability to embark on scalable programs across provinces and succeed in effecting change at the front line. This has supported our growth and positive working environment, enabling clinicians to thrive in their practice. Evidence is not only at our fingertips, but also actively used in practice, supported by leadership in all roles.

CASE STUDY

ST. MICHAEL'S HOSPITAL BPSO EXPERIENCE

St. Michael's Hospital (SMH) is a 459-bed, inner city, academic health sciences center fully affiliated with the University of Toronto. The hospital employs over 6,000 staff including 1,887 registered nurses and 52 nurse practitioners. The hospital provides tertiary and quaternary services in cardiovascular surgery, neurosurgery, inner city health, and therapeutic endoscopy. It is one of two Level 1 adult trauma centers in Greater Toronto. SMH was founded by the Sisters of Saint Joseph in 1892 with the mission of taking care of the sick and poor of Toronto's inner city.

EMBEDDING EVIDENCE-BASED PRACTICE INTO THE CULTURE

Our RNAO BPSO Designation journey enabled evidence-based practices to become embedded and sustained into the fabric of nursing practice at SMH. BPSO work is evident throughout the organization from our corporate communication and professional development offerings to corporate priority planning and direct-care activities. The transition from BPSO candidate to Designate was a smooth, seamless process due, in part, to the strong foundation laid during our candidacy work. Nursing has embraced the importance of evidence-based practices and has continued to engage in further BPG implementation, sustainability, and spread activities since BPSO Designation.

The BPSO Designation team now concentrates its efforts on developing and supporting corporate processes and structures to sustain, spread, and initiate BPG uptake. Since our quest for BPSO Designation began in 2009, we have successfully initiated 33 BPGs; of those, 6 have most recently been implemented, 13 have been initiated and sustained; and 14 have been sustained and spread to new areas. Approximately 30% of our staff from 37 different clinical care areas are recognized as BPG Champions based on their knowledge and leadership in BPG uptake. See Table 8.1 for a detailed list of BPGs that have been implemented at SMH.

TABLE 8.1   BPGS THAT HAVE BEEN IMPLEMENTED AT SMH, AND THEIR STATUS—IMPLEMENTED, SUSTAINED, OR SPREAD

NUMBER	RNAO BEST PRACTICE GUIDELINE	STATUS
	Establishing Therapeutic Relationships (RNAO, 2002c)	Spread
	Professionalism in Nursing (RNAO, 2007)	Spread
	Workplace Health, Safety, and Wellbeing of the Nurse (RNAO, 2008b)	Spread
	Crisis Intervention (RNAO, 2002b)	Spread
	Strengthening and Supporting Families Through Expected and Unexpected Events (RNAO, 2002f)	Spread
	Nursing Management of Hypertension (RNAO, 2005d)	Sustained
	Stroke Assessment Across the Continuum (RNAO, 2005e)	Sustained
	Developing and Sustaining Safe Effective Staffing and Workload Practices (RNAO, 2005b)	Sustained
	Integrating Smoking Cessation into Daily Nursing Practice (RNAO, 2003c)	Sustained
	Woman Abuse: Screening, Identification and Initial Response (RNAO, 2005f)	Spread
	Breastfeeding Best Practices Guidelines for Nurses (RNAO, 2003a)	Spread
	Embracing Cultural Diversity in Health Care: Developing Cultural Competence (RNAO, 2003b)	Spread
	Interventions for Post-Partum Depression (RNAO, 2005c)	Sustained
	Promotion of Continence Using Prompted Voiding (RNAO, 2002e)	Sustained
	Screening for Delirium, Dementia and Depression in Older Adults (RNAO, 2010d)	Spread
	Assessment and Management of Foot Ulcers for People with Diabetes (RNAO, 2013a)	Sustained
	Assessment and Device Selection for Vascular Access (RNAO, 2004)	Sustained
	Client Centred Care (RNAO, 2002a)	Spread
	Prevention of Falls and Fall Injuries in Older Adults (RNAO, 2002d)	Spread
	Caregiving Strategies for Older Adults with Delirium, Dementia and Depression (RNAO, 2010b)	Spread
	Risk Assessment and Prevention of Pressure Ulcers (RNAO, 2010c)	Sustained
	Promoting Safety: Alternative Approaches to the Use of Restraints (RNAO, 2012b)	Spread
	Preventing and Managing Violence in the Workplace (RNAO, 2009c)	Sustained

continues

TABLE 8.1   BPGS THAT HAVE BEEN IMPLEMENTED AT SMH, AND THEIR STATUS—IMPLEMENTED, SUSTAINED, OR SPREAD   (CONTINUED)

NUMBER	RNAO BEST PRACTICE GUIDELINE	STATUS
	Assessment and Management of Pain (RNAO, 2009a)	Spread
	Care and Maintenance to Reduce Vascular Access Complications (RNAO, 2005a)	Sustained
	Strategies to Support Self-Management in Chronic Conditions (RNAO, 2010e)	Sustained
	Assessment and Care of Adults at Risk for Suicidal Ideation and Behaviour (RNAO, 2010a)	Sustained
	Preventing and Mitigating Nurse Fatigue in Health Care (RNAO, 2011b)	Implemented
	Developing and Sustaining Interprofessional Health Care (RNAO, 2009b)	Implemented
	Care Transitions (RNAO, 2014a)	Implemented
	Delirium, Dementia and Depression in Older Adults: Assessment and Care (RNAO, 2016a)	Implemented
	Person-and Family-Centred Care (RNAO, 2015)	Implemented
	End-of-Life Care During the Last Days and Hours (RNAO, 2011a)	Implemented

Embedding evidence-based practice into our culture and daily work processes is a result of six collective strategic efforts, including:

1. Aligning BPSO work with organizational strategic objectives and priorities

2. Evolving governance structures, infrastructure, and mechanisms

3. Communicating updates and sharing achievements

4. Evaluating our impact

5. Spreading and sustaining BPGs

6. Leveraging external funding and partnership opportunities

ALIGNING BPSO WORK WITH ORGANIZATIONAL STRATEGIC OBJECTIVES AND PRIORITIES

BPG implementation is purposefully aligned with the SMH strategic objectives and priorities. During our initial candidacy period, the BPSO deliverables were embedded in the annual corporate goals and objectives. Since that time, ongoing BPSO implementation and evaluation work has been aligned not only with our corporate strategic objectives and priorities, but further aligned with the Corporate Strategic, Quality Improvement, and Interprofessional Strategic Plans and the Senior Friendly Hospital Initiative.

Quality patient care has always been a priority for nursing at SMH; however, the RNAO BPSO Designation created an opportunity to be explicit in communicating that nursing's priority at SMH was to provide consistent, quality patient care through evidence-based knowledge. Supported by nursing leadership, nurses identified BPGs that they believed would best address potential gaps in quality care on their local units. The BPSO Steering Committee recommended three foundational corporate BPGs that all clinical units would implement. These were: 1) *Establishing Therapeutic Relationships* (RNAO, 2002c); 2) *Professionalism in Nursing* (RNAO, 2007); and 3) *Workplace Health, Safety and Wellbeing of the Nurse* (RNAO, 2008b).

EVOLVING GOVERNANCE STRUCTURES, INFRASTRUCTURE, AND MECHANISMS

Since its selection as a BPSO, SMH has evolved its governance structures and infrastructure (e.g., positions and resources) to ensure that oversight and professional practice support are available to meet the BPSO requirements.

GOVERNANCE

Currently, BPSO activities are part of the responsibilities of the Nursing Advisory Council (NAC) and its various subcommittees. NAC is accountable to the Chief Nursing and Health Disciplines Executive as the BPSO Executive Sponsor who supports the integration of best practices into the daily operations and priorities of the organization. This high-level sponsorship enables linkages with clinical research, nursing practice, and education. SMH also established a steering committee in 2015 to lead the selection of BPG indicators to report to NQuIRE, a new requirement to maintain the BPSO Designation. The membership reflected key stakeholders in practice, education, and research, as well as management and data systems.

PROFESSIONAL PRACTICE INFRASTRUCTURE

Changes to the infrastructure of the professional practice portfolio were also made to respond to the requirements to maintain BPSO Designation. The portfolio includes a full-time position responsible for supporting the integration and sustainability of Best Practice Guidelines into daily practice. Also included is a part-time data analyst role for Professional Practice to develop processes and audit tools to support BPG evaluation at the local and corporate levels and support our NQuIRE commitments.

MECHANISMS

Over the last 8 years, several mechanisms were designed and delivered to provide learning and capacity-building opportunities for direct-care nurses, such as communities of practice, boot camps, booster sessions, and assigned mentors. Other mechanisms included fellowships and financial support for release time for nurses to participate in these offerings and lead implementation and dissemination of their respective BPG projects.

COMMUNICATING UPDATES AND SHARING ACHIEVEMENTS

Over the last 8 years, in keeping with BPSO deliverables, the Professional Practice team has also made it a top priority to profile BPSO activities, Champions, and teams who lead the work to acknowledge and recognize achievements in efforts to keep BPSO momentum across the organization. Key communication strategies associated with BPSO Designation and implementation of BPGs are listed in Table 8.2. Further, we have published aspects of our implementation processes and outcomes in scholarly and professional journals (Santiago & Smith, 2015; Thomas et al., 2016; Wannamaker, Michelsen, & Santiago, 2015).

TABLE 8.2 COMMUNICATION AND DISSEMINATION OF BPSO WORK AND IMPLEMENTATION OF BPGS

MECHANISM	DESCRIPTION
Shining the Light on St. Michael's BPSO Achievements	An annual BPSO newsletter intended to highlight some of SMH's best practice achievements with examples of how our nursing teams are implementing, evaluating, and sustaining RNAO BPGs
Nursing Week—Poster Gallery Walk Internal Media Nursing Rounds Professional Practice Scenario of the Month	BPSO activities are continuously profiled through regular nursing columns in internal media, nursing week events, nursing rounds, internal intranet, and the "Professional Practice Scenario of the Month," ensuring our BPSO Designation and activities remain at the forefront of SMH.
BPSO Symposium	A corporate BPG showcasing opportunity with oral and poster presentations
Standing Ovations	Standing ovations were first introduced at our BPSO Symposium in November 2010. The BPSO Project Management Team and SMH executives travel to the clinical areas where BPGs have been implemented. Local-level clinicians present their BPG implementation activities and receive thanks and a standing ovation for their accomplishments.
BPSO Intranet	Our BPSO intranet site was developed and continually updated and includes all the components of our BPSO work.
BPSO Poster and BPSO Pins	As part of our designation celebration, we created a poster that highlighted each BPG implementation team with a team photo and a brief description of their successes to date, along with key messages from SMH executives. Each nurse received a copy of the poster and a BPSO pin to commemorate our BPSO Designation.
BPG Nurse Champion and Mentor Pins	During the annual SMH Nursing Week BPG Sustainability Poster Gallery Walk event, BPG Nurse Champions and Mentors are awarded a pin to recognize and celebrate their role in implementing and evaluating BPGs in their respective areas.

EVALUATING IMPACT

We have evaluated implementation of BPGs since the BPSO candidacy period both corporately and at local unit/team levels using research, quality-improvement, and program evaluation methods. A few key evaluation activities are highlighted.

NQUIRE

A select number of BPGs are being monitored and evaluated through NQuIRE. The steering committee is following a systematic approach to the BPG indicator selection process. Each indicator within the RNAO BPG data dictionaries (DD) was assessed by our steering committee based on the following considerations: 1) alignment with corporate/programmatic initiatives or priorities; 2) current data-collection activities (processes and sites); 3) matching of definitions and timing; 4) planned data-collection activities; 5) current and future feasibility; 6) data owners and partners; and 7) type of measure.

The following are five BPG indicators that were selected using this process: 1) "Minutes to receive pain medication" (*Assessment and Management of Pain*); 2) "Treated with courtesy and respect" corporate-wide (*Client Centered Care*); 3) "Falls rate" (*Prevention of Falls in*

Older Adults); 4) "Exclusive breastfeeding rate"; and 5) "Formula supplementation rate" (*Breastfeeding*).

CARE UTILIZING EVIDENCE (CUE) AND CUE-QI (QUALITY IMPROVEMENT) INITIATIVES

The CUE dashboard is a corporate audit and feedback mechanism that shares BPG-related outcome and process data with direct-care nursing staff. It has become a valuable way for clinicians and unit managers to see the impact of their care on patients, stay on track, monitor for trends, and identify opportunities for ongoing improvement through regular review and follow-up (Jeffs, 2014; Jeffs et al., 2014).

In addition, a series of research studies has been carried out exploring patient safety, nurse and organizational outcomes, and experiences associated with an integrated approach to BPG implementation. The results clearly demonstrate the positive relationships between client and provider outcomes and clinical and HWE BPG implementation in our organization (Beswick, Westell, Sweetman, Mothersill, & Jeffs, 2013; Jeffs, 2014; Jeffs, Acott, Simpson, et al., 2013; Jeffs, Beswick, Acott, et al., 2014; Jeffs, Beswick, Campbell, et al., 2013; Jeffs, Beswick, Lo, et al., 2013; Jeffs, Cardoso, et al., 2013; Jeffs, Lo, Beswick, & Campbell, 2013; Jeffs, Sidani, et al., 2013; Jeffs et al., 2012).

SPREADING AND SUSTAINING BPGS AT ST. MICHAEL'S HOSPITAL

A set of strategies has been developed (see Table 8.3) for spreading and sustaining BPGs into daily workflow processes and functions.

TABLE 8.3 SPREAD AND SUSTAINABILITY STRATEGIES

STRATEGIES	DESCRIPTION
Sustainability Community of Practice	Monthly BPG Sustainability Communities of Practice meetings to exchange experiences and knowledge.
Sustainability Workshops	Expanded 6-hour workshop is targeted at Sustainability Evaluation Fellows and others in leadership positions. Prerequisite to attendance is completed evaluation plans and associated Plan-Do-Study-Act cycling.
BPG Sustainability Template	This template is circulated bi-annually to all clinical areas as a mechanism to report back to Nursing Professional Practice on BPG implementation, evaluation, and sustainability activities. This becomes part of an organization-wide report to track BPG-related activities at the local and corporate levels.

LEVERAGING EXTERNAL FUNDING AND PARTNERSHIP OPPORTUNITIES

Integral to our successful ongoing BPSO Designation have been the opportunities to leverage external funding and partnerships. This includes use of research funding to evaluate BPG impact. We have been active participants with the Nursing Best Practices Research Centre (NBPRC) and are also involved in BPG development and review teams and BPSO applicant selection panels.

LESSONS LEARNED

Our BPSO is a large site with over 2,000 registered nurses and related stakeholders. Making minor practice changes is a challenge, let alone a major change in culture that the BPSO Designation entailed. Some of the key lessons learned that were and continue to be critical to our BPSO successes include:

- Develop and use plans throughout

- Engage direct-care staff in planning, implementing, leading, disseminating, and evaluating

■ Use multiple innovative strategies to initiate, sustain, and boost

■ Develop and engage Champions at all levels

■ Align strategically with overall organizational priorities

■ Involve the senior leadership team

FUTURE PRIORITIES

Into the future, we continue to build capacity and support Champion/team development and success through:

■ Offering a monthly BPG Community of Practice

■ Establishing a formal BPG Nurse Champion mentorship model

■ Providing BPG Nurse Champions with protected time to lead BPG initiatives

SMH will continue to align BPSO activities—including the spread, sustainability, and adoption of new RNAO BPGs—with other corporate priorities. We will also continue to contribute to RNAO's NQuIRE database, routinely assess newly published BPG data dictionaries, and seek opportunities to leverage NQuIRE reports and processes with other corporate priorities.

Through these BPG initiatives and others, SMH is able to make strides toward ensuring our patients and their families are receiving the highest-quality care possible and are safe throughout their healthcare journey with us.

CONCLUDING PERSPECTIVES FROM THE BPSO ORGANIZATIONAL LEADERS

In this chapter, nursing leaders from five BPSOs representing all sectors and ranging from early to recent cohorts have shared their BPSO story. Each has described the motivation to become a BPSO, getting started, successes and challenges, overall organizational impact, what BPSO looks like in their organizations today, as well as future perspectives. In summary:

■ Toronto Public Health has reshaped its nursing and interprofessional teams to focus on evidence-based practice and nursing leadership through the development of Best Practice Guideline Champions and storytelling.

■ Bluewater Health, a community hospital, has "hardwired" its organization with Best Practice Guidelines, including the *Person-and Family-Centred Care* BPG, and has set the stage for a patient-oriented cultural revolution.

■ The North Bay Nurse Practitioner-Led Clinic has used the BPSO Designation to connect with community stakeholders to build a strong interprofessional team through the use of BPGs to guide practice in a consistent way.

■ Bayshore Home Health has spread the Best Practice Guidelines across the nation and maximized their impact within the community and home care sector through interprofessional evidence-based practice and use of evidence-based nursing order sets.

■ St. Michael's Hospital, a large acute-care setting, has implemented numerous Best Practice Guidelines to create and sustain a "tsunami" of evidence-based practice across its entire organization.

CONCLUSION

New BPSO challenges and successes are yet to be experienced in our organizations and in yours. One thing we know for sure is that nursing leaders need to be committed to maximizing the impact of Best Practice Guidelines on both patient/client outcomes and nursing practice. There is no need to approach this work on your own. Connect with the other nursing leaders in your region, your province, your country, and the world. Becoming part of the international BPSO movement can be a transformational step for your organization. Connect with the Registered Nurses' Association of Ontario to explore how you can begin your own BPSO journey. Share ideas, innovations, and resources. Know that patients, families, employees, volunteers, physicians, and donors are counting on you to lead . . . and to get it right. We must be curious. We must be compassionate. We must be courageous!

KEY MESSAGES

Although there were significant differences in our healthcare sectors, geographical locations, and organizational size and complexity, there were commonalities for nursing leaders across all five organizations. The authors of this chapter believe that it may be helpful to readers to consider these alignments. All are shared through the perspective of the firsthand experiences of those who have been or are currently immersed in this incredible work, with the intent of maximizing success.

- It is essential to *ignite the desire* to become a Best Practice Spotlight Organization (BPSO) across the organization, including your board of directors. The Senior Leadership Team must be visibly supportive and committed to this goal. It is important to use existing committees and departmental structures as platforms and levers for the work.

- It is critical to *align the decision* to proceed to becoming a BPSO with your Mission Statement, current Strategic Plan, and Quality Plan. *Don't wait for your next Strategic Plan or next Quality Plan. Start where you are. Work with what you have.* Look at your Quality Plan to see where your targets are related to the Best Practice Guidelines. Assess the environment and timing. What else is happening? *It's ideal if there is an appetite, a pull, a gap, and strategic structures in place.* Begin by choosing the specific Best Practice Guidelines (BPG) that will have the most impact, significance, and appeal to get started. *Look for early wins.* You will have noticed through our stories in this chapter that each of our organizations selected the BPGs that would give them the early traction needed for knowledge transfer, translation, and eventual impact.

- *Clarify that this is not a project.* The BPGs must align with the current goals of the board, executive, directors, managers, and educators. It is critical for this to become the *real* work and part of your regular workflows, not an add-on. Fulfilling your care philosophy *is* your mission. This work has a beginning and no end.

- *Set a realistic budget.* There are positions you may need to create, training and development on BPGs to provide, expenses to back-fill positions so staff can attend the training, events to plan, and reasons for celebration(s).

- *This work takes feet on the ground, yours, and other senior leaders.* We need to be seen, and our supportive voices need to be heard. Get out there. See for yourself. Talk with patients, clients, and families (mostly listen). Set aside the time. Ask questions. Find out what is real. Create opportunities for dialogue with direct-care interdisciplinary staff, physicians, the chair of quality committee of the board, managers, and directors. Be appreciative. Become the face of the BPSO work.

- *Open the Best Practice Champion opportunity to interprofessional staff.* They are eager to learn and to step into this work. The inclusivity also supports collaborative practice as outlined in the *Developing and Sustaining Interprofessional Health Care* BPG (RNAO, 2013b) and enhances quality outcomes. Set and communicate practice expectations for scope and role. Involve human resources, clinical educators, union leadership, managers, and directors. Being a Champion is not an easy task. Let them know they have your support.

- *Take advantage of all RNAO supports* to build capacity in evidence-based clinical excellence, implementation science, and leadership, as wonderful opportunities for direct-care staff and others.

- *Assign a Best Practice Lead* as the point-person for all BPGs and Champions. Have the right person in the role. The candidate is typically a master's-prepared nurse with a passion for the work. This person needs to exude an energy that excites people and invites them into the best-practice experience.

- *Form alliances with Community College/University health program(s).* Include the students and faculty in orientation and celebrations. These young professionals are our future.

- *Leverage resources* such as your Corporate Communications Team (if you have one) or RNAO to help tell your stories and cover your progress and celebrations. They'll take photos, help with presentations, include stories in communications, help with branding of the work, and make sure that publications include information related to BPSO. Keep your local media and local politicians informed about the work you are doing.

- *Believe that your people want to do meaningful work,* have purpose, make a positive difference, and feel part of things. Acknowledge that they know best what needs to change. Use your nursing leadership role and influence to insist that movement forward requires patients, clients, and families to be involved. This is not up for debate. It is non-negotiable.

- *Know that your RNAO coach is a wise strategic and operational partner* with you. Attend RNAO events. Get involved. Present at RNAO educational events. Tell your stories. Publish the work your organization is doing.

REFERENCES

Beswick, S., Westell, S., Sweetman, S., Mothersill, C., & Jeffs, L. (2013). Being more conscientious, collaborative and confident in addressing patients' fears and anxieties: Nurses' perspectives. *Nursing: Research and Reviews, 3,* 119–124.

Capacity Review Committee. (2006). *Revitalizing Ontario's public health capacity: The final report of the Capacity Review Committee.* Retrieved from http://tools.hhr-rhs.ca/index.php?option=com_mtree&task=att_download&link_id=5976&cf_id=68&lang=en

Choosing Wisely Canada. (n.d.). *Choosing wisely campaign.* Retrieved from http://www.choosingwiselycanada.org/

College of Nurses of Ontario. (2017). *Nurse Practitioner* [Practice Standard]. Toronto, ON: College of Nurses of Ontario.

Community Health Nurses of Canada. (2015). *Leadership competencies for public health practice in Canada*. Retrieved from https://www.chnc.ca/en/competencies

Flodgren, G., Parmelli, E., Doumit, G., Gattellari, M., O'Brien, M. A., Grimshaw, J., . . . Eccles, M. P. (2011). Local opinion leaders: Effects on professional practice and health care outcomes. *Cochrane Database of Systematic Reviews, 11*, Article No. CD000125.

Health Canada. (2003). *Learning from SARS: Renewal of public health in Canada*. Retrieved from http://www.phac-aspc.gc.ca/publicat/sars-sras/pdf/sars-e.pdf

Jeffs, L. (2014). Insights from staff nurses and managers on unit-specific nursing performance dashboards. *BMJ Quality & Safety, 23*(12), 1001–1006.

Jeffs, L., Acott, A., Simpson, E., Campbell, H., Irwin, T., Lo, J., . . . Cardoso, R. (2013). Enhancing nurse surveillance, accountability, and patient safety: The value of bedside shift reporting. *Journal of Nursing Care Quality, 28*(3), 226–232.

Jeffs, L., Beswick, S., Acott, A., Simpson E., Cardoso, R., Campbell H., & Irwin, T. (2014). Patients' views on bedside nursing handover: Creating a space to connect. *Journal of Nursing Care Quality, 29*(2), 149–154.

Jeffs, L., Beswick, S., Campbell, H., Lo, J., Byer, C., & Ferris, E. (2013). Hospital nurses' perceptions associated with implementing multiple guidelines: A qualitative study. *Journal of Nursing Education and Practice, 3*(2), 31–40.

Jeffs, L., Beswick, S., Lo, J., Campbell, H., Ferris, E., & Sidani, S. (2013). Defining what evidence is, linking it to patient outcomes, and making it relevant to practice: Insights from clinical nurses. *Applied Nursing Research, 26*(3), 105–109.

Jeffs, L., Beswick, S., Martin, K., Campbell, H., Rose, D., & Ferris, E. (2012). Quality nursing care and opportunities for improvement: Insights from patients and family members. *Journal of Nursing Care Quality, 28*(1), 76–84.

Jeffs, L., Cardoso, R., Beswick, S., Acott, A., Simpson, E., Campbell, H., . . . Ferris, E. (2013). Enablers and barriers to implementing bedside reporting: Insights from nurses. *Canadian Journal of Nursing Leadership, 26*(3), 39–52.

Jeffs, L., Lo, J., Beswick, S., & Campbell, H. (2013). Implementing an organization-wide quality improvement initiative: Insights from project leads, managers and frontline nurses. *Nursing Administration Quarterly, 7*(3), 222–230.

Jeffs, L., Lo, J., Beswick, S., Chuun, A., Lai, Y., Campbell, H., & Ferris, E. (2014). Enablers and barriers to implementing unit-specific nursing performance dashboards. *Journal of Nursing Care Quality, 29*(3), 200–203.

Jeffs, L., Sidani, S., Rose, D., Espin, S., Smith, O., Martin, K., . . . Ferris, E. (2013). Using theory and evidence to drive measurement of patient, nurse, and organizational outcomes of professional nursing practice. *International Journal of Nursing Practice, 19*(2), 141–148.

Jennings, L., O'Neil, B., Bossy, K., Dodman, D., & Campbell, J. (2016). The story of Emily. *Patient Experience Journal, 3*(1), 146–152.

Joint Task Group on Public Health Human Resources. (2005, October). *Building the public health workforce for the 21st century: A pan Canadian framework for public health human resources planning*. Retrieved from http://publications.gc.ca/collections/collection_2008/phac-aspc/HP5-12-2005E.pdf

Kitson, A. L. (2009). The need for systems change: Reflections on knowledge translation and organizational change. *Journal of Advanced Nursing, 65*(1), 217–228.

Maher, L., Gustafson, D., & Evans, A. (2010). NHS Sustainability Model. Retrieved from http://www.institute.nhs.uk/sustainability

Ministry of Health and Long-Term Care (MOHLTC). (2008). Ontario Public Health Standards. Retrieved from http://www.health.gov.on.ca/en/pro/programs/publichealth/oph_standards/docs/ophs_2008.pdf

National Research Corporation. (2015, October). *Bluewater Health provides exemplary access to care through a patient-centred culture*. Retrieved from http://www.bluewaterhealth.ca/documents/159/CS%20Bluewater%20Health%20FINAL.pdf

Ontario Agency for Health Protection and Promotion (Public Health Ontario). (2015). *Planning health promotion programs: Introductory workbook* (4th ed.). Toronto, ON: Queen's Printer for Ontario.

Ontario Hospital Association. (n.d.). *Inspiring improvement: Hospital successes in strengthening hospital-physician relationships*. Toronto, ON: Ontario Hospital Association.

Ploeg, J., Skelly, J., Rowan, M., Edwards, N., Davies, B., Grinspun, D., . . . Downey, A. (2010). The role of nursing best practice champions in diffusing practice guidelines: A mixed methods study. *Worldviews on Evidence-Based Nursing, 7*(4), 238–251. doi: 10.1111/j.1741-6787.2010.00202.x.

Public Health Agency of Canada (PHAC). (2012). *What is the population health approach?* Retrieved from http://www.phac-aspc.gc.ca/ph-sp/approach-approche/index-eng.php

Registered Nurses' Association of Ontario (RNAO). (2002a). *Client centred care*. Toronto, ON: Registered Nurses' Association of Ontario.

Registered Nurses' Association of Ontario (RNAO). (2002b). *Crisis intervention*. Toronto, ON: Registered Nurses' Association of Ontario.

Registered Nurses' Association of Ontario (RNAO). (2002c). *Establishing therapeutic relationships*. Toronto, ON: Registered Nurses' Association of Ontario.

Registered Nurses' Association of Ontario (RNAO). (2002d). *Prevention of falls and fall injuries in the older adult.* Toronto, ON: Registered Nurses' Association of Ontario.

Registered Nurses' Association of Ontario (RNAO). (2002e). *Promotion of continence using prompted voiding.* Toronto, ON: Registered Nurses' Association of Ontario.

Registered Nurses' Association of Ontario (RNAO). (2002f, 2006 Supplement). *Supporting and strengthening families through expected and unexpected life events.* Toronto, ON: Registered Nurses' Association of Ontario.

Registered Nurses' Association of Ontario (RNAO). (2003a). *Breastfeeding Best Practice Guidelines for nurses.* Toronto, ON: Registered Nurses' Association of Ontario.

Registered Nurses' Association of Ontario (RNAO). (2003b). *Embracing cultural diversity in health care: Developing cultural competence.* Toronto, ON: Registered Nurses' Association of Ontario.

Registered Nurses' Association of Ontario (RNAO). (2003c). *Integrating smoking cessation into daily nursing practice.* Toronto, ON: Registered Nurses' Association of Ontario.

Registered Nurses' Association of Ontario (RNAO). (2004). *Assessment and device selection for vascular access.* Toronto, ON: Registered Nurses' Association of Ontario.

Registered Nurses' Association of Ontario (RNAO). (2005a). *Care and maintenance to reduce vascular access complications.* Toronto, ON: Registered Nurses' Association of Ontario.

Registered Nurses' Association of Ontario (RNAO). (2005b). *Developing and sustaining safe effective staffing and workload practices.* Toronto, ON: Registered Nurses' Association of Ontario.

Registered Nurses' Association of Ontario (RNAO). (2005c). *Interventions for postpartum depression.* Toronto, ON: Registered Nurses' Association of Ontario.

Registered Nurses' Association of Ontario (RNAO). (2005d). *Nursing management of hypertension.* Toronto, ON: Registered Nurses' Association of Ontario.

Registered Nurses' Association of Ontario (RNAO). (2005e). *Stroke assessment across the continuum.* Toronto, ON: Registered Nurses' Association of Ontario.

Registered Nurses' Association of Ontario (RNAO). (2005f). *Woman abuse: Screening, identification and initial response.* Toronto, ON: Registered Nurses' Association of Ontario.

Registered Nurses' Association of Ontario (RNAO). (2006). *Collaborative practice among nursing teams.* Toronto, ON: Registered Nurses' Association of Ontario.

Registered Nurses' Association of Ontario (RNAO). (2007). *Professionalism in nursing.* Toronto, ON: Registered Nurses' Association of Ontario.

Registered Nurses' Association of Ontario (RNAO). (2008a). *Oral health: Nursing assessment and intervention.* Toronto, ON: Registered Nurses' Association of Ontario.

Registered Nurses' Association of Ontario (RNAO). (2008b). *Workplace health, safety, and wellbeing of the nurse.* Toronto, ON: Registered Nurses' Association of Ontario.

Registered Nurses' Association of Ontario (RNAO). (2009a). *Assessment and management of pain* (3rd ed.) Toronto, ON: Registered Nurses' Association of Ontario

Registered Nurses' Association of Ontario (RNAO). (2009b). *Developing and sustaining interprofessional health care.* Toronto, ON: Registered Nurses' Association of Ontario.

Registered Nurses' Association of Ontario (RNAO). (2009c). *Preventing and managing violence in the workplace.* Toronto, ON: Registered Nurses' Association of Ontario.

Registered Nurses' Association of Ontario (RNAO). (2010a). *Assessment and care of adults at risk for suicidal ideation and behaviour.* Toronto, ON: Registered Nurses' Association of Ontario.

Registered Nurses' Association of Ontario (RNAO). (2010b). *Caregiving strategies for older adults with delirium, dementia and depression.* Toronto, ON: Registered Nurses' Association of Ontario.

Registered Nurses' Association of Ontario (RNAO). (2010c). *Risk assessment and prevention of pressure ulcers.* Toronto, ON: Registered Nurses' Association of Ontario.

Registered Nurses' Association of Ontario (RNAO). (2010d). *Screening for delirium, dementia and depression in the older adult.* Toronto, ON: Registered Nurses' Association of Ontario.

Registered Nurses' Association of Ontario (RNAO). (2010e). *Strategies to support self-management in chronic conditions: Collaboration with clients.* Toronto, ON: Registered Nurses' Association of Ontario.

Registered Nurses' Association of Ontario (RNAO). (2011a). *End-of-life care during the last days and hours.* Toronto, ON: Registered Nurses' Association of Ontario.

Registered Nurses' Association of Ontario (RNAO). (2011b). *Preventing and mitigating nurse fatigue in health care.* Toronto, ON: Registered Nurses' Association of Ontario.

Registered Nurses' Association of Ontario (RNAO). (2012a). *Facilitating client centred learning.* Toronto, ON: Registered Nurses' Association of Ontario.

Registered Nurses' Association of Ontario (RNAO). (2012b). *Promoting safety: Alternative approaches to the use of restraints.* Toronto, ON: Registered Nurses' Association of Ontario.

Registered Nurses' Association of Ontario (RNAO). (2012c). *Toolkit: Implementation of Best Practice Guidelines* (2nd ed.). Toronto, ON: Registered Nurses' Association of Ontario.

Registered Nurses' Association of Ontario (RNAO). (2013a). *Assessment and management of foot ulcers for people with diabetes* (2nd ed.). Toronto, ON: Registered Nurses' Association of Ontario.

Registered Nurses' Association of Ontario (RNAO). (2013b). *Developing and sustaining interprofessional health care: Optimizing patients/clients, organizational, and system outcomes.* Toronto, ON: Registered Nurses' Association of Ontario.

Registered Nurses' Association of Ontario (RNAO). (2013c). *Developing and sustaining nursing leadership.* Toronto, ON: Registered Nurses' Association of Ontario.

Registered Nurses' Association of Ontario (RNAO). (2013d). *Managing and mitigating conflict in health-care teams.* Toronto, ON: Registered Nurses' Association of Ontario.

Registered Nurses' Association of Ontario (RNAO). (2014a). *Care transitions.* Toronto, ON: Registered Nurses' Association of Ontario.

Registered Nurses' Association of Ontario (RNAO). (2014b). *Preventing and addressing abuse and neglect of older adults: Person-centred, collaborative, system-wide approaches.* Toronto, ON: Registered Nurses' Association of Ontario.

Registered Nurses' Association of Ontario (RNAO). (2014c). *Primary prevention of childhood obesity* (2nd ed.). Toronto, ON: Registered Nurses' Association of Ontario.

Registered Nurses' Association of Ontario (RNAO). (2015). *Person-and family-centred care.* Toronto, ON: Registered Nurses' Association of Ontario.

Registered Nurses' Association of Ontario. (2016a). *Delirium, dementia and depression in older adults: Assessment and care* (2nd ed.). Toronto, ON: Registered Nurses' Association of Ontario.

Registered Nurses' Association of Ontario (RNAO). (2016b). *Intra-professional collaborative practice among nurses.* Toronto, ON: Registered Nurses' Association of Ontario.

Santiago, C., & Smith, O. (2015). My story: Humanizing the critical care experience. *The Canadian Journal of Critical Care Nursing, 26*(2), 33.

Thomas, A., Murray, M. A., Jeffs, L., Lonnelly, S., Marticorena, R. M., & Wald, R. (2016). Are you SURE about your vascular access? Exploring factors influencing vascular access decisions with chronic hemodialysis patients and their nurses. *Canadian Association of Nephrology Nurses and Technologists Journal, 26*(2), 21–28.

Toronto Public Health. (2011). *The impact of the Best Practice Spotlight Organization candidacy on Toronto Public Health.* Toronto, ON: Toronto Public Health.

Toussaint, J., Gerard, R., & Adams, E. (2010). *On the mend: Revolutionizing healthcare to save lives and transform the industry.* Cambridge, MA: Lean Enterprise Institute.

Wannamaker, K., Michelsen K. C., & Santiago, C. (2015). Ticket to ward: Transitioning patients from MSICU to inpatient areas. *The Canadian Journal of Critical Care Nursing, 26*(2), 33.

Young, R. A., Roberts, R. G., & Holden, R. J. (2017). The challenges of measuring, improving, and reporting quality in primary care. *Annals of Family Medicine, 15*(2), 175–182. doi: 10.1370/afm.201.

ENHANCING THE EVIDENCE-BASED NURSING CURRICULUM AND COMPETENCE IN EVIDENCE-BASED PRACTICE

JoAnne MacDonald, PhD, MN, RN
Amalia Silva-Galleguillos, MSc, RN
Olga Lucía Gómez Díaz, MA(Ed), RN
Irmajean Bajnok, PhD, MScN, BScN, RN

LEARNING OBJECTIVES

After reading this chapter, you will be able to:

- Define academic Best Practice Spotlight Organizations

- Describe processes for becoming an academic Best Practice Spotlight Organization

- Understand how Best Practice Guideline (BPG) integration in the undergraduate nursing curriculum enhances student learning about evidence-based practice

- Outline teaching-learning strategies to enhance nursing student learning about BPGs

- Identify supports for successful integration of BPGs in the academic setting

- Discuss strategies for overcoming challenges to integrate and sustain BPG integration in curriculum

- Delineate ways to measure the success of integrating BPGs in academic settings

- Consider how academic Best Practice Spotlight Organizations contribute to a program of research in academic institutions

INTRODUCTION

The purpose of this chapter is to introduce academic Best Practice Spotlight Organizations (academic BPSO) and describe how the quality of undergraduate nursing education and graduate nurse competence in evidence-based practice (EBP) is enhanced through the integration of the Registered Nurses' Association of Ontario's (RNAO) Best Practice Guidelines (BPG) in the curriculum. Academic BPSOs focus on integrating BPGs into nursing curricula to better prepare students for EBP, enhancing patient and family outcomes. This chapter is relevant to all those involved in the education and mentoring of undergraduate nurses, including educators in academic settings, nurses and managers in practice settings, and members of the interprofessional healthcare team with whom nurses collaborate for person and family care.

Integration of BPGs into undergraduate and graduate nursing curricula can greatly facilitate the academic sector's efforts to close the theory-practice gap. Since the BPG Program's inception, RNAO has engaged nursing faculty in supporting the use of BPGs in the nursing curricula. For example, RNAO partnered with various schools of nursing in a series of projects to demonstrate the process and impact of integrating select BPGs into the curriculum. The resulting program enhancements provided current evidence to inform the curriculum, and also demonstrated to students the research and evidence base of nursing, through the BPGs. These projects highlighted the need for a resource for faculty and staff development educators that would incorporate lessons learned and provide a guide, much like the RNAO Implementation Toolkit (2012c), targeted to faculty and focused on integration of BPGs into the curriculum. Such a guide—the *Educator's Resource: Integration of Best Practice Guidelines* (RNAO, 2005)—was subsequently developed with extensive involvement of faculty and service-setting educators from inception to publication and dissemination. Since its publication, numerous faculty and service-setting educators have accessed the resource to inform their use of BPGs in teaching activities.

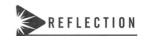 **REFLECTION**

As an educator in an academic or service setting, how do you see yourself using a clinical Best Practice Guideline to reinforce nursing as a knowledge profession?

The formal involvement of academic settings in the BPSO Designation began in 2009 with Trent/Fleming School of Nursing in Ontario leading the way for the establishment of what would become a growing cohort of international academic BPSOs. In 2013, St. Francis Xavier University Rankin School of Nursing, Nova Scotia, began its candidacy as Canada's first national academic BPSO. These BPSOs are now located in universities in 10 countries—Belgium, Canada, Chile, China, Colombia, Italy, Jamaica, Portugal, Qatar, and Spain. Regardless of their geographic location, academic BPSOs are committed to enriching the professional practice of graduate nurses, enhancing evidence-based cultures, and ultimately improving person and family care.

This chapter draws on the experiences of three national and international academic BPSOs: the Rankin School of Nursing St. Francis Xavier University (StFX) in Nova Scotia, Canada; the Universidad de Chile Nursing Department in Santiago de Chile; and the Universidad Autonoma de Bucaramanga Nursing Program (UNAB) in Bucaramanga, Colombia.

C A S E   S T U D Y

Founded in 1853, StFX is one of Canada's oldest universities located in Nova Scotia, Canada. Rooted in values of integrity, dignity, truth, and respect for all, StFX is known for its reputable undergraduate experience and for the excellence of its teaching, research, and service. StFX has a rich tradition of social justice and leadership, a mission for service, and is home to the world-renowned Coady International Institute and National Collaborating Centre for the Determinants of Health. The school of nursing was established in 1926 and is an innovative leader in nursing education, research, community engagement, and collaborative partnerships locally, provincially, nationally, and globally. This Nova Scotian school of nursing was accepted as a BPSO in December 2013.

The Universidad de Chile was founded in 1842 and is the largest, oldest, and amongst the three top institution of higher education in the country. The University of Chile is a public university and fosters leadership and innovation in sciences and technologies and in the humanities and the arts through its teaching, development, and outreach, with special emphasis on research and postgraduate studies. It promotes a prepared, critical citizenship embracing a social conscience and ethical responsibility.

It espouses the values of tolerance, pluralism, and equity; intellectual independence and freedom of thought; as well as respect, promotion, and preservation of diversity in all areas of its work. In 1906, the School of Nursing was founded and was the first school for nurses in both the state and in South America. This Chilean school of nursing became a BPSO in December 2011 (Silva-Galleguillos, 2015, 2016).

The Autonomous University of Bucaramanga (UNAB) is a private, not-for-profit institution located in the city of Bucaramanga, Department of Santander, Colombia. UNAB is rooted in the values of democracy, independence, and liberty. It is committed to excellence of its academic programs, strong academic and administrative support processes, and ongoing accreditation of the institution. Its programs adhere to the Guidelines for Higher Education in Colombia (LAW 266, 1996) that promote accessibility and quality in higher education within the global context. The nursing program was founded in 2008 and seeks to innovate within the nursing profession, through an international program that responds to the needs of both the country and the world. This Colombian school of nursing became a BPSO in October 2014.

In this chapter, we will first introduce the candidacy and designation of academic BPSOs. The purpose and process of becoming a BPSO is presented, and the integration of BPGs into curricula is described in detail. We discuss reinforcing supports and overcoming challenges for sustained change, as well as measuring the success of BPG integration in the academic setting. The chapter concludes with a discussion of the role of academic BPSOs in research. When applicable, similarities or distinctions are made between academic and health service BPSOs.

FROM CANDIDACY TO DESIGNATION

The BPSO Designation aims to support BPG implementation and evaluation at the organizational (meso) level (RNAO, 2017a). To achieve designation, academic BPSOs must go through the same rigorous application and candidacy process as health service organizations (RNAO, 2017a). With the support of RNAO, academic BPSOs commit to a 3-year candidacy period during which they build institutional capacity for curriculum innovation, integrate BPGs into theoretical and practice-based courses, and formalize related evaluation and research. Academic institutions that achieve these goals by the end of the 3-year qualifying period become Designated academic BPSOs. The focus of Designate BPSOs shifts from establishing, planning, and implementing the curriculum innovation to sustaining the existing BPGs in the curriculum and integrating additional ones. Designates also focus on sustaining BPG use by student nurses in the care of persons and families, mentoring other academic BPSOs, and engaging in research related to implementation science.

PURPOSE OF ACADEMIC BPSOs

Educators in schools of nursing are charged with ensuring that their graduating nursing students are prepared to apply the best evidence for safe, high-quality, and effective healthcare. Yet, new nurses frequently believe they are not adequately prepared to integrate scientific evidence into their daily practice (Dawley, Rosen Bloch, Dunphy Suplee, McKeever, & Scherzer, 2011; Finotto, Carpanoni, Casadei Turroni, Camellini, & Mecugni, 2013). Nurse leaders also question the ability of graduating nurses to understand evidence-based practice (Nursing Executive Center, 2008). Scholars further argue that nursing students' education in class is often far removed from the realities experienced during clinical practice (Florin, Ehrenberg, Wallin, & Gustavsson, 2012; Jones, 2007). Furthermore, students experience more support to use and apply research during their classroom instruction compared to their clinical practice experiences (Florin et al., 2012).

Academic BPSOs are leading a curriculum innovation that uses BPGs to address this evidence preparation and readiness gap amongst new nurses.

Unlike the implementation of BPGs in health service settings, where recommendations become actionable at the bedside, BPGs in academic BPSOs serve a different yet critical purpose. In the academic setting, BPGs serve as a foundational tool for teaching and preparing nursing students for evidence-based practice. BPGs are threaded into all theoretical and practice-based courses as a way for students to learn about how to make evidence–based decisions for nursing practice, effecting better person and family outcomes.

In each course, applicable BPGs are used to support student learning about how to identify, assess, select, apply, and evaluate evidence. For example, pressure injuries (RNAO, 2016a), vascular access (RNAO, 2008), and end-of-life care (RNAO, 2011a) BPGs guide student learning about clinical management issues. BPGs related to breastfeeding (RNAO, 2003), safe sleep (RNAO, 2014b), and woman abuse (RNAO, 2012d) are valuable to population-focused courses such as paediatrics or women's health. Substance use (RNAO, 2015b), suicide (RNAO, 2009a), pain management (RNAO, 2013a), and hypertension (RNAO, 2009b) BPGs are beneficial to specialty-based courses such as mental health or medical-surgical nursing, while health-promoting BPGs, such as prevention of childhood obesity (RNAO, 2014a) and management of chronic disease (RNAO, 2010), support public health and community-based courses.

The experience of the three schools of nursing is that the BPGs can be used in many ways throughout the curriculum. For example, the *Person-and Family-Centred Care* BPG (RNAO, 2015c) serves to guide student learning about people's experience of health and the role of family in health, which is foundational to all nursing practice and thus applicable to all nursing courses. In some cases, a BPG can inform the overall design of a course. The *Establishing Therapeutic Relationships* BPG (2006b), for instance, has impacted course design in a number of ways. It is used by academic BPSOs to organize course content that aims to support nursing students' development of requisite knowledge and capacities for establishing and engaging in therapeutic relationships. It is also used to complement specific courses in the mental health component of the curriculum. System and Healthy Work Environment BPGs are used to design courses focused on the health, safety, and well-being of the nurse.

Moreover, the authors also found that the System and Healthy Work Environment BPGs (RNAO, 2017c) have a critical role in nursing education. Learning how to work in intra- and interprofessional teams (RNAO, 2006a, 2013b, 2016b), managing conflict (2012b), and developing cultural competence (2007a) and leadership (2013c) are examples of the Healthy Work Environment BPGs that support the development of professional practice as part of the Professionalism BPG (RNAO, 2007b) amongst nursing students. Essentially, all 41 clinical (RNAO, 2017b) and 12 system and healthy environment BPGs (RNAO, 2017c) have a place in a broad range of diverse nursing courses. Thus, in academic BPSOs, BPGs are an integrated component of a curriculum that serves to prepare future nurses for professional, evidence-based practice.

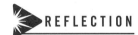

REFLECTION

What are the benefits to practice, education, nurses, students, and patients when both service and academic settings become designated as BPSOs?

Finally, as part of evidence-based practice competencies (Melnyk, Gallagher-Ford, Long, & Fineout-Overholt, 2014), it is important that students are aware of the elements of implementation science as they use BPGs, observe their uptake by clinicians, and collaborate to initiate sustained BPG use over time in clinical settings. This is an important component of the curriculum, especially in those academic BPSOs with graduate programs. Using RNAO's BPGs and related implementation resources in both the theory and practicum components of their curriculum, the University of Antwerp in Belgium has found that through the academic BPSO Designation, it has been able to strengthen its graduate degree curriculum in relation to implementation science.

"The BPSO Designation and related work with our faculty and students has strengthened the evidence-based practice component of our curriculum, in particular implementation science. Our graduate students are now learning and leading in this area in their workplaces."

–Prof. Dr. Peter Van Bogaert, PhD, RN
BPSO Lead
Professor, Nursing and Midwifery Sciences
Centre for Research and Innovation in Care (CRIC)
University of Antwerp, Belgium—BPSO Direct-Academic

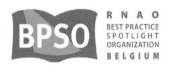

BECOMING AN ACADEMIC BEST PRACTICE SPOTLIGHT ORGANIZATION

The process of becoming a BPSO engages academic institutions in a systematic planned change strategy. A *planned change strategy* is the deliberate design and implementation of an innovation. According to Field and colleagues, "conceptual frameworks are recommended as a way of applying theory to enhance implementation efforts" (Field, Booth, Ilott, & Gerrish, 2014, p. 1). RNAO's process of moving BPGs into practice is informed by the Knowledge-to-Action framework (Graham et al., 2006), composed of two components: knowledge creation and an action cycle. The action phase of the Knowledge-to-Action framework is particularly useful for managing change. The use of this framework, illustrated in Figure 9.1, is shown to be effective for guiding the integration of evidence into undergraduate nursing education (Stacey et al., 2009).

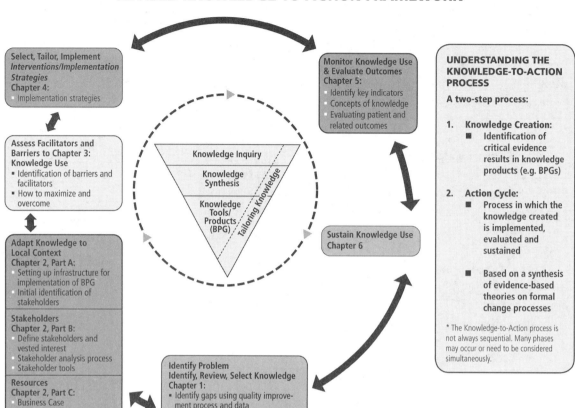

REVISED KNOWLEDGE-TO-ACTION FRAMEWORK

Adapted from "Knowledge Translation in Health Care: Moving From Evidence to Practice."
S. Straus, J. Tetroe, and I. Graham. Copyright 2009 by Blackwell Publishing Ltd. Adapted with permission.

FIGURE 9.1 Knowledge-to-Action framework as depicted in *Toolkit: Implementation of Best Practice Guidelines* (RNAO, 2012c).
© Registered Nurses' Association of Ontario. All rights reserved. Used with permission.

The academic BPSO trajectory also benefits from a whole-system approach. This approach assumes that integrating BPGs into curriculum is part of a broader system, inclusive of facilitators and barriers and system dynamics (MacDonald, Edwards, Davies, Marck, & Read Guernsey, 2012). Change within this system is "multi-level, non-linear and multi-directional, with sustainable system adaptations" (Edwards & Grinspun, 2011, p. 4). From this lens, integrating BPGs into a curriculum involves a holistic approach that considers what is happening with students and educators, the academic institution, the health service organizations and its providers, the broader health system, and beyond, to other external systems. Throughout this chapter, reference will be made to action phases of the Knowledge-to-Action framework and to whole-system approaches, which were used whether in Canada, Chile, or Colombia.

BUILDING A CULTURE OF EVIDENCE

A key step in the BPSO Designation is building a culture of evidence. A culture of evidence is the set of values, beliefs, and norms related to the uptake of evidence-informed clinical, management, and academic decision-making (Fineout-Overholt & Melnyk, 2005). Building a culture of evidence begins with establishing the relevance of being an academic BPSO. Within the action phase of the Knowledge-to-Action framework, the initial stage is to establish the relevance of the curriculum innovation. Identifying how the integration of BPGs contributes to the strategic direction of the academic institution can inspire interest for change. Strategic goals—such as enriching educators' pedagogy, enhancing students' competence in evidence-based practice, and creating a program of research related to the learning and application of evidence in nursing education—are supported with the integration of BPGs in the curriculum.

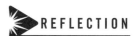

REFLECTION

What rationale would you use to convince your faculty colleagues and administrative leadership to become an academic BPSO?

Educators and students may also be receptive to deliberately integrating BPGs into their teaching and practice. For instance, knowing that the uptake of BPGs at the bedside lends credibility to decisions about client care may encourage consistent application of accepted standards of care (Friedman et al., 2009; RNAO, 2005), discourages the use of interventions that have little effect and/or cause harm (RNAO, 2005), and ultimately has the potential to improve evidence-based practice, health system, and client outcomes (Athwal et al., 2013; Graham & Harrison, 2005; Prentice et al., 2009; Rempel & Mc-Cleary, 2012; RNAO, 2011b). Another important motivator for introducing a curriculum innovation is educators' recognition of gaps in the curriculum. Curricular reviews are one way to expose areas where teaching and learning about evidence can be strengthened, opening opportunities for integrating BPGs into the curriculum. In addition, having key stakeholders such as educators, students, and practitioners engaged in the change process is a critical component to gaining buy-in and creating cultures of evidence (Missal, Schafer, Halm, & Schaffer, 2010; RNAO, 2012c).

The RNAO *Educator's Resource: Integration of Best Practice Guidelines* (2005, p. 9) presents a framework shown in Figure 9.2 to guide integration of BPGs into learning events at all levels of the curriculum. Whether used for the curriculum as a whole, a course, or a specific lesson, this framework helps guide integration of BPGs into related learning events or components of the program.

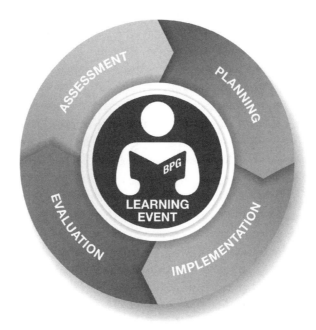

FIGURE 9.2   Framework for Integration of Best Practice Guidelines into learning events (adapted from RNAO, 2005a, p. 9).

ESTABLISHING STRUCTURAL SUPPORTS

Establishing structural supports is another key step in becoming an academic BPSO. Structural supports include the processes and resources necessary to engage in the planned change. Within the action phase of the Knowledge-to-Action framework, planning for change within the local context is an essential building block for change and includes identifying stakeholders, developing an action plan, and securing resources. From a whole-systems perspective, the successful integration of BPGs in curricula includes communicating and engaging multiple stakeholders and establishing structural supports across the system.

IDENTIFYING STAKEHOLDERS

The identification of stakeholders who can potentially influence the curriculum innovation is essential. *Stakeholders* include those who are directly or indirectly affected by the implementation of BPGs in the curriculum or those who have a vested interest in the curricular change (RNAO, 2012c). Understanding stakeholder interests, decision power, plans, and relationships informs the influence, supports, and barriers they may yield when integrating BPGs into the curriculum. Common stakeholders involved in curriculum innovations include nurse educators, students, senior academic administration, health service providers and interdisciplinary teams, regulatory bodies, and accreditation bodies. However, depending on the local context, stakeholders vary amongst academic institutions and yield varying degrees of influence and support. Thus, each academic institution should conduct a stakeholder analysis. Details for conducting a stakeholder analysis are available through the RNAO Implementation Toolkit (RNAO, 2012c).

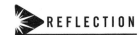 **REFLECTION**

You are considering the integration of BPGs in your academic unit. Conduct a preliminary stakeholder analysis. Describe each stakeholder's level of support and influence.

DEVELOPING AN ACADEMIC BPSO ACTION PLAN

The development of an action plan is part of the structural supports required by all BPSOs and, as outlined in the RNAO Implementation Toolkit (RNAO, 2012c), a critical aspect of moving knowledge into action. For BPSOs, an action plan supports the structured methodology and planned change approaches necessary for sustained BPG use, whether in practice or academia. In academic BPSOs, action plans identify the goals, objectives, and activities that direct changes necessary to integrate RNAO BPGs throughout the curriculum and to achieve the BPSO Designation requirements. Table 9.1 shows an example of an academic BPSO Action Plan with excerpts of goals, objectives, and related activities.

In this example, the *goals* set out the broad results that the academic BPSO aims to achieve. The goals shown in this sample plan related to capacity building, integration, and research were common amongst the three academic BPSOs profiled in this chapter. The *objectives* are shorter-term results representing the stepping stones that will lead to the achievement of the goals. Objectives for the first year of the BPSO related to Goal #1 are shown in the sample plan. The objectives are modified as the academic BPSO continues to progress toward achievement of its overall goals. Examples of objectives for Goal #1 for the second year are included as well in the plan shown here. The *activities* represent the actions that will be taken to successfully achieve the objectives. The sample plan includes activities related to the objectives for the first year for Goal #1.

TABLE 9.1   ACADEMIC BPSO ACTION PLAN (EXCERPTS) FOR INTEGRATING BPSOS INTO CURRICULUM AND ACHIEVING BPSO DELIVERABLES

GOALS	OBJECTIVES	ACTIVITIES	LEAD FACULTY	TIMELINES	MONITORING AND EVALUATION
1. To enhance capacity for the uptake of BPGs by students, nurse educators and faculty, and health service providers	**YEAR 1** 1. A sustainable infrastructure exists, which supports the integration of BPGs into curriculum and the development of a program of research related to integration of BPGs into curriculum. 2. Support is gained from key academic and health service provider stakeholders who will advance and champion the integration of BPGs into curriculum. 3. Resources are secured that support BPG integration into curriculum. **YEAR 2** 1. A local network of BPG Champions is established and composed of academic and health service provider stakeholders committed to implementing BPGs into nursing curriculum. 2. A collection of human and financial resources exists that supports BPG integration in curriculum and uptake in clinical practice settings. 3. BPGs are an integrated component of the academic BPSO's theoretical courses and clinical practice experiences.	1. An academic BPSO steering committee Terms of Reference document is developed. 2. Potential members are identified and invited to form the academic BPSO's steering committee inclusive of both academic and health service provider members. 3. Dedicated funding is secured for training and other initiatives that support achievement of academic BPSO's goals.			

continues

TABLE 9.1   ACADEMIC BPSO ACTION PLAN (EXCERPTS) FOR INTEGRATING BPSOS INTO CURRICULUM AND ACHIEVING BPSO DELIVERABLES (CONTINUED)

GOALS	OBJECTIVES	ACTIVITIES	LEAD FACULTY	TIMELINES	MONITORING AND EVALUATION
2. To integrate BPGs in theoretical courses and clinical practice experiences					
3. To establish a BPG program of research led by the School of Nursing in partnership with other stakeholders					

Determining who is responsible for the actions to be taken, the timelines, and the measures to evaluate progress toward achieving the plan are also key elements of an action plan. Exemplar action plan templates are available on the RNAO website as part of the RNAO Implementation Toolkit (RNAO, 2012c).

ESTABLISHING AN INFRASTRUCTURE

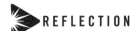
REFLECTION

What key elements of implementation science as reflected in the Knowledge-to-Action framework are most critical in your setting? How would you see yourself using the model to initiate curriculum change to integrate BPGs?

All three academic BPSOs paid attention to the establishment of an infrastructure in their plans for the curriculum innovation. As noted in the exemplars above, a key infrastructural component is a steering committee to provide the oversight of BPG integration into the curriculum. Steering committees often include curriculum committee coordinators or chairs, other faculty, students, and health service providers. Having a dedicated academic lead who holds accountability for leading the academic BPSOs is also essential. In most academic BPSOs, depending on the size, the curriculum coordinator or program head often assumes this responsibility. However, it is imperative that there is visible support from the program head, and that the BPSO lead has dedicated time to devote to this role.

Champions to mentor, educate, persuade others (Edwards & Grinspun, 2011; Ploeg et al., 2010), and initiate various components of the curriculum innovation are also an important part of the infrastructure. These Champions are particularly relevant at the initial stage of the curriculum innovation, as early adopters influence the attitudes and facilitate stakeholder engagement (RNAO, 2012c). For all academic BPSOs, Champion development is a key start-up activity. Champions can assume a team lead role in the integration of a BPG across the curriculum or the integration of several BPGs across a level of the program. In many academic BPSOs, students have been part of the Champion network (Beijing University of Chinese Medicine, School of Nursing; University of Antwerp, School of Nursing; University of West

Indies School of Nursing). The intent is to create a network of stakeholders to promote the coordination and continuity of integration of BPGs across the curriculum.

Other infrastructure required includes educational, financial, and in-kind resources. *Educational resources* encompass curriculum support tools such as BPG-related instructional and student assessment tools. In some cases, *financial resources* may be needed to support educational training or to support dissemination activities. *In-kind resources* and non-cash forms of support include, for example, the coverage of costs by the university for printing Champion workbooks, or provision of the venue for training sessions.

INTEGRATING BPGS INTO THE CURRICULUM

A key goal of academic BPSOs is the integration of BPGs into theoretical and practice-based courses. Within the action phase of the Knowledge-to-Action framework, achieving this integration is accomplished by executing the action plan. Moreover, "change is more likely to occur with more planned and focused interventions" (Graham et al., 2006, p. 21). Key strategies to integrate BPGs into curriculum include developing multilevel learning objectives and designing teaching and learning strategies. In addition, in all academic BPSOs, the integration of BPGs becomes a standing item on the curriculum committee agenda, for regular meetings, and in particular at major curriculum review and revision sessions.

DESIGNING MULTILEVEL BPG-RELATED LEARNING OBJECTIVES

Learning objectives in academic BPSOs feature BPG competencies that students will gain through their nursing education. BPG-related learning outcomes, required at multiple levels of the program, facilitate their integration throughout the curriculum. At the program level, learning objectives refer to broad knowledge, judgment, skill, and attitude competencies expected of students by program end. Given that evidence-based practice is a common undergraduate-level competence expected of nursing students, BPG-related learning objectives are an easy addition to nursing curricula.

At the course level, BPG-related learning objectives provide a guide for identifying the specific BPG knowledge, skills, attitudes, and judgment competences students will gain by the end of the course. In an introductory course, examples of class-level learning objectives include, but are not limited to:

- Students gain increased knowledge about BPGs.

- Students are able to select BPGs relevant to practice.

- Students are able to provide rationale for BPGs selected.

- Students are able to select recommendations to guide person- and family-centred care.

- Students are able to provide rationale for recommendations selected.

- Students integrate BPG recommendations into plans of care for persons and families.

Building on this foundational learning, educators throughout the program tailor course-level learning objectives to align with specific course content. For instance, an appropriate course-level learning objective for a public health course is:

"Students gain competence in the use of health-promoting Best Practice Guidelines."

Each of the academic BPSOs showcased here designed learning opportunities that enabled students to gradually build competence and confidence in the use of BPGs. Their work reflects a systematic integration that began with an introduction to BPGs, followed by repeated exposure to the range of BPGs and their application with increased detail and complexity, as students progress from a novice to an expert (Benner, Sutphen, Leonard, Day, & Shulman, 2010) in BPG-related undergraduate-level competence.

Course-level learning objectives provide the scaffolding for more specific content-related, class-level learning objectives. Based on the assumption that students gradually gain proficiency (Benner et al., 2010), educators create learning pathways that require students to build on abstract principles about BPGs to refine and expand their evidence-based practice through repetition and increasingly complex experiences. Continuing with the example above, educators tailor class-level learning objectives to align with course-level objective content. Toward achievement of the above course-level objective, the class-level learning objectives refer to specific health promoting BPGs such as: "Students have increased knowledge about the *Primary Prevention of Childhood Obesity* BPG (RNAO, 2014a)"; or "Students integrate recommendations from the *Strategies to Support Self-Management in Chronic Conditions: Collaboration with Clients* BPG (RNAO, 2010) into plans of care for persons and families."

The deliberate design of learning objectives at all levels of the program directs students to systematically gain knowledge and skills in evidence-based nursing, which become an embedded component of their nursing practice.

DEVELOPING BPG-RELATED TEACHING AND LEARNING STRATEGIES

The academic BPSOs use a range of teaching and learning strategies to integrate BPGs into theoretical and practice-based courses. Christie, Hamill, and Power (2012) specifically argue that nursing students need to be able to value the relevance, authority, and utility of evidence for patient care by embedding learning in both academic and practice-based settings. Thus, integrating BPGs requires a complement of teaching and learning strategies in both theoretical and practice-based courses. As research has demonstrated, teaching and learning about BPGs must also go beyond static methods of teaching to include interactive methods that engage learners (Friedman et al., 2009). For example, at the Beijing University School of Nursing academic BPSO (see Chapter 14, *Overcoming Context and Language Differences: BPSO Trailblazers in China),* with the integration of BPGs into the curriculum, there have been numerous changes in teaching and learning strategies to include use of video, role-playing, simulation, and generally a move to less didactic teaching methods. Many of these changes were inspired by the integration of the *Facilitating Client Centred Learning* BPG (RNAO, 2012a) into the curriculum, which precipitated faculty to apply much of the evidence and some of the recommendations to their teaching methodologies.

LECTURES

Lectures provide a means for students to get a broad understanding about BPGs. Lectures can contribute to student understanding about the rigorous process used to develop BPGs and their various recommendations. These include *practice recommendations,* or the "statements that guide care based on available research evidence, or on the consensus of experts from best available anecdotal and experiential evidence in the absence of research" (RNAO, 2012c, p. 19). Students can also gain understanding about *organizational and system recommendations,* or the "statements of conditions required for a practice setting that enable the successful implementation of best practice guidelines" (RNAO, 2012c, p. 19), and educational recommendations, or "statements of educational requirements and educational approaches/strategies for the introduction, implementation and sustainability of best practice guidelines" (RNAO, 2012c, p. 19). Students can also grasp the scope and types of evidence that inform the recommendations through lectures.

INTERACTIVE CLASSROOM ACTIVITIES

Engaging students through interactive classroom activities provides a way for them to gather additional information, conduct problem-solving, and share or articulate knowledge gained. Having students work together to complete an assessment of an RNAO BPG using the AGREE II Tool (Brouwers et al., 2010) is one example of an interactive classroom activity that requires students to navigate through a BPG, encouraging them to become more familiar with a guideline and standards for guideline development. The use of case studies creates opportunities for students to examine and apply BPG recommendations in plans of care. Simulation and role-playing can also be used to encourage students to develop skills in planning the application of BPG recommendations or to articulate rationale for selecting specific BPGs in a plan of care. At the University of West Indies School of Nursing BPSO in Jamaica, faculty revised their simulation laboratory teaching-learning guides to incorporate all the clinical BPGs as they relate to critical knowledge and skills reinforced through simulated teach-back sessions. At the Beijing University School of Nursing BPSO, faculty use videos and role-playing to teach concepts of the pain management (RNAO, 2013a) and client-centred learning BPGs (RNAO, 2012a).

PRE- AND POST-CLINICAL CONFERENCE DISCUSSIONS

Pre- and post-clinical conference discussions provide students with opportunities to critically think through the application of BPG recommendations in their plans of care, consider modifications based on the clinical and patient context, defend the clinical decisions they made, and evaluate the outcome of BPG-related nursing interventions. Students can also focus on investigating how practice setting policies and procedures align with best practice evidence. Featuring a BPG as a focal point for discussion during a pre- or post-clinical conference also helps students to identify potential areas for practice change and consider how such change could be initiated.

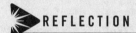 **REFLECTION**

What teaching and learning strategies are used in your setting to support students' understanding and their application of research evidence in practice? How can these strategies be used to integrate BPGs into theoretical courses and into practice-based courses?

ACCESS TO BPG-RELATED RESOURCES

Creating access to BPG-related resources is also essential to supporting student learning about BPGs. Citing BPGs as key course references and including RNAO's BPG implementation support tools are common in academic BPSOs. BPGs are a standard part of student readings, starting in the first year of the nursing program and continuing until graduation. Learning Management Systems (LMS) provide a means to organize these BPG resources and provide BPG-related links for easy access. The use of the RNAO BPG App (http://rnao.ca/bpg/pda/app) further enables students to access content from all RNAO guidelines, whether they are in the classroom or at the bedside.

ASSIGNMENTS AND TESTS

BPG-related assignments provide another means for students to reflect upon, visualize the application of, and critique BPGs. Students may incorporate BPGs into learning plans or write a reflective journal related to a BPG important to their area of nursing practice. Developing plans of care that include pertinent BPGs is a common expectation in academic BPSOs. Tests or exam questions provide an opportunity for students to demonstrate critical thinking and judgment related to BPGs.

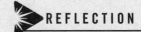

REFLECTION

How could clinical assignments for students in various years of the curriculum be structured to assist in the application of BPGs in the clinical setting across sectors?

REINFORCING SUPPORTS AND OVERCOMING CHALLENGES FOR SUSTAINED CHANGE

Another critical stage of the action cycle is assessment of the conditions or factors that can influence the outcome of integrating BPGs into a curriculum. According to Graham et al. (2006), those who plan change "control the variables that increase or decrease the likelihood of the occurrence of change" (p. 20). Dependent upon local context, these conditions and factors can serve as facilitators that promote the success of integration or barriers that interfere with integration. Academic BPSOs look to reinforce the conditions or factors that will support BPG integration, while taking steps to mediate or eliminate those conditions and factors that interfere with integration plans. From a whole-systems perspective, the successful integration of BPGs in curricula includes anticipating those variables and developing and adapting plans based on context.

Provincial, national, or even international initiatives can serve to support a decision related to BPG integration. Initiatives such as academic reviews, changes to licensing examinations, and changes to the migration policy for health professionals may arouse interest in new curriculum innovations such as BPG integration and becoming a BPSO. For instance, a provincial review of nursing education in Nova Scotia, Canada, by the Department of Health and Wellness included a recommendation that schools of nursing "identify and implement a set of common, best-practice guidelines across the schools and with clinical partners" (Cruickshank & Ells, 2014, p. 27). In the case of Colombia, BPG integration in nursing curricula was a partial response to changes in the professional regulations, requiring schools of nursing to prepare future nurses for critical and reflective decision-making. In the case of Italy, it was faculty-driven, to strengthen evidence-based practice in the curriculum and also to be consistent with its hospital service partner that was becoming a service BPSO. In Portugal, the Atlantica University Nursing Department was motivated by the desire to strengthen its own curriculum and lead and role-model evidence-based education and practice in the country.

Successful curricular innovations align with the mission, vision, values, and overall strategic directions of academic institutions and schools of nursing. Common to higher education institutions is a quest to provide quality education that will prepare graduates to serve and contribute to society. All academic BPSOs are strengthening their contributions to this quest through the integration of BPGs in nursing education. This curricular innovation serves to develop a community of nurses who use the most current and rigorous evidence that assists with clinical decision-making and encourages consistent high-quality care of persons and families.

The capacity for stakeholders to meet the demands required for planning and integrating BPGs into their everyday educational practice also impacts the outcomes of BPG implementation. Adequate knowledge is necessary for success, while lack thereof can impede progress. As in health service BPSOs (RNAO, 2012c), resistance to change in the academic setting can stem from lack of knowledge or misinformation. Consistent with all academic and service BPSOs, the three nursing schools featured in this chapter found that providing information and training sessions through the Champions program is the best way to address knowledge gaps. With knowledge, access to resources and supports, academic BPSO mentors, and initial successes, administrators and educators come to realize that the academic BPSO Designation is the most effective way for students to learn the research base of nursing practice and actually experience it through active use of BPGs. It is also an effective way to align the entire program with best evidence in nursing and healthcare and foster an integrated curriculum.

With many opportunities for faculty engagement in all aspects of BPG development, uptake, and evaluation, faculty gain avenues for scholarly contributions. Educators may be concerned about time constraints or including additional content into curricula that are already overloaded. Educators resisting change for these reasons can be made aware of how BPGs may easily be integrated into specific courses and that BPGs are an effective tool to gain competence in evidence-based practice. Creating a map that depicts how BPGs can be threaded throughout the curriculum is also useful. Many of these implementation strategies, from managing challenges and barriers to designing EBP- and BPG-integrated curricula, are outlined in the *Educators' Resource: Integration of Best Practice Guidelines* (RNAO, 2005).

A unique challenge for academic BPSOs is the need to secure opportunities for students to apply BPG competences in the practice setting. Health service organizations and practicing nurses have varied knowledge and experience related to BPG implementation. In some cases, health service organizations are also BPSOs with ample experience, while other organizations and their health service providers may be unfamiliar with or not using BPGs or evidence-based practice.

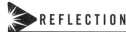
REFLECTION

Consider how academic institutions and health services work together to support students' evidence-based learning and practice. What are some ways such a partnership and the BPSO Designation could be used to strengthen or improve students' use of BPGs and staff's use of BPGs?

Maintaining positive relationships with health service partners is critical to the quality of the student learning experience in the practice setting. Sharing curriculum outcomes, including with health service partners as external members of curriculum committees, and providing education or workshops about BPGs can facilitate collaborative approaches for student and staff learning. In some cases, academic institutions (such as those in Belgium, Canada, Chile, China, Colombia, Jamaica, and Spain) were the impetus for the formation of health-service and academic partnerships, which simultaneously implement BPGs. In Italy, academic and service partners applied to be BPSOs at the same time, planning to implement the same BPGs in the same timeframes, with both organizations benefitting from joint training and preparation activities. These partnerships result in collaborative work on BPG implementation and curriculum integration, creating a synergy that maximizes learning for students and evidence-based practice for staff. The opportunity allows students to see how evidence, as learned in the classroom, is applied in practice. The following quote from the academic and service BPSOs in Jamaica attests to the mutual benefits of service academic partnerships in the BPSO Designation process.

> *"The BPSO Designation has assisted us to strengthen our curriculum framework through integration of BPGs in many courses, and to provide our students and faculty with research-based resources to support nursing as a knowledge profession. It has also been mutually beneficial to both UWISON and the University Hospital of West Indies to work together as BPSOs, focused on the same BPGs. Our students see BPGs being used in practice, which strengthens the focus of evidence-based practice in nursing."*

—Steve Weaver, PhD, MPH, BScN, RN
Head of School, UWISON
Director, WHO Collaborating Centre for Nursing and Midwifery Development in the Caribbean
BPSO Sponsor

—Eulalia Kahwa, PhD, BScN (hon), RN
Senior Lecturer and Graduate Program Coordinator
The University of West Indies School of Nursing (UWISON), Mona

—Mrs. Claudett James, MScHA, BScN, RN, RM, JP
Senior Director, Nursing
University Hospital of the West Indies
Jamaica

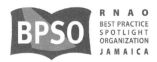

BPG INTEGRATION IN ACADEMIA: MEASURING SUCCESS

Evaluation of nursing education (Institute of Medicine [IOM], 2011; Kitson, Wiechula, Conroy, Muntlin Athlin, & Whitaker, 2013) and practice (Hanrahan et al., 2015) is a standard for quality, excellence, and innovation. Moreover, the three featured schools of nursing recognize that evaluating the outcomes of nursing education and practice makes nurses' contributions to health outcomes more visible (RNAO, 2012c). Within the action phase of the Knowledge-to-Action framework, evaluation is necessary to determine whether the action taken made a difference. Equally important is planning for sustainability of successful actions.

The effective achievement of educational innovations, such as BPG integration in nursing curricula, relies on quality evaluation that demonstrates the contributions of the new educational practice. Approaches to evaluation should begin when planning the curriculum innovation. An evaluation plan serves as a bridge between the planned innovation and the expected outcomes by making explicit the goals, objectives, planned activities, what will be monitored, the use of the evaluation results, and for what audience (Centers for Disease Control and Prevention's Office on Smoking and Health and Division of Nutrition, Physical Activity, and Obesity, 2011). As part of the planning process, collecting baseline data is of prime importance to serve as a comparison with subsequently acquired data.

The evaluation plan should derive from an evaluation framework to guide questions, outcome indicators, and data sources and their collection methods. As with the evaluation of BPG implementation in health service organizations (RNAO, 2012c, 2015a), Donabedian's (1988) evaluation framework can similarly guide the evaluation of academic BPSO actions. The Donabedian evaluation framework is conceptualized into three categories: structure, process, and outcome.

DONABEDIAN EVALUATION FRAMEWORK

Structure measures quantify aspects within the teaching and learning environment, including the classroom and practice setting. Structure measures are inclusive of the resources (e.g., equipment, placement opportunities); the attributes of educators (e.g., knowledge, skills, attitudes, judgment); and program structure (e.g., curriculum model, learning objectives).

Process measures quantify how teaching-learning transpires. Examples of process measures include pedagogical approaches and the quality of the teaching and learning experience, including its appropriateness, acceptability, consistency, and accuracy.

Outcome measures quantify the end points of the education innovation. While outcome measures resulting from BPG implementation in health service organizations focus on person and family health outcomes, the focus of measures linked to the integration of BPGs in curriculum is on learner outcomes. More specific measures of learner outcomes are conceptualized in Kirkpatrick's (1994, 2007) Four Level Training Model, illustrated in Figure 9.3. This model depicts measures related to reactions, learning, behaviours, and educational and healthcare system change. Relevant learner outcomes are students' appropriation of critical and reflexive thinking, their acquisition of theoretical knowledge, their application in practice, and their sustained application in the practice setting following graduation.

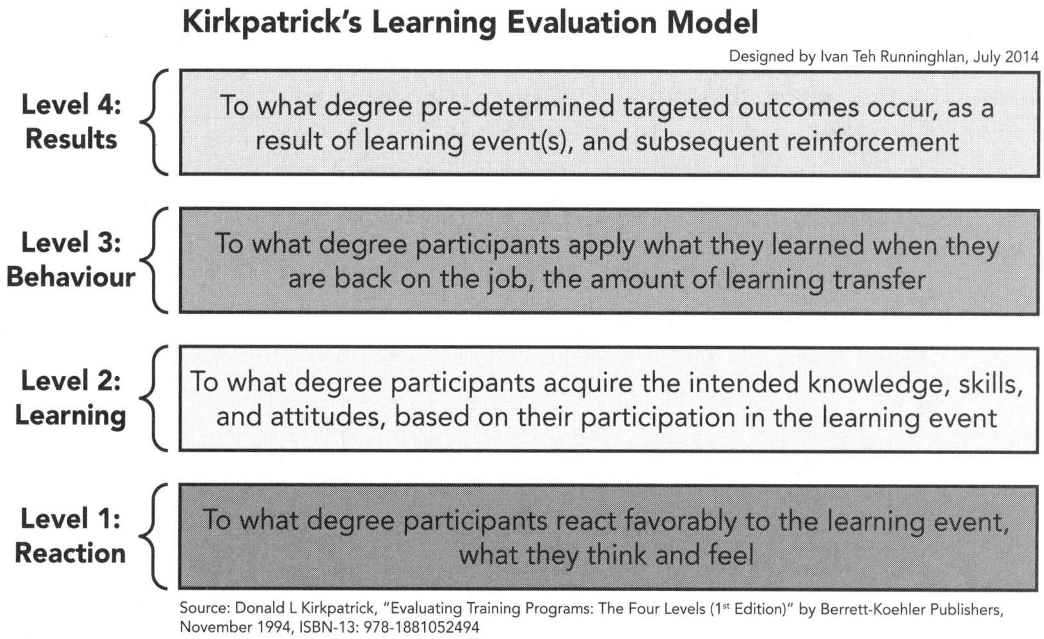

Kirkpatrick's Learning Evaluation Model

Designed by Ivan Teh Runninghlan, July 2014

Level 4: Results { To what degree pre-determined targeted outcomes occur, as a result of learning event(s), and subsequent reinforcement

Level 3: Behaviour { To what degree participants apply what they learned when they are back on the job, the amount of learning transfer

Level 2: Learning { To what degree participants acquire the intended knowledge, skills, and attitudes, based on their participation in the learning event

Level 1: Reaction { To what degree participants react favorably to the learning event, what they think and feel

Source: Donald L Kirkpatrick, "Evaluating Training Programs: The Four Levels (1st Edition)" by Berrett-Koehler Publishers, November 1994, ISBN-13: 978-1881052494

FIGURE 9.3 Kirkpatrick's Four Level Model for Evaluating Training Programs.
Reprinted with permission of the publisher. From *Evaluating Training Programs: The Four Levels*, © 1994 by Donald Kirkpatrick, Berrett-Koehler Publishers, Inc., San Francisco, CA. All rights reserved. www.bkconnection.com

To determine the impact of the BPSO Designation on the curriculum, academic BPSOs are utilizing various evaluation methods based on course and class-level objectives, as well as the goals and activities of their BPSO action plans. Reflecting Kirkpatrick's (1994, 2007) learning evaluation model, as depicted in Figure 9.3, these approaches to evaluation for students include measurement of:

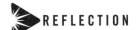

REFLECTION

How do the Kirkpatrick and Donabedian models of evaluation compare? What are their similarities and differences? What benefit is there to using both models in education evaluation related to integration of BPGs in the curriculum?

- Knowledge, through testing that incorporates information about evidence-based practice (EBP) in general and about each of the specific RNAO BPGs studied

- Attitudes, through attention to the students' ability to seek out and inquire about supporting evidence for practice

- Application, through observation of students' use of RNAO BPGs in patient care and written care plans, student discussions pre- and post-clinical experience, and written reflections

- Broader impacts on patients and the organization, through observation of changes in patient outcomes, and the student's ability to discuss BPGs and or lead change in the workplace related to EBP

During curriculum meetings and overall end-of-semester reviews, faculty examine the impact of BPGs on the curriculum and how and to what extent EBP and BPGs have been incorporated. In the schools of nursing featured in this chapter, specific evaluation plans have been developed from the outset that enable measurement of EBP and RNAO BPG competence in students, as well as faculty integration of EBP and RNAO BPGs throughout the overall curriculum, each program year, and each course.

Evaluation research related to the integration of BPGs in undergraduate nursing curriculum is in its infancy, with few specific, observable, and measurable markers to monitor and track progress and accomplishments attributable to the use of BPGs to enhance learning about evidence-based practice. This gap contributes to the challenges experienced by RNAO's Nursing Quality Indicators for Research and Evaluation (NQuIRE) comprehensive data system (see Chapter 16, *Evaluating BPG Impact: Development and Refinement of NQuIRE*) in identifying and defining appropriate education indicators. In partnership with the academic BPSOs, the development of educational indicators is progressing and will undoubtedly break new ground for nursing academia. Identified indicators will be included in the NQuIRE data system, and academic BPSOs will join health services organizations in collecting, analyzing, and reporting comparative data arising from the integration of BPGs in undergraduate nursing curricula.

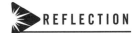

REFLECTION

Describe how academic BPSOs can determine the impact of BPGs on the curriculum and how the BPSO Designation might enhance the relationship amongst teaching, practice, and research.

SUPPORTING EVIDENCE-BASED EDUCATION THROUGH RESEARCH

Some scholars argue that teaching and research are "analogous practices with a common essential goal: the advancement of learning and knowledge" (Light & Calkins, 2015, p. 345). Others suggest that "good research is a prerequisite for good teaching, and the quality of teaching relies heavily on the instructors' ability to create as well as communicate knowledge" (Bak & Kim, 2015, p. 845). Educators who use their research as part of the course material introduce students to the most updated knowledge and expose them to current concepts, ideas, and solutions to real-life, practical health problems. "Conversely, teaching may enrich research by encouraging professors to clarify their thinking and describe their reasoning to new audiences" (Bak & Kim, 2015, p. 845). All three academic BPSOs in this chapter are engaged in evidence-based and BPG-related research. Educators lead programs of research with other academic departments, service organizations, government partners, and students related to the development, implementation, evaluation, and dissemination of BPGs. Creating such research opportunities aligns with universities' common strategic priority to enhance research clusters and engage students in faculty research.

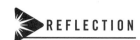

REFLECTION

Identify ways in which the research agenda in a school of nursing can be enriched through integration of BPGs in the curriculum and the BPSO Designation.

CONCLUSION

Academic BPSOs support the intent of schools of nursing to develop a community of nurses who think critically, engage effectively in problem-solving, and use the most current and rigorous evidence to ensure the public receives the best possible nursing care. Figure 9.4 reflects the pride of the Atlantica Higher School of Health Sciences as an Academic BPSO. BPGs are a tool for teaching and learning about evidence that has international applicability. Alongside other forms of evidence, their integration into curricula provides a solid way for students to gain competence in identifying, implementing, evaluating, and critiquing best practice and its application in the care of persons and families. Academic BPSO Designation as a curriculum innovation that embraces BPG integration throughout the curriculum requires a deliberate planned change that includes capacity building, stakeholder analysis, management of facilitators and barriers, quality evaluation, and plans for sustainability. Academic BPSOs provide a means to engage academe and health services in their common goals to prepare students for evidence-based practice; to support sustained evidence-based practice in the workplace and thus close the service-academic gap; and to establish programs of research for enhanced evidenced-based teaching, learning, and practice.

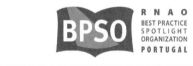

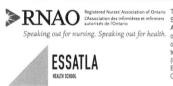

FIGURE 9.4 Atlantica Higher School of Health Sciences Academic BPSO.

KEY MESSAGES

- In the academic setting, Best Practice Guidelines serve as a foundational tool for teaching and preparing nursing students for evidence-based practice.

- The Registered Nurses' Association of Ontario's (RNAO) Best Practice Spotlight Organization Designation engages academic institutions in a dynamic and planned change strategy leading to the establishment, implementation, and sustained integration of Best Practice Guidelines in the curriculum.

■ Key strategies to integrate Best Practice Guidelines into curricula include developing multilevel learning objectives and designing teaching and learning strategies.

■ The successful integration of Best Practice Guidelines in curricula requires anticipating factors and conditions that can increase or decrease the likelihood of the curriculum innovation. It also necessitates adapting integration plans to the local context.

■ Evaluation research related to the integration of BPGs in undergraduate nursing curriculum is in its infancy, with a need to develop specific, observable, and measurable indicators to monitor and track progress and accomplishments attributable to the use of Best Practice Guidelines in curricula.

■ Academic BPSOs engage in evidence-based and BPG-related research that can advance both learning and knowledge development.

■ The quality of nursing education and undergraduate and graduate nurse competence in evidence-based practice is enhanced through the integration of BPGs in curricula.

REFERENCES

Athwal, L., Marchuk, B., Laforet-Fliesser, Y., Castanza, J., Davis, L., & LaSalle, M. (2013). *Adaptation of a Best Practice Guideline to strengthen client-centered care in public health. Public Health Nursing, 31*(2),134–143. doi: 10.1111/phn.12059

Bak, H., & Kim, D. (2015). Too much emphasis on research? An empirical examination of the relationship between research and teaching in multitasking environments. *Research in Higher Education, 56*(8), 843–860. doi: 10.1007/s11162-015-9372-0

Benner, P., Sutphen, M., Leonard, V., Day, L., & Shulman, L. S. (2010). *Educating nurses: A call for radical transformation.* San Francisco, CA: Jossey-Bass.

Brouwers, M., Kho, M., Browman, G., Cluzeau, F., Feder, G., Fervers, B., . . . Makarski, J. on behalf of the AGREE Next Steps Consortium. (2010). AGREE II: Advancing guideline development, reporting and evaluation in healthcare. *Canadian Medical Association Journal, 182*(18), E839–E842. doi: 10.1503/cmaj.090449

Centers for Disease Control and Prevention's Office on Smoking and Health and Division of Nutrition, Physical Activity, and Obesity. (2011). *Developing an effective evaluation plan: Setting the course for effective program evaluation.* Retrieved from https://www.cdc.gov/obesity/downloads/cdc-evaluation-workbook-508.pdf

Christie, J., Hamill, C., & Power, J. (2012). How can we maximize nursing students' learning about research evidence and utilization in undergraduate, preregistration programmes? *Journal of Advanced Nursing, 68*(12), 2789–2801. doi: 10.1111/j.1365-2648.2012.05994.x

Cruickshank, C., & Ells, G. (2014). *Building our future: A new collaborative model for undergraduate nursing education in Nova Scotia.* Halifax, NS: Nova Scotia Department of Health and Wellness.

Dawley, K., Rosen Bloch, J., Dunphy Suplee, P., McKeever, A., & Scherzer. G. (2011). Using a pedagogical approach to integrate evidence-based teaching in an undergraduate women's health course. *Worldviews on Evidence-Based Nursing, Second Quarter, 8*(2), 116–123. doi: 10.1111/j.1741-6787.2010.00210.x

Donabedian, A. (1988). The quality of care. How can it be assessed? *Journal of American Medical Association, 260*(12), 1743–1748.

Edwards, N., & Grinspun, D. (2011). Understanding whole systems change in healthcare: The case of emerging evidence-informed nursing. Final report for CHSRF REISS Program #RC2-1266-06. Ottawa, ON: Canadian Health Services Research Foundation.

Field, B., Booth, A., Ilott, I., & Gerrish, K. (2014). Using the Knowledge to Action Framework in practice: A citation analysis and systematic review. *Implementation Science, 9*(172). doi: 10.1186/s13012-014-0172-2

Fineout-Overholt, E., & Melnyk, B. (2005). Building a culture of best practice. *Nurse Leader, 3*(6), 26–30. doi: 10.1016/j.mnl.2005.09.007

Finotto, S., Carpanoni, M., Casadei Turroni, E., Camellini, R., & Mecugni, D. (2013). Teaching evidence-based practice: Developing a curriculum model to foster evidence-based practice in undergraduate student nurses. *Nurse Education in Practice, 13*(5), 459–465. doi.org/10.1016/j.nepr.2013.03.021

Florin, J., Ehrenberg, A., Wallin, L., & Gustavsson, P. (2012). Educational support for research utilization and capability beliefs regarding evidence-based practice skills: A national survey of senior nursing students. *Journal of Advanced Nursing, 68*(4), 888–897. doi: 10.1111/j.1365-2648.2011.05792.x

Friedman, L., Engelking, C., Wickham, R., Harvey, C., Read, M., & Whitlock, K. B. (2009). The EDUCATE Study: A continuing education exemplar for clinical practice guideline implementation. *Clinical Journal of Oncology Nursing, 13*(2), 219–230. doi:10.1188/09.CJON.219-230

Graham, I., & Harrison, M. (2005). EBN users' guide: Evaluation and adaptation of clinical practice guidelines. *Evidence-Based Nursing, 8*, 68–72. doi: 10.1136/ebn.8.3.68

Graham, I. D., Logan, J., Harrison, M. B., Straus, S. E., Tetroe, J., Caswell, W., . . . Robinson, N. (2006). Lost in knowledge translation: Time for a map? *Journal of Continuing Education in the Health Professions, 26*, 13–24.

Hanrahan, K., Wagner, M., Matthews, G., Stewart, S., Dawson C., Greiner, J., . . . Williamson, A. (2015). Sacred cow gone to pasture: A systematic evaluation and integration of evidence-based practice. *Worldviews on Evidence-Based Nursing, 12*(1), 3–11.

Institute of Medicine (IOM). (2011). *The future of nursing: Leading change, advancing health.* Washington, DC: National Academies Press.

Jones, A. (2007). Putting practice into teaching: An exploratory study of nursing undergraduates' interpersonal skills and the effects of using empirical data as a teaching and learning resource. *Journal of Clinical Nursing, 16*(12), 2297–2307. doi: 10.1111/j.1365-2702.2007.01948.x

Kirkpatrick, D. L. (1994). *Evaluating training programs: The four levels.* San Francisco, CA: Berrett-Koehler.

Kirkpatrick, D., & Kirkpatrick, J. (2007). *Implementing the four levels: A practical guide for effective evaluation of training programs.* San Francisco, CA: Berrett-Koehler.

Kitson, A., Wiechula, R., Conroy, T., Muntlin Athlin, A., & Whitaker, N. (2013). *The future shape of the nursing workforce: A synthesis of the evidence of factors that impact on quality nursing care.* Adelaide, South Australia: School of Nursing, University of Adelaide.

LAW 266. (1996, January 25). Why the nursing profession in Colombia is regulated and other provisions. Official Gazette No. 42.710, of February 5, 1996. Retrieved from https://www.global-regulation.com/translation/colombia/6403967/why-the-nursing-profession-in-colombia-is-regulated-and-other-provisions.html

Light, G., & Calkins, S. (2015). The experience of academic learning: Uneven conceptions of learning across research and teaching. *Higher Education, 69*(3), 345–359. doi: 10.1007/s10734-0-14-9779-0

MacDonald, J., Edwards, N., Davies, B., Marck, P., & Read Guernsey, J. (2012). Priority setting and policy advocacy by nursing association: A scoping review and implications using a socio-ecological whole systems lens. *Health Policy, 107*(1), 31–43.

Melnyk, B. M., Gallagher-Ford, L., Long, L. E., & Fineout-Overholt, E. (2014). The establishment of evidence-based practice competencies for practicing registered nurses and advanced practice nurses in real-world clinical settings: Proficiencies to improve healthcare quality, reliability, patient outcomes and costs. *Worldviews on Evidence-Based Nursing, 11*(1), 5–15.

Missal, B., Schafer, K., Halm, M., & Schaffer, M. (2010). A university and health care organization partnership to prepare nurses for evidence-based practice. *Journal of Nursing Education, 49*(8), 456–461.

Nursing Executive Center. (2008). Bridging the preparation-practice gap, Volume I: Quantifying new graduate nurse improvement needs. Retrieved from http://www.advisory.com/Research/Nursing-Executive-Center/Studies/2008/Bridging-the-Preparation-Practice-Gap-Volume-I

Ploeg, J., Skelly, J., Rowan, M., Edwards, N., Davies, B., Grinspun, D., . . . Downey, A. (2010). The role of nursing best practice champions in diffusing practice guidelines: A mixed methods study. *Worldviews on Evidence-Based Nursing, 7*(4), 238–251. doi: 10.1111/j.1741-6787.2010.00202.x

Prentice, D., Ritchie, R., Crandall, J., Harwood, L., McAuslan, D., Lawrence-Murphy, J., & Wilson, B. (2009). Implementation of a diabetic foot management Best Practice Guideline (BPG) in hemodialysis units. *The CANNT Journal, 19*(4), 20–24.

Registered Nurses' Association of Ontario (RNAO). (2003). *Breastfeeding: Best Practice Guidelines for nurses.* Toronto, ON: RNAO. Retrieved from http://rnao.ca/sites/rnao-ca/files/Breastfeeding_Best_Practice_Guidelines_for_Nurses.pdf

Registered Nurses' Association of Ontario (RNAO). (2005). *Educators' resource: Integration of Best Practice Guidelines.* Toronto, ON: RNAO. Retrieved from http://rnao.ca/bpg/guidelines/resources/educators-resource-integration-best-practice-guidelines

Registered Nurses' Association of Ontario (RNAO). (2006a). *Collaborative practice among nursing teams.* Toronto, ON: RNAO.

Registered Nurses' Association of Ontario. (RNAO). (2006b). *Establishing therapeutic relationships.* Toronto, ON: RNAO.

Registered Nurses' Association of Ontario (RNAO). (2007a). *Embracing cultural diversity in health care: Developing cultural competence.* Toronto, ON: RNAO.

Registered Nurses' Association of Ontario (RNAO). (2007b). *Professionalism in nursing.* Toronto, ON: RNAO.

Registered Nurses' Association of Ontario (RNAO). (2008). *Assessment and device selection for vascular access.* Toronto, ON: RNAO.

Registered Nurses' Association of Ontario (RNAO). (2009a). *Assessment and care of adults at risk for suicide ideation and behaviour.* Toronto, ON: RNAO.

Registered Nurses' Association of Ontario (RNAO). (2009b). *Nursing management of hypertension.* Toronto, ON: RNAO.

Registered Nurses' Association of Ontario (RNAO). (2010). *Strategies to support self-management of chronic conditions: Collaboration with clients.* Toronto, ON: RNAO.

Registered Nurses' Association of Ontario (RNAO). (2011a). *End-of-life care during the last days and hours.* Toronto, ON: RNAO.

Registered Nurses' Association of Ontario (RNAO). (2011b). *Prevention of falls and fall injuries in the older adult.* Toronto, ON: RNAO.

Registered Nurses' Association of Ontario (RNAO). (2012a). *Facilitating client centred learning.* Toronto, ON: RNAO.

Registered Nurses' Association of Ontario (RNAO). (2012b). *Managing and mitigating conflict in health-care teams.* Toronto, ON: RNAO.

Registered Nurses' Association of Ontario (RNAO). (2012c). *Toolkit: Implementation of Best Practice Guidelines* (2nd ed.). Toronto, ON: RNAO.

Registered Nurses' Association of Ontario (RNAO). (2012d). *Woman abuse: Screening, identification, and initial response.* Toronto, ON: RNAO.

Registered Nurses' Association of Ontario (RNAO). (2013a). *Assessment and management of pain* (3rd ed.). Toronto, ON: RNAO.

Registered Nurses' Association of Ontario (RNAO). (2013b). *Developing and sustaining interprofessional health care: Optimizing patient, organizational, and system outcomes.* Toronto, ON: RNAO.

Registered Nurses' Association of Ontario (RNAO). (2013c). *Developing and sustaining nursing leadership.* Toronto, ON: RNAO.

Registered Nurses' Association of Ontario (RNAO). (2014a). *Primary prevention of childhood obesity* (2nd ed.). Toronto, ON: RNAO.

Registered Nurses' Association of Ontario (RNAO). (2014b). *Working with families to promote safe sleep for infants 0–12 months of age.* Toronto, ON: RNAO.

Registered Nurses' Association of Ontario (RNAO). (2015a). 2014–2015 Best Practice Spotlight Organization (BPSO) impact survey: Summary of survey results. Toronto, ON: RNAO.

Registered Nurses' Association of Ontario (RNAO). (2015b). *Engaging clients who use substances.* Toronto, ON: RNAO.

Registered Nurses' Association of Ontario (RNAO). (2015c). *Person- and family-centred care.* Toronto, ON: RNAO.

Registered Nurses' Association of Ontario (RNAO). (2016a). *Assessment and management of pressure injuries for the interprofessional team* (3rd ed.). Toronto, ON: RNAO.

Registered Nurses' Association of Ontario (RNAO). (2016b). *Intra-professional collaborative practice among nurses* (2nd ed.). Toronto, ON: RNAO.

Registered Nurses' Association of Ontario (RNAO). (2017a). Best Practice Spotlight Organization (BPSO). Retrieved from http://rnao.ca/sites/rnao-ca/files/RNAOBPSOFactSheetApril2017.pdf

Registered Nurses' Association of Ontario (RNAO). (2017b). Clinical guidelines. Retrieved from http://rnao.ca/bpg/guidelines/clinical-guidelines

Registered Nurses' Association of Ontario (RNAO). (2017c). Healthy work place environment guidelines. Retrieved from http://rnao.ca/bpg/guidelines/hwe-guidelines

Rempel, L., & McCleary, L. (2012). Effects of the implementation of a breastfeeding Best Practice Guideline in a Canadian public health agency. *Research in Nursing & Health, 35*(5), 435–449. doi: 10.1002/nur.21495

Silva-Galleguillos, A. (2015). Implementación de guías de buenas prácticas clínicas elaboradas por Registered Nurses' Association of Ontario en curriculum de en Enfermería Universidad de Chile. *MedUNAB, 17*(3), 182–189.

Silva-Galleguillos, A. (2016). Formación por competencias en Enfermería. Experiencia de la Universidad de Chile. *MedUNAB, 19*(2), 134–141.

Stacey, D., Higuchi, K., Menard, P., Davies, B., Graham, I., & O'Connor, A. (2009). Integrating patient decision support in an undergraduate nursing curriculum: An implementation project. *International Journal of Nursing Education Scholarship, 6*(1), Article 10.

SCALING UP, SCALING OUT, AND SCALING DEEP: SYSTEM-WIDE IMPLEMENTATION

SCALING UP AND OUT: SYSTEM-WIDE IMPLEMENTATION INITIATIVES

Heather McConnell, MAE(Ed), BScN, RN
Sabrina Merali, MN, RN
Sheila John, MScN, BScN, RN
Susan McNeill, MPH, RN
Irmajean Bajnok, PhD, MScN, BScN, RN

LEARNING OBJECTIVES

After reading this chapter, you will be able to:

- Identify the key factors that influence scaling up and out of evidence-based practices, and why each is important in creating sustained change

- Understand the multifaceted strategies that have been utilized to achieve system-wide engagement in evidence-based practice as illustrated through three case studies highlighting RNAO implementation initiatives

- Describe the role of RNAO's evidence-based guidelines in scaling activities within nursing, the healthcare system, and beyond

- Gain appreciation for the role of Champions knowledgeable about change and spread processes as well as about the content of the change

- Outline how partnerships can be leveraged to scale out to increase exposure and scale up to influence policy

- Define how leadership at all levels can impact scaling up and out of innovations

- Express how delivery of the innovation through building networks, developing capacity, adapting to local context, and integrating with the current system impact scaling up, scaling out, and scaling deep

INTRODUCTION

Using diffusion theory that reflects principles of scaling up and scaling out, this chapter outlines key factors that influence the successful spread of evidence-based practices, education, and policy from organizational to regional, provincial, and national levels, with impact on all sectors. The three case studies presented illustrate RNAO's use of these principles in selected implementation projects, focused on mental health and addiction, smoking cessation, and falls prevention initiatives and the resulting effect on sustained practice and policy changes. Specifically, a systematic spread methodology; access to clear, credible, evidence-based resources known to be effective; identification of related implementation enablers; capacity development; and engagement of administrative and clinical leaders and collaboration with partners all contribute to the effective scaling up and out of evidence in practice, leading to sustained use across levels and in all sectors of the health system.

SCALING: THE GOAL OF DIFFUSION AND INNOVATION

Over the last decade there has been growth in the implementation literature exploring how practice innovations can be deliberately spread across the system to enhance health outcomes. In part, this is due to an increasing recognition that despite the development of innovative products, practices, and programs within the system, they have not always achieved their full impact due to challenges with scaling up (Mangham & Hanson, 2010). Much of the emerging research in the area of scaling up is focused on public health interventions and large-scale global health programs, and there are many definitions of scaling up in the literature. However, common elements include a description of *scaling up* as a series of processes to introduce innovations with demonstrated effectiveness and with the aim of improving coverage and equitable access to the innovation(s) (Edwards, 2010).

In the health sector, *scaling up* has been defined in some cases to mean expanding coverage of an intervention (Mangham & Hanson, 2010) and in other cases to mean "efforts to increase the impact of innovations successfully tested in pilot or experimental projects so as to benefit more people and to foster policy and program development on a lasting basis" (Simmons, Fajans, & Ghiron, 2007, p. viii). This latter definition reflects the typology to scaling presented by Moore and Riddell (2015) and includes *scaling up* (expanding coverage), *scaling out* (altering the policies, laws, and standards), and *scaling deep* (changing the norms). In order to maximize benefits from implementation efforts, it is critically important to consider all three aspects of scaling when diffusing innovations. In this chapter, we differentiate amongst scaling up, out, and deep, where it is important to emphasize specific activities targeted to expansion, policy impact, and sustainment.

SCALING UP: KEY CONSIDERATIONS

Edwards (2010, p. 12) explored the elements that affect the scale-up of programs through examining both effective and ineffective scaling up experiences. The challenges identified in ineffective initiatives can be grouped into six categories:

- Underestimating the resources required for scaling up

- Political and policy naivety

- Lack of attention to issues of sustainability and scaling up during early efforts to test or implement innovation uptake

- An over-emphasis on either the vertical or the horizontal spread of innovations

- Inattention to spatial elements of scaling up

- Inattention to the demand side of scaling up

Edwards (2010) put forward a typology for innovations relevant to public health practice according to their potential for scaling up. She classified these innovations as: 1) discrete innovations; 2) mixed component and multilevel innovations; and 3) paradigmatic innovations. *Discrete interventions* are those that are well-defined and have also been referred to as direct interventions (Policy Brief, 2010). They are considered for scale-up because their efficacy and effectiveness have been demonstrated, and their implementation initially appears to be straightforward. Some examples of this type of innovation within public health include vaccinations and micronutrient fortification and fluoride in drinking water.

The second category—mixed component and multilevel innovations—involves many interrelated components (intersecting set of innovations) that are targeted at more than one system level. These innovations tend to be more complex, less prescriptive, less structured, and have components that must work synergistically to achieve the intended benefits. Components of these interventions need to be adapted to both the target population and the context in which they are being introduced, while maintaining the elements of the intervention that have proven to be effective. In addition, elements of these innovations may diffuse organically, for example, through a social movement. Examples of this type of innovation are seen in the fields of tobacco control, heart health, childhood obesity prevention, and workplace safety (Edwards, 2010, p. 9).

The final category described by Edwards (2010) is paradigmatic innovations. These innovations involve a new way of thinking about issues, how we understand them, what might be possible solutions, and who should be involved in determining and implementing the solutions. Examples include utilizing a social determinants of health lens in an upstream approach to programs and considering health in all policies in an effort to achieve population health. This typology of innovations helps those working to scale up programs to consider the features of the innovation and the factors that may impact on the scaling up process. In some ways this innovations typology is akin to the scaling typology—scaling up, out, and deep (Moore & Riddell, 2015)—with the exception that Moore and Riddell assert that in all scaling initiatives, regardless of size, cultural impact is critical to make them stick. In other words, the deeper the scaling, the better.

SCALING UP SUCCESSFULLY

In determining how best to approach scaling of an innovation, Yamey (2011) offers a useful framework based on a review of the literature, personal experiences, and the experiences of "scale-up experts" in the global development field. Through this examination of key themes in the emerging science of large-scale change in global health, Yamey (2011) identified the following factors that explain successful scale-up:

■ **Attributes of the intervention**—Recognized as valuable, easy to use, and evidence-based

■ **Leadership and governance**—Involve leadership at all levels and foster commitment to scaling up and out

■ **Get buy-in**—The adopters engage a range of key stakeholders and implementers in the target community

■ **Delivery strategy**—Tailor the scale-up approach to the local community, using diffusion and social network theories, cascade and phased approaches, adaptation to the local context, and integration into the local system

■ **Measurement and evaluation**—Build in evaluation and incorporate lessons learned

The three case studies that follow illustrate many aspects of both the Edwards (2010) typology of innovations and the typology of scaling by Moore and Riddell (2015) and demonstrate how the elements of Yamey's (2011) scaling framework were addressed to ensure success. The innovations being scaled up in these implementation projects all fall within the mixed component and multilevel category, founded on evidence-based practices proven to be effective, as synthesized in the relevant RNAO BPGs. The approaches to scaling reflect scaling up, scaling out, and scaling deep through the multiple methods used and the degree of community engagement. In addition, many of Yamey's (2011) themes will be evident in unique ways in each of these examples of scaling up initiatives and highlighted as to their impact.

CASE STUDY

MENTAL HEALTH AND ADDICTION INITIATIVE

The Ontario Ministry of Health and Long-Term Care's (Ministry) Methadone Task Force was established in April 2006 in response to an increase in opioid prescribing and misuse and the need for accessible, equitable, and timely Methadone Maintenance Treatment (MMT) services for opioid addiction in Ontario. Following extensive deliberation by the Task Force based on expert, scientific, and experiential evidence, the report was released in 2007 (Ministry of Health and Long-Term Care [MOHLTC], 2007). It included 26 recommendations addressing nursing and other healthcare disciplines and outlined elements necessary for accessible, comprehensive, and integrated MMT services in Ontario. Subsequently, the RNAO was funded to develop a Best Practice Guideline entitled *Supporting Clients on Methadone Maintenance Treatment* (RNAO, 2009b) and to support its uptake through awareness raising, education, and capacity building. This was in response to one of the report's recommendations directed toward RNAO due to its strong reputation for excellence in the area of policy and evidence-based practice guideline development, dissemination, and evaluation.

Following RNAO's publication of the guideline in 2009, the guideline development Expert Panel identified the need for additional guidelines and resources for nurses and other healthcare providers to effectively support Ontarians with mental health and addiction needs. Through continued advocacy for this population, RNAO received additional funding from the Ministry and launched the RNAO Mental Health and Addiction Initiative (the "Initiative") in 2010. Since then, the Initiative has served as a key resource in Ontario to support nurses and other healthcare providers in effectively working with people who use substances and need assistance with mental health.

SYSTEMATIC IMPLEMENTATION METHODOLOGY

In 2013, to better understand the needs and gaps within the Mental Health and Addiction system, RNAO sponsored an in-depth environmental scan to inform the development of a 5-year comprehensive strategy to guide the work of the Initiative. The findings from the scan concluded that nurses needed support in all sectors and across the continuum of care that could be addressed through implementation of guidelines specific to mental health and addiction. Other priorities in mental health and addiction included strengthening the practice/policy interface with BPG development and uptake, enhancing capacity in nurses through undergraduate nursing programs across Canada and professional development opportunities, and developing evidence-based resources for nurses and other health disciplines to support their practice.

RNAO crafted a conceptual model (see Figure 10.1) that provides direction for the systematic implementation methodology utilized by the Initiative to spread and scale up addiction and mental health best practices. The Initiative incorporates the key elements of access to evidence-based guidelines and implementation supports; capacity building related to knowledge, skills, and attitudes; and collaboration with partners and supportive stakeholders to aid in scaling up, out, and deep.

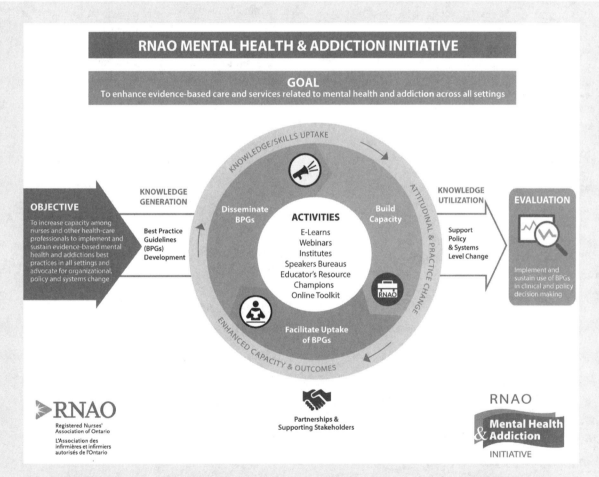

FIGURE 10.1   RNAO Mental Health and Addiction Initiative conceptual model.
© Registered Nurses' Association of Ontario. All rights reserved.

ACCESS TO EVIDENCE-BASED TOOLS (DISSEMINATION OF BPGS AND IMPLEMENTATION RESOURCES)

RNAO has over 15 years of experience developing Best Practice Guidelines and supporting effective dissemination and knowledge uptake at the practice, education, and policy levels. To date, multiple BPGs have been used to impact system-level change related to mental health and addiction. For example, the practice recommendations contained in the guideline *Engaging Clients Who Use Substances* (RNAO, 2015a) form the core curriculum for all RNAO professional development programs related to addiction. The education recommendations from this BPG, along with those from the following BPGs with a mental health and addiction focus—*Person- and Family-Centred Care* (RNAO, 2015b); *Establishing Therapeutic Relationships* (RNAO, 2006a); *Facilitating Client Centred Learning* (RNAO, 2012a); *Crisis Intervention* (RNAO, 2006b); and *Enhancing Healthy Adolescent Development* (RNAO, 2010a)—supported RNAO's work with the Canadian Association of Schools of Nursing (CASN) and faculty across Canada in the development of Entry-to-Practice Mental Health and Addiction Competencies. Moreover, the policy recommendations inform RNAO's advocacy work related to harm reduction, decreasing health inequities, and provision of improved access to integrated and collaborative care for clients who use substances. All the above-mentioned BPGs as well as others focused on mental health and addiction—such as *Interventions for Postpartum Depression* (RNAO, 2005a); *Assessment and Care of Adults at Risk for Suicidal Ideation and Behaviour* (RNAO, 2009a); and *Woman Abuse: Screening, Identification and Initial Response* (RNAO, 2012c)—have been used to inform capacity building and practice, education, and policy initiatives.

The Mental Health and Addiction home page on the RNAO site (www.RNAO.ca/mentalhealth) serves as a one-stop shop for nurses, other healthcare providers, and the public to access the many evidence-based resources developed by RNAO and provided to promote knowledge translation and exchange at the provincial, national, and international level. These resources include: self-directed e-Learning modules, educational videos, a Youth Mental Health and Addiction Champion (YMHAC) Toolkit (which supports mental health promotion and resiliency amongst youth), educator guides (to support best practices consistent with mental health and addiction core competencies), regular knowledge-exchange webinars, nursing order sets (technology-enabled implementation supports), decision trees, and "pocket guides" as reminder prompts to support BPG implementation. Various other communication channels targeted to local, national, and international stakeholders are used to support dissemination, including partnerships, social media, presentations, publications, and mental health campaigns such as the Canada-wide Bell Let's Talk (Bell Canada, 2017).

CAPACITY DEVELOPMENT

Given the prevalence of mental illness across the age spectrum and the relationships amongst mental health, illness, addiction, and other related conditions, it is assured that nurses in all practice settings will care for clients with mental health and illness challenges (Nadler-Moodie, 2010). The Initiative builds capacity amongst nurses to utilize evidence-based best practices and tools when working with individuals with needs in mental health and addiction.

UNDERGRADUATE NURSING PROGRAMS

A key priority for the Initiative, in partnership with the Canadian Federation of Mental Health Nurses (CFMHN), is to support faculty to ensure the undergraduate nursing curriculum provides an integrated focus on evidence-based addiction and mental health content. The intent is to enhance students' ability to address mental health and addiction needs with clients in all settings.

Related to this priority, RNAO worked with CASN and other national stakeholders in developing a national consensus-based framework of essential discipline-specific entry-to-practice mental health and addiction competencies and indicators, which were published by CASN in 2015 as the *Entry-to-Practice Mental Health Competencies for Undergraduate Nursing Education in Canada* (CASN, 2015). The competencies ensure integration of core content related to mental health and addiction into nursing curriculum and are used by CASN along with other competencies and standards when accrediting schools of nursing.

RNAO was also engaged in a partnership with CASN to determine strategies to disseminate the competencies and ensure their uptake. This resulted in collaboration in the development of the RNAO *Nurse Educator Mental Health and Addiction Resource* (RNAO, 2017a) endorsed by CASN and mapped against the CASN mental health and addiction competencies. The document is available in hard copy and online and has been disseminated to schools of nursing across Canada. Multistakeholder capacity-building events and supports have been established to facilitate uptake of this valuable resource.

ENGAGEMENT OF CHAMPIONS

As discussed in Chapter 4, *Forging the Way With Implementation Science*, RNAO has invested in the training, engagement, and mobilization of Best Practice Champions. As a key strategy within this Initiative, a tailored Champions program has been established to address not only the principles of implementing practice change, but also clinical content related to mental health and addiction. To date, the program has trained over 1,400 nurses and other healthcare providers to lead the uptake of evidence-based practices in this clinical area. To support ongoing capacity development for these Champions, RNAO partners with other local and national stakeholders to provide monthly webinars on topics relevant to the field, which have a wide reach locally, nationally, and internationally.

A unique application of the Champions approach in the MHA Initiative is evident in the RNAO Youth Mental Health and Addiction Champions (YMHAC) program. It is an innovative and empowering strategy for creating awareness amongst youth about mental health, illness, and substance use. This program utilizes elements of the Best Practice Champions Network and has been conceptualized as peer-led, multicomponent, and involving multistakeholders.

In the YMHAC program, building on the principle of peer leadership, youth leaders work with their local public health unit, district school boards, and schools to mentor youth Champions in planning, delivering, and evaluating local engagement strategies. The program helps shift attitudes from a focus on mental illness toward mental health promotion, and also draws on the strength of nurses and educators working in partnership with youth to create positive, resilient school communities.

The overwhelming success of the initiative, from 2013 to 2015, was enabled by RNAO's collaborative leadership; provision of evidence-based BPGs and implementation strategies; and the partnerships that were nurtured amongst RNAO, public health, school boards, and school mental health and staff supports. To foster sustainment following the project timeframe, RNAO created the YMHAC Toolkit (http://ymhac.rnao.ca) in English and French and is working with key stakeholders in education and health to enable widespread implementation of the YMHAC program across schools in Ontario communities.

COLLABORATIVE PARTNERSHIPS

The Initiative is based on a collaborative approach that engages partners (nursing and healthcare stakeholders) committed to the goal of enhancing mental health and addiction services and improving outcomes. Partners that influence practice, policy, and education change include government at the policy and special program levels, the public health system and education systems, mental health nurse special interest groups at the national and local levels, and national standard setting bodies. These partnerships within and beyond the health sector are vital to the Initiative, in particular to the scaling out and scaling deep of the RNAO BPGs for MHA. Partnerships not already highlighted are outlined in Table 10.1.

TABLE 10.1   COLLABORATIVE PARTNERSHIPS AND RELATED ACTIVITIES IN THE MHA INITIATIVE

PARTNER	PARTNERSHIP ACTIVITIES
Ministry of Health and Long-Term Care (MOHLTC)	RNAO has provided input and support to Ontario's 10-year mental health and addiction strategy, entitled *Open Minds, Healthy Minds*, through various consultations.
	RNAO supported related initiatives such as the need for specialized Mental Health and Addiction Nurses working in schools across Ontario; bolstering province-wide training with RNAO-led Institutes; promoting networking and partnership of nurses with other professionals (such as the school mental health ASSIST leads and integration with public health nurses); and also actively participating on the Ministry's Mental Health and Addiction Nurse Reference Group to further the expansion and sustainability of the nurses' role.
Provincial Opiate Workgroup (POWG)	RNAO is an active member of the Ontario POWG, a group of Ministry-funded agencies and initiatives that work toward reducing duplication of services, increasing knowledge exchange, and streamlining collaboration on various initiatives. Through this workgroup, RNAO has partnered with Centre for Addiction and Mental Health (CAMH) and the Ontario Pharmacy Association to conduct monthly webinars on emerging topics in the area of addiction, including the release of Naloxone for mass distribution.
Ontario Coalition for Child and Youth Mental Health	This coalition consists of education, social service, health, and justice-based organizations and works diligently to advocate for better child and youth mental health services. Through its involvement with the YMHAC program and this coalition, the Initiative has been able to meet with various Ministries to advocate for strengthening mental health care and education systems.
Specialty Nursing Interest Groups	RNAO leverages the expertise and experiences of its Mental Health Nurses Interest Group and Ontario Correctional Nurses Interest Group to learn about gaps in services and potential opportunities to inform their advocacy efforts.
Canadian Centre on Substance Use and Addiction (CCSA)	RNAO also partners with CCSA, a national organization that provides leadership on these issues in Canada. RNAO and CCSA have collaborated on a number of activities to raise awareness and gain a deeper understanding of matters pertaining to substance use.

SUMMARY

Key overall impacts of the Initiative include:

- Mental Health and Addiction (MH&A) has a higher priority on the Ontario Health Agenda

- Spread of Best Practice Guidelines to secondary education with the YMHAC Program

- Spread of Best Practice Guidelines to post-secondary education with the collaboration at the national level related to entry-to-practice mental health and addiction competencies and related tools for faculty

- Enhanced focus on youth mental health and addiction in public health

- Increased capacity of nurses and other clinicians in MH&A care and service

- Reduced stigma related to MH&A in both the education and health sectors

A number of aspects of scaling up, out, and deep have been demonstrated through this case study:

- The Initiative enables scaling up by extending the BPGs and their uptake into the area of Mental Health and Addiction, influencing practice, education, and policy and extending into the education sector, involving nonclinicians.

■ The capacity-building focus contributes to scaling up and scaling deep, in particular for clinicians in relation to mental health and addiction practice changes.

■ The engagement of Champions demonstrates use of a diffusion and network strategy in the spread of best practices.

■ The nature of the Champions program and network targeted to youth in the school system influenced changes in attitudes about mental health.

■ Engagement of stakeholders as partners in all aspects of the program has enabled sustained spread or scaling deep.

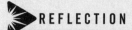

REFLECTION

What impact do you think engagement of Champions had on the scaling up of this work in clinical practice and undergraduate nursing education? How might the outcomes have been different without the targeted development of capacity in Champions?

CASE STUDY

TOBACCO INTERVENTION INITIATIVE

The RNAO Tobacco Intervention (TI) Initiative is a prime example of how scaling up and out can be achieved with the right vision, plan, resources, and strategies. The vision for the TI Initiative was conceptualized in 2008 as a way to help Ontarians stop tobacco use by leveraging RNAO's BPGs and the leadership of public health nurses to support clients on their quit journey. This vision shaped the Initiative's goals, which include:

■ Support the role of nurses working in a variety of healthcare settings across Ontario to reduce the prevalence of tobacco use amongst all Ontarians and increase the number of smokers who quit

■ Promote the role of public health nurses (PHN) as leaders in the area of tobacco control and reduce the of the number of Ontarians who smoke by utilizing TI best practices to increase TI capacity in nurses and other healthcare workers, and stimulate organizational policy change

■ Build, strengthen, and support nursing capacity across a variety of healthcare sectors to utilize TI best practices through knowledge transfer, knowledge exchange, role-modeling, and mentoring as supported by a TI Champions Network

■ Maximize initiative outcomes through strengthening and building partnerships and working in collaboration with key nursing and other healthcare stakeholders, organizations, groups, and initiatives focused on tobacco cessation locally, provincially, and nationally

Based on these goals, since 2008, RNAO has partnered with the Ontario Ministry of Health and Long-Term Care and other members of the Tobacco Free Ontario collaborative to facilitate spread of BPGs in all healthcare sectors. RNAO's role focuses on its specific TI BPG-implementation activities targeted to nurses (and other healthcare professionals and organizations) to impact spread. The RNAO TI Initiative has grown exponentially over the past 10 years; however, at its core remain the evidence-based recommendations from the BPG *Integrating Smoking Cessation into Daily Nursing Practice* (RNAO, 2007) and more recently the revised guideline *Integrating Tobacco Interventions into Daily Practice* (2017b). The TI Initiative utilizes a multipronged approach to support a systematic implementation methodology. Each prong represents a core pillar, which provides direction and guidance to the Initiative (see Figure 10.2).

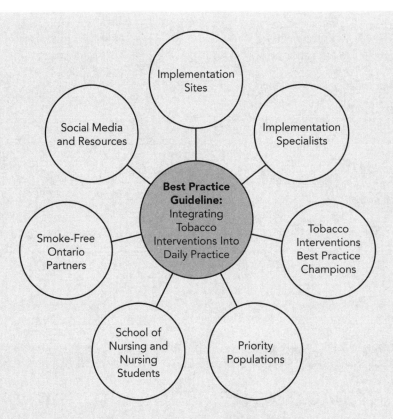

FIGURE 10.2 RNAO's Tobacco Intervention Initiative's multipronged approach.
© Registered Nurses' Association of Ontario. All rights reserved.

To highlight RNAO's approach to the spread and scaling up of this Initiative, the following pillars will be discussed in detail as they relate to the elements of scaling up and out described previously in this chapter:

- **Implementation sites** (adapting to local context and capacity building)

- **Schools of nursing and nursing students** (capacity building, engagement of implementers and partnerships)

- **TI Best Practice Champions and the TI Champions Network** (capacity building and engagement of implementers)

- **Social media and resources** (access to evidence-based resources)

- **Evaluation** (systematic methodology)

- **Partnerships and collaborations** (partnerships)

IMPLEMENTATION SITES

Since its inception with three public health units as implementation sites in 2008, over 45 healthcare organizations have partnered with RNAO to implement the BPG on smoking/tobacco cessation. This approach has provided opportunities for these organizations (public health units, primary care settings, community settings, hospitals, and academic institutions) to develop capacity in guideline implementation and tobacco cessation interventions. Capacity development is achieved through the support of an RNAO Tobacco Intervention Specialist and an onsite Champions workshop. Support from a TI Specialist is provided to staff at the implementation site based on the results of an organizational needs assessment and may involve consultation on planning, implementation, and evaluation and/or sustainability of practice change. Results of these activities include: smoking cessation identified as a priority program, specific smoking cessation interventions adapted for the community level, and organizational policy change. The *Toolkit: Implementation of Best Practice Guidelines* (RNAO, 2012b), as described in Chapter 4, provides the framework for these consultations. The Champions Workshop focuses on evidence-based tobacco use interventions and how to access numerous evidence-based resources.

SCHOOLS OF NURSING AND NURSING STUDENTS

Recognizing the importance of basic education for nurses to enhance TI knowledge and skill within the nursing profession, RNAO looked to spread this concept to schools of nursing by influencing the undergraduate nursing education curriculum. RNAO's *Nursing Faculty Education Guide (NFEG): Tobacco Use and Associated Health Risks* (RNAO, 2010b) was created to develop the nursing faculty's capacity to integrate tobacco intervention best practices into nursing curriculum. Using principles of effective spread, the guide was based on the advice of an advisory committee of faculty and other stakeholders, best evidence in curriculum design, and the RNAO TI Best Practice Guideline.

To enhance uptake and sustained use as part of the scaling process, the *Education Guide,* consisting of practical tools and resources to facilitate uptake, was distributed to 157 schools of nursing across the country, targeting deans, directors, and nursing faculty leaders. It is available (in English and French) for free download on the TobaccoFreeRNAO website (http://tobaccofreernao.ca/en/NFEG).

As part of the spread strategy, faculty representatives act as Champions/leaders/facilitators in integrating the NFEG resource at their academic institution. They seek, create, and coordinate opportunities to promote integration of tobacco cessation into the curriculum; develop and mentor others to support knowledge transfer (KT) of the *Education Guide* within the curriculum; network and raise awareness about TI resources, including RNAO's BPG; and serve as a resource to the faculty for KT related to TI and as a link to RNAO. RNAO also hosted nursing faculty working group meetings focused on the clinical aspects of TI, the *Education Guide,* and other resources, and from this, with widespread interest amongst nursing faculty across the country, an online community forum for networking is now active.

TI BEST PRACTICE CHAMPIONS

Since 2008, the TI Initiative has provided a total of 80 TI Champion workshops across Canada to over 5,500 nurses, other healthcare providers, and students to develop capacity in individual practitioners. Workshops are founded on the principles of adult education pedagogy and address knowledge, skills, and attitudes of participants in relation to their role in TI. Teaching methodologies include knowledge application sessions, role-playing, patient stories, and networking to foster integration of tobacco cessation interventions in daily practice in all health sectors.

Overall, the TI Champion workshops have been extremely successful in developing evidence-based knowledge and best practices essential for nurses and other healthcare professionals to effectively intervene with smokers. Each workshop educates TI Champions on how to implement the BPG into their practice settings, including education on brief intervention strategies, motivational interviewing techniques, and a focused and goal-directed client-centered counselling style. Participants have also gained knowledge of how to promote the use of TI best practices amongst their colleagues and how to engage with key stakeholders both within and beyond their organization. The TI Champions Network provides opportunities for ongoing sharing, collaboration, continuing education offerings, and networking to help nurses and other health professionals sustain integration of TI in daily practice.

SOCIAL MEDIA AND WEB-BASED RESOURCES

A comprehensive communication strategy and dissemination plan enhances the spread of activities and resources that support the TI Best Practice Champions in TI interventions and implementation activities. The social media and web-based presence of the TI Initiative is outstanding and consists of a number of elements outlined here:

- Regular social media messaging draws attention to online evidence-based resources and print materials.

- The TobaccoFreeRNAO website serves as a central hub for all TI communications, events, and tools, with people from over 191 countries accessing the site to date. All print and social media information is branded with the TobaccoFreeRNAO logo as shown in Figure 10.3.

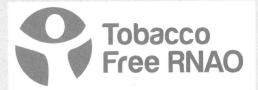

FIGURE 10.3 TobaccoFreeRNAO logo.
© Registered Nurses' Association of Ontario.
All rights reserved.

- TobaccoFreeRNAO has a steady presence on Twitter, with over 650 current followers.

- TI eLearning modules are popular and widely used resources amongst nurses, nursing students, and other healthcare providers. Over 3,225 individuals have completed the five TI eLearning modules to enhance their capacity in tobacco cessation interventions. These modules address helping clients quit, health professionals who smoke, mental illness and addiction and TI, TI for commercial tobacco use in indigenous populations, and TI in pre- and postnatal women.

- Knowledge exchange webinars on the integration of evidence-based tobacco cessation strategies into daily practice are interactive, archived following the session, and available through TobaccoFreeRNAO.ca.

- A virtual TI Community of Practice is hosted by RNAO on its online platform, a free professional networking website dedicated to communication and sharing of resources amongst those implementing best practices worldwide (http://communities.rnao.ca/smoking-cessation/). The "Resource Library" section includes a selection of tools shown to be effective in implementing evidence-based tobacco cessation interventions (http://tobaccofreernao.ca/en/rnao-resources).

EVALUATION

Evaluation is an important and consistent part of the TI Initiative and continues to be instrumental in highlighting the impact of the RNAO TI Best Practice Guideline in directing the evidence-based individual and organizational-level activities that are part of the TI Initiative. Through evaluation, we have learned the critical role nurses play as leaders in tobacco control and the impact of the TI Champions Network in supporting nurses to engage in TI best practices in their workplace settings. RNAO has partnered with the Ontario Tobacco Research Unit (OTRU) to plan and conduct the comprehensive evaluation which provides feedback enabling us to examine the impact of the Initiative and gain deeper insight into its successes, barriers, strategies, and critical learnings to sustain, spread, and scale up TI best practices in various settings across the country.

PARTNERSHIPS AND COLLABORATIONS

RNAO has formed strong partnerships with Smoke-Free Ontario–funded programs, other tobacco cessation projects, and initiatives related to chronic diseases and special populations. The aim of these partnerships is to ensure the successful integration, mobilization, and utilization of established services and programs for tobacco control in order to increase awareness and reach of the support and services available through the TI Initiative. These partnerships are mutually beneficial, as cross-promotion of each other's resources allows for spread and enhances impact.

NATIONAL SPREAD: PAN-CANADIAN TOBACCO INTERVENTION INITIATIVE

The success of this project at the provincial level spurred Canada's federal government to provide funding to RNAO over a 3-year period to replicate the TI Initiative and scale up to the national level in Canada, targeting all jurisdictions. Similar to the Ontario-based Initiative, the National Initiative focused on knowledge transfer, in particular related to the RNAO TI BPG, and mobilization of networks and increased use of existing services and programs to build capacity for tobacco interventions amongst nurses and other healthcare professionals.

The National Tobacco Intervention Initiative proved to be a huge success, with over nine provinces and territories involved, 40 workshops facilitated across Canada, and over 1,000 healthcare providers trained as TI Champions. The BPG was translated for use by a First Nations site that sparked further scaling up in northern First Nations communities. RNAO's current TI social media and web presence, discussed earlier in this chapter, helps these sites to sustain their work, and the Champion Network engages these Champions from the national sites.

SUMMARY

Key impacts of the TI Initiative include:

- TI and Tobacco Use Prevention Programs have a higher priority focus in Public and Community Health across Canada

- Policy changes in public health unit implementation sites reinforce TI and smoking-prevention programming

- Spread of Best Practice Guidelines into nursing education through integration of TI into undergraduate nursing curricula and the engagement of faculty and students as Champions

- Increased capacity of nurses and other clinicians in TI in a variety of populations across Canada, and adoption of brief TI intervention strategies into daily practice for nurses in all sectors

- Accessibility to evidence-based resources to support smoking cessation, TI, and prevention strategies for clinicians, students, and the public

- Networks for Champions and other professionals engaged in TI in their daily practice

- National acknowledgement of the TI Initiative for implementation across Canada

A number of aspects of scaling up, out, and deep have been demonstrated through this case study:

- The Initiative enables scaling up by extending the Tobacco Intervention BPG and related resources to all sectors in health and post-secondary education in nursing.

- The focused work with the Implementation Sites has resulted in scaling up and scaling out as organizational policy and planning incorporates TI, including prevention.

- The focus on capacity building for clinicians contributes to scaling up and scaling deep in relation to incorporating TI interventions into their daily practice.

- The engagement of Champions demonstrates use of a variety of delivery strategies (including diffusion and networking and train the trainer approaches) in the spread of best practices related to TI.

- The nature of the Champion program curriculum focuses on scaling deep and influences changes in attitudes of nurses and other clinicians about their role in TI, their competency, and effective ways to integrate these practices into their daily workflow.

- Engagement of stakeholders as partners in all aspects of the program has enabled sustained spread or scaling deep.

- The consistent inclusion of a comprehensive evaluation has enabled the TI Initiative to build on lessons learned, which has influenced scaling success.

- Scaling up was demonstrated in the nationwide spread, and the program components influenced both scaling out and scaling deep at the national level.

▶ REFLECTION

What are the differences in approach to the integration of evidence-based content in the undergraduate nursing curriculum in Case Study 1 and Case Study 2? Which elements of these approaches do you predict will have the most long-term impact on scaling up?

PREVENTION OF FALLS AND INJURY FROM FALLS IN THE OLDER ADULT

In 2002, RNAO published the first edition of a Best Practice Guideline, *Prevention of Falls and Fall Injuries in the Older Adult* (hereafter referred to as Falls BPG). At the time, falls were identified as a major focus for healthcare organizations, given that about 50% of residents in long-term care were falling each year; 7% of falls-related hip fractures were fatal; and falls contributed to pain, suffering, and a major economic burden on the healthcare system (RNAO, 2002).

In 2007, Safer Healthcare Now! (SHN!), a signature program of the Canadian Patient Safety Institute (CPSI), identified falls as a critical patient safety issue and fall prevention as a national patient safety priority (MacLaurin & McConnell, 2011). SHN!'s mandate is to reduce preventable adverse events across healthcare settings in Canada through the implementation of evidence-based interventions. Given RNAO's leadership on the topic of fall prevention, its evidence-based Falls BPG, and its expertise in knowledge translation and implementation science, CPSI approached RNAO to be the Intervention Lead for SHN!'s national Falls Prevention Intervention (MacLaurin & McConnell, 2011).

In 2008, a formal partnership between SHN! (CPSI) and RNAO was launched, and the two organizations embarked on a collaboration that would impact patient safety and healthcare practices for the next decade. This work involved a systematic approach to implementing practice change through quality-improvement science, access to evidence-based resources, capacity development at the individual and organizational level, and collaboration with national partners.

NATIONAL COLLABORATIVE ON FALLS PREVENTION IN LONG-TERM CARE (2008–2009)

The National Collaborative on Falls Prevention in Long-Term Care (hereafter referred to as the LTC Collaborative) was the inaugural initiative undertaken by the SHN!/RNAO partnership. The LTC Collaborative was conducted from May 2008 to May 2009 and involved teams of five to seven interdisciplinary staff members representing 32 long-term care homes from across Canada.

The overarching goal of the LTC Collaborative was to reduce falls and injury from falls in LTC homes across Canada by 40% over a 1-year period, and the objectives were to provide:

- A dynamic, interactive learning experience that incorporates quality improvement and falls prevention theory, techniques, and tools to assist improvement teams in reaching their falls and injury prevention goals

- A forum for improvement teams to learn from faculty and exchange various approaches to quality improvement that they can test at the local level

- An opportunity for LTC improvement teams to participate in, and learn about, a Breakthrough Series Collaborative methodology that they can then utilize for other quality-improvement initiatives

SYSTEMATIC IMPLEMENTATION METHODOLOGY

The curriculum of the LTC Collaborative was informed by the second edition of the RNAO BPG *Prevention of Falls and Fall Injuries in the Older Adult* (2005b) and by theoretical models for change based in the quality-improvement literature. A conceptual model, the Falls Intervention Model, was developed to visually represent key evidence-based concepts from the RNAO guideline (see Figure 10.4). A *Change Package* was developed to operationalize best practices for the LTC Collaborative and guide the work of the teams (RNAO & SHN!, 2008). It highlighted four key change concepts: 1) design systems to avoid mistakes; 2) improve workflow; 3) manage variation; and 4) change the environment.

The Breakthrough Series Collaborative methodology (see Figure 10.4), a well-established approach within the quality-improvement world (Institute for Healthcare Improvement [IHI], 2003), was used to structure each learning session.

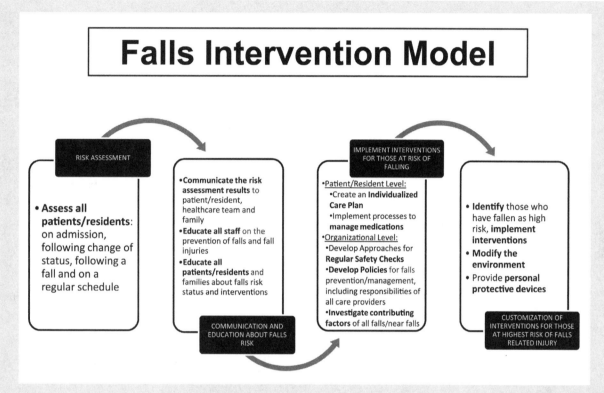

FIGURE 10.4 Falls Intervention Model.
Reprinted from *Journal of Safety Research, 42*(6), MacLaurin, A., & McConnell, H., Utilizing quality improvement methods to prevent falls and injury from falls: Enhancing resident safety in long-term care, p. 11. Copyright 2011, with permission from Elsevier.

ELEMENTS OF THE LTC COLLABORATIVE

The LTC Collaborative included an interprofessional expert faculty and LTC teams recruited from across Canada to participate in the LTC Collaborative, which involved three in-person learning sessions and a closing session in sites spanning the country. Consistent with the collaborative model, between each learning session was an "Action Period" where teams conducted small tests of change using Plan-Do-Study-Act (PDSA) cycles based on the Model for Improvement (Langley et al., 2009), received extensive support and feedback from quality-improvement advisors and members of the falls faculty, and were encouraged to network with other teams within the LTC Collaborative. Monthly teleconferences and an online Community of Practice (COP) for sharing ideas and resources were utilized to engage teams and build capacity in falls prevention strategies.

In the spirit of quality improvement, teams collected data on key process indicators such as: percentage of residents with completed fall risk assessments, percentage of risk assessments following status change, percentage of at-risk residents with intervention plans, and outcome indicators such as falls per 1,000 resident days and percentage of harmful falls. In addition, data were collected on a balancing measure, percent of restraint use, to ensure that falls interventions were not contributing to problems in other areas. The multiple structures and processes of the LTC National Collaborative are illustrated in Figure 10.5.

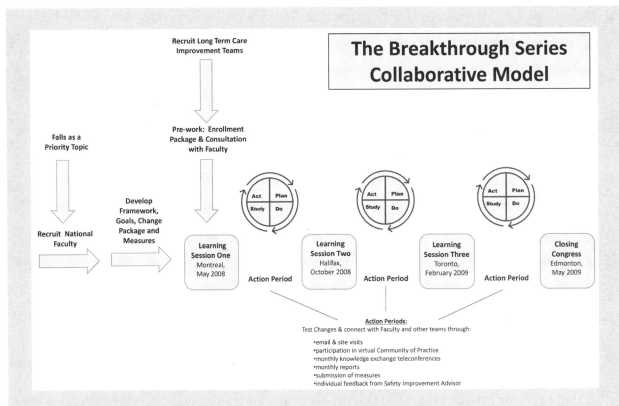

FIGURE 10.5 The Breakthrough Series Collaborative Model used for the National Collaborative on Falls Prevention in Long-Term Care (2008–2009). Reprinted with permission from the Canadian Patient Safety Institute.

OUTCOMES OF THE LTC COLLABORATIVE

Overall, the LTC Collaborative proved to be highly successful. Teams were fully engaged and found the process of learning from each other and sharing successes an effective way to support practice change within their long-term care homes. According to the evaluation results, the greatest improvements were noted in all three process measures, indicating that practice changes were being integrated with work processes in the participating homes. Furthermore, there was a notable decline in restraint use in those homes that submitted these data. Outcome measures were promising, with 16% of the LTC homes achieving or exceeding the goal of 40% reduction in a 1-year period. For other homes, the trends were positive; however, it was determined that more time would be required to scale out and deep, to embed and sustain practice changes before these outcome measures would be achieved. Further support of LTC homes was offered through a subsequent initiative led by RNAO through its partnership with SHN!—the Virtual Learning Collaborative.

VIRTUAL LEARNING COLLABORATIVE (2010–2011)

The National Virtual Learning Collaborative (Virtual Collaborative) built on the experience of the LTC Collaborative but using exclusively web-based technology to deliver a flexible and practical approach to learning, sharing, and networking. The initiative took place over an 8-month period and included many of the same elements of the LTC Collaborative. Virtual technologies were used to actively engage participants during and between meetings (e.g., webinars for learning sessions, including in-session chatting, question and answer sessions, virtual break-out rooms, and an online Community of Practice).

To guide the work of the quality-improvement teams, RNAO collaborated with SHN! on the development of another evidence-based resource entitled *Reducing Falls and Injury from Falls—Getting Started Kit* (hereafter the Falls GSK), which addressed interdisciplinary falls prevention initiatives in home care, acute care, and long-term care (SHN! & RNAO, 2010). This user-friendly resource was based on the recommendations from RNAO's guideline *Prevention of Falls and Fall Injuries in the Older Adult* (RNAO, 2005b), quality-improvement methodology, and contributions from expert faculty.

Figure 10.6 provides an overview of the structure of the Virtual Collaborative, using the same Breakthrough Series Collaborative methodology applied in the LTC Collaborative.

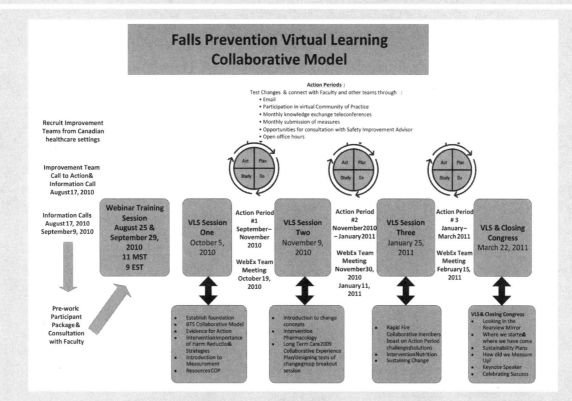

FIGURE 10.6   Falls Prevention Virtual Learning Collaborative Model.
Reprinted from *Journal of Safety Research, 42*(6), MacLaurin, A., & McConnell, H., Utilizing quality improvement methods to prevent falls and injury from falls: Enhancing resident safety in long-term care, p. 11.
Copyright 2011, with permission from Elsevier.

OUTCOMES OF THE VIRTUAL COLLABORATIVE

The response to the Virtual Collaborative exceeded expectations. Over 47 organizations, representing 74 improvement teams, participated from a variety of sectors, including LTC, home care, acute care, rehabilitation, and mental health, with most Canadian provinces and territories represented. The findings were similar to those of the initial LTC Collaborative, in relation to practice change based on best evidence; however, in this instance, 26.8% of the participating teams reached the target of 40% improvement in reduction in falls causing injury (MacLaurin & McConnell, 2011).

The Virtual Collaborative initiative demonstrated that technology was an effective tool in scaling up and out,

resulting in major practice change in falls prevention in all sectors, and it enabled greater access to expert resources and peers. With the view that greater emphasis on sustained practice change would show greater impact on resident and patient outcomes, the partners collaborated on a third initiative focused on sustainability: the Falls Facilitated Learning Series.

FALLS FACILITATED LEARNING SERIES (2011–2012)

The Falls Facilitated Learning Series (Learning Series) focused on sustainability of falls prevention interventions within practice settings. The purpose of the Learning Series was to help teams within healthcare organizations evaluate their existing falls prevention programs for sustainability and to strengthen the uptake, spread, and integration of evidence-based best practices throughout the organization. Participating teams submitted baseline and follow-up data on the key process and outcome indicators used in other initiatives, with the goal of demonstrating a 20% improvement in these measures and sustaining the gains for 3 consecutive months. The Learning Series was rooted in evidence from RNAO's Falls BPG and quality-improvement theory, and resources developed for the previous initiatives, including the

Change Package and the *Getting Started Kit,* were utilized in conjunction with a new resource developed by RNAO, the *Sustainability Workbook* (SHN! & RNAO, 2011).

The *Sustainability Workbook* was grounded in implementation science, sustainability theory, change theory, and quality-improvement methodology. It provided teams with structured activities before learning sessions and focused questions during "action periods" to help them apply evidence within their practice. Figure 10.7 provides an overview of the structure of the Learning Series.

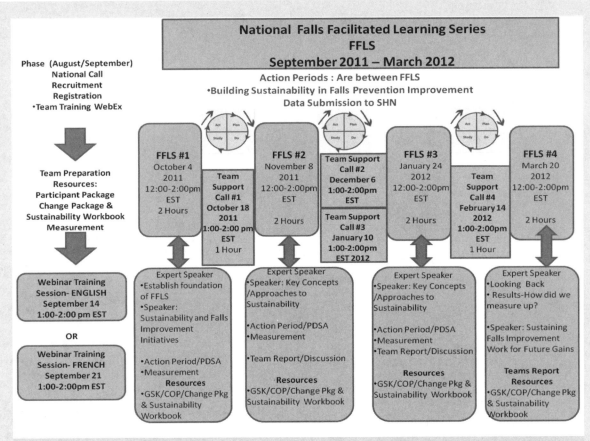

FIGURE 10.7 National Falls Facilitated Learning Series.
Reprinted with permission from the Canadian Patient Safety Institute.

OUTCOMES OF THE LEARNING SERIES

Engagement in this initiative again exceeded SHN! and RNAO's expectations, with 41 teams participating in the Learning Series, representing provinces and territories across Canada and including acute care, home care, LTC, and mental-health settings. According to data submitted by participating teams, gains were noted across all three healthcare sectors, with improvements in the percentage of patients with completed assessments or screening on admission, and percentage of patients with a document-ed plan in place to reduce falls risk. Furthermore, 25% of home care, 55% of long-term care, and 69% of acute care settings also noted reductions in falls causing injury.

MAINTAINING MOMENTUM AND EXPANDING REACH

Following these successful spread, scale-up, and scale-out initiatives—which advanced from in-person to entirely virtual, and from a focus on LTC to the inclusion of all sectors, and resulting in the development of three evidence-based resources informed by the RNAO Falls BPG—RNAO has continued its partnership with CPSI as the national Falls Prevention Intervention Lead. The role of the Intervention Lead involves building capacity and supporting the uptake of falls-prevention best practices through sharing knowledge and expertise in falls preven-tion and implementation science, creating and updating evidence-based resources, and expanding the network of organizations engaged with fall prevention work. Table 10.2 provides a summary of these activities to date.

TABLE 10.2   FALLS PREVENTION INTERVENTION LEAD ACTIVITIES (2013–PRESENT)

ACTIVITY	DESCRIPTION
2013 2nd edition Falls GSK published	The Falls GSK was revised in collaboration with an interprofessional Pan-Canadian expert faculty. The GSK was published in English and French and disseminated through a national webinar and extensive national networks through RNAO and CPSI.
2013–2016 National Calls	One-hour knowledge exchange webinars facilitated by members of the Falls Faculty offered two to three times throughout the year. A range of topics engage a national audience and include using "positive deviance" and "frontline ownership" to support innovation in falls prevention, lessons learned from videos capturing fall events, and emerging research on appropriate footwear to wear in winter conditions.
2013–2014 Development of a falls audit tool	Over 14 months, RNAO collaborated with CPSI and Alberta Health Services to develop, pilot test, and implement the falls audit tool, informed by best practices outlined in the Falls GSK. The purpose of the tool was to support organizations to assess the quality of their falls-prevention and injury-reduction practices and determine areas requiring quality improvement.
2015 National Audit Month	A series of virtual orientation sessions were held for quality-improvement teams across Canada in home care, acute care, and long-term care to explain the falls audit tool and prepare for National Audit Month in April 2015. The audit event included 162 participating sites representing 3,499 records. Aggregated results provide a snapshot of the falls-prevention processes across Canada and were disseminated through a national webinar to participating teams. Organizations are using lessons learned from audit data to maximize strengths and address areas for quality improvement, and they are encouraged to continue to audit falls.
2015–2016 Home Care Safety Falls Prevention Virtual Improvement Collaborative	RNAO contributed expertise related to falls-prevention best practices to a Virtual Improvement Collaborative developed for the home care sector. This initiative was co-led by CPSI, the Canadian Home Care Association, and the Canadian Foundation for Healthcare Improvement and involved teams from five home care organizations from across the country.

continues

TABLE 10.2   FALLS PREVENTION INTERVENTION LEAD ACTIVITIES (2013–PRESENT)   CONTINUED

ACTIVITY	DESCRIPTION
2015– Present Fall Prevention Month	RNAO and CPSI have collaborated with over 10 diverse organizational partners across Canada to develop, disseminate, and evaluate an online toolkit and other resources to support Pan-Canadian activities in recognition of Fall Prevention Month, held annually in November.
2017 RNAO Falls BPG, 3rd edition, published	The scope of this evidence-based Best Practice Guideline has been expanded to support fall prevention across the spectrum of care and amongst all adults (18 years and older) who are at risk of falls.
2017 *Falls Getting Started Kit,* 3rd edition	This edition of the Falls GSK reflects the same evidence summaries that informed the 3rd edition of RNAO's Falls BPG. The revisions have been focused on updating the evidence, and this work has been completed in collaboration with an interprofessional national faculty of falls experts.

Key impacts of the Falls Prevention Initiative include:

- Extensive spread of the Falls BPG through use of a quality-improvement approach and extension to a virtual methodology

- A successful partnership between RNAO and CPSI that used evaluation feedback and evolving technology to adapt and shape the Falls Prevention Initiative to advance spread and impact process and outcomes

- Sustained use of the Falls BPG across the country, with positive results, augmented by tools such as the RNAO Falls BPG, the collaborative curriculum, the *Change Package,* the *Getting Started Kit,* and the *Sustainability Workbook*

- Increased capacity of nurses and other clinicians in falls prevention, quality improvement, outcomes evaluation, and sustainability

- Accessibility to evidence-based resources, including expert faculty and peers, to support falls prevention activities

- Major changes in practice in all sectors across Canada with outcome improvements on falls and injury from falls

A number of aspects of scaling up, out, and deep have been demonstrated through this case study:

- Massive scaling up by extending the Falls Collaborative across the country and maximizing participation through technology

- Scaling out and deep facilitated by access to expert faculty, peer participants, and use of the quality-improvement and collaborative models

- Delivery strategies include networking, integrated approaches with quality-improvement initiatives, and local adaptation to various sectors

- The focused virtual work with the implementation sites has resulted in scaling up and scaling out as organizational policy and planning incorporates falls prevention

- The capacity building focus for clinicians in various sectors through the in-person and virtual sessions, and the key evidence-based resources, contribute to scaling up and scaling deep in relation to integrating falls-prevention strategies into daily practice

- The attention to evaluation as part of quality improvement has enabled participating sites to build on lessons learned, influencing scaling deep

◤ REFLECTION

Thinking about all three case studies, what is the contribution of committed partnerships to advancing evidence-based practices in efforts to scale up?

CONCLUSION

The three case studies in this chapter show the phenomenal success RNAO is achieving—first in designing and delivering context-specific BPG-implementation interventions to meet the qualities of effective scaling, and second in addressing the full typology of scaling—scaling up, out, and deep.

In the first case study, the use of a conceptual model incorporating all aspects of Yamey's (2011) framework sets the stage for impressive scaling in the health and education sectors at practice, policy, and cultural levels. The framework guides the systematic implementation methodology, used in the MH&A Initiative. Here we see how the elements of the framework, including access to evidence-based resources, capacity development opportunities, the engagement of Champions, and collaborative partnerships result in scaling up, out, and deep of RNAO's evidence-based guidelines. These guidelines focused on mental health and addiction impact health-service delivery, organizational policy, secondary and post-secondary education, and the social service system. The case study demonstrates scaling deep through discussion of impacts on values and culture in the school system, in particular related to stigma and mental health amongst youth.

The second case study demonstrates the use of a multipronged strategy that informs a systematic implementation methodology and leverages mutually beneficial partnerships. This facilitates scaling of the smoking and tobacco-cessation BPG recommendations up, out, and deep to impact local and national target groups. The evidence-based resources, capacity development opportunities (both self-directed and facilitator supported), and the engagement of Champions in a range of roles and sectors aid in the scaling and spread activities in TI. Here we gain an appreciation for how scaling deep is fostered in the Champion curriculum and the supports provided to implementation sites and to the Champions Network. Scaling up and out are particularly evident in the deliberate integration of tobacco-cessation interventions within nursing program curricula and the impacts on organizational TI-related policies in all sectors.

The third case study shows how RNAO's 15-year commitment to support healthcare providers, teams, and organizations in implementing best practices to prevent falls and fall injuries has spread country-wide, engaging organizations across the spectrum of care. It is an outstanding exemplar of successful scaling up, out, and deep. The partnership between RNAO and CPSI—together with expert falls faculty and in some cases other organizational stakeholders—shaped dynamic initiatives that engage quality-improvement teams and provide opportunities for capacity building. Best evidence, use of implementation science and quality-improvement methodologies, and committed partnerships were keys to the spread and scaling up of the fall prevention initiatives. With the attention to sustainment, and ongoing audit and feedback in particular, there is also strong evidence of scaling deep.

These diverse cases demonstrate the typology of scaling in three areas of health and healthcare that provide challenges for practitioners, policymakers, administrators, educators, and the public alike—mental health and addiction, smoking and tobacco cessation, and falls prevention. As illustrated in these exemplars, RNAO has leveraged its evidence-based BPGs and other resources, as well as a systematic implementation methodology and context-specific delivery approaches, to realize effective scaling.

Effective scaling up has meant extensive exposure in healthcare and beyond; effective scaling out has impacted policy and organizational priorities; and effective scaling deep has helped create cultures that sustain and spread evidence-based practices in each area. Through its BPG Program, for almost two decades RNAO has been committed to closing the theory-practice gap in a way that will create lasting change with ripple effects for providers, clients, organizations, and the system. These cases demonstrate how well this is being realized.

KEY MESSAGES

- Successful scaling up, out, and deep of implementation initiatives requires attention to the evidence, the process, and individual/organizational capacity development.

- Champions at all levels are key to implementation of practice change and scaling up of proven approaches.

- Systematic implementation methodologies provide guidance and direction to project teams working to scale implementation up, out, and deep.

- Committed partners, with mutual goals for improving practice, can support the uptake and scaling of evidence-based practices in service and academic organizations.

REFERENCES

Bell Canada. (2017). *Bell Let's Talk toolkit*. Retrieved from http://letstalk.bell.ca/en/toolkit

Canadian Association of Schools of Nursing (CASN). (2015). *Entry-to-practice mental health competencies for undergraduate nursing education in Canada*. Retrieved from http://www.casn.ca/2015/11/entry-to-practice-mental-health-and-addiction-competencies-for-undergraduate-nursing-education-in-canada/

Edwards, N. (2010). Scaling-up health innovations and interventions in public health: A brief review of the current state-of-the-science. A commissioned paper for the inaugural *Conference to Advance the State of the Science and Practice on Scale-up and Spread of Effective Health Programs*, Washington, DC, July 6–8.

Institute for Healthcare Improvement (IHI). (2003). *The breakthrough series: IHI's collaborative model for achieving breakthrough improvement*. IHI Innovation Series white paper. Boston, MA: Institute for Healthcare Improvement.

Langley, G., Moen, R., Nolan, K., Nolan, T., Norman, C., & Provost, L. (2009). *The improvement guide. A practical approach to enhancing organizational performance* (2nd ed.). San Francisco, CA: John Wiley & Sons, Inc.

MacLaurin, A., & McConnell, H. (2011). Utilizing quality improvement methods to prevent falls and injury from falls: Enhancing resident safety in long-term care. *Journal of Safety Research, 42*(6), 525–535.

Mangham, L. J., & Hanson, K. (2010). Scaling up in international health: What are the key issues? *Health Policy and Planning, 25*(2), 85–96.

Ministry of Health and Long-Term Care (MOHLTC). (2007). *Report of the Methadone Maintenance Treatment Practices Task Force*. Retrieved from http://www.health.gov.on.ca/fr/common/ministry/publications/reports/methadone_taskforce/methadone_taskforce.pdf

Moore, M., & Riddell, D. (2015). Scaling out, scaling up, scaling deep: Advancing systemic social innovation and the learning processes to support it. *Journal of Corporate Citizenship, 58*, 67–84. doi: 10.9774/GLEAF.4700.2015.ju.00009

Nadler-Moodie, M. (2010). Psychiatric emergencies in med-surg patients: Are you prepared? *American Nurse Today, 5*(5), 23–28.

Policy Brief. (2010). Scaling up nutrition: A framework for action. *Food and Nutrition Bulletin, 31*(1), 178–186.

Registered Nurses' Association of Ontario (RNAO). (2002). *Prevention of falls and fall injuries in the older adult*. Toronto, ON: Registered Nurses' Association of Ontario.

Registered Nurses' Association of Ontario (RNAO). (2005a). *Interventions for postpartum depression*. Toronto, ON: Registered Nurses' Association of Ontario.

Registered Nurses' Association of Ontario (RNAO). (2005b). *Prevention of falls and fall injuries in the older adult* (2nd ed.). Toronto, ON: Registered Nurses' Association of Ontario.

Registered Nurses' Association of Ontario (RNAO). (2006a). *Establishing therapeutic relationships*. Toronto, ON: Registered Nurses' Association of Ontario.

Registered Nurses' Association of Ontario (RNAO). (2006b). *Crisis intervention*. Toronto, ON: Registered Nurses' Association of Ontario.

Registered Nurses' Association of Ontario (RNAO). (2007). *Integrating smoking cessation into daily nursing practice*. Toronto, ON: Registered Nurses' Association of Ontario.

Registered Nurses' Association of Ontario (RNAO). (2009a). *Assessment and care of adults at risk for suicidal ideation and behaviour*. Toronto, ON: Registered Nurses' Association of Ontario.

Registered Nurses' Association of Ontario (RNAO). (2009b). *Supporting clients on methadone maintenance treatment*. Toronto, ON: Registered Nurses' Association of Ontario.

Registered Nurses' Association of Ontario (RNAO). (2010a). *Enhancing healthy adolescent development*. Toronto, ON: Registered Nurses' Association of Ontario.

Registered Nurses' Association of Ontario (RNAO). (2010b). *Nursing faculty education guide: Tobacco use and associated health risks*. Retrieved from http://tobaccofreernao.ca/en/NFEG

Registered Nurses' Association of Ontario (RNAO). (2012a). *Facilitating client centred learning*. Toronto, ON: Registered Nurses' Association of Ontario.

Registered Nurses' Association of Ontario (RNAO). (2012b). *Toolkit: Implementation of Best Practice Guidelines* (2nd ed.). Toronto, ON: Registered Nurses' Association of Ontario.

Registered Nurses' Association of Ontario (RNAO). (2012c). *Woman abuse: Screening, identification and initial response*. Toronto, ON: Registered Nurses' Association of Ontario.

Registered Nurses' Association of Ontario (RNAO). (2015a). *Engaging clients who use substances*. Toronto, ON: Registered Nurses' Association of Ontario.

Registered Nurses' Association of Ontario (RNAO). (2015b). *Person- and family-centred care*. Toronto, ON: Registered Nurses' Association of Ontario.

Registered Nurses' Association of Ontario (RNAO). (2017a). *Nurse educator mental health and addiction resource*. Retrieved from www.rnao.ca/bpg/initiatives/mhai

Registered Nurses' Association of Ontario (RNAO). (2017b). *Integrating tobacco interventions into daily practice*. Retrieved from www.rnao.ca/bpg/guidelines/integrating-tobacco-interventions-daily-practice

Registered Nurses' Association of Ontario (RNAO) and Safer Healthcare Now! (SHN!). (2008). *National collaborative on the prevention of falls in long-term care: Change package*. Retrieved from https://tools.patientsafetyinstitute.ca/Communities/falls/Shared%20Documents/National%20Falls%20Collaborative%202008/Change%20Package/Change%20Package.pdf

Safer Healthcare Now! (SHN!) and Registered Nurses' Association of Ontario (RNAO). (2010). *Reducing falls and injury from falls—Getting started kit*. Retrieved from http://www.saferhealthcarenow.ca/EN/Interventions/Falls/Pages/default.aspx

Safer Healthcare Now! (SHN!) and Registered Nurses' Association of Ontario (RNAO). (2011). *Falls facilitated learning series—Sustainability workbook*. Retrieved from https://tools.patientsafetyinstitute.ca/Communities/falls/Shared%20Documents/Falls%20Facilitated%20Learning%20Series%202011/FFLS%20Session%201-%20October%204,%202011.%20SAPC%201-%204%20octobre/Sustainability%20Workbook%20Final.pdf

Simmons, R., Fajans, P., & Ghiron, L. (Eds.). (2007). *Scaling up health service delivery: From pilot innovations to policies and programmes*. Geneva, CH: World Health Organization Press.

Yamey, G. (2011). Scaling up global health interventions: A proposed framework for success. *PLoS Med, 8*(6), e1001049. doi:10.1371/journal.pmed.1001049

11

EVIDENCE-BASED PRACTICE IN LONG-TERM CARE

Carol Holmes, MN, RN, GNC(C)
Suman Iqbal, MSN/MHA, RN, CON(C)
Bahar Karimi, MN, MHSc(HA), RN, CHE
Heather McConnell, MA(Ed), BScN, RN
Irmajean Bajnok, PhD, MScN, BScN, RN

LEARNING OBJECTIVES

After reading this chapter, you will be able to:

- Describe the multifaceted approach and strategies (awareness raising, engagement, capacity development, implementation, integration, evaluation) utilized in scaling up the BPG Program and BPSO Designation to create evidence-based practice cultures in LTC homes

- Identify the impact of the Long-Term Care Best Practices Program (LTC BPP) on resident, provider, and organizational outcomes

- Discuss the approach taken by RNAO to leverage the BPSO Designation within the LTC BPP

- Describe the impact of the organizational (meso) level LTC-BPSO Designation on successful guideline uptake as illustrated in a case example

- Understand how adaptation of an innovation can support scaling up across the LTC sector

INTRODUCTION

The Registered Nurses' Association of Ontario's (RNAO's) *Long-Term Care Best Practices Program* (LTC BPP) represents an example of scaling up of evidence-based practice to the system level in the long-term care (LTC) sector. Mangham and Hanson (2010) describe *scaling up* as a set of processes used in introducing an innovation, that has been effective elsewhere, to a new setting. In this case, RNAO spread the use of BPGs and the Best Practice Spotlight Organization (BPSO) Designation throughout the long-term care sector using various processes and strategies that considered both the policy and cultural contexts of the sector (Mangham & Hanson, 2010).

This chapter chronicles the development of the LTC BPP and highlights key aspects of implementation science and the evidence-based resources instrumental in scaling up this program, leading to positive outcomes for residents and their families, providers, and the sector itself.

BACKGROUND AND HISTORY

Canada has a large and growing community residential care sector that includes a range of living options for people, primarily older adults, needing nursing, personal care, and other therapeutic and support services. The terminology used to describe these residential care settings varies across the country. In some provinces they include lodges, assisted living, supportive housing, and nursing and personal care homes (Canadian Institute for Health Information [CIHI], 2017). In Ontario, these residential care facilities are called long-term care (LTC) homes, specifically to denote the home-like environment that they are designed to emulate. There are approximately 627 publicly funded, licensed, and inspected LTC homes (including 78,052 resident care beds) that provide care for adults in the province (Ministry of Health and Long-Term Care [MOHLTC] Ontario, 2016).

Registered nursing staff in Ontario LTC homes account for 26% of the total resident care hours provided. Registered nurses provide 9% of those hours and registered practical nurses provide 17% of the total hours. Other professional care staff providing expert family, social, activation, nutritional, and physical care, such as social workers, activation therapists, dieticians, physiotherapists, and occupational therapists, provide another 8% of the total resident care hours. Specialized care staff, such as nurse practitioners, infection control specialists, and clinical nurse specialists, provide a small portion of the direct resident care hours (0.27%). The vast majority of direct-care staff in Ontario LTC homes are unregulated personal support workers, and they provide 65% of the total resident care hours (Ontario Association of Non-Profit Homes and Services for Seniors, 2015).

In the late 1990s and early 2000s, in an effort to increase the quality of care in Ontario's LTC sector, the Ontario Government invested resources to address priority care issues. Given its emerging and already highly successful clinical Best Practice Guideline (BPG) Program, RNAO was approached by the Ministry of Health and Long-Term Care (MOHLTC) to develop and disseminate select nursing BPGs on topics such as pressure ulcer prevention and treatment and falls prevention and management for use by the LTC sector and beyond.

In 2005, the Long-Term Care Best Practice Co-ordinator (LTC BPC) role was introduced in Ontario through a 3-year pilot project, the Long-Term Care Best Practices Initiative (Initiative), managed and funded by the Ontario MOHLTC and led by RNAO. The goal of the newly established Initiative was to promote the dissemination and uptake of nursing BPGs in the LTC sector, advance the awareness and use of BPGs in LTC homes, and enhance the care of LTC home residents (Nursing Health Services Research Unit [NHSRU], 2007a).

This Initiative was evaluated through the Nursing Health Services Research Unit (NHSRU), a collaborative endeavour of the University of Toronto and McMaster University. Using a two-phase approach, the evaluation examined the processes used in phase 1, and the impact of the Initiative at the organizational (LTC home) level in phase 2. Feedback from stakeholders in phase 1 revealed that the LTC BPC role was viewed as a very positive force in increasing the awareness and uptake of BPGs (NHSRU, 2007a). In phase 2, stakeholders indicated that the implementation of the BPGs in the participating LTC homes was beginning to have a positive impact on resident care and outcomes, particularly in the areas of falls prevention, skin and wound care, and continence (NHSRU, 2007b). This was significant at the time because these care areas included three of the top four areas of risk and concern (as identified by the sector) in the care of LTC home residents.

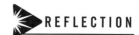

REFLECTION

From your experience, what are some of the challenges of introducing evidence-based practice in long-term care settings, and what types of supports do you think would be most helpful?

Two key recommendations to the MOHLTC from the evaluation of the pilot Initiative included (NHSRU, 2007b):

■ Provide sustainable funding for the Initiative while continuing to evaluate the impact of the implementation of BPGs on LTC resident, health provider, and system outcomes

■ Consider increasing the number of LTC BPCs in the province (from the original eight) to enhance the opportunity for better resident outcomes resulting from evidence-based practice in LTC homes across the province

Following the success of the 3-year pilot project, the Initiative was formalized in 2008 as an ongoing government-funded program, with an increase in the number of BPCs to 14 (one for each healthcare region in the province) and additional education and management support. RNAO was asked to lead this program in recognition of its cutting-edge work in BPG development and implementation, expertise in project management, and in-depth knowledge of the sector. In 2009, the program was awarded the *Health Minister's Award of Excellence* at the provincial *Innovations in Health Care Expo*, acknowledging its innovative approach to improving quality and patient safety in LTC homes.

PROGRAM INFRASTRUCTURE

Following the formalization and expansion of the program, its philosophical underpinnings were refined to include a vision, mission, set of values, and a guiding framework. This infrastructure enabled and supported the work of the program team and in particular the BPCs, whose role was further developed based on the early work of the pioneer BPCs.

VISION, MISSION, AND VALUES

The vision, mission, and values gave the program a clear focus and direction and fostered a shared understanding of the program's vision amongst the team and stakeholders across the LTC sector. They have been updated regularly in keeping with evaluation data and context changes. Table 11.1 delineates these aspects of infrastructure.

TABLE 11.1   MISSION, VISION, VALUES OF THE LTC BEST PRACTICES PROGRAM (RNAO, 2008)

Mission	The mission of the Long-Term Care Best Practices Program is to enhance the quality of care for residents in LTC homes and facilitate a culture of evidence-based practice through the implementation of the Best Practice Guidelines by direct-care staff in LTC homes.
Vision	BPGs will be implemented and successfully sustained throughout the long-term care sector for the benefit of residents and their families, providers, the organization, and the system.
Values	Successful BPG implementation will be achieved through collaboration and partnerships by: involving key stakeholders throughout the process, sharing of resources, learning through dialogue, ongoing evaluation and reflection, and developing plans for sustainability.

THE GUIDING FRAMEWORK

The guiding framework consists of six strategies and was developed to operationalize the mission, vision, and values, and reflect principles of implementation science as embedded in the RNAO *Toolkit: Implementation of Best Practice Guidelines* (2012b). These strategies guide the BPG implementation and knowledge-translation work of the Long-Term Care Best Practice Coordinators and other program team members as they support EBP in the LTC Sector. See Figure 11.1.

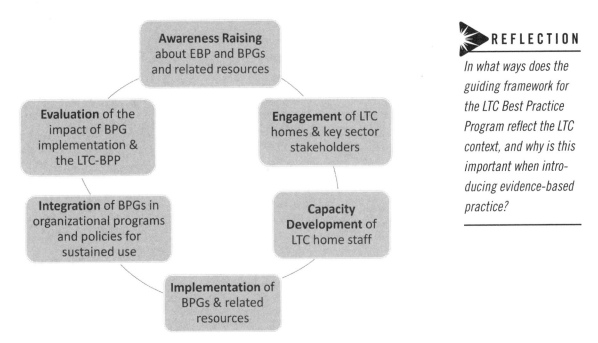

> **▶ REFLECTION**
>
> *In what ways does the guiding framework for the LTC Best Practice Program reflect the LTC context, and why is this important when introducing evidence-based practice?*

FIGURE 11.1   The six-strategy guiding framework of the LTC Best Practices Program.

THE LTC BEST PRACTICE COORDINATORS

The BPCs are experts in the care of older persons, the LTC sector, and implementation science strategies. They engage with LTC home leaders, nurse practitioners, and direct-care staff to establish and adopt practices based on RNAO clinical BPG recommendations. Thus, the BPCs are catalysts in the provision of evidence-based care to LTC home residents and their families. Their role includes the following activities:

■ Seek, create, and coordinate opportunities to promote the use of evidence-based best practices in LTC homes

■ Collaborate in the development of a plan for the local implementation of RNAO BPGs in LTC homes, including strategies to facilitate their sustainability and spread

■ Promote and support capacity development and knowledge transfer related to evidence-based practice within LTC homes

■ Provide support for best practice implementation and integration of best practices in legislated LTC required care and service programs and mandatory quality-improvement plans

The role of the BPCs can be more specifically delineated through a description of each of the six strategies in the guiding framework.

AWARENESS RAISING

Awareness raising is a strategy used by the LTC BPCs to focus the attention of LTC leaders and staff on evidence-based practice (EBP), the RNAO BPGs, related implementation resources applicable to clinical care of LTC home residents, and the RNAO Healthy Work Environment (HWE) BPGs (see Chapter 3, *Creating Healthy Workplaces: Enabling Clinical Excellence*) that support workplace improvements. The LTC BPCs use numerous approaches, such as newsletters, brochures, electronic mailings, meetings with LTC home leaders and staff, and exhibits at various events including workshops and conferences, to raise awareness about the BPGs and program resources. All of the approaches used are designed to encourage LTC home staff to be aware of evidence-based practice, become engaged with the program, and use BPGs in practice.

ENGAGEMENT

Engaging LTC home leaders and their staff with the program through the regional LTC BPCs is a very important strategy to advance homes toward using BPGs in day-to-day practice. LTC BPCs establish and facilitate individual and group meetings in LTC homes and develop networking groups of LTC home staff and other provincial LTC stakeholder groups who are implementing similar BPGs. Communities of practice focusing on a specific clinical practice issue (e.g., falls prevention, oral health) at the local and provincial levels are one example of a purposeful approach to engagement that has been effective in supporting BPG implementation in LTC homes.

CAPACITY DEVELOPMENT

Capacity includes the organizational and technical abilities, knowledge and skills, as well as relationships, attitudes, and values that enable organizations, groups, and individuals to carry out the necessary functions to achieve their development goals over time. Stakeholders are individuals or groups who have an interest in and are affected by, or can effect, a practice change (Baker et al., 1999; Legare, 2009). They play an important role in any change initiative and need to be involved throughout the process. The systematic use of RNAO clinical and HWE BPGs assists LTC homes in developing capacity at the individual staff level and within the sector.

To increase capacity in evidence-based practice and implementation science in LTC, there are varied strategies used including a program to develop LTC Best Practice Champions, a clinical fellowship program, and professional development offerings. In addition, given the importance of leadership at all levels in supporting and sustaining evidence-based practice, RNAO provides education and support to LTC leaders through professional development. For example, the *League of Excellence for LTC* is an interactive educational program developed by the LTC BPP; it is designed to enhance LTC leaders' ability to develop, integrate, evaluate, and sustain evidence-based programs and quality-improvement initiatives in Ontario LTC homes. Two primary resources developed by the LTC BPC Program that are widely used in the sector are presented in the following section.

KEY PROGRAM RESOURCES

Long-Term Care Best Practices Toolkit, 2nd edition

The *LTC Toolkit*, 2nd edition (www.ltctoolkit.rnao.ca) is a free online repository of evidence-based resources that support BPG implementation and LTC program planning and evaluation (RNAO, 2015a). Topics included were based on the expressed needs of the LTC homes and were identified through regular provincial surveys and ongoing contact with the LTC BPCs. All topics are associated with one or more of RNAO's clinical and/or HWE BPGs. Related implementation resources that support evidence-based practice in LTC are sourced for each topic, based on specific criteria. To be included in the *LTC Toolkit*, a resource/tool must reflect applicable legislative and regulatory requirements, be applicable to LTC, be evidence-based, and be available on the web at no cost or very minimal cost to users. To date, thousands of unique users from around the world, including practitioners, faculty, and students, have accessed this resource.

The Nursing Orientation eResource for LTC

This is a popular, evidence-based eResource (http://ltcorientationeresource.rnao.ca/) that includes comprehensive information to prepare nurses and others to work in and or understand the context of LTC. It includes four knowledge domains—professional, role, clinical, and organizational—and links nurses with the best available online resources and learning activities from reputable provincial and national organizations and select RNAO clinical and HWE BPGs. Each knowledge domain contains several learning modules, each of which includes an introduction to the topic and various "activities to do" and "resources to review" (Holmes & Warner, 2013).

The eResource provides a self-directed approach to learning based on a self-assessment of learning needs using an embedded checklist and planning tool. It is designed to enhance LTC home nursing orientation programs and to introduce users to evidence-based sources of information applicable to LTC that can help answer practice questions as they arise. While the e-Resource was designed for nurses new to LTC, it is also accessed by hundreds of experienced nurses to expand their knowledge and other healthcare professionals, students, and faculty as a source of evidence-based information about the sector (Holmes & Warner, 2013).

IMPLEMENTATION

Although LTC home leaders and direct-care staff strive to provide safe, high-quality, integrated, and evidence-based care, practice change using the best evidence does not happen quickly. Introducing best evidence into day-to-day practice requires a planned change process, with attention to both "hard" (technical) and "soft" (people) areas (Sarayreh, Khudair, & Barakat, 2013). Haines (2007) recognized the importance of garnering internal motivation for change toward a clear vision of the future. His model includes a focus on the experience of the individual, which is predictable as one moves from the current practice to the future desired state, which he depicts through a rollercoaster model. Successful implementation of practice change relates to the culture of the organization, including the leadership capacity, motivation, and resources to pursue clinical excellence.

The LTC BPCs guide implementation of BPGs through use of the Knowledge-to-Action (KTA) framework (Straus, Tetroe, & Graham, 2013), which enables a structured, systematic approach to implementation of best evidence in LTC homes. The KTA framework is described in detail in RNAO's user-friendly *Toolkit: Implementation of Best Practice Guidelines* (2012b). An important aspect of the BPC's role is helping to initiate the structured process to move knowledge (evidence) into practice. They start their work with homes using a gap analysis, linking this approach to the first phase of the KTA Cycle: *"Identify Problem: Identify, Review, and Select Knowledge"* (see Figure 11.2).

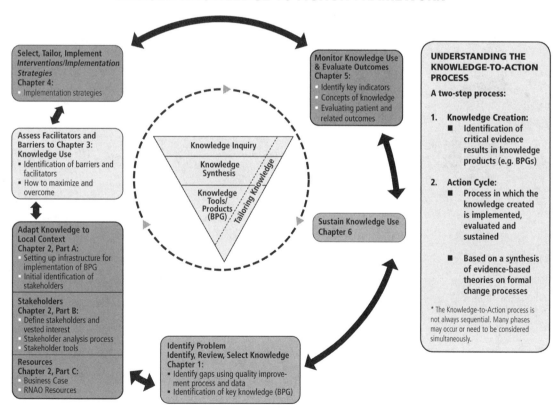

Adapted from "Knowledge Translation in Health Care: Moving From Evidence to Practice."
S. Straus, J. Tetroe, and I. Graham. Copyright 2009 by Blackwell Publishing Ltd. Adapted with permission.

FIGURE 11.2 Knowledge-to-Action framework as depicted in *Toolkit: Implementation of Best Practice Guidelines* (RNAO, 2012b).

The gap analysis is led by the LTC BPCs in partnership with the LTC home leaders and is a process for comparing current practice within an LTC home with evidence-based best practice recommendations in the selected BPGs to determine the following:

■ Existing practices and processes that are currently implemented and are supported by evidence in the BPG—this information is useful to reinforce practice strengths

■ Recommendations that are currently partially implemented in practice or implemented in specific areas of the LTC home—these would be good first targets for change efforts

■ Recommendations that are not currently being met

■ Recommendations that are not applicable to the practice setting

The team, along with internal and external stakeholders, carries out these comparisons, and at the same time also determines:

■ Facilitators to the process and any barriers to implementation, which may include staffing, skill mix, budget, workload issues, and staff knowledge and motivation

■ The timeframes related to specific actions and people or departments that can support the change effort

■ Links with other practices and programs in the LTC home

■ Existing resources and education that the LTC home can access

Table 11.2 illustrates an example of a gap analysis for one recommendation in the RNAO *Prevention of Falls and Fall Injuries in the Older Adult* BPG (2005, 2011) that will help the team determine areas of the recommendation that are met, partially met, and not met, and enable them to focus their actions.

TABLE 11.2   EXAMPLE OF A GAP ANALYSIS FOR ONE RECOMMENDATION

RNAO Best Practice Guideline Recommendations	Met	Partially Met	Unmet	Notes (Examples of what to include: is this a priority, information on current practice, possible overlap with other programs or partners)
Practice Recommendation: Assessment 1.0 Assess fall risk on admission. (Level 1b Evidence)		X		Discussed the risk assessment tool used on admission to determine if the staff is knowledgeable about the risk factors associated with falls and if risk assessments are completed within 24 hours of admission. Staff asked if the past fall history could be available at admission. Staff identified from latest Quality Improvement reports that 40% of admissions have a staff-completed falls risk assessment. Action plan: Select and use a consistent tool for falls risk assessment on all units, and complete 100% of the time within 24 hours of admission.

Benefits of conducting a gap analysis include (RNAO, 2012b):

- Identifying strengths in current practice

- Focusing on needed practice change based on best evidence, with attention to priority areas that may be most easily addressed

- Determining barriers and facilitators, resource requirements, selection of implementation strategies, and evaluation approaches

- Agreeing on next steps, such as development of infrastructure to support BPG implementation, stakeholder engagement

- Increasing likelihood of sustained practice change through involving staff in a candid discussion of current practice and how to plan for practice changes

The LTC Best Practice Program focuses on supporting LTC homes, within the context of their available resources, to develop and carry out their plans to implement BPGs. Support is provided, primarily though the expertise of the LTC BPCs, who use consultative and coaching approaches while working with LTC leaders and Champions to apply change-management principles in adopting clinical and HWE best practices.

> **REFLECTION**
>
> *How would you introduce the gap analysis and tool to your colleagues in your setting? In what ways does this process facilitate change management related to uptake of BPGs?*

INTEGRATION

Adoption of clinical and HWE BPGs in LTC homes is compatible with the LTC regulations and requirements for service programs, policies, procedures, clinical care, and workplace practices. This, along with the systematic, inclusive approaches used in implementation, helps to sustain BPG uptake across the sector. LTC BPCs provide expert consultation to LTC home leaders and staff in maintaining a focus on EBP through leveraging regulatory requirements, quality-improvement initiatives, orientation, performance appraisal, and ongoing evaluation and follow-up.

EVALUATION

Evaluation is a critical component of the role of the BPC in their BPG implementation work with the LTC homes. Through full integration of BPGs into required care and service programs and mandatory quality-improvement plans (QIP), the impact of BPG implementation can be measured. LTC homes are mandated to monitor and report on Resident Assessment Instrument-Minimum Data Set (RAI-MDS) quality indicators on a quarterly basis. Several of the LTC quality indicators are publicly reported, and they are important sources of information used by the LTC BPP to gauge the BPG uptake and impact on resident care and workplace outcomes. Staff leads are helped to assess the approaches taken, and their results, to inform subsequent work in relation to the next BPG to be implemented.

LTC BEST PRACTICE GUIDELINES PROGRAM EVALUATION

In April 2014, a two-phase program evaluation, focusing on program structures and processes (phase 1) and program outcomes (phase 2), was carried out by an external evaluator. It included an examination of the entire program across Ontario and implementation activities within individual homes where that information was useful in gleaning promising practices related to overall program delivery.

KEY EVALUATION QUESTIONS (SOURCE: MCGUIRE ASSOCIATES, 2014)

The key evaluation questions for phase 1 and phase 2 of the LTC BPP evaluation were:

1. To what extent was the LTC BPP implemented as planned?

2. Were the recommendations from the pilot project evaluation implemented? Why or why not? What changes have occurred?

3. To what extent did the services and resources provided to LTC homes through the program meet their needs and expectations?

4. What effect did the program have on the use of evidence-based practice in LTC homes?

5. Which of the strategies used by the program contributed most toward LTC homes moving forward in the use of evidence-based practices?

The key questions directed the type and focus of data collection and the data analysis. Results from phase 1 of the program evaluation were very positive, indicating a steady increase in awareness about the program amongst long-term care homes, and strong agreement that services and resources were very useful and making a difference in the homes. Recommendations included strengthening data collection and monitoring processes, in particular striving for consistency and reliability in approaches to gathering and analyzing monitoring data and using it for program planning and reporting.

The results from phase 2 showed that the nature of the relationship between the BPCs and the LTC home in the awareness-raising and implementation phases of the guiding framework was critical in moving the LTC home to BPG uptake. This reinforced the need for consistent coaches and the importance of retaining BPCs in the role over time. In addition, it was clear that in early stages of adoption, homes required much more interaction and support, while those in the later stages of BPG uptake could maintain their work with regular but less-intensive coaching sessions (McGuire Associates, 2015).

IMPACT OF THE PROGRAM ON THE LONG-TERM CARE SECTOR

Included here are two examples from the field as to how specific BPGs were implemented and the impact they have had on resident, provider, and organizational outcomes.

EXTENDICARE HALIBURTON

Extendicare Haliburton, Ontario, Canada, working with its LTC BPC, successfully implemented the RNAO BPG *Promoting Safety: Alternative Approaches to the Use of Restraints* (2012a) across the entire LTC home. The results were spectacular—the facility reduced restraint use from 15.9% to zero over a 2-year period. Implementation activities were based on the three types of recommendations in the BPG and included:

- Revising and implementing a set of behavioural assessment and organizational policies, based on the organizational recommendations

- Developing and implementing care plans, based on the practice recommendations

- Educating staff by developing them as Best Practice Champions to lead practice change, based on the education recommendations

The home's restraint-free practices were shared with new residents, their families, and staff. Residents and family members appreciated understanding how the home's policies were supported by evidence-based recommendations from the RNAO BPG. The team at Extendicare Haliburton committed to providing quality, person-centered care (RNAO, 2012a), and that meant everyone including residents and families understood the benefits of alternative approaches to the use of restraints without compromising resident safety (Wood, 2017). Figure 11.3 depicts restraint use over time at Extendicare Haliburton after implementation of the *Promoting Safety: Alternative Approaches to the Use of Restraints* BPG (2012a) as compared to restraint use regionally, provincially, and nationally.

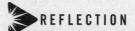

REFLECTION

What factors do you feel contributed to the excellent outcomes experienced by this LTC home in relation to the adoption of the Alternative Approaches to Use of Restraints BPG?

Trend Over Time: Restraint Use in Long-Term Care (Percentage)
Website location: https://yourhealthsystem.cihi.ca/hsp/indepth?lang=en#/indicator/043/4/O99187/

Comparator	2011–12	2012–13	2013–14	2014–15	2015–16
Canada	13.4	11.2	9.6	8.6	7.4
Ontario	13.9	11.0	8.9	7.4	6.0
Central East LHIN	12.1	9.3	7.9	6.7	5.3
Extendicare — Haliburton	15.9	2.9	0.8	0.0	0.0

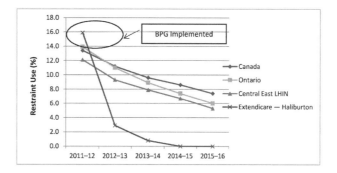

FIGURE 11.3 Organization restraint use over time compared to the region, province, and country.
Source: *Your Health System: Restraint Use in Long-Term Care Details for Extendicare Ontario,* CIHI, 2016. Used with permission of Extendicare Haliburton.

CASE STUDY

TILBURY MANOR

Tilbury Manor is a 75-resident LTC home in Tilbury, Ontario that implemented Best Practice Guidelines to improve resident care and create a healthy work environment. The interprofessional team used several gap-analysis tools to review current practices in relation to the BPG recommendations and created action plans to improve resident outcomes in the required programs (falls prevention and management, skin and wound care, continence care and bowel management, and pain management). Existing policies, resident care practices, and documentation were reviewed to determine the extent to which screening, assessment, and re-assessment tools aligned with RNAO BPGs. From November 2014 to June 2015, Tilbury Manor implemented practice changes based on the recommendations from 12 RNAO BPGs. *Senior Care Canada* magazine featured Tilbury Manor as a cover story for its nomination for the *Ontario Long-Term Care Association's Leadership Excellence Award* in 2015. The article shares their journey in maintaining best practices by "organizing and empowering staff to find solutions" (Patten, 2017).

Program teams, led by nurses and supported by the LTC BPCs, were established to promote practice changes and improve resident outcomes. Each leader was responsible for training and educating staff, implementing practice changes, and evaluating their effectiveness, based on the KTA model as outlined in the RNAO Implementation Toolkit (2012b). Results of chart audits, nursing care reviews, and scores measuring key RAI-MDS indicators of quality in LTC used in many parts of Canada were monitored and regularly reported to the Director of Care to promote continuity and ensure sustainability of practice changes. Within one reporting cycle (fiscal quarter), the RAI-MDS indicators (see Figure 11.4) showed considerable improvements that have been sustained for over 2 years (Le & Faubert, 2016).

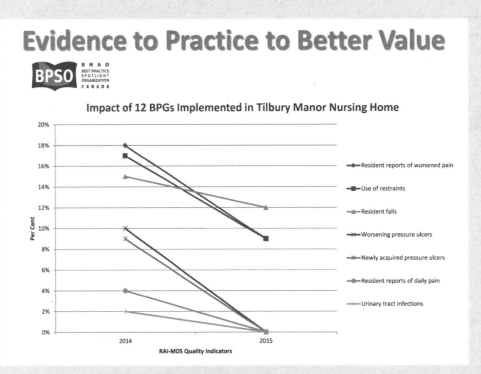

FIGURE 11.4 Impact of 12 BPGs implemented in Tilbury Manor.
Source: Tilbury Manor RAI-MDS quality indicators November 2014 to June 2015.
Implementation of 12 RNAO BPGs improved resident outcomes for seven Resident Assessment Instrument-Minimum Data Set (RAI-MDS) quality indicators. Used with permission.

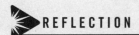

REFLECTION

What are the benefits of monitoring, measuring, and sharing client health outcomes with staff in achieving and sustaining quality care?

FURTHER SCALING UP THROUGH ADAPTATION OF THE RNAO BEST PRACTICE SPOTLIGHT ORGANIZATION DESIGNATION

Once the LTC BPP was soundly established, and considerable effort was spent in building individual capacity related to evidence-based practice and developing a network of Champions within the sector, RNAO turned to spreading its successful organizational implementation strategy—the Best Practice Spotlight Organization Designation (see Chapter 6, *Best Practice Spotlight Organization: Implementation Science at Its Best*)—across the LTC sector by incorporating it into the LTC BPP as the LTC-BPSO. The BPSO Designation, established in 2003, gives organizations the opportunity to formally implement BPGs in partnership with RNAO and was adapted to be consistent with the LTC context.

PURPOSE AND ADAPTATIONS OF THE BPSO DESIGNATION TO LONG-TERM CARE

Through a formal partnership with RNAO, LTC homes create evidence-based cultures in their organizations through the systematic implementation and evaluation of multiple RNAO BPGs over a 3-year period, after which they are designated as LTC-BPSOs. The objectives of the LTC-BPSO Designation are to (RNAO, 2016):

- Establish dynamic, long-term partnerships with LTC settings that focus on making an impact on resident care through supporting knowledge-based nursing practice

- Demonstrate creative strategies for successfully implementing nursing BPGs at the individual and organizational level

- Establish and adopt effective and consistent approaches to evaluate implementation activities utilizing appropriate structure, process, and outcome indicators

- Integrate effective strategies for system-wide dissemination of guideline implementation and outcomes, particularly targeted to LTC

To adapt the BPSO Designation to the LTC sector, an open consultation was held with LTC home leaders to discuss their contextually related challenges and needs in implementing RNAO's BPGs. The program was tailored to provide committed support to the LTC-BPSO homes while maintaining the integrity of the BPSO Designation. The LTC BPCs serve as formal coaches to the LTC-BPSO leadership teams and provide consultation services up to the equivalent of 1 day a week over the initial 3-year predesignation period. LTC-BPSOs work collaboratively with RNAO, and both commit human and financial resources to support achievement of program deliverables.

ORGANIZATIONAL COMMITMENT

The request-for-proposal (RFP) process for the LTC-BPSO began in 2014. As opposed to the 3-year intake of the other Ontario BPSOs, the RFP for LTC-BPSOs is issued annually, and intake has been maintained for 4 successive years since 2014. The increased frequency was established in response to the early positive outcomes achieved by LTC-BPSO predesignate homes and the demand expressed by LTC homes across the province to participate in this meso-level BPG implementation program. In 2017, the first LTC-BPSOs achieved designation. To date, there are 29 LTC-BPSOs—providing care to 3,750 residents—with more planned to come each year.

COLLABORATIVE ROLE OF THE LTC-BPSO COACH AND LTC-BPSO LIAISON

The LTC-BPSO Coach is an RNAO LTC BPC, who supports the LTC-BPSO in the systematic implementation, evaluation, and sustainability of the RNAO BPGs identified by the LTC-BPSO. The LTC-BPSO Coach works directly with the LTC-BPSO Liaison, a staff member of the LTC-BPSO who coordinates implementation and evaluation activities. The coach provides consultation, teaching, support, and role-modeling, using the RNAO Implementation Toolkit (2012b) as a guide to implementation science and through holistic facilitation processes of enabling individuals, teams, and organizations to change (Harvey et al., 2002).

DELIVERABLES

The key requirement for participating LTC-BPSOs is to implement and/or expand the implementation of a minimum of three RNAO clinical BPGs from a select list of BPGs that support quality resident care, are highly relevant to the care of LTC home residents, and are included in legislated required programs for which RNAO has a BPG. At minimum, one of the three clinical guidelines must be implemented across the entire LTC home, while the others may be implemented within specific resident care areas. All BPGs selected must be implemented by the end of the second year, and at least one guideline must be fully implemented in the first year. In year three, the focus is on evaluation and sustainability and preparing for LTC-BPSO Designation.

CAPACITY BUILDING

Consistent with the expectations for all BPSOs, LTC-BPSOs are required to engage at least 15% of caregiving and management staff as RNAO Best Practice Champions over the span of the 3-year predesignation period. The intent is to develop capacity amongst a cohort of direct-care staff, including registered nursing staff, to support guideline implementation and evaluation. In addition, there are requirements for other capacity-building activities, such as attendance at RNAO learning institutes and other professional development offerings related to evidence-based practice and implementation science.

DISSEMINATION

As a way of consolidating, reinforcing, and acknowledging their work, organizations are required to share their key lessons learned, resources developed, and achievements with the LTC sector and the wider healthcare community. In keeping with the resources available in the sector, LTC-BPSOs have a number of in-person and web-based options for disseminating their work. In addition, a minimum of one manuscript is to be submitted for publication in a peer-reviewed or non-peer-reviewed journal by the end of the 3-year predesignation period.

MONITORING AND EVALUATION

As is the case for all BPSOs, mandatory participation in the RNAO international indicator data system, Nursing Quality Indicators for Reporting and Evaluation (NQuIRE) (see Chapter 16, *Evaluating BPG Impact: Development and Refinement of NQuIRE*), is a key deliverable for the LTC-BPSO Designation. NQuIRE collects data on human resource structural indicators, and process and resident outcome indicators. This participation is formalized through a signed agreement with RNAO outlining responsibilities related to monitoring and evaluation requirements, data security, and data sharing. LTC-BPSOs work with the NQuIRE team to select quality indicators related to the guidelines identified for implementation and appropriate to the LTC sector, and data are collected on a monthly basis on these indicators and submitted to the NQuIRE data system. The LTC-BPSOs can retrieve their reports and are required to submit them in progress reports to RNAO, along with results of other regular quality-improvement monitoring activities related to the implementation of each BPG.

SUSTAINING AND SPREADING

At the end of the 3-year LTC-BPSO predesignation period, assuming all deliverables are met, the LTC-BPSO attains "LTC-BPSO Designate" status. This is a renewable designation every 2 years, pending achievement of ongoing requirements consistent with an evidence-based LTC organization continuing to enhance, expand, and spread implementation of best practices. BPSO Designates become mentors to other new LTC-BPSOs at the local, national, and international levels.

SUMMARY OF THE BPSO SCALING UP INITIATIVE

The LTC-BPSO has been a resounding success in creating a culture of evidence-based practice in LTC settings and in improving resident outcomes, particularly in those consistently challenging areas of care for older persons such as wound care, chronic pain, falls, and urinary incontinence. The formula of soundly developed evidence-based practice guidelines and related resources, expert coaches, dedicated organizations that have committed resources, a systematic methodology, and a focus on evaluation and sustainability has meant that long-term care settings have embraced evidence-based practice. This has resulted in unprecedented outcomes in many cases for residents, staff, organizations, and the system.

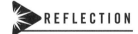

REFLECTION

Why is it so important to tailor programs to the local context, in this case the long-term care context? How do you think this tailoring contributed to the BPSO Designation's success in LTC?

THE IMPACT OF LTC-BPSO AT ST. PETER'S RESIDENCE

St. Peter's Residence at Chedoke (SPR) is a nonprofit LTC home for 210 residents in Hamilton, Ontario, Canada and is part of the Thrive Group. In 2013, SPR responded to the first LTC-BPSO request for proposals. Many factors led senior leaders to recognize the opportunity in pursuing the LTC-BPSO Designation and its focus on evidence-based practice. Ontario LTC homes are required to meet the regulations of the LTC Homes Act, 2007 (Queen's Printer for Ontario, 2007) and to submit annual QIPs that are publicly reported.

The changing resident population within the LTC sector also challenges homes to meet the needs of the residents with complex health conditions, including mental health issues and psychosocial and behavioural symptoms of dementia. Residents, families, and substitute decision-makers are increasingly better informed and expect excellent care and customer service for which they hold the healthcare team accountable. At SPR, Resident and Family Councils are highly involved in decision-making and hold the team accountable for ensuring care and service meets and/or exceeds legislated standards. As LTC homes struggle with limited resources and funding, finding efficiencies (through the use of best practices, developing staff capacity and knowledge, and empowering staff members) is essential.

Leading innovation and enhancing versatility are two of the values of the Thrive Group organizations. As such, the decision to partner with the RNAO as an LTC-BPSO and support SPR in implementing BPGs and making practice changes to improve resident outcomes was consistent with both the values and the current goals and challenges of the sector.

GETTING STARTED

As part of the application process and based on a participatory approach, the SPR team chose one HWE and five clinical BPGs to implement during the 2014–2017 3-year predesignation period. The BPGs implemented included:

- *Client Centred Care* (RNAO, 2006); *Person- and Family-Centred Care* (RNAO, 2015b)

- *Assessment and Management of Pain* (RNAO, 2002, 2007 Supplement, 2013a)

- *Preventing and Addressing Abuse and Neglect of Older Adults: Person-Centred, Collaborative, System-Wide Approaches* (RNAO, 2014)

- *Prevention of Falls and Fall Injuries in the Older Adult* (RNAO, 2005, 2011 Supplement)

- *Promoting Safety: Alternative Approaches to the Use of Restraints* (RNAO, 2012a)

- *Developing and Sustaining Nursing Leadership* (2nd ed.) (RNAO, 2013b)

SPR is committed to the mission, vision, and values of the Thrive Group, ensuring that clients, employees, and all other stakeholders receive excellent quality services. Organizational values include teamwork, honesty, respect, innovation, versatility, and excellence. The LTC-BPSO Program and its focus on evidence-based practice were seen as a way to promote innovation and practice excellence.

At SPR, staff are consistently encouraged and supported to commit to continuous learning and development, always moving forward and building highly efficient programs and services. The rationale for engaging in the LTC-BPSO included: enhancing required care and service programs, empowering nursing staff, increasing the engagement of all disciplines in decision-making, and enhancing collaboration and teamwork. It was also anticipated that this work would inspire a sense of ownership and pride in all staff, encourage shared responsibility and sustainment of desired changes to improve resident care, and address the common barriers to knowledge translation in LTC.

SPR's goals for the LTC-BPSO were as follows:

- Enhance staff knowledge in implementing BPGs

- Review and revise resident care programs related to falls, restraint use, and pain

- Increase awareness of and prevent abuse and neglect to ensure the safety of residents

- Share knowledge and learn from peers to improve nursing services

- Develop staff capacity to engage in BPG implementation

- Review and identify the quality indicators aligned with BPGs selected for implementation

- Develop quality-improvement plans, and evaluate and enhance programs, policies, and processes to achieve improved outcomes for residents, families, and staff

One of the first steps in the predesignation experience was to appoint an LTC-BPSO Liaison and an internal steering committee accountable to the senior leadership team. Operating in an advisory capacity, the committee was responsible for laying the foundation for change and implementing the strategies outlined in the Knowledge-to-Action framework and the *Toolkit: Implementation of Best Practice Guidelines* (RNAO, 2012b; Straus et al., 2013).

The steering committee was highly involved: participating in regular meetings chaired by the LTC-BPSO Liaison, making sure the BPSO remained a priority, contributing to decision-making, and reporting on (as well as providing recognition and acknowledgement of) milestones met. Staff interest in becoming RNAO Best Practice Champions grew far beyond the initial target group of nurses. Participation levels amongst quality-improvement committee members were also high. Both Champions and committee members were responsible for program development and evaluation; annual review of policies and programs; and ensuring best practices through conducting gap analysis, implementation of practices changes, facilitating education, and conducting audit and feedback.

PRACTICE CHANGES AND RESIDENT OUTCOMES

Through the implementation of the BPGs, significant changes to practice were established. The team achieved this by using organizational policy and education recommendations in the relevant BPGs to revise policies and procedures, improve or develop new structures, provide education, and create new tools and processes. These changes included areas related to the clinical and HWE BPGs and spread to other areas of care and services. Some examples include the implementation of recommendations from HWE BPGs within the home's Joint Health and Safety Committee, Employee Wellness program, and Transportation program.

RAI-MDS quality indicators data demonstrated sustained improvement in resident outcomes in all BPGs implemented. For example, the number of resident falls decreased from 21.2% to 16.7% from June 2015 to April 2017 and continues to drop. In conjunction with a decrease in falls, simultaneously an improvement in the percentage of residents in daily physical restraints fell from 2.1% to 0.6% in the same timeframe.

BENEFITS TO THE ORGANIZATIONS, LTC SECTOR, AND SYSTEM

The most significant change through this process was the culture shift in using evidence in practice and sustaining practice change. SPR is recognized by the community for key achievements associated with the LTC-BPSO Designation, which include but are not limited to the following:

- A national journal published a manuscript called *Transformational Leadership at the Point of Care: Approaches and Outcomes in a Long-Term Care Setting* (Karimi, Mills, Clavert, & Ryckman, 2017).

- As part of the implementation of the nursing leadership BPG, SPR developed an internal mentorship program for staff. A poster on the mentorship program was presented at a national nursing conference.

- SPR continues to be invited to present at multiple conferences and events and to mentor other LTC homes with BPG implementation, Champion development, and leadership at the point of care.

- SPR is a member of an international working group with multiple universities to develop a research agenda to understand how to sustain the culture of EBP.

▶ REFLECTION

Consider how engagement of the SPR LTC Home as a BPSO impacted their uptake of BPGs and contributed to positive outcomes for residents, staff, and the organization as a whole. Do you think that SPR is an evidence-based organization?

CONCLUSION

The LTC Best Practices Initiative was formalized as a program under the management of the RNAO in 2008 following a successful 3-year pilot project. Since that time, it has grown to become an extremely successful example of a scaling up strategy that has served to create evidence-based practice cultures and deliver improved clinical outcomes. Through the LTC Best Practices Program, and in particular with the work of the Best Practice Coordinators focused on building individual and organizational capacity, more LTC homes are now expecting all categories of staff to use evidence in their decision-making and have established this as the "modus operandi" for both regulated and unregulated staff members.

Furthermore, scaling up of the specific meso-level BPG implementation strategy, the BPSO Designation, was made possible through its adaptation to the LTC sector. The LTC-BPSO Designation, now spreading rapidly in this sector, has shown considerable promise in improving outcomes for residents and their families; enhancing the quality of care provided by nursing and other staff; and inspiring staff to embrace evidence-based practice, leading to a cultural shift in the sector.

KEY MESSAGES

- Multifaceted approaches—at the individual (micro), organizational (meso), and systems (macro) levels—are necessary to enable the scaling up of practice change within a sector.

- Implementation of BPGs in the LTC sector can have a significant positive impact on resident, provider, and organizational outcomes.

- Meso-level BPG implementation programs, such as the BPSO Designation, that are based on implementation science principles can be successfully adapted and scaled up to address the context of specific sectors, in this case, LTC.

REFERENCES

Baker, C., Ogden, S., Prapaipanich, W., Keith, C. K., Beattie, L. C., & Nickleson, L. (1999). Hospital consolidation: Applying stakeholder analysis to merger life cycle. *Journal of Nursing Administration, 29*(3), 11–12.

Canadian Institute for Health Information (CIHI). (2016). Your health system: Restraint use in long-term care details for Extendicare Ontario. Retrieved from https://yourhealthsystem.cihi.ca/hsp/indepth;jsessionid=eSApTV8b+-JOTqGIIoSQcpE+j.yhs?lang=en#/overall/O99187/4/

Canadian Institute for Health Information (CIHI). (2017, May 31). Canadian Institute for Health information. Retrieved from https://www.cihi.ca/en/access-data-and-reports

Haines Centre for Strategic Management. (2007). The natural cycles of life and change. Retrieved from http://hainescentre.com/rollercoaster/

Harvey, G., Loftus-Hills, A., Rycroft-Malone, J., Titchen, A., Kitson, A., McCormack, B., & Seers, K. (2002). Getting evidence into practice: The role and function of facilitation. *Journal of Advanced Nursing, 37*(6), 577–588.

Holmes, C., & Warner, N. (2013). RNAO's new nursing orientation e-Resource for long-term care. *Long Term Care,* 12–14.

Karimi, B., Mills, J., Clavert, E., & Ryckman, M. (2017). Transformational leadership at the point of care: Approaches and outcomes in a long-term care setting. *Canadian Nursing Home,* 4–7.

Le, S., & Faubert, B. (2016, Winter). Tilbury Manor implements Best Practice Guidelines to improve resident care and create a healthy work environment. *Best Practices in Long-Term Care,* 1–2. Retrieved from http://rnao.ca/sites/rnao-ca/files/LTC_BPP_Newsletter_Winter_2016_FINAL.pdf

Legare, F. (2009). Assessing barriers and facilitators to knowledge use. In S. Straus, J. Tetroe, & I. D. Graham (Eds.), *Knowledge translation in health care: Moving from evidence to practice* (pp. 83–93). Oxford, UK: Wiley-Blackwell/BMJI Books.

Mangham, I. J., & Hanson, K. (2010). Scaling up in international health: What are the key issues? *Health Policy and Planning, 25*(2), 85–96.

McGuire Associates. (2014). *Long-term care best practices program: Phase I evaluation report.* Mississauga, ON: McGuire Associates.

McGuire Associates. (2015). *Long-term care best practices program: Phase II evaluation report.* Mississauga, ON: McGurie Associates.

Ministry of Health and Long-Term Care (MOHLTC) Ontario. (2016). *Long-term care utilization report.* Toronto, ON: Ministry of Health and Long-Term Care.

Nursing Health Services Research Unit (NHSRU). (2007a). *Promoting awareness & uptake of Best Practice Guidelines in long-term care: A process evaluation—Summary of phase I finding.* Toronto, ON: Nursing Health Services Research Unit.

Nursing Health Services Research Unit (NHSRU). (2007b). *Promoting awareness and uptake of best practices in long-term care— An impact evaluation.* Toronto, ON: Nursing Health Services Research Unit.

Ontario Association of Non-Profit Homes and Services for Seniors. (2015). *The need is now: Addressing understaffing in long-term care—Provincial budget submission.* Toronto, ON: Association of Non-Profit Homes and Services for Seniors.

Patten, L. (2017). Organizing and empowering staff to find solutions. *Senior Care Canada, Third Quarter 2017,* 6–8.

Queen's Printer for Ontario. (2007). *Long-Term Care Homes Act, 2007, S/O. 2007, c.8.* Retrieved from https://www.ontario.ca/laws/statute/07l08

Registered Nurses' Association of Ontario (RNAO). (2002, 2007 Supplement). *Assessment and management of pain.* Toronto, ON: Registered Nurses' Association of Ontario.

Registered Nurses' Association of Ontario (RNAO). (2005, 2011 Supplement). *Prevention of falls and fall injuries in the older adult.* Toronto, ON: Registered Nurses' Association of Ontario.

Registered Nurses' Association of Ontario (RNAO). (2006). *Client centred care.* Toronto, ON, Canada: Registered Nurses' Association of Ontario.

Registered Nurses' Association of Ontario (RNAO). (2008, November). *Best Practices in Long-Term care.* Toronto, ON: Registered Nurses' Association of Ontario. Retrieved from http://rnao.ca/sites/rnao-ca/files/Newsletter_-_Fall_2008.pdf

Registered Nurses' Association of Ontario (RNAO). (2012a). *Promoting safety: Alternative approaches to the use of restraints.* Toronto, ON: Registered Nurses' Association of Ontario.

Registered Nurses' Association of Ontario (RNAO). (2012b). *Toolkit: Implementation of Best Practice Guidelines* (2nd ed.). Toronto, ON: Registered Nurses' Association of Ontario.

Registered Nurses' Association of Ontario (RNAO). (2013a). *Assessment and management of pain* (3rd ed.). Toronto, ON: Registered Nurses' Association of Ontario.

Registered Nurses' Association of Ontario (RNAO). (2013b). *Developing and sustaining nursing leadership* (2nd ed.). Toronto, ON: Registered Nurses' Association of Ontario.

Registered Nurses' Association of Ontario (RNAO). (2014). *Preventing and addressing abuse and neglect of older adults: person-centred, collaborative, system-wide approaches.* Toronto, ON: Registered Nurses' Association of Ontario.

Registered Nurses' Association of Ontario (RNAO). (2015a). *Long-term care best practices toolkit* (2nd ed.). Retrieved from http://ltctoolkit.rnao.ca/

Registered Nurses' Association of Ontario (RNAO). (2015b). *Person- and family-centred care.* Toronto, ON: Registered Nurses' Association of Ontario.

Registered Nurses' Association of Ontario. (2016, December 7). *LTC - Best Practice Spotlight Organization designation request for proposals.* Retrieved from Registered Nurses' Association of Ontario: http://rnao.ca/sites/rnao-ca/files/RNAO_LTC-BPSO_Cohort_D_-_FINAL.pdf

Sarayreh, B., Khudair, H., & Barakat, E. (2013). Comparative study: The Kurt Lewin of change management. *International Journal of Computer and Information Technology, 2*(4), 627–629.

Straus, S., Tetroe, J., & Graham, I. (Eds.). (2013). *Knowledge translation in health care* (2nd ed.). Oxford, UK: Wiley-Blackwell.

Wood, C. (2017, Winter). Alternatives to the use of restraints: A long-term care home's experience. *Best practices in long-term care,* p. 5. Retrieved from http://rnao.ca/sites/rnao-ca/files/LTC_BPP_Newsletter_Winter_2017_Feb_3.pdf

INSPIRING AND MANAGING IMPLEMENTATION ON A GLOBAL SCALE

RNAO'S GLOBAL SPREAD OF BPGS: THE BPSO DESIGNATION SUSTAINABILITY AND FIDELITY

Irmajean Bajnok, PhD, MScN, BScN, RN
Doris Grinspun, PhD, MSN, BScN, RN, LLD(hon), Dr(hc), O.ONT
Valerie Grdisa, PhD, MS, BScN, RN

LEARNING OBJECTIVES

After reading this chapter, you will be able to:

- Describe the key factors that have contributed to widespread diffusion of RNAO's evidence-based guidelines

- Identify how the Best Practice Spotlight Organization (BPSO) Designation is critical to RNAO's diffusion of Best Practice Guidelines (BPG) at the meso and macro levels

- Differentiate between a BPSO Direct and BPSO Host, and relate the models to diffusion of innovation theory, sustainability, and fidelity

- Outline key strategies that are used to ensure fidelity of the BPSO Designation as it is operationalized in different contexts worldwide

- Discuss the elements of an effective Training of Trainers (TOT) Model and how these are reflected in RNAO's International BPSO TOT Model

INTRODUCTION

As discussed in previous chapters, RNAO developed a signature program devoted to impacting the practice of nurses through use of best evidence to improve patient outcomes. RNAO's Best Practice Guidelines (BPG) Program, launched in 1999, produces rigorously developed, evidence-based guidelines that translate the latest and best research knowledge into tools for ready use by clinicians. At the same time, RNAO leads a program of diffusion and implementation of these guidelines in practice and academia and helps users evaluate the outcomes. Over the years, various strategies have been utilized to support dissemination and spread of this work, such that RNAO's BPGs are recognized as a global movement in healthcare (Health Council of Canada, 2012; Grinspun, Melnyk, & Fineout-Overholt, 2014; Bajnok, Grinspun, Lloyd, & McConnell, 2015; Gardner, 2010; Grinspun, Lloyd, Xiao, & Bajnok, 2015; Jordan, 2005).

This chapter discusses why RNAO's BPG Program has sustained change and how it has achieved extensive global diffusion. We compare and contrast Rogers' (2003) main elements with key aspects of RNAO's BPG Program that have been central to its success. In doing so, we discuss the program's spread, sustainability, and fidelity—all critical attributes to consider in any large-scale global initiative. We highlight opportunities and challenges and how RNAO is addressing these now and into the future to strengthen the qualities that have propelled the BPG Program into a global movement in evidence-based practice (EBP). This is particularly important to others who seek to influence spread in a program that, like RNAO's BPG Program, has been adopted in different service sectors and academia, geographic locations, contexts, and cultures around the world.

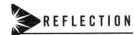 **REFLECTION**

As you read this chapter, consider how involvement of a professional association has influenced the success of the evidence-based practice movement around the world.

ROGERS' DIFFUSION OF INNOVATION AND RNAO'S BPG PROGRAM SUCCESS

Diffusion of innovation is an age-old challenge, first recognized as a sociological concept in the late-18th century and expanded in the area of rural sociology in the mid-19th century (Kinnunen, 1996). Everett Rogers, a professor of rural sociology, advanced the phenomenon through an extensive synthesis of research in this area and published his theory of the adoption of innovation in a groundbreaking publication, *Diffusion of Innovations* (Rogers, 1962). Since then, he has revised the model of diffusion over time (Rogers and Shoemaker, 1971; Rogers, 1983; Rogers, 1995), with the last iteration published in 2003 (Rogers, 2003). It has also been further refined and expanded to fields other than sociology (Berwick, 2003; Greenhalgh, Robert, Bate, Macfarlane, & Kyriakidou, 2005; Meyer, 2004).

Diffusion remains an ongoing quest for those aspiring to advance uptake of new ideas, especially at the systems level (Greenhalgh et al., 2004). In healthcare, diffusion of innovation has been identified as an urgent challenge that is in serious need of attention (Melnyk, 2017). Archie Cochrane first pointed to the negative impact of not integrating evidence into practice in his most influential 1973 publication, *Effectiveness and Efficiency*, where he strongly criticized the lack of reliable evidence behind many of the commonly accepted healthcare interventions at the time. Over 40 years have passed, and it continues to be of grave concern that new knowledge generation at breakneck speed by world-class healthcare researchers is yet to be adopted into daily use by healthcare practitioners (Berwick, Godfrey, & Roessner, 1991, 2002; Grinspun et al., 2014; Melnyk, 2017; Van Achterberg, Schoonhoven, & Grol, 2008).

THE ELEMENTS OF DIFFUSION: FACTORS AND CHARACTERISTICS

Rogers (2003) discusses four factors that influence spread of an innovation:

- The innovation itself

- The means of communication

- Time

- The social system

Rogers (2003) also identifies six characteristics of innovations that determine between 49% and 87% of the variation in their adoption:

- Relative advantage

- Compatibility with existing values and practices

- Degree of complexity and ease of use

- Trialability

- Visible results

- Transferability

Figure 12.1 depicts these factors and characteristics.

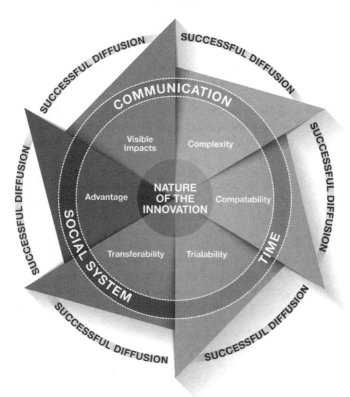

FIGURE 12.1   Model of diffusion of innovation theory, adapted by RNAO from Rogers (2003).
Used with permission.

RNAO's BPG Program, including its most transformative meso-level implementation strategy—the BPSO Designation—are discussed next, paralleling our success to Rogers' key elements of innovation spread and uptake.

THE INNOVATION ITSELF

According to Rogers (2003) and others (Greenhalgh et al., 2004, 2005), the nature of the innovation is a critical factor in its adoption. Those involved in implementation science need to embed the characteristics of successful innovations—relative advantage, compatibility, complexity, trialability, visible results, and transferability—in their planning and implementation efforts. The BPG Program, as a successful innovation, exemplifies these characteristics (Health Council of Canada, 2012).

Advantage

First, Rogers (1983) indicates innovations that demonstrate perceived efficiencies, or show some *advantage* compared to the current system, are likely to be met with less resistance. In the case of the BPGs, these have been perceived as highly advantageous to healthcare organizations and health professionals in all roles to address needed quality improvements. This has been validated by our early adopters in Chapter 7, as well as by others (Jeffs, Lo, Beswick, & Campbell, 2013). With the BPGs, and the related supports offered by RNAO, adopters have a tangible program, evidence-based tools, and a systematic methodology (RNAO, 2012) to tackle the implementation of best evidence and solve some of the thorniest issues in healthcare—pressure injuries, falls, pain, smoking cessation, and breastfeeding rates (Athwal et al., 2014; Gifford et al., 2016; Jennings, O'Neil, Bossy, Dodman, & Campbell, 2016; Johnson-Bhatti, Case, & Shaikh, 2017; Rempel & McCleary, 2012). The evidence behind the key BPG recommendations clearly demonstrates the desired outcomes (advantages) for patients, health providers, and the system.

Compatibility

Rogers' (2003) second characteristic of *compatibility*, how the innovation relates to the pre-existing system, is evident in the BPGs and how the recommendations are structured for implementation. Given that the guidelines include recommendations addressing practice, education, and organizational policy (Grinspun et al., 2014), it is likely that some of these structures, processes, and practices are already in place. Through a gap analysis, a method of analyzing what is already being carried out as compared to the recommended best practices (RNAO, 2012), BPG implementation teams identify what they are doing that matches best practice and what they need to do (Patten, 2017). Invariably, some recommendations are already being implemented, either fully or partially, creating a "we can do it" attitude. Based on their assessment, a guide for what is to be maintained, strengthened, or newly implemented can be developed (Bajnok et al., 2015; Grinspun et al., 2015). This makes the new knowledge compatible with the current system, "makes sense" to both managers and clinicians, and eases the uptake of BPGs (Rogers, 2003). The three types of recommendations also provide a blueprint for how change in practice can be successful with appropriate policy supports and targeted education.

Moreover, another compatibility factor for direct-care nurses, the real targets for the BPGs, is that this innovation focuses on "what they do"—their work with patients. In many cases, innovations in healthcare sorely lack any relevance to the direct-care nurse. That is never the case with BPGs, and these clinicians love it.

Complexity

Third, innovations theory reinforces that the new product must not be too complex and/or it must be easy to learn about. *Complexity*, especially in the absence of visible learning resources, is a major barrier to change (Heath & Heath, 2010). In keeping with this characteristic, RNAO focuses on making evidence-based practice meaningful, easy, and enjoyable to learn. BPG Champion programs are hosted and facilitated around the province of Ontario and have also been delivered in numerous sites across Canada. RNAO invited nurses to engage in the BPG Champion workshops and attracted the innovators and early adopters (Rogers, 2003). These Champions enthusiastically embrace new knowledge, are ambassadors of the change with their peers, and know how to convey the information in ways that can be easily understood (Ploeg et al., 2010).

In 2002, RNAO published its first Implementation Toolkit, which was revised in 2012; it is a highly popular resource that embodies implementation science principles (RNAO, 2002, 2012) and incorporates a step-by-step process to BPG implementation. In 2003, RNAO inaugurated its world-renowned BPG Learning Institute, a 5-day event packed with knowledge transfer, opportunities for application, and network building. The Institute uses dynamic, engaging teaching methodologies and adult learning principles that make learning about EBP and BPGs very meaningful, effective, and fun.

Trialability

Rogers' (2003) fourth characteristic is *trialability* of the innovation, wherein the target just wants to test it out, have a taste, or take a small step. In this regard, organizations are coached by RNAO to get started with the first BPG and to "try it out" on one unit or with one team, then revise and refine from there. Champions are encouraged to work with one peer at a time, helping them understand what evidence-based practice and BPG implementation could mean for their patients and also to their own sense of satisfaction as a nurse (Ploeg et al., 2010). RNAO has a number of communication channels (newsletters, networks, webinars, knowledge-exchange teleconferences) through which organizations can share the results of their trials and lessons learned, and further diffuse the innovation.

Visible Impact

Fifth, a good innovation should *show results*, which is incredible fuel to continue and sustain the innovation (Rogers, 2003). RNAO requires a focus on evaluation right at the outset in implementation of the BPGs (RNAO, 2012). Organizations are helped to identify baseline data so they can gauge their progress. We also encourage realistic goal setting, recognizing that practice change in healthcare has a history of taking up to 17 years (Morris, Wooding, & Grant, 2011). We help staff focus on small steps of change (Grol, Wensing, Eccles, & Davis, 2013; Heath & Heath, 2010; Kotter, 2012), beginning with provider awareness, knowledge, practice change, and then patient outcomes.

With such a focus on the clinical domain of nursing, nurses are invigorated about their practice, have language from the BPGs with which to explain their work, and feel increasing confidence in understanding the knowledge base of their profession and the evidence behind their interventions. Once these results and more improvements are evident to BPG adopters, including higher rates of retention; less variability in care resulting in cost savings; and better outcomes for patients, such as reduced falls and falls injuries (Davies, Edwards, Ploeg, & Virani, 2008; Ireland, Kirkpatrick, Boblin, & Robertson, 2013), adoption becomes an imperative.

Rogers (2003) also discusses the visibility of the innovation or how tangible it is. In order to make the BPGs more tangible, all education sessions and resources define a BPG, so there is clear understanding about what a BPG is (Jeffs, Beswick, Lo, Campbell, Ferris, & Sidani, 2013). Furthermore, in the initial stages of uptake, although RNAO had developed a state-of-the-art BPG website, we were strongly encouraged by the innovators who first used them to have hard copies of the BPGs. They indicated that it was important for nurses to be able to hold a BPG in their hands and have BPGs available to pick up and use.

Transferability

The sixth characteristic of an effective innovation, *transferability*, or use be-yond the initial purpose, is important to mention here because of its impact with the BPG innovation. This last characteristic can also be seen as the degree to which the innovation will spill over into other situations and can be reinvented for other uses (Rogers, 1962, 2003). In the case of the BPGs, there are numerous other impacts that result from engagement in the BPG Program, and three are highlighted in the following discussion.

First, the RNAO Implementation Toolkit (2002) and its second edition (2012), and the many knowledge-translation strategies learned by clinicians as part of implementation science, are useful in other endeavours related to working in the rapidly changing healthcare system. This meant that nurses were more frequently identified to lead other change initiatives in their workplaces. The Implementation Toolkit has also become a teaching resource used by faculty in academic settings. Second, with the advent of BPG Champions, BPG Leaders, and the many opportunities for nurses to be involved with and engaged in BPG development and implementation networks, there has been rapid growth of leadership capacity in the nursing profession. Mid-career nurses in particular have welcomed this for the many career-en-hancement opportunities it brings. Third, because many of the BPG recommendations address other members of the interprofessional team, it eases interprofessional relationships and fosters interprofes-sional care (McKeown, Woodbeck, & Lloyd, 2014).

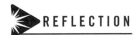
REFLECTION

How have you experienced the characteristics of an innovation as applied to RNAO's BPGs? How has this contributed to diffusion of BPGs in your workplace?

Summary of Characteristics of the Innovation

RNAO's BPGs meet the characteristics of a successful innovation. Some characteristics are innate to the innovation, such as the magnetic clinical focus of the guidelines. Others are by design, as RNAO creates approaches to guideline development, implementation, and evaluation that make BPGs "diffusion-friendly" resources.

Rogers' (2003) work reinforces the need for innovations to meet the above characteristics; however, the nature of the innovation alone is not sufficient for sustained uptake, as there are still the factors of communication of the innovation, the timeframe, and the social system, which must all be considered. These three factors are addressed next in relation to RNAO's successful diffusion of its BPGs.

COMMUNICATION

Communication is extremely important to move the idea about an innovation into the system through various means of information-sharing and promoting its value. According to diffusion theory, two stages of communication are necessary—one that is more general and widespread through mass media, and the other that is more targeted and usually person to person. This helps the potential adopter move from awareness to evaluation of the innovation, and eventually to uptake (Ghoshal & Bartlett, 1988; Rogers, 1983, 2003).

RNAO built powerful communication channels to advance its BPG innovation. The BPG development process itself is a communication channel because it involves a broad range of stakeholders, from the Expert Panel to the reviewers of the draft guideline prior to publication, and the wide dissemination of the guideline once published both in hard copy and on the web.

The BPGs are RNAO branded, prominently featuring the names of the Expert Panel members and all stakeholder reviewers and including photographs of direct-care nurses in practice situations. This serves to both acknowledge all that have contributed, adding to our collective identity (a term discussed in Chapter 1 and later in this chapter), as well as to advance program spread. Various forms of mass communication—to all nurses, other healthcare providers, and stakeholders including government leaders and the public—are used, including RNAO's *Registered Nurse Journal* (Punch, 2016); online newsletter; media releases; news stories; publications; presentations at local, national, and international events; and ongoing learning opportunities that always feature the BPGs.

For example, each year during Nursing Week, RNAO co-hosts in partnership with BPSOs a series of media events to showcase nursing leadership in evidence-based practice, featuring the impact of BPG implementation on patients and families (RNAO, 2015b, 2016a, 2017b). RNAO and healthcare organizations implementing BPGs are also very present in the media, through regular submissions of letters to the editor that respond to key healthcare issues such as breastfeeding, dementia, diabetes, pain management, and sudden infant death syndrome. In this way, important information is provided to the public about best practices related to the respective issue and how nurses are using them with demonstrated results (Bajnok, 2008; Brundage, 2008; Virani, 2007).

Furthermore, RNAO uses its commanding media presence to host press events when initiating and/or releasing specific BPGs with high public interest, such as the elder abuse BPG (RNAO, 2014) and the supervised injection services BPG (RNAO, 2016b). Our BPSOs around the world have learned to use the media as an influential communication channel to reinforce nursing as a knowledge profession making strong contributions to positive health outcomes. In Beijing, China, the launch of their BPSOs was publicized on both of their websites in order to showcase this milestone for nursing (China Care Management, 2015; School of Nursing, Beijing University of Chinese Medicine, 2017). In Colombia, a BPSO Audit was profiled in the media (Vanguardia, 2017).

Person-to-person communication channels are also involved including Champions, Expert Panel members, coaches, BPSO leaders, and RNAO partners, all of whom engage in peer-to-peer communication about available guidelines and their use and impact. The professional association status of RNAO provides ready outreach to all members through chapters and regions and to those members of other like organizations. Through these means, RNAO's BPGs have become known as credible tools that are rigorously developed and easy to use, with proven results (Davies et al., 2008).

TIME

In all diffusion activity, time is a critical factor. Rogers (2003) discusses it as the *rate of adoption*, basically how long it takes to move from awareness to uptake and full use, and also from when the product is first marketed until it can be readily available. As identified in the early exploration of the phenomenon of diffusion, uptake can happen over a long period after introduction of the innovation (Ryan & Gross, 1943). However, RNAO has learned that in most cases with release of a particular BPG, readiness soon follows, and in fact in many cases it is already apparent. RNAO's focus—since the inception of the program—on critical clinical issues in nursing and healthcare as a guide to BPG development priorities greatly influences readiness and therefore uptake (Grinspun, Virani, & Bajnok, 2002).

RNAO is fully aware of the need to be nimble when organizations are ready to adopt BPGs, and we make them highly accessible on the website and in hard copy. Implementation Toolkits are dispatched to sites on request, and BPG Champions trained, with follow-up from RNAO to keep the momentum. Other aspects of time have to do with the BPG development process, which has been reduced sharply from 24 months to 14 months. Once a BPG that reflects a major issue in healthcare is launched in the development phase, there is keen interest in its availability by nurses and other stakeholders. In our case, the shorter the development time the greater the readiness for uptake and successful diffusion.

The passage of time has been most evident in the international uptake of BPGs. Through various networks and communication channels such as the RNAO BPG website, international conferences, and publications, nurses in other countries began to adopt the BPGs in their work and were ready to become Best Practice Spotlight Organizations (BPSO) when that opportunity became available.

THE SOCIAL SYSTEM

The final factor is the social system, or the set of interrelated units that are engaged in joint problem-solving to accomplish a common goal (Rogers, 1983; Strang & Soule, 1998). Rogers maintains that the values and culture of the social system will impact the degree and speed of uptake of an innovation (Rogers, 1983, 2003). Basically, the social system is a gatekeeper and accepts or rejects innovations based on values and norms. RNAO's profile as a professional association of registered nurses, nurse practitioners, and nursing students, and a credible, successful advocate for quality, evidence-based healthcare in the system, means it understands the nursing and healthcare social systems well.

The fact that an organization such as RNAO committed to lead this work for the profession in Ontario is embraced by nursing and health systems. The social system on all levels is addressed by RNAO in the BPG development and implementation work. For example, from the outset, the BPG user targets were broad, with recommendations developed for practitioners, educators, administrators, organizations, and system policy-makers. Therefore, the guidelines encourage full engagement of all elements of the social system. In addition, RNAO actively encourages opinion leaders, Champions, and other BPG leaders in organizations to conduct stakeholder analyses in order to determine the degree of support for and influence in the adoption of the BPG innovation (Baker et al., 1999; Legare, 2009). All of these activities reinforce how the social system is a facilitator in relation to diffusion of the BPGs.

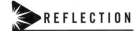 **REFLECTION**

Can you identify how RNAO successfully used diffusion theory in its plans for BPG development, dissemination, and support for uptake?

The narrative above provided an in-depth analysis of the RNAO BPG Program and its BPGs using Rogers' (2003) key factors that influence the spread of an innovation. Included is a discussion of the specific characteristics of successful innovations as they apply to the program and BPGs, as the innovation. The analysis of the BPG Program using the *factors of diffusion* is presented in summary form for the reader in Table 12.1. In Table 12.2, a summary of how the RNAO BPGs and the BPSO Designation reflect the *characteristics of successful innovations* is presented.

TABLE 12.1 COMPARING RNAO'S BPG PROGRAM TO ROGERS' (2003) FACTORS OF DIFFUSION

ROGERS' DIFFUSION OF INNOVATION THEORY: FACTORS THAT INFLUENCE SPREAD	RNAO BPG PROGRAM AND BPGS
The innovation is an idea, or entity, or practice perceived as being new by the unit of adoption—individual or organization or other unit (Rogers, 1983).	▪ The RNAO BPG Program with evidence-based BPGs, as the innovation, was a new entity in the nursing profession in the early 2000s, requiring practice change. See Table 12.2 for an outline of how this innovation reflects the characteristics for successful diffusion or what now is coined as spread.
Adopters are individuals, and/or organizations, or parts or all of a social system (Meyer, 2004). In Rogers' (1983) theory they are categorized, according to the timing and degree of adoption, as innovators, early adopters, early majority, late majority, and laggards.	▪ Adopters are individuals (micro level) attracted through the BPG Champion Network and our powerful communication channels. Many are innovators and early adopters who champion the BPGs to others in various categories of adoption—early majority, late majority, and laggards (Rogers, 1983). ▪ Other adopters, attracted through the BPSO Designation, are BPSO organizations at the meso level and BPSO Host organizations at the macro level.

Communication channels are the means by which the adopters learn about the innovation and are a must if diffusion is to occur (Ghoshal & Bartlett, 1988; Rogers, 1983).	▪ The BPG development process:
	   ▪ The BPG launch
	   ▪ Expert Panel
	   ▪ Stakeholders
	   ▪ BPG release once published, and wide dissemination
	
	 ▪ Mass communication to all nurses, other stakeholders, and the public through RNAO's *Registered Nurse Journal;* online newsletter; media releases; news stories; scholarly publications; presentations at local, national, and international events; and ongoing learning opportunities featuring BPGs
	
	 ▪ Inclusion of all BPG and related resources on the easily accessible RNAO website, available at no cost
	
	 ▪ Person-to-person communication channels involving Champions, Expert Panel members, coaches, BPSO leaders, and RNAO partners engaging in peer-to-peer communication
	
	 ▪ Professional association status of RNAO and ready outreach to all members through chapters and regions, and to members of other like organizations

Time is an element in diffusion, and usually passage of time is necessary for diffusion.	▪ Organizations express readiness for the innovation, given key communication channels used. ▪ RNAO reduced time from initiation to release for guideline development in response to readiness (BPG development time reduced from 24 months to 14 months and less). ▪ RNAO is responsive—Toolkits are dispatched to sites, on request, and Champions are trained. ▪ Passage of time has influenced worldwide dissemination of all BPGs across all sectors, including governments and academia.

continues

TABLE 12.1 COMPARING RNAO'S BPG PROGRAM TO ROGERS' (2003) FACTORS OF DIFFUSION (CONTINUED)	
ROGERS' DIFFUSION OF INNOVATION THEORY: FACTORS THAT INFLUENCE SPREAD	**RNAO BPG PROGRAM AND BPGS**
The social system is the context of the adopter, including internal and external influences, values, and norms (Rogers, 1983; Strang & Soule, 1998).	■ The social system is a facilitator in relation to diffusion of the BPGs. ■ RNAO's status as a powerful and evidence-based professional association gives it a sound understanding of the nursing and health and healthcare systems, inspiring respect for the BPG Program. ■ The social system on all levels is addressed by RNAO BPG development and implementation—BPG user targets are broad, with recommendations developed for practitioners, educators, administrators, organizations, and system policymakers. ■ Guidelines encourage full engagement of all elements of the social system. ■ RNAO actively encourages opinion leaders, Champions, and other leaders to conduct stakeholder analyses.

BPSO DESIGNATION: SUCCESSFUL DIFFUSION AT THE ORGANIZATIONAL LEVEL

In order to speed up the rate of diffusion of BPGs and ensure sustainability, RNAO began to formally target organizations as adopters and shifted its energies for implementation to the meso (organizational) level with the creation of the Best Practice Spotlight Organization (BPSO) Designation. RNAO's intent with BPSOs is to embed EBP into the culture of an organization, thereby sustaining BPG use in a way not possible with a focus only on individuals. BPG Champions, competent ambassadors of EBP, have provided feedback that their work is not enough to effect sustained change in practice, education, and policy at the meso level in a timely manner.

As outlined in Chapter 6, *Best Practice Spotlight Organization: Implementation Science at Its Best*, BPSOs are organizations that are selected by a request-for-proposal application process to partner directly with RNAO (through a formal signed Agreement) to implement multiple clinical guidelines. These are called BPSO Direct organizations. Some of the guidelines selected by BPSOs must be implemented at the unit/team level and others at the organizational level, truly engaging the entire organization. Very specific deliverables expected of the BPSOs relate to: establishing an infrastructure, building capacity in EBP and implementation science, implementing the guidelines, dissemination of implementation efforts, results and outcomes, evaluation, regular meetings with RNAO and peer BPSOs, and biannual reports to RNAO (Bajnok et al., 2015).

This formalized organizational meso level knowledge-translation strategy commenced in 2003, and every 3 years RNAO accepts a new cohort of BPSOs in Ontario, Canada, with the most recent cohort launched in 2018. The LTC BPSO Designation tailored to this sector has some differences in BPSO intake time and other parameters as discussed fully in Chapter 11, *Evidence-Based Practice in Long-Term Care*. Beginning with nine Canadian spotlights, the BPSO Designation has expanded in Canada and since 2012 opened its doors to the world, encompassing today more than 100 BPSOs representing over 550 healthcare and academic organizations. This indicates the massive growth in 15 years, since each BPSO can represent a number of organizations either as part of a corporation, a recent amalgamation, a Canada-wide health service incorporating several provincial jurisdictions, or a whole country as is the case in Spain (for the latter, see Chapter 13, *BPSO Host: A Model for Scaling Out Globally*). The numbers of healthcare providers and organizations using BPGs and the number of BPSOs worldwide have clearly reached a critical mass (Rogers, 2003).

The first cohort of BPSOs that eagerly stepped forth to partner with RNAO to create and sustain evidence-based cultures (Bajnok et al., 2015; Higuchi, Davies, Edwards, Ploeg, & Virani, 2011; Higuchi, Davies, & Ploeg, 2017) were spurred on by their BPG Champions, who themselves were innovators and early adopters. These organizations represented large acute care settings in Toronto and northern Ontario, and also two large home health settings and one large rehabilitation hospital (see Chapter 7, *The BPSO Pioneers: Creating, Sustaining, and Expanding Evidence-Based Cultures Through the BPSO Designation*). All had substantial numbers of nurses, were looking to create meaningful work for their staff, and were prepared to target resources to knowledge translation for quality improvement to achieve better patient outcomes. These pioneers, most of whom have retained their designation over the past 15 years, demonstrate sustainability above the norm (Davies, Tremblay, & Edwards, 2010; Higuchi, Downey, Davies, Bajnok, & Waggott, 2013). They have also paved the way and have become exceptional mentors to novice BPSOs, a much-needed strategy in EBP implementation (Grinspun et al., 2014; Melnyk, 2007, 2014; Stetler, Richie, Rycroft-Malone, & Charns, 2014).

From acute care teaching hospitals to large home healthcare organizations, the BPSOs have spread throughout the health sectors, including community hospitals, public health, primary care, and long-term care, as well as academic settings (Bajnok et al., 2015). In fact, to support the ever-growing cohort of academic BPSOs, RNAO developed the *Educator's Resource* (2005), much like the Implementation Toolkit initially developed in 2002, to be used as a guide to integrate BPGs throughout the curriculum, address change challenges, align teaching methodology with BPG integration, and evaluate outcomes. Moreover, RNAO has collaborated with faculty to develop resources for undergraduate nursing curricula to support integration of specific BPGs such as the *Nurse Educator Mental Health and Addiction Resource* (RNAO, 2017a) and *Nursing Faculty Education Guide (NFEG): Tobacco Use and Associated Health Risks* (RNAO, 2010).

The approach to diffusion of the BPSO Designation and its rapid uptake around the world reflect Rogers' diffusion theory in ways similar to uptake of the BPGs. Table 12.2 summarizes the discussion of the BPG Program and the BPSO Designation in relation to Rogers' (2003) theory of diffusion and shows how each meet the six characteristics of a successful innovation.

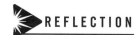 **REFLECTION**

How do the characteristics of the BPSO Designation link to diffusion theory? How did attention to this theory help overcome potential challenges of organizational adoption of evidence-based practice?

TABLE 12.2   APPLICATION OF ROGERS' (2003) CHARACTERISTICS OF SUCCESSFUL INNOVATIONS TO RNAO BPGS AND THE BPSO DESIGNATION

CHARACTERISTIC OF SUCCESSFUL INNOVATIONS (ROGERS, 2003)	BPGS AS AN INNOVATION	BPSO DESIGNATION AS AN INNOVATION
Advantage	■ Advantageous to healthcare organizations and staff working to address quality improvements ■ Offers a tangible program, evidence-based tools, and a systematic methodology (RNAO, 2012) to use in tackling the implementation of best evidence ■ Tools are now available to solve issues in healthcare—pressure injuries, falls, pain, smoking cessation, and breastfeeding. ■ Evidence in BPGs demonstrates the potential advantages to the users and, ultimately, the patients.	■ The BPSO Designation provides a tangible program to support organization-wide implementation of EBP, and taking action to resolve some key healthcare issues. ■ Evidence-based BPGs and implementation resources, including systematic methodology for implementation, are perceived as advantageous to the organizations. ■ The BPSOs engage and involve nurses directly in leading evidence-based solutions for clinical issues through BPG implementation.
Compatibility	■ Gap analysis helps determine what is being done right and gives information for development of a plan increasing compatibility with current work. ■ The three types of recommendations provide a blueprint for how change in practice can be successful with appropriate policy supports and focused education. ■ Compatible with direct-care nurses, this innovation is focused on "what they do," their work with patients, and is welcomed.	■ Given that the BPSO Designation bundles numerous approaches based on implementation science, it simplifies the knowledge transfer and BPG implementation, influencing the speed of uptake and further aiding diffusion across health sectors and borders. ■ The formal Agreement with RNAO clearly identifies the supports available from RNAO and expectations of the organizations. ■ RNAO hosts webinars in advance of BPSO application due dates to provide information. ■ The BPSO Orientation Program brings clarity to the BPG implementation and evaluation processes.
Complexity	■ Focus on making EBP meaningful, easy, and enjoyable to learn ■ BPG Champion programs are hosted and facilitated. ■ The Champions are also ambassadors of the change with their peers and can simplify information for them. ■ RNAO's Implementation Toolkit was developed, which embodies implementation science and incorporates a step-by-step process to BPG implementation.	■ BPSO applicants are expected to have had some success already in BPG implementation. ■ Many organizations have a critical mass of BPG Champions. ■ The BPSO activities provide an approach organizations are committed to carrying out for quality patient care according to their vision, mission, and values. ■ BPSOs identify BPGs that align with their priorities and quality-improvement challenges, within the parameters of the BPSO Agreement.

CHARACTERISTIC OF SUCCESSFUL INNOVATIONS (ROGERS, 2003)	BPGS AS AN INNOVATION	BPSO DESIGNATION AS AN INNOVATION
Complexity (continued)	■ RNAO inaugurated the Clinical BPG Learning Institute, which makes learning this innovation very accessible, fun, and effective, through sound content and engaging, participatory, action-oriented methodology.	■ Opportunities for mentoring from other BPSOs and the peer collaboration and support in each cohort of BPSOs reduces complexity and helps address challenges.
Trialability	■ Organizations are coached by RNAO to get started with the first BPG and to "try it out" on one unit or with one team, then revise and refine and take next steps. ■ Champions are encouraged to work with one peer at a time and help them to understand what EBP and BPG implementation could mean. ■ RNAO set up communication channels so organizations can share the results of their trials, and lessons learned, and widen the spread.	■ Although the BPSO signs a formal Agreement, there is an option to end the Agreement. ■ The 3-year timeframe, along with RNAO supports and peer support throughout the BPSO qualifying period and following qualification as a BPSO Designate, helps organizations to address issues one step at a time. ■ There is opportunity for an extension of the predesignation period should an organization require it.

Tangible innovation and visible impacts	■ To make BPGs more tangible, all education sessions and resources provide a discussion of BPGs, what they are, why they are important, and how to use them.
	
	■ In the initial stages of uptake, RNAO produced hard copies of the BPGs so nurses could hold a BPG in their hands and have them available to pick up and use.
	
	■ RNAO encourages a focus on evaluation at the outset in implementation of the BPGs.
	
	■ Organizations are helped to identify baseline data so they can gauge their progress.
	
	■ Realistic goal setting is encouraged.
	
	■ Small steps of change are a focus, beginning with provider awareness, knowledge, practice change, and then patient outcomes.
		■ The BPSO Model includes a focus on several areas to ensure robust evaluation of the BPG implementation efforts by BPSOs, including:
		
		  ■ Submission of data to NQuIRE (RNAO's data system), as well as through assessment of structures, processes, and patient outcomes
		
		  ■ Monthly knowledge-exchange sessions with peer BPSOs, regular reporting to RNAO, and requirements for dissemination all contribute to visible outcomes from the innovation.
		
		  ■ Biannual reporting into RNAO's myBPSO, which is the online reporting system
		
		  ■ Secondary data analysis of other health system data repositories to complement NQuIRE data analysis
		
		  ■ This supports triangulation of quantitative and qualitative data within the different analytic approaches in our framework to respond to various research and evaluation questions, methods, and methodologies. (See Chapter 16, *Evaluating BPG Impact: Development and Refinement of NQuIRE*)

continues

TABLE 12.2   APPLICATION OF ROGERS' (2003) CHARACTERISTICS OF SUCCESSFUL INNOVATIONS TO RNAO BPGS AND THE BPSO DESIGNATION (CONTINUED)

CHARACTERISTIC OF SUCCESSFUL INNOVATIONS (ROGERS, 2003)	BPGS AS AN INNOVATION	BPSO DESIGNATION AS AN INNOVATION
Tangible innovation and visible impacts (continued)	■ Early results are shared widely through communication channels. ■ For nurses: They are invigorated about their practice, have language from the BPGs with which to explain their work, and feel increasing confidence in understanding the knowledge base of their profession and evidence-based interventions. ■ For patients: They experience better outcomes such as reduced falls and fall injuries. ■ For organizations: They report increased retention of nurses and less variability in care, resulting in cost savings.	■ Evaluation is a key component of BPSO deliverables, both through submission of data to NQuIRE (RNAO's data system), as well as through assessment of structures, processes, and patient outcomes.
Usefulness in other situations	■ Numerous other transferable impacts from this innovation: ■ Nurses and others learn about change management and practice change. ■ Nurses assume leadership roles in other change initiatives. ■ Faculty use implementation resources in teaching. ■ Broad leadership capacity building for nurses and other clinicians ■ Career boost for mid-career nurses ■ Stronger interprofessional relationships and interprofessional care	■ The expectations related to the BPSO Program enhance professional practice, interprofessional practice, and the organizational profile as an EBP culture. ■ Increased engagement and morale of nurses and other clinicians ■ There are strong links between BPSO and accreditation success, and BPSOs in LTC incorporate their BPG implementation efforts and outcomes in their required Quality Improvement Plans submitted to the government to support funding. ■ BPSOs in all sectors, and especially in hospitals, home care, and LTC, are achieving top scores in quality improvements and financial efficiencies. ■ BPSO enrollment has assisted several hospitals secure their Magnet status.

BPSO HOST MODEL: SUCCESSFUL DIFFUSION AT THE MACRO GLOBAL LEVEL

The creation of the BPSO Host Model was the next step in RNAO's approach to diffusion, from micro-level diffusion with the BPG Champion Network, to meso-level diffusion with the BPSO Direct Model, to macro-level diffusion with the BPSO Host Model. RNAO was spurred onto the development of the BPSO Host Model by the great enthusiasm shown by nurse leaders in Spain regarding RNAO's work in policy and evidence-based guidelines and our active implementation through the BPSO Designation. The vision of RNAO leadership to extend the BPSO Designation to incorporate satellite sites around the world (BPSO Host Model), with Spain as the first innovator BPSO Host, was the springboard to a rapid global spread. From this beginning in Spain in 2012 (Grinspun, 2011; Albornos-Munoz, González-María, & Moreno-Casbas, 2015), other BPSO Hosts have been established in Australia, Italy, Peru, and Chile. Logos from some of these Hosts are included in Figure 12.2. In addition, RNAO continues using the BPSO Direct Model to establish centers of evidence-based practice in countries like Belgium, China, Colombia, Nova Scotia (Canada), Portugal, and Jamaica, some of which will in time become BPSO Hosts and extend the spread throughout their jurisdictions.

The evidence-based practice movement, led by RNAO and impacting nursing and healthcare on a global level, has affected practice change, policies at organizational and systems levels, the image of nursing, the scope of practice of nurses, governance and decision-making structures, and monitoring and evaluation of outcomes. From Canadian BPSOs in public health, primary care, hospitals, home care, and long-term care, to service organizations and academic institutions in Australia, Belgium, Chile, China, Colombia, Italy, Jamaica, Peru, Portugal, Qatar, and Spain, there has been a sustained shift in how care is delivered and how students are taught. This has bolstered the degree of nursing pride and satisfaction and strengthened the status and place of nursing on the healthcare team (RNAO, 2015a).

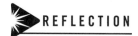

REFLECTION

What other examples can you think of where change in practice has influenced the organization or system more broadly? How do you think involvement of a professional association and its partnerships influenced the changes generated by the BPSO global spread?

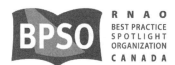 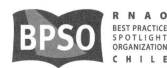 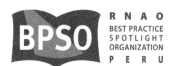

FIGURE 12.2   Logos from BPSO Hosts in Canada, Chile, and Peru.

MAXIMIZING SPREAD WHILE MAINTAINING BPG PROGRAM AND BPSO FIDELITY

As we enable global spread, RNAO is paying close attention to the systems and processes necessary to ensure BPSO fidelity. Mowbray, Holter, Teague, and Bybee (2003) define *fidelity* as the degree to which program delivery is consistent with the program model as planned by the developers. Carroll et al. (2007), in crafting a conceptual framework for implementation fidelity, purport that attention to fidelity is critical in being able to determine program impacts and prevent inaccurate conclusions about a program's effectiveness. They reinforce the importance of this, stressing that program fidelity affects how well it succeeds.

There is general agreement (Dane & Schneider, 1998; Durlak & DuPre, 2008; Dusenbury, Brannigan, Falco, & Hanson, 2003; Fagan, Hanson, Hawkins, & Arthurs, 2008) that fidelity implementation can be measured through a review of the following components that should be part of all program evaluation. These components are:

- **Adherence**—How well the program meets the requirements

- **Exposure**—The extent of program delivery, how widespread it is

- **Quality of delivery**—Its ability to reflect program standards and values to a high degree

- **Participant responsiveness**—The extent of engagement, level of interest, belief in usefulness of the program, and enthusiasm

- **Program differentiation**—The distinctiveness of each component of the program, including those with most impact

Alternatively, in recognizing the concepts of fidelity and fit and their inherent tensions (Castro, Barrera, & Martinez, 2004), Chambers, Glasgow, and Stange (2013) discuss the importance of dynamic sustainment that acknowledges evolution of EBP interventions over time and contexts, and they assert that dynamic sustainability is necessary in order to respond to contextual realities and keep programs relevant to the users. Chambers et al. (2013) reinforce the need for program targets to be able to contribute to the program and co-create some aspects to ensure relevance and sustainability within the program parameters.

These are all critical considerations in the ongoing expansion and spread of the BPSO Designation and present challenges that RNAO's program of quality assurance and fidelity has kept in focus, including:

- Ensuring the BPSO Designation remains consistent in all aspects: when RNAO acts as the BPSO Host; when an organization outside RNAO acts as a BPSO Host; when BPSOs are overseen by BPSO Hosts in other jurisdictions

- Balancing continued contextual relevance, along with sustainment and fidelity

- Maintaining communication channels to keep BPSO Hosts and RNAO BPSO Direct organizations informed about changes in the BPSO Designation

- Fostering a collective identity amongst all BPSO organizations as part of a global evidence-based practice movement

Each aspect of the fidelity process is designed to meet one or more of the four goals identified above. As discussed at the outset of this book, a key success factor of RNAO's program and especially of its BPSOs is that it has created a sense of *collective identity*, which is a major influencer of sustainability, fidelity, and accelerated diffusion (see Chapter 1, *Transforming Nursing Through Knowledge: The Conceptual and Programmatic Underpinnings of RNAO's BPG Program*). Collective identity of the BPSOs reflects the values of the BPSO Designation. It is expressed through the intense pride organizations have in being a BPSO and part of the global EBP movement through sustained implementation of RNAO BPGs and ongoing evaluation and dissemination of their impact. Collective identity is evident in:

■ The display of the logo on organizational materials

■ Open sharing and building of new tools and approaches together across borders

■ Dissemination of outcomes in presentations and publications

■ Ready agreement to be part of all aspects of the program—whether it be guideline development, implementation, evaluation, teaching, mentoring, or auditing

■ The intense work by all BPSOs to make use of best evidence better and better for patients

This section discusses the various ways RNAO has addressed fidelity of the BPSO Designation as it expands and spreads. They encompass approaches that enable dynamic sustainment (Chambers et al., 2013) of a quality EBP initiative that impacts effective guideline uptake across global contexts, and address each of the five components discussed above. The quality assurance and fidelity assessment components incorporate: 1) the BPSO Orientation Program; 2) the Certified BPSO Orientation Trainer process; 3) the audit and feedback requirement; 4) the NQuIRE Data System and MyBPSO Reports; 5) the use of technology to provide education and consultation; 6) approaches to translation; and 7) ongoing program requirements.

These are all apparent when measuring fidelity, in particular the components of quality and participant responsiveness.

THE BPSO ORIENTATION PROGRAM

The 5-day BPSO Orientation Program provides foundational knowledge and skills to the identified group of stakeholders and Champions who will lead the BPSO process in their organization, including specific BPG implementation. This Orientation Program is based on the RNAO Implementation Toolkit (2012), uses several examples of successful BPG implementation and achievements of BPSOs, and consists of curriculum components based on the Knowledge-to-Action framework (Straus, Tetroe, & Graham, 2013). It serves as the training program for BPSO Sponsors, BPSO Leads, and Champion Leaders, who in turn train BPG Leads and Champions in a workshop targeted to their roles in accomplishing BPSO deliverables including BPG implementation.

All BPSOs and BPSO Hosts begin their BPSO Designation work with the Orientation Program, which is delivered in a consistent manner in all settings. Where possible, participants from different BPSOs attend the orientation together, contributing to their collective identity as BPSOs. RNAO leads the orientation for its BPSO Direct organizations as well as new BPSO Host organizations and provides ongoing support according to the BPSO Agreement. Once fully oriented, BPSO Hosts plan and lead the orientation for BPSOs in their own jurisdictions and continue with the follow-up monitoring and support.

Participants receive a workbook prepared by RNAO, complete with objectives, content, handouts, application exercises, and reference material for each session. The teaching methodology (as critical as the content) is built on a model of sustainable capacity building and includes personal goal setting, critical knowledge exchange, engagement, application exercises reflecting their context, network building, individual and group leadership opportunities, and action planning. For many nurses outside of North America, these sessions introduce an entirely new approach to teaching and learning and build knowledge and understanding, and ability to apply theory, as well as confidence and skill in articulating the rationale for evidence-based practice and the value and impact of nursing.

The BPSO Orientation Program is led by RNAO International BPSO Coaches—as *BPSO Master Trainers*. In the case of orientation for BPSO Hosts, the BPSO Orientation Program incorporates a train-the-trainer process at the outset, wherein RNAO trains the BPSO Host Lead as a *Certified BPSO Host Master Trainer* for future delivery of the program to continue capacity development and BPSO spread in their jurisdiction. For new BPSO Direct organizations, the RNAO BPSO Master Trainers, BPSO Host Master Trainers, and/or a *Certified BPSO Orientation Trainer* (CBOT) conduct their orientation. CBOTs are registered nurses who meet set criteria and undergo training with the Master Trainer, be it RNAO or the BPSO Host. More details about the RNAO International BPSO Training of Trainers Model are discussed later in this chapter.

The Training of Trainers Model for BPSO Hosts benefits both the BPSO initiative in that country and the overall BPSO Program. Not only does the country-specific initiative build on a partnership model and extend RNAO resources, it also contributes to capacity development and the collective identity of BPSOs, working collaboratively with each other.

BPSO AUDIT AND FEEDBACK REQUIREMENT

The Cochrane Effective Practice and Organization of Care (EPOC) group defines *audit and feedback* as a synopsis of clinical behaviours of health practitioners related to their care, over a specific timeframe, in order to modify such behaviours according to a standard (Grimshaw, Eccles, Lavis, Hill, & Squires, 2012). The synopsis may result from observed practice, outcomes, and/or written records, and include recommendations and action plans (Grimshaw et al., 2012). In exploring effective interventions to improve health outcomes, Grimshaw et al. (2012) analyzed key Cochrane reviews of professional behaviour change strategies, including audit and feedback. They identified that important elements of effective audit and feedback are: an objective standard, provision of feedback with recommendations, and an action plan. Grimshaw and colleagues (2012) concluded that audit and feedback are useful tools because up to almost a third of the time, professionals rate their performance at levels higher than actual (Adams, Soumerai, Lomas, & Ross-Degnan, 1999). Audit and feedback, by exposing this discrepancy, can stimulate behaviour change. In more in-depth secondary analyses of these systematic reviews, Ivers and colleagues (2014) verified these findings and asserted that audit and feedback indeed works.

Consistent with these views related to motivating professional behaviour change, RNAO's attention to BPSO quality includes an annual audit of the BPSO in years two and three of the prequalifying period. Through the required audit and feedback processes, site visits are made to the BPSO Hosts and BPSO Directs. The BPSOs are informed in advance that the visit will take place within a mutually agreed upon timeframe. They are advised that we expect to observe evidence of the required deliverables as outlined in the BPSO Agreement. These deliverables include infrastructure, capacity building, BPG implementation, dissemination, and evaluation, as well as in-time practice and/or teaching observations according to the recommendations contained in the selected BPGs. Specific audit tools have been developed for BPSO Hosts, as well as Direct Service and Academic BPSOs, which reflect the BPSO Agreement deliverables and serve as criteria for the audit. The audit tools guide the BPSO audit visit and assist in determining strengths and areas for growth for provision of timely feedback to BPSOs. BPSO Hosts conduct audits with their BPSO Directs; RNAO audits the BPSO Directs for which it is responsible, as well as all the BPSO Hosts.

During the onsite audit, an initial meeting is held and presentations are made by the BPSO or BPSO Host reflecting major aspects of the cultural shift that has taken place over the past year. In service BPSO audits, this meeting is attended by key organizational stakeholders including senior management, the BPSO Lead, specific BPG Champions, and other leaders, all of whom have a role to play in the presentation. Visits are then made to specific units/teams where BPGs are being implemented, and the auditors observe practice situations and speak with nurses, physicians, other members of the team, and patients. If students and faculty are part of the audited unit or team, they participate as well. This type of visit can take from 3 to 4 days depending on the size of the BPSO and number of units and teams involved. When an academic BPSO is audited, the same process is used involving senior academic administration, BPSO Leads, faculty, and students, and observations are made of the curriculum, teaching materials, and teaching-learning situations.

Consistent with the recommendations of Ivers et al. (2014) and Grimshaw et al. (2012), relative to an effective audit and feedback process, the visit concludes with a final opportunity for the organization to review highlights, followed by a presentation from the auditors. The auditors present a summary of the strengths and necessary improvements according to the criteria, and recommendations for follow-up are outlined and discussed. Within a 2-week period, the BPSO receives a written summary with the recommendations that are to be addressed by the BPSO in a plan of action. Coaching and monitoring continues, and progress is measured through regular meetings, biannual reports, and future audits.

NQUIRE DATA SYSTEM AS A FIDELITY AND QUALITY ASSURANCE STRATEGY

RNAO's focus on a consistent means of evaluation of BPG implementation through NQuIRE (see Chapter 16, *Evaluating BPG Impact: Development and Refinement of NQuIRE*) also acts as a quality assurance strategy (Grinspun et al., 2015). All BPSOs are required to submit data on quality indicators defined in data dictionaries for the NQuIRE international data system. Human resource structural indicators are submitted for the BPSO and implementation sites, as are the evidence-based process and outcome indicators specific to each BPG. Regular communication with BPSOs, and review of the NQuIRE results in the biannual report submissions to RNAO, ensure that BPSOs are consistent in their focus on key interventions and in how they measure both practice changes and BPG impacts. NQuIRE is enabling RNAO, BPSO Hosts, and BPSO Direct organizations to review implementation across jurisdictions or units and teams, which helps identify trending of outcomes that can lead to further opportunities for quality-improvement practices.

USE OF TECHNOLOGY TO PROVIDE EDUCATION AND CONSULTATION

In an effort to better prepare local, national, and international BPSOs, RNAO devised a boot camp methodology to exchange knowledge on critical aspects of the BPG Program and BPSO Designation. These include face-to-face interactive sessions attended by Ontario BPSOs in person and virtual boot camps organized for national and international BPSOs. Such sessions have provided information about the NQuIRE data system, guidance for selecting indicators and submitting data, and the opportunity to troubleshoot problems and to have hands-on experience using the NQuIRE demonstration site. This mode of interactive education serves as another means to ensure consistent approaches to data submission that meet the quality standards. It also provides opportunities for BPSOs to meet via interactive web-conferencing platforms. It is important in our focus on global uptake that we offer similar education, coaching, and feedback opportunities to local, national, and international partners, and build collective identity amongst BPSOs.

APPROACHES TO TRANSLATION

Currently, RNAO has a formal translation process that guides the translation of BPGs and various resources and supports into a variety of languages. The process includes a signed Agreement between RNAO and the organization sponsoring the translation, stipulating their responsibilities for funding the initial translation, and our mutual engagement in reverse translation and other validating processes. An ever-critical aspect of quality control is accurate translation of the evidence-based tools that reflects the evidence and the intent of the recommendations and is consistent with language and cultural nuances.

ONGOING BPSO DESIGNATION REQUIREMENTS AND OPPORTUNITIES

The stringent requirements to become a BPSO Designate and to retain the Designation, as outlined in Chapter 6 and highlighted throughout this chapter, are also key factors that impact program fidelity. These requirements ensure program consistency and fidelity. Opportunities for meetings and interactive reviews of processes and outcomes, including NQuIRE outcomes, contribute to BPSOs' understanding of the program requirements and RNAO's ability to monitor that the BPSOs have met the requirements. BPSOs have a wealth of opportunities to be informed about and engaged in aspects of BPG development, implementation, and evaluation. They may contribute as BPG development Expert Panel members; stakeholder reviewers of guidelines, implementation tools, indicators, and other program proposals; and members of advisory committees.

Table 12.3 summarizes the goals of RNAO's process of measuring implementation fidelity and the key components relevant to each goal.

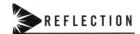

REFLECTION

How will attention to quality assurance and fidelity of the BPG implementation and the BPSO Designation assist in building nursing as a knowledge profession, and creating evidence-based cultures the world over?

TABLE 12.3 GOALS OF RNAO'S PROCESS OF MEASURING IMPLEMENTATION FIDELITY AND THE KEY COMPONENTS RELEVANT TO EACH GOAL

GOAL OF FIDELITY	KEY FIDELITY PROGRAM COMPONENTS TO ADDRESS GOAL
Ensure the BPSO Designation remains consistent in all aspects when RNAO acts as the BPSO Host; when an organization outside RNAO acts as a BPSO Host; when BPSOs are overseen by BPSO Hosts in other jurisdictions	■ BPSO Orientation Program ■ Certified BPSO Orientation Program Trainer ■ Regular knowledge exchange meetings amongst RNAO and BPSOs organized by country, region, designation status, and/or type or model of BPSO ■ RNAO's annual audit and feedback process with the BPSO when RNAO acts as the Host, and of the BPSO Host with selected visits to BPSOs ■ Annual audit and feedback process conducted by BPSO Host ■ Review of reports including NQuIRE and myBPSO reports ■ Translation process
Balance continued contextual relevance, along with sustainment and fidelity	■ Formal and informal opportunities to provide feedback ■ Sharing of context-related strategies in meetings, reports ■ Opportunities to be stakeholders, reviewers, and/or give input to BPGs, BPG development process, implementation tools, BPG evaluation, NQuIRE, BPSO Agreements ■ Membership on advisory committees related to major program elements, development, implementation, and evaluation ■ Audit site visits to see context and how BPSO is relevant in the context
Maintain communication channels to keep BPSO Hosts informed about changes in the BPSO Designation; and monitor achievements	■ RNAO website ■ Connection with RNAO Coach and regular meetings and knowledge exchange sessions with RNAO and BPSOs ■ BPG Newsletter ■ Regular reports with discussion ■ Similar processes carried out by BPSO Hosts with their BPSOs—website, newsletter, meetings, and reporting ■ Several knowledge tools to assist in understanding specific BPGs and their application, including webinars, eLearning programs, BPG quick reference guides, NQUIRE updates, and overall reporting requirements
Cultivate a collective identity amongst all BPSOs as part of a global evidence-based practice movement	■ BPSO is a partnership. ■ Collective meetings with all BPSOs ■ Annual international BPSO symposium ■ Regional BPSO events ■ CBOT and Network ■ Certified BPSO auditor (CBA) and Network ■ Use of BPSO logo ■ BPSO Communities of Practice ■ Mentorship opportunities ■ Technology-supported learning opportunities

THE FUTURE

The future for the RNAO BPGs and BPSO Designation holds much promise. With the BPSO Designation currently in 12 countries and several others in the application phase, the RNAO BPGs are well recognized as quality knowledge products that are positively transforming the nursing profession and its clinical, educational, and managerial practices. The program's impact in service and academic organizations consistently demonstrates improvements in education, patient, organizational, and health system outcomes. The enthusiastic BPG use by nurses in all roles and sectors, other health professionals, faculty and students, as well as policymakers has cemented the strong credibility of RNAO's BPGs and its BPSO Program. Added to this is the ongoing media attention that has served to spread the success of this program. The rapid growth of the BPSO Designation as a successful knowledge transfer strategy across various contexts has brought new strengths and important challenges to the BPSO Designation. Within this perspective, some of the future considerations are discussed next.

BPSO DESIGNATION AS A PARTNERSHIP INSPIRING COLLECTIVE IDENTITY

As the BPSO Models expand and mature, RNAO's role will be to continue to partner with BPSOs, to examine what is working well, what needs to be strengthened, and what needs to evolve to ensure effective evidence-based care around the world, through a high-quality BPG Program and BPSO Designation. The BPSO Model presents an opportunity for capacity development in the nursing profession from the perspective of evidence-based practice. Furthermore, in the process, countries around the world have learned many strategies related to policy development, political advocacy, and honing collaborative partnerships with other professional and healthcare bodies, and governments.

There are a number of emerging supports that will need to be tested and contextualized to fit the variety of systems and cultures that are part of the burgeoning BPSO Designation worldwide. Mentoring has been identified in the literature as a significant support (Melnyk, 2007, 2014), and based on RNAO's experience, it enhances quality in both the mentor and mentee organizations. More international mentors will be identified and supported into the future, as technology is harnessed to expand and create new knowledge-sharing links, which connect individuals and organizations for mutual learning.

Collective identity is a term discussed in detail in Chapter 1, *Transforming Nursing Through Knowledge: The Conceptual and Programmatic Underpinnings of RNAO's BPG Program*. RNAO will continue to set the standard to inspire and nurture the program's collective identity in all forms of knowledge exchange, wherein BPSOs build on their relationships and expertise to learn from each other and together with RNAO build the BPSO movement. For example, academic BPSOs in Belgium, Canada, Chile, China, Colombia, Italy, Jamaica, Peru, Portugal, and Spain are teaching us how to best integrate BPGs throughout the curriculum. The Academic BPSOs around the world are helping us build better evaluation strategies of BPG impact on faculty, student, and patient outcomes, which will soon be part of the NQuIRE data system. The onsite visits, including RNAO's in-person audit and feedback processes, were first introduced in our international BPSOs and in 2016 became part of the requirements for Ontario's BPSOs.

The more our international BPSOs have a voice in the processes of developing evidence-based cultures, the more the co-created structures and processes will contribute to a collective identity and dynamic sustainment, yielding better outcomes for our patients at home and abroad. Real and sustained growth of the nursing profession globally will only happen when all nurses have equal voices in shaping the destiny of our profession as evidence-based, client-centred, and equal partners on the interprofessional team. This is being realized through the BPSO Designation that is experiencing continued spread, dynamic sustainment, and robust fidelity.

BPG TRANSLATION

As the development of BPSOs around the world accelerates, so too must the systems of translation to see that BPGs are accurately translated into different languages. Spread in regions and countries will facilitate this, as the presence of several BPSOs in an area that communicate in a similar language will mean additional skills and resources to engage in the process. Translation teams—including RNAO staff and members of the BPSO organizations who can work to synchronize language, healthcare, and cultural differences—will be more and more important as expansion occurs.

BPSO SPREAD, SUSTAINABILITY, AND QUALITY MONITORING THROUGH TRAINING TRAINERS

Critical to the spread of the BPGs and BPSOs is RNAO's philosophy and capacity to extend its knowledge, skills, and resources widely beyond its own milieu. As described in Chapter 1 and Chapter 18, *Scaling Deep to Improve People's Health: From Evidence-Based Practice to Evidence-Based Policy*, such capacity has been fuelled by RNAO's strong standing as a professional association with a network of members in chapters and interest groups, an activist membership, and strong relations with like organizations. RNAO's formal dissemination channels and extensive use of technology provide a robust springboard for the BPG Program to build upon, with a roster of educational opportunities that serve audiences across the globe. Chapter 4, *Forging the Way With Implementation Science*, details a few of these capacity-building opportunities.

Consistent with the concept of purposeful evolution discussed in Chapter 1, RNAO has honed additional spread, sustainability, and quality-monitoring approaches: the *Certified BPSO Host Master Trainer*, *Certified BPSO Orientation Trainer*, and the *Certified Auditor* that are part of the emerging RNAO Training of Trainers Model. These approaches are integral to global scaling within a context of promoting a dynamic BPSO Designation that spreads, sustains, ensures fidelity, and serves to manage finite resources. What follows is an overview of the *Certified BPSO Host Master Trainer*, *Certified BPSO Orientation Trainer*, and the *Certified Auditor*.

CERTIFIED BPSO HOST MASTER TRAINER

Certified BPSO Host Master Trainers (CBHMT) are registered nurses from BPSO Hosts who have worked closely with an RNAO Master Trainer in the Certified BPSO Orientation Trainer role, training BPSO Sponsors, BPSO Leads, and Champion Leaders in their BPSO Directs. CBHMTs are familiar with the BPSO Orientation materials and teaching methodologies. They work independently in their jurisdictions with their BPSO Directs. Monitoring of this role by RNAO occurs through the reporting, knowledge transfer, and audit requirements of the BPSO Host, which includes ongoing assessment of the CBHMT role.

CERTIFIED BPSO ORIENTATION TRAINER

As briefly discussed earlier, Certified BPSO Orientation Trainers (CBOT) are registered nurses who meet set criteria including: Champion experience in a BPSO, skill in training, and experience in working with international populations. They are nominated from BPSO Designate organizations and once selected, receive the BPSO Orientation Program for review and discussion. They then partner with an RNAO BPSO Master Trainer or a BPSO Host Master Trainer to co-lead orientation sessions until they demonstrate proficiency to be certified. After the Orientation Program, CBOTs commit to working with BPSOs as they achieve the required deliverables and work with Master Trainers in delivering the BPSO Orientation Program to new BPSOs.

The involvement of more CBOTs from each of the BPSO countries and creation of a Certified BPSO Trainer Network will enhance this approach to quality assurance for budding BPSOs all over the world, and also sharpen the work in the trainers' BPSOs. Moreover, this cross-pollination of best evidence will enhance healthcare globally. The impacts of a Certified BPSO Trainer Network merit investigation, and the best practices in selecting and training trainers, and maintaining trainer skill levels, need to be developed over time. The involvement of BPSO Hosts in developing CBOTs and expanding the Certified Trainer Network will be increasingly necessary.

CERTIFIED BPSO AUDITOR

Certified BPSO Auditors (CBA) are registered nurses from BPSOs who have worked with an RNAO International BPSO Coach in conducting service and academic audits using RNAO's audit tools with specific feedback and follow-up processes. Previous discussion in this chapter outlined the BPSO audit process and its effectiveness internationally as means of providing feedback, a critical component of guideline implementation and sustainment. The future will bring more requirements for RNAO and BPSO Hosts to conduct audits around the world and increase the need for Certified BPSO Auditors (CBA) from across jurisdictions and the creation of a CBA Network, much like the Certified BPSO Trainers Network. The TOT Model, explained next, will be central to this process.

TRAINING OF TRAINERS MODEL (TOT)

To establish a clear process for training of trainers such as CBOTs and CBAs, as well as the additional knowledge leaders to ensure BPSO quality and fidelity, RNAO has developed the International BPSO Training of Trainers (TOT) Model. The literature supports some of the obvious benefits of the TOT Model for individuals, organizations, trainers, and trainees alike, including: more rapid diffusion, direct access to local communities, understanding of contextual issues, local collaboration, and cost benefits (Assemi, Mutha, & Hudmon, 2007; Hiner et al., 2009; Rajapakse, Neeman, & Dawson, 2013; Yarber et al., 2015).

TRAINING PROGRAMS KEY COMPONENTS

Key components of the most effective approaches to training programs have been identified in the literature based on research of local and global programs, as detailed:

- Careful selection of candidates (Hiner et al., 2009)

- Provision of a workbook and/or specific tools (Assemi et al., 2007; Baron, 2006; Rajapakse et al., 2013)

- Supervised hands-on experience and group work (Hiner et al., 2009; Yarber et al., 2015)

- Teach-back opportunities (Hiner et al., 2009; Yarber et al., 2015)

- Focus on content as well as methodology of instruction (Assemi et al., 2007; Baron, 2006; Hiner et al., 2009; Rajapakse et al., 2013)

- Connection with local structures (Hiner et al., 2009; Rajapakse et al., 2013)

- Evaluation and feedback (Assemi et al., 2007; Baron, 2006; Hines et al., 2009)

- Creation of a TOT network (Baron, 2006; Yarber et al., 2015)

RNAO's TOT Model meets all the above criteria, and given its clear link to the specific set of deliverables required in the BPSO Designation, unlike many TOT programs, where most trainees never replicate the program (Hahn, Noland, Rayens, & Christie, 2002), in our case those trained actually deliver. RNAO's aim is to multiply its effects the world over through a TOT Model that cascades through several tiers of trainers and trainees, including RNAO BPSO Master Trainers, BPSO Host Master Trainers, Certified BPSO Orientation Trainers, BPSO Sponsors, BPSO Coaches, Champion Leaders, BPSO Leads, Champions, and BPG Leads.

Figure 12.3 shows the tiered approach to the TOT Model, whereas Figure 12.4 defines each of the tiers in the model and explains their linkages, evident in the BPSO Designation activities. Both are explained in the narrative after the figures.

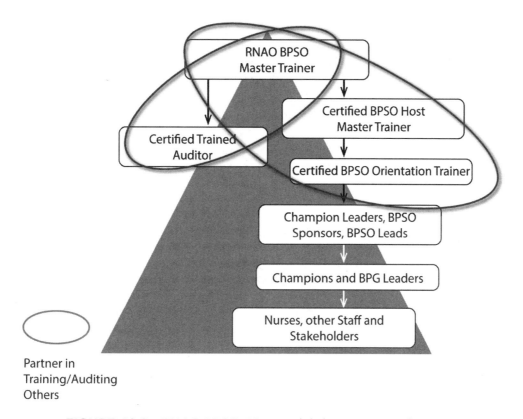

FIGURE 12.3 RNAO BPSO TOT Model showing tiers of training.

RNAO BPSO Training of Trainers Model

| System Tier Certified BPSO Host Master Trainers | System Tier Certified BPSO Orientation Trainers | Organization Tier BPSO Sponsor, BPSO Lead, Champion Leader | Unit Tier Champions, BPG Leaders |

RNAO BPSO MASTER TRAINERS LEAD and MONITOR the Training Processes

Certified BPSO Host Master Trainer
- RN from BPSO Host
- Trained as a CBOT
- Worked closely with *RNAO BPSO Master Trainer*
- Conducted BPSO Orientation Program
- Familiar with content and methodologies
- Trains *CBOTs in their BPOS Directs*

Certified BPSO Orientation Trainers
- RN with BPSO experience
- Trained by RNAO BPSO Master Trainer in two BPSO Orientation Program sessions
- Competent in: content presentation; application exercises; discussion and Q&A sessions; session *BPSO Sponsor* opening & debriefing; teaching methodologies
- Trains *Champion Leaders*

BPSO Sponsor
- Nursing Head in BPSO
- Supports *BPSO Lead*

BSPO Lead
- Nurse who completed BPSO Orientation Program
- Leads the BPSO Designation in the organization

Champion Leaders
- Completed the BPSO Orientation Program
- Part of overall BPSO team
- Helps train *Champions* and *BPG Leaders* in training workshops

Champions
- Nurses and others in the BPSO
- Trained in the Champion Workshop
- Part of the Champion Network
- Promote BPG uptake with peers

BPG Leaders
- Champions knowledgeable about a specific BPG
- Work with team to implement BPG in clinical setting, or integrate in academic setting

FIGURE 12.4 RNAO BPSO TOT Model with an explanation of each tier of the model.

As can been seen in Figures 12.3 and 12.4, the TOT Model begins with the training of BPSO Sponsors, BPSO Leads, and Champion Leaders by RNAO International BPSO Coaches who are the BPSO Master Trainers. The RNAO BPSO Master Trainers select the candidates for certification based on specific criteria and work with them side by side to prepare them to fulfill the role of the Certified BPSO Trainer or Certified BPSO Auditor.

As mentioned earlier, the BPSO Host Model presents another opportunity for training the trainer. In these situations, the RNAO BPSO Master Trainer will train a BPSO Host Master Trainer, who in turn can train Certified BPSO Trainers as well as organization-tier leaders.

These Champion Leaders in turn train Champions and BPG leaders at the unit tier, using a similar methodology in a shortened course. The Champions and BPG Leaders have clear roles in working with nurses, other staff, and stakeholders. Nurses and others who have received training wear their titles of Champion Leader, BPSO Lead, Champion, and BPG Leader with pride.

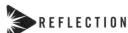

REFLECTION

How does RNAO's International BPSO TOT Model influence engagement of staff in all roles in the BPSOs?

CONCLUSION

This chapter provides an overview of how RNAO has used diffusion theory in its approaches to the spread of BPGs and the adoption of the BPSO Designation around the globe. The RNAO BPG Program, including the BPSO Designation juxtaposed against diffusion theory (Rogers, 2003), demonstrates how and why the innovations and the processes used by RNAO are effective. Such processes include BPG development through to dissemination and creation of robust, systematic, evidence-based implementation processes, and establishment of the NQuIRE data system and BPSO-NQuIRE Evaluation Model.

The creation of the BPSO Designation through both the Direct and Host Models has greatly enhanced BPG dissemination and added a robust global component to RNAO's work in evidence-based practice. Undoubtedly, it has been a strong factor in the speed of uptake and sustainment of evidence-based practice. The system-wide impacts of BPG implementation and creation of evidence-based cultures have resulted in changes in practice and education in Canadian healthcare settings and the international BPSOs. These results, augmented by an effective Training of Trainers Model developed by RNAO and used around the world, enable faster program spread and sustainability, as well as effective use of resources.

Finally, with rapid growth and uptake, close attention is given to fidelity. RNAO has and will continue to build its quality-assurance program, increasingly involving BPSOs. The strong quality-improvement strategies that are currently in use have a number of benefits that all BPSOs have experienced. Knowledge exchange, cross-country sharing, and growing better together are signature values of the BPG Program and foundational to the collective identity that we have built as BPSOs.

KEY MESSAGES

- Both the widespread implementation of RNAO BPGs and uptake of the BPSO Designation reflect key elements of the theory of diffusion.

- The BPSO Designation, both the BPSO Direct and BPSO Host Models, has positively impacted the quality of educational, clinical, and managerial practices and outcomes. It has also directly influenced enrichments in scope of practice, nurse-to-nurse and nurse-physician communication and collaboration, standards of practice excellence, the image of nursing and nurses, patient-centred care, organizational policy, and closing the research-to-practice gap.

- The BPSO Host Model supports "in country" capacity development in the area of EBP and has enabled RNAO to maximize diffusion and sustainability of the BPG Program and BPSO Designation at the global level, while ensuring effective use of resources.

- A standardized BPSO Orientation Program, certified trainers, annual in-person audits, and ongoing requirements and opportunities have enabled RNAO to maximize spread, sustainability, and BPSO Designation fidelity.

- The RNAO BPSO TOT Model augments the human resources necessary to support global spread of the BPSO Designation, while at the same time contributes to engagement in uptake and sustained use of BPGs.

■ The collective identity of BPSOs around the world has contributed to dynamic spread, sustainability, and fidelity of the program.

■ The future includes a focus on expanding and spreading resources to meet the global demand for the BPSO Designation. Increased engagement with BPSOs as full partners will build on the program's strengths, tackle areas for improvement, and extend cross-border communication and knowledge exchange through technology.

REFERENCES

Adams, A. S., Soumerai, S. B., Lomas, J., & Ross-Degnan, D. (1999). Evidence of self-report bias in assessing adherence to guidelines. *International Journal for Quality in Health Care, 11*(3), 187–192. doi: 10.1093/intqhc/11.3.187

Albornos-Munoz, L., González-María, E., & Moreno-Casbas, T. (2015). Best Practice Guidelines implementation in Spain: Best practice spotlight organizations. *Med UNAB, 17*(3), 163–169.

Assemi, M., Mutha, S., & Hudmon, K. S. (2007). Evaluation of a train-the-trainer program for cultural competence. *American Journal of Pharmaceutical Education, 71*(6), 110.

Athwal, L., Marchuk, B., Laforêt-Fliesser, Y., Castanza, J., Davis, L., & LaSalle, M. (2014). Adaptation of a Best Practice Guideline to strengthen client-centered care in public health. *Public Health Nursing Volume, 31*(2), 134–143.

Bajnok, I. (2008, May 6). Re "It beats sucking up to teacher" [Letter to the Editor]. *Toronto Star.*

Bajnok, I., Grinspun, D., Lloyd, M., & McConnell, H. (2015). Leading quality improvement through Best Practice Guideline development, implementation, and measurement science. *MedUNAB, 17*(3), 155–162.

Baker, C., Ogden, S., Prapaipanich, W., Keith, C. K., Beattie, L. C., & Nickleson, L. (1999). Hospital consolidation: Applying stakeholder analysis to merger life cycle. *Journal of Nursing Administration, 29*(3), 11–12.

Baron, N. (2006). The 'TOT': A global approach for the training of trainers for psychosocial and mental health interventions in countries affected by war, violence and natural disasters. *Intervention, 4*(2), 109–126.

Berwick, D. M. (2003). Disseminate innovations in health care. *The Journal of the American Medical Association, 289*(15), 1969–1975.

Berwick, D. M., Godfrey, A .B., & Roessner, J. (1991). *Curing health care: New strategies for quality improvement.* Hoboken, NJ: John Wiley & Sons.

Berwick, D. M., Godfrey, A. B., & Roessner, J. (2002). *Curing health care: New strategies for quality improvement* (2nd ed.). Hoboken, NJ: John Wiley & Sons.

Brundage, A. (2008, June 16). Check your blood sugar [Letter to the editor]. *The Toronto Sun.*

Carroll, C., Patterson, M., Wood, S., Booth, A., Rick, J., & Balain, S. (2007). A conceptual framework for implementation fidelity. *Implementation Science 2:* 40–49.

Castro, F. G., Barrera, M. Jr., & Martinez, C. R. Jr. (2004). The cultural adaptation of prevention interventions: Resolving tensions between fidelity and fit. *Prevention Science, 5*(1), 41–45.

Chambers, D. A., Glasgow, R. E., & Stange, K. C. (2013). The dynamic sustainability framework: Addressing the paradox of sustainment amid ongoing change. *Implementation Science, 8,* 117. doi: 10.1186/1748-5908-8-117

China Care Management. (2015, July 24). The first RNAO-BPSO evidence-based nursing research center in China is located in Beijing University of Traditional Chinese Medicine, will build a local nursing practice guide (translated). Retrieved from https://mp.weixin.qq.com/s/e4MrXwAS4_rHVKKjeTROqA

Cochrane AL. Effectiveness and efficiency: Random reflections on health services. London: Nuffield Provincial Hospitals Trust; 1973.

Dane, A. V., & Schneider, B. (1998). Program integrity in primary and early secondary prevention: Are implementation effects out of control? *Clinical Psychology Review, 18*(1), 23–45.

Davies, B., Edwards, N., Ploeg, J., & Virani, T. (2008). Insights about the process and impact of implementing nursing guidelines on delivery of care in hospitals and community settings. *BMC Health Services Research, 8,* 29. http://doi.org/10.1186/1472-6963-8-29

Davies, B., Tremblay, D., & Edwards, N. (2010). Sustaining evidence-based practice systems and measuring the impacts. In D. Bick & I. D. Graham (Eds.), *Evaluating the impact of implementing evidence based practice* (pp. 165–188). Oxford, UK: STTI/Wiley-Blackwell.

Durlak, J. A., & DuPre, E. P. (2008). Implementation matters: A review of research on the influence of implementation on program outcomes and the factors affecting implementation. *American Journal of Community Psychology, 41*(3–4), 237–350.

Dusenbury, L., Brannigan, R., Falco, M., & Hanson, W. B. (2003). A review of research on fidelity of implementation: Implications for drug abuse prevention in school settings. *Health Education Research*, *18*(2), 237–256. https://doi.org/10.1093/her/18.2.237

Fagan, A. A., Hanson, K., Hawkins, J. D., & Arthurs, M. W. (2008). Bridging science to practice: Achieving prevention program implementation fidelity in the community youth development study. *American Journal of Community Psychology*, *41*(3–4), 235–249.

Gardner, D. (2010). A passion for improving health care: An interview with Doris Grinspun. *Nursing Economics*, *28*(2), 126–129.

Ghoshal, D. S., & Bartlett, C. (1988). Creation, adoption and diffusion of innovations by subsidiaries of multinational corporations. *The Journal of International Business Studies*, *19*(3), 372.

Gifford, W., Davies, B., Rowan, M., Egan, M., Lefebre, N., & Brehaut, J. (2016). Understanding audit and feedback to support falls prevention and pain management in home health care. *Home Health Care Management and Practice*, *28*(2), 79–95.

Greenhalgh, T., Robert, G., Bate, P., Macfarlane, F., & Kyriakidou, O. (Eds.). (2005). *Diffusion of innovations in health service organizations: A systematic literature review*. Maldne, MA: Blackwell.

Greenhalgh, T., Robert, G., Macfarlane, F., Bate, P., Kyriakidou, O., & Peacock, R. (2004). Storylines of research in diffusion of innovation: A meta-narrative approach to systematic review. *Social Science and Medicine*, *61*(2), 417–430.

Grimshaw, J. M., Eccles, M. P., Lavis, J. M., Hill, S. J., & Squires, J. E. (2012). Knowledge translation of research findings. *Implementation Science*, *7*, 50. https://doi.org/10.1186/1748-5908-7-50

Grinspun, D. (2011). Guías de practica clínica y entorno laboral basados en la evidencia elaboradas por la Registered Nurses' Association of Ontario (RNAO). *Enfermeria Clinica*, *21*(1): 1–2.

Grinspun, D., Lloyd, M., Xiao, S., & Bajnok, I. (2015). Measuring quality of evidence-based care: NQuIRE—Nursing Quality Indicators for Reporting and Evaluation data-system. *Med UNAB*, *17*(3), 170–175.

Grinspun, D., Melnyk, B. M., & Fineout-Overholt, E. (2014). Advancing optimal care with rigorously developed clinical practice guidelines and evidence-based recommendations. In B. M. Melnyk & E. Fineout-Overholt (Eds.), *Evidence-based practice in nursing and health care: A guide to best practice* (3rd ed.) (pp. 182–201). Philadelphia, PA: Wolters Kluwer.

Grinspun, D., Virani, T., & Bajnok, I. (2002). Nursing Best Practice Guidelines: The Registered Nurses' Association of Ontario project. *Hospital Quarterly*, *5*(2), 56–60.

Grol, R., Wensing, M., Eccles, M., & Davis, D. (2013). *Improving patient care: The implementation of change in health care* (2nd ed.). London, UK: John Wiley & Sons.

Hahn, E. J., Noland, M. P., Rayens, M. K., & Christie, D. M. (2002). Efficacy of training and fidelity of implementation of the life skills training program. *Journal of School Health*, *72*(7), 282–287. doi: 10.1111/j.1746-1561.2002.tb01333.x

Health Council of Canada. (2012). *Understanding clinical practice guidelines: A video series primer*. Retrieved from https://healthcouncilcanada.ca/files/CPG_Backgrounder_EN.pdf.pdf

Heath, C., & Heath, D. (2010). *Switch: How to change things when change is hard*. New York, NY: Random House.

Higuchi, K. S., Davies, B. L., Edwards, N., Ploeg, J., & Virani, T. (2011). Implementation of clinical guidelines for adults with asthma and diabetes: A three-year follow-up evaluation of nursing care. *Journal of Clinical Nursing*, *20*(9–10), 1329–1338. doi: 10.1111/j. 1365-2702.2010.03590.x

Higuchi, K. S., Davies, B., & Ploeg, J. (2017). Sustaining guideline implementation: A multisite perspective on activities, challenges and supports. *Journal of Clinical Nursing*, 1–12. doi: 10.1111/jocn.13770

Higuchi, K. S, Downey, A., Davies, B., Bajnok, I., & Waggott, M. (2013). Using the NHS Sustainability framework to understand the activities and resource implications of Canadian nursing guideline early adopters. *Journal of Clinical Nursing*, *22*(11–12), 1707–1716.

Hiner, C. A., Mandel, B. G., Weaver, M. R., Bruce, D., McLaughlin, R., & Anderson, J. (2009). Training-of-trainers model in a HIV counseling and testing program in the Caribbean Region. *Human Resources for Health*, *7*, 11.

Ireland, S., Kirkpatrick, H., Boblin, S., & Robertson, K. (2013). The real world journey of implementing fall prevention best practices in three acute care hospitals: A case study. *Worldviews on Evidence-Based Nursing*, *10*(2), 95–103.

Ivers, N. M., Grimshaw, J. M., Jamtvedt, G., Flottorp, S., O'Brien, M. A., French, S. D., . . . Odgaard-Jensen, J. (2014). Growing literature, stagnant science? Systematic review, meta-regression and cumulative analysis of audit and feedback interventions in health care. *Journal of General Internal Medicine*, *29*(11), 1534–1541. http://doi.org/10.1007/s11606-014-2913-y

Jadad, A. R., Cook, D. J., Jones, A., Klassen, T. P., Tugwell, D., Moher, M., . . . Moher, D. (1998). Methodology and reports of systematic review and meta-analyses: A comparison of Cochrane reviews with articles published in paper-based journals. *JAMA*, *280*(3), 278–280.

Jeffs, L., Beswick, S., Lo, J., Campbell, H., Ferris, E., & Sidani, S. (2013). Defining what evidence is, linking it to patient outcomes, and making it relevant to practice: Insights from clinical nurses. *Applied Nursing Research*, *26*(3), 105–109.

Jeffs, L., Lo, J., Beswick, S., & Campbell, H. (2013). Implementing an organization-wide quality improvement initiative: Insights from project leads, managers and frontline nurses. *Nursing Administration Quarterly*, *7*(3), 222–230.

Jennings, L., O'Neil, B., Bossy, K., Dodman, D., & Campbell, J. (2016). The story of Emily. *Patient Experience Journal, 3*(1), 146–152.

Johnson-Bhatti, G., Case, A., & Shaikh, S. (2017). Raising the bar: Putting evidence into practice. *Senior Care Canada* (3rd Quarter), 14–15.

Jordan, Z. (2005, Oct/Dec). Turning challenges into opportunities. *PACEsetterS, 2*(4), 6–11.

Kinnunen, J. (1996). Gabriel Tarde as a founding father of innovation diffusion research. *Acta Sociologica, 39*(4), 431–442. doi: 10:1177/000169939603900404

Kotter, J. P. (2012). *Leading change.* Boston, MA.: Harvard Business Review Press.

Legare, F. (2009). Assessing barriers and facilitators to knowledge use. In S. Straus, J. Tetroe, & I. D. Graham (Eds.), *Knowledge translation in health care: Moving from evidence to practice* (pp. 83–93). Oxford, UK: Wiley-Blackwell/BMJI Books.

McKeown, L. L., Woodbeck, H. H., & Lloyd, M. (2014). A journey to improve oral care with best practices in long-term care. *Canadian Journal of Dental Hygiene, 48*(2), 51–53.

Melnyk, B. M. (2007). The evidence-based practice mentor: A promising strategy for implementing and sustaining EBP in healthcare systems. *Worldviews on Evidence-Based Nursing, 4*(3), 123–125.

Melnyk, B. M. (2014). Building cultures and environments that facilitate clinician behaviour change to evidence-based practice: What works? *Worldviews on Evidence-Based Nursing, 11*(2), 79–80.

Melnyk, B. M. (2017). The difference between what is known and what is done is lethal: Evidence-based practice is a key solution urgently needed. *Worldviews on Evidence-Based Nursing, 14*(1), 3–4.

Meyer, G. (2004). Diffusion methodology: Time to innovate. *Journal of Health Communication: International Perspectives, 9*(S1), 61.

Morris, Z. S., Wooding, S., & Grant, J. (2011). The answer is 17 years, what is the question: Understanding time lags in translational research. *Journal of the Royal Society of Medicine, 104*(12), 510–520. http://doi.org/10.1258/jrsm.2011.110180

Mowbray, C. T., Holter, M. C., Teague, G. B., & Bybee, D. (2003). Fidelity criteria: Development, measurement, and validation. *American Journal of Evaluation, 24*(3), 315–340. doi: 10.1016/S1098-2140(03)00057-2

Patten, L. (2017). Organizing and empowering staff to find solutions. *Senior Care Canada* (3rd Quarter), 6–8.

Ploeg, J., Skelly, J., Rowan, M., Edwards, N., Davies, B., Grinspun, D., . . . Downey, A. (2010). The role of nursing best practice Champions in diffusing practice guidelines: A mixed methods study. *Worldviews on Evidence-Based Nursing, 7*(4), 238–251.

Punch, D. (2016). Doing more for the 3Ds. *Registered Nurse Journal, 28*(6), 12–17.

Rajapakse, B. N., Neeman, T., & Dawson, A. H. (2002). The effectiveness of a 'Train the Trainer' Model of resuscitation education for rural peripheral hospital doctors in Sri Lanka. *PLoS ONE, 8*(11), e79491. https://doi.org/10.1371/journal.pone.0079491

Registered Nurses' Association of Ontario (RNAO). (2002). *Toolkit: Implementation of Best Practice Guidelines.* Toronto, ON: Registered Nurses' Association of Ontario.

Registered Nurses' Association of Ontario (RNAO). (2005). *Educator's resource: Integration of Best Practice Guidelines.* Toronto, ON: Registered Nurses' Association of Ontario.

Registered Nurses' Association of Ontario (RNAO). (2010). *Nursing faculty education guide: Tobacco use and associated health risks.* Retrieved from http://tobaccofreernao.ca/en/NFEG

Registered Nurses' Association of Ontario (RNAO). (2012). *Toolkit: Implementation of Best Practice Guidelines* (2nd ed.). Toronto, ON: Registered Nurses' Association of Ontario.

Registered Nurses' Association of Ontario (RNAO). (2014, June 13). *Recommendations for first comprehensive nursing guideline on elder abuse released today.* Retrieved from http://rnao.ca/news/media-releases/2014/06/13/recommendations-first-comprehensive-nursing-guideline-elder-abuse-rel

Registered Nurses' Association of Ontario (RNAO). (2015a). *2014–2015 Best Practice Spotlight Organization Impact Survey: Summary of survey results.* Retrieved from http://rnao.ca/sites/rnao-ca/files/FINAL_RNAO-BPSO_Impact_Survey_from_Printer.pdf

Registered Nurses' Association of Ontario (RNAO). (2015b, May 4). *Health-care professionals mark Nursing Week by showcasing excellence in evidence-based patient care.* Retrieved from http://rnao.ca/news/media-releases/2015/05/04/health-care-professionals-mark-nursing-week-showcasing-excellence-evi

Registered Nurses' Association of Ontario (RNAO). (2016a, May 4). *Nurses share their successes and challenges during National Nursing Week (May 9–15).* Retrieved from http://rnao.ca/news/media-releases/2016/05/04/nurses-share-their-successes-and-challenges-during-national-nursing-w

Registered Nurses' Association of Ontario (RNAO). (2016b, July 14). *RNAO celebrates approval of supervised injection services by launching Best Practice Guideline.* Retrieved from http://rnao.ca/news/media-releases/2016/07/14/rnao-celebrates-approval-supervised-injection-services-launching-best

Registered Nurses' Association of Ontario (RNAO). (2017a). *Nurse educator mental health and addiction resource.* Retrieved from www.rnao.ca/bpg/initiatives/mhai

Registered Nurses' Association of Ontario (RNAO). (2017b, May 25). *Nurses stand proud during Nursing Week.* Retrieved from http://rnao.ca/news/nurses-stand-proud-during-nursing-week

Rempel, L. A., & McCleary, L. (2012). Effects of the implementation of a breastfeeding Best Practice Guideline in a Canadian public health agency. *Research in Nursing & Health, 35*(5), 435–449. doi:10.1002/nur.21495

Rogers, E. M. (1962). *Diffusion of innovations.* New York, NY: Free Press.

Rogers, E. M. (1983). *Diffusion of innovations* (3rd ed.). New York, NY: Free Press.

Rogers, E. M. (1995). *Diffusion of innovations.* New York, NY: Free Press.

Rogers, E. M. (2003). *Diffusion of innovations* (5th ed.). New York, NY: Free Press.

Rogers, E. M., & Shoemaker, F. F. (1971). *Communication of innovations: A cross-cultural approach* (2nd ed.). New York, NY: Free Press.

Ryan, B., & Gross, N. (1943). The diffusion of hybrid seed in two Iowa communities. *Rural Sociology, 8*(1), 15–24.

School of Nursing, Beijing University of Chinese Medicine. (2017, August 18). *Canada Ontario Registered Nurses Association BPSO evidence-based care and methods training campaign video.* Retrieved from http://huli.bucm.edu.cn/tzggsy/41572.htm

Stetler, C. B., Richie, J. A., Rycroft-Malone, J., & Charns, M. P. (2014). Leadership for evidence-based practice: Strategic and functional behaviour for institutionalizing EBP. *Worldviews in Evidence-Based Nursing, 11*(4), 219–226.

Strang, D., & Soule, S. (1998). Diffusion in organizations and social movements from hybrid corn to poison pills. *Annual Review of Sociology, 24*, 265–290.

Straus, S., Tetroe, J., & Graham, I. (Eds.). (2013). *Knowledge translation in health care* (2nd ed.) Oxford, UK: Wiley-Blackwell.

Van Achterberg, T., Schoonhoven, L., & Grol, R. (2008). Nursing implementation science: How evidence-based nursing requires evidence-based implementation. *Journal of Nursing Scholarship, 40*(4), 302–310.

Vanguardia. (2017, August 17). *Visita.* Retrieved from http://m.vanguardia.com/entretenimiento/sociales/407800-visita

Virani, T. (2007, June 12). Nurses help prevent falls [Letter to the editor]. *The Peterborough Examiner.*

Yarber, L., Brownson, C. A., Jacob, R. R., Baker, E. A., Jones, E., Baumann, C., . . . Brownson, R. C. (2015). Evaluating a train-the-trainer approach for improving capacity for evidence-based decision making in public health. *BMC Health Services Research, 15*, 547. http://doi.org/10.1186/s12913-015-1224-2

13

BPSO HOST: A MODEL FOR SCALING OUT GLOBALLY

Teresa Moreno-Casbas, PhD, MSc, RN, FEAN
Esther González-María, PhD, MSc, RN
Laura Albornos-Muñoz, BSc

LEARNING OBJECTIVES

After reading this chapter, you will be able to:

- Identify how the BPSO Host Model has addressed evidence-based practice gaps internationally

- Describe the multifaceted strategies for knowledge translation developed and used under the BPSO Host Model

- Outline the impact of the BPSO Designation in different health system contexts

INTRODUCTION

Evidence-based practice is considered a methodological paradigm that serves as a reference for common criteria to be used in clinical decision-making. In this context, the Nursing and Healthcare Research Unit (Investén-isciii) and the Spanish Centre for Evidence Based Nursing and Healthcare applied to become a BPSO (Best Practice Spotlight Organization) Host, to initiate the BPSO Designation at the national level. This chapter describes the organization of the BPSO Host Model in Spain, as well as the strategies and process used in its development. The BPSO Designation in Spain currently has two active cohorts, one of BPSOs initiated in 2012 and designated in 2015, and a second cohort of BPSO candidates initiated in 2015. The next cohort of BPSO candidates will start in 2018. The BPSO Designation is demonstrated to have an impact on health structures, organizational challenges, and process and patient outcomes. Overall, the participating organizations have achieved a change in culture, shifting to one that is oriented to evidence.

NURSING CARE IN THE SPANISH HEALTH SYSTEM

Spain's 17 regions, or autonomous communities (CCAA), are part of the Spanish National Health System, which is configured as a coordinated group of health services of the Administration of the State and Health Services of the CCAA. The National Health System integrates all of the health provisions and functions that, according to the law, are the responsibility of the national authorities, while transferring other areas to the CCAA. Therefore, the central government has authority over the basic legislation, which affects the entire Spanish population and the coordination of the responsibilities of the CCAAs. The major aspects of the central government's responsibilities include health financing, pharmaceutical policy, international policies, as well as everything related to the education of specialist professionals.

Meanwhile, the CCAA are competent in subsidiary financing and legislation; the deployment of public health in their territory; the organization of their health system; and aspects regarding accreditation, planning, purchase, and provision of services.

The Spanish National Health System is characterized by its universal integration; it is publically financed through taxes and provides integral care to the population. It has a specific portfolio of services, including the co-payment of nonhospital pharmaceutical prescriptions and a system of evaluation. It is decentralized in the CCAA and organized in levels: mainly primary care, specialized care (hospital), and long-term care. In 2012, the Royal Decree-Law 16/2012 introduced into law severe cuts to the Spanish National Health System. In 2015, the Spanish National Health System (NHS) had a total of 164,385 nurses, being the largest group of health professionals, with a ratio of 1.5 nursing professionals for every physician. Hospitals employ the highest number of professionals—77,446 physicians and 134,743 nurses—while the primary care level employs 34,900 physicians and 29,642 nurses. The ratio of professionals per 1,000 inhabitants remains stable, with almost 0.6 professionals per 1,000 inhabitants in primary care, and 2.9 per 1,000 inhabitants in hospital care.

Within the Spanish health system, nurses hold an important role in the delivery of health services in primary care and in hospitals. Efforts to systematize the transfer of best available evidence into nursing clinical practice are common country-wide across hospital and service delivery settings, led by different institutions. However, in the early 2000s, the use of evidence-based guidelines in practice was found to vary considerably, contributing to undue differences in the quality of services delivered.

THE SPANISH EXPERIENCE OF IMPLEMENTING RNAO BPGS

The Spanish National Nursing and Healthcare Research Unit (Investén-isciii) belongs to the Institute of Health Carlos III, the main Public Biomedical Research Entity at the national level. One of the objectives is to incorporate nursing research into daily clinical practice.

Our concern was the variability in nurses' clinical practice within our national health system and its influence on safety and the quality of services provided. Approaches to evaluation of nursing practices were not comparable across regions, or even across institutions, which constrained the ability to systematically monitor service delivery. Previous efforts to increase and sustain the use of evidence-based guidelines in the delivery of health services in Spain had relatively limited success. In spite of this, Spanish nurses perceive knowledge translation as a priority (Comet-Cortés et al., 2010).

In 2010, as a means to both address variations in care delivery and quality of care and to improve service quality, the Nursing and Healthcare Research Unit formally partnered with the Registered Nurses' Association of Ontario (RNAO) to influence and evaluate the uptake of nursing BPGs across healthcare organizations, to enable practice excellence and positive client outcomes. The Nursing and Healthcare Research Unit became a Best Practice Spotlight Organization (BPSO) Host, responsible for overseeing the implementation of RNAO's BPSO Designation in Spain (Grinspun, 2011).

To reach clinical professionals, depending on each regional health system, our first strategy was to have the support of the Spanish Centre for Evidence Based Nursing and Healthcare. This is a nationwide center, established in 2004 and led by the Institute of Health Carlos III through the Spanish Nursing and Healthcare Research Unit, with 16 regions participating. The Collaborating Centre aims to promote and support the synthesis, transfer, and utilization of evidence through identifying feasible, appropriate, meaningful, and effective healthcare practices to assist in the improvement of healthcare outcomes globally. The Spanish BPSO Host is coordinated by the national Nursing and Healthcare Research Unit (Investén-isciii) and the Spanish Centre for Evidence Based Nursing and Healthcare (www.evidenciaencuidados.es).

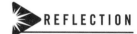

REFLECTION

How does this context impact the BPSO Designation process in Spain? What kinds of strengths and challenges are apparent that may have to be addressed in the BPG implementation process?

BUILDING A SUCCESSFUL INITIATIVE

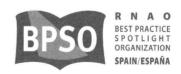

RNAO Best Practice Guidelines focus on nursing care and integrate not only practice recommendations, but also education, organization, and policy recommendations. BPGs are thus aligned with the Spanish National Quality Plan (Plan de Calidad para el Sistema Nacional de Salud), which addresses quality from practice, education, and policy perspectives (Ministerio de Sanidad, Política Social e Igualdad, 2010). In addition, RNAO has experience with BPG implementation through: hosting a number of BPSO cohorts in Ontario,

Canada; developing and using an evidence-based implementation tool (RNAO, 2012); and providing training and ongoing support. The conditions in Spain were also favourable, as the Spanish BPSO Host is supported by two strong and prestigious structures, very well known by Spanish nurses and other stakeholders.

The Spanish BPSO Designation is based on four key strategies:

- **Translation of BPGs into Spanish**—Investén-isciii signed an agreement with RNAO to translate RNAO's Best Practice Guidelines for use in the Spanish context, and in partnership with RNAO established the criteria for quality guidelines translation.

- **Dissemination**—RNAO provides online access to BPSO Designation information. BPSO launches promoted through the media and marketing of informative sessions are means to draw attention to the opportunity of participating. BPSOs in Spain are called "Centros Comprometidos con la Excelencia en Cuidados" (CCEC).

- **Implementation and evaluation**—The Spanish BPSO Host launched the first call for proposals through a competitive application process to select healthcare settings in Spain for implementing the RNAO's BPGs and evaluating the results (Ruzafa-Martínez et al., 2011). The approach is nursing-led and multidisciplinary, multipronged in strategy, context-specific, and involves a wide range of stakeholders. The RNAO (2012) *Toolkit: Implementation of Best Practice Guidelines* guides the process with a train-the-trainer approach, selection of recommendations to be implemented, a 3-year schedule of planned implementation activities, and monitoring by measuring process and outcome results for patients.

> ►**REFLECTION**
>
> *Consider how the four key strategies that are part of the BPSO Host plan reflect the Knowledge-to-Action framework and successful change processes.*

- **Sustainability**—As the regional host for Spain, Investén-isciii supports the maintenance and scaling-up of BPG implementation, and creating a national network of BPSOs to join the international BPSO network overseen by RNAO.

OUR FIRST COHORT

Out of 33 organizations responding to the call, eight health-care settings (involving 11 sites, providing care to 1.3 million of people) were selected. They are located in seven different regions and include hospitals as well as primary healthcare centers.

The BPSOs selected are:

- Centro de Salud Ponferrada II (G.A. P. Bierzo)
- Complejo Hospitalario de Universitario de Albacete
- Hospital Clínico San Carlos
- Hospital Doctor José Molina Orosa
- Hospital Medina del Campo
- Hospitales de Sierrallana y Tres Mares (G.A.E. Áreas de Salud Torrelavega-Reinosa)
- Hospital Rafael Méndez de Lorca junto con la Universidad de Lorca
- Hospital Universitario Vall d'Hebrón

As one of the BPSO Leads said:

"To be selected [as a BPSO] it's a very important motivation to change our nursing practices and to demonstrate that small organizations can do big things."

—Mª Angeles González; G.A. P. Bierzo

Overall, the BPSOs implemented 10 BPGs, according to the needs at each institution.

The most-selected BPGs were:

- *Ostomy Care and Management* (RNAO, 2009)
- *Prevention of Falls and Fall Injuries in the Older Adult* (RNAO, 2011)
- *Breastfeeding Best Practice Guidelines for Nurses* (RNAO, 2003)
- *Assessment and Management of Pain* (RNAO, 2013)

"When guidelines were not aligned with areas of improvement identified by nurses and other professionals, they were not so innovative and engaging as they are when there is alignment."

—Mª Luz Fernández; Hospitales de Sierrallana y Tres Mares

From 2012 to 2014, BPSO candidates engaged and trained health practitioners in implementing the selected guidelines, reviewing and updating protocols and procedures, monitoring and evaluating their utilization, and reporting data to the Nursing and Healthcare Research Unit and RNAO (Albornos-Muñoz, González-María, & Moreno-Casbas, 2015; González-María, 2014; World Health Organization [WHO], 2015). Upon successfully attaining all of the deliverables, they earned their BPSO Designation in 2015. Designated organizations continue to receive support from the National Unit for Nursing Research and RNAO, and renew their designation every 2 years, based on successful achievement of required deliverables.

While organizations receive considerable support from the BPSO Host (the Nursing and Healthcare Research Unit), they are ultimately responsible for ensuring the implementation of guidelines within their own organization. Each organization is required to designate an overall BPSO Designation leader, the BPSO Lead, as well as a leader for each guideline to be implemented. In addition, all senior management within the organization must sign the BPSO Agreement with the National Unit for Nursing Research to demonstrate widespread managerial support for becoming a BPSO. A group of health practitioners is selected by organizations to become Champions for each guideline; it is up to organizations how many are recruited, as long as they fulfill the minimum of 15% of nursing staff stipulated in the Agreement. Champions are trained by the National Unit for Nursing Research on BPG implementation and how to motivate peers to utilize BPGs in practice.

Training was provided through a train-the-trainer model, whereby a group of guideline Champions is appointed at each participating institution and receives a weeklong, formal training program on implementing the RNAO guidelines, motivating practitioners to use guidelines, and monitoring performance. Additional training is offered annually because building staff capacity is recognized as an ongoing process that continually needs updating. Champions are then responsible for training health practitioners in their respective organizations and supervising adherence to guidelines.

For the evaluation component of the program, "Data Dictionaries" have been developed to document and report on the Nursing Quality Indicators, which are specifically related to each BPG and used to assess RNAO BPG implementation.

As BPSO Host, we provide considerable support to our BPSO Directs in a number of ways. Besides the initial training of BPSO leaders, there is continuous follow-up to guide the implementation and monitoring process. Monthly meetings, regular review and feedback on evaluation results, and annual audits provide windows to understanding the progress of each BPSO, enabling us to support them on their specific needs. This relationship of follow-up and exchange is highly acknowledged by BPSO leaders:

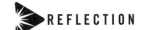

REFLECTION

In your view, what factors in the implementation process spurred the remarkable uptake of BPSO by organizations, the full engagement of nurses, and the sustained interest in this work across Spain? How could these factors be replicated in your setting?

"Many things are new for us, but we don't feel alone; the support from the BPSO Host helps us to keep focused so we don't lose direction."

—Emma Alonso; Hospital Doctor José Molina Orosa

In addition, we promote knowledge exchange between BPSOs, encouraging networking between and amongst organizations with similar characteristics implementing similar BPGs.

"We were not used to working with health organizations belonging to different regional health systems; this approach gives a new perspective and is a powerful tool."

—Pilar Pérez; Hospital Universitario Vall d'Hebrón

OUR SECOND COHORT

In late 2014, a second open call for BPSO candidates was issued, and 10 out of 60 organizations, representing 70 healthcare sites across Spain, were selected to begin implementation in 2015. The selected BPSO candidates are:

- Hospital Universitario Donostia
- Complejo Hospitalario de Navarra
- Área de Salud de Menorca

- Consorcio HUAV-HSM-Facultad enfermería Lleida

- Hospital Universitario Puerto Real

- Complejo Hospitalario Universitario de Granada

- Organización Sanitaria Integrada Debabarrena

- Centro de Salud José María Llanos

- Gerencia de Atención Integrada de Alcázar de San Juan

- Hospital Valle de Nalón

At this time, 16 BPGs are currently being implemented, taking into account both cohorts. Figure 13.1 shows the distribution of BPSOs in both cohorts in Spain, with the figures in the bold representing Cohort 2. Figure 13.2 shows the complete list of selected BPGs, as well as how many BPSOs in each cohort are implementing each one, with the figures in bold representing Cohort 2. All in all, 19,100 health professionals in 193 units are involved in the BPSO initiative in Spain. They have 1,200 Champions, and they are working with thousands of collaborators. Together they collect data on 35,983 patients and serve a population of 4,478,050.

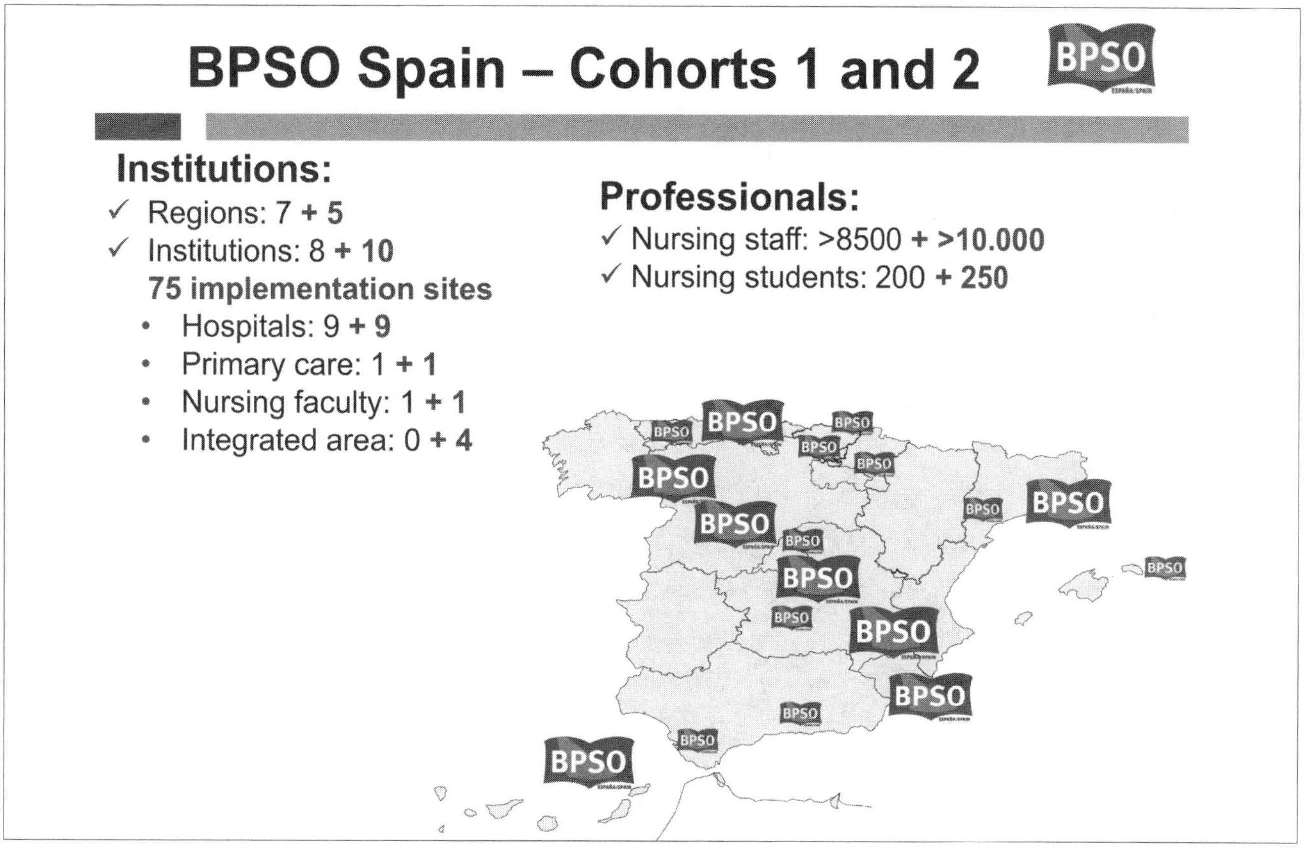

FIGURE 13.1   BPSO cohorts 1 and 2 in Spain.
Used with permission.

BPSO Spain – Cohorts 1 and 2

Best Practice Guidelines Implemented (15)

✓ Prevention of **Falls** and Fall Injuries (6 + 5)
✓ Care and Management of Ostomy (6 + 3)
✓ **Breastfeeding** (5 + 4)
✓ Assessment and Management of **Pain** (4 + 1)
✓ **Stroke** Assessment Across the Continuum of Care (2 + 1)
✓ Assessment & Management of **Foot Ulcers** for People with **Diabetes** (2 + 0)
✓ Reducing **Foot Complications** for People with **Diabetes** (1 + 1)
✓ Subcutaneous **Administration of Insulin** in Adults with Type 2 **Diabetes** (+ 1)
✓ Integrating **Smoking Cessation** into Daily Nursing Practice (+ 2)
✓ Supporting & Strengthening Families Through Expected and Unexpected Life Events (+ 1)
✓ **Primary Prevention** of **Childhood Obesity** (1 + 1)
✓ **Person- and Family-Centered** Care (+ 2)
✓ Risk Assessment and **Prevention** of **Pressure Ulcers** (+ 5)
✓ Assessment and Device Selection for **Vascular Access** (1 + 3)
✓ Assessment and Care of Adults at Risk for **Suicidal Ideation and Behaviour** (+ 1)
✓ **Healthy Work Environments** (5)

FIGURE 13.2 BPGs implemented by BPSO cohorts 1 and 2 in Spain.
Used with permission.

While the characteristics of the organizations in the new cohort differ from the first one, the feelings of leaders and Champions continue to be encouraging. The following quotes represent their outstanding successes.

"It's so amazing to observe how three organizations who previously worked separately are working together for a common objective ..."

–Mercè Folguera and Josep María Gutiérrez; Consorcio HUAV-HSM-Facultad enfermería Lleida

"Champions are developing actions unthinkable one year ago."

–Cristina Torres; Organización Sanitaria Integrada Debabarrena

▶ REFLECTION

How do you think Cohort 2 benefitted from the experiences of the first cohort? What did the BPSO Host do to encourage this?

OVERALL STRATEGIES

Table 13.1 depicts a summary of the common strategies carried out by BPSOs.

TABLE 13.1	COMMON STRATEGIES FOR EFFECTIVE BPSO IMPLEMENTATION	
AREAS	**OBJECTIVES**	**ACTIVITIES**
Training	▪ Design and deliver continuous training in implementation methodology ▪ Design and deliver continuous training in relation to guideline topics	▪ Design different modalities of training (online, face to face, express) ▪ Develop training plans for guidelines ▪ Involve Champions
Implementation	▪ Develop the operations of implementation teams in relation to the selection and adoption of recommendations ▪ Establish an action plan developed by healthcare professionals of units ▪ Collect and mobilize implementation strategies suggested by units, and disseminate to all groups ▪ Increase adherence to recommendations ▪ Follow up and support implementation teams on the development of strategies	▪ Assess modalities (by subgroups, etc.) ▪ Establish different mechanisms for implementation (e.g., pilot vs. recommendations) ▪ Establish different mechanisms for communication ▪ Assess barriers and strategies ▪ Strategize for professional compensation
Exchange Sessions	▪ Meet periodically to discuss successes, challenges, and strategies with the healthcare professionals of the units ▪ Create external alliances ▪ Participate in a wider network of external groups (regional, etc.)	▪ Facilitate systems for meetings and communication ▪ Plan and schedule meetings ▪ Promote multicenter studies, clinical residency, exchanges, etc.
Evaluation Planning	▪ Evaluate using a common method ▪ Minimize variability amongst evaluators ▪ Provide systematic and multilevel feedback ▪ Maintain a continuous system for evaluation and improvement	▪ Develop documentation manuals and mechanism of translation to electronic records ▪ Develop a coordination plan for evaluation and feedback ▪ Identify new indicators to evaluate
Dissemination	▪ Ensure multilevel dissemination of the project	▪ Create a dissemination group ▪ Design a dissemination plan that include different processes and channels

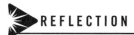

REFLECTION

Consider how you might use the implementation strategy chart presented above. What strategies would work well in your setting and why?

EVALUATION PROCESS

Evaluation is one of the key pillars of the program. The information obtained allows the Host to know the degree of implementation, as well as the impact on patients' health. The systematized feedback to different stakeholders is one of the most appreciated mechanisms amongst those involved.

> *"Evaluation and feedback at the unit level are an essential element. Champions who participate on the evaluation team share results with their colleagues and contribute to development of new solutions for improvements."*
>
> –Lucía Gárate; Hospital Universitario Donostia

RNAO's Nursing Quality Indicators for Reporting and Evaluation (NQuIRE) provides the evaluation mechanism and process to monitor BPG implementation by BPSOs. To adapt evaluation to country requirements, the Spanish BPSO Host developed a specific database, CarEvID, to measure the structure, process, and outcomes of BPG implementation in Spanish organizations. Together, RNAO and the Spain BPSO Host have analyzed the minimum data set applicability and established procedures to transfer data from the national nursing database CarEvID to the international platform NQuIRE.

Similar to NQuIRE, the CarEvID database integrates indicators at three levels to provide comparative reports. The first level is composed of *structure data*, which includes nursing hours, model of care delivery, and organizational profile of the institution and unit level. Structure indicators have been internationally defined as to reflect staffing and other human resource–type data that should be collected at the level of the implementation site. The second level includes the minimum data set of *process and outcomes-based quality indicators*, currently related to 16 Best Practices Guidelines. Forty-two process and 30 outcome indicators are part of the common minimum data set and are evaluated internationally following the same definition of indicators, variables records, and procedures. At the third level, *national or local data* are collected and processed. These outcome and process indicators present specificities, such as being part of national programs, not being included in national records, or following different collection procedures.

All BPSOs collect baseline data from the month prior to their official beginning as BPSO candidates. Data are collected subsequently during the last 5 days of every month, except for low prevalent cases, such as ostomy, in which case all patients are measured. Descriptive analysis of variables is carried out by CarEvID.

CarEvID includes more than 8,000 records related to falls prevention, 3,000 records of assessment and management of pain, 1,500 records related to breastfeeding, 700 records related to ostomy care, and 200 records related to stroke assessment. This database is perceived by the BPSOs as an important way to network:

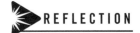

REFLECTION

How can the evaluation data shown in this chapter be best used to spread the BPSO Designation and sustain the efforts of the early cohorts in Spain?

"Use of common indicators, measured in the same way, reinforces our ability to learn from each other in the network."

–Pilar Rodríguez; Hospital Medina del Campo

In terms of impact, currently 18 facilities in Spain contribute to the growing NQuIRE database, which can now be used to show impact of implementation. The international component is one of the keys to success:

"The possibility of international benchmarking increases the credibility of the program for the managerial boards that have to sustain it."

–Dolores Quiñoz; Complejo Hospitalario Universitario de Granada

OVERALL IMPACT

There are many areas where we can observe the impact of the BPSO Designation in Spain.

- New organizational structures have been created or promoted, which serve to embed evidence-based culture into the organization.

- More than 3,200 nurses and other healthcare professionals have training in implementation and/or specifically in each BPG's recommended interventions. Their training has resulted in: the harmonization of interventions, the development or update of evidence-based protocols, the promotion of patient education, and the evaluation of international BPSO indicators using an electronic platform.

- One of the most important results is the harmonization of records. Because clinical records are established at a regional level, any change influences all healthcare organizations, thus potentially resulting in a wide spread of BPG implementation in the future.

- Some of the major findings include the improvement of process and outcome indicators. Falls prevention, ostomy care, and breastfeeding were three of the most frequently selected guidelines, by eleven BPSOs, nine BPSOs, and nine BPSOs respectively. Their results in relation to these guidelines showed significant improvements when comparing baseline measures to the 3rd-year post-implementation data as indicated below:

    - Registration of falls prevention assessment (69.4% vs. 80%)

    - Ostomy preoperative assessment and education (31.6% vs. 46%)

    - Preoperative ostomy marking (16% vs. 54%)

    - Reduction of falls (2.2% vs. 1.78%)

    - Improvement of exclusive breastfeeding at discharge (60% vs. 81%)

    - Exclusive breastfeeding at 6 months (29.7% vs. 40.3%)

Scholarly and scientific contributions are another area of success for BPSO participants. In addition to increased participation by Champions in congress and other scientific events, BPG implementation has become a prominent area of study for master's and PhD students currently involved as Champions in clinical BPSOs. The collaborative BPSO network is now being used, amongst other means, to develop research projects. While published research results related to Spain's implementation of BPGs are not yet available, data collection that is currently taking place will allow for outcomes to be evaluated and analyzed.

> *"When we engaged with RNAO in the BPGs implementation program we were very optimistic regarding success, but we never thought it would have such a strong impact."*
>
> –Spanish BPSO Host team; Investén-isciii/Spanish Centre for Evidence Based Nursing and Healthcare

To sum it up succinctly, the overall impact has included:

- Improved access and adherence to BPG-specific evidence-based tools developed for nurses, other health professionals, and patients/caregivers, enabling more comprehensive care

- Improved patient satisfaction

- Introduction of risk assessments for prevention of health issues such as falls and pressure injury, with planning and development involving the interprofessional team, contributing to better uptake and greater satisfaction

- Improvement of records completion

- Establishment of nursing sensitive indicators

- Better coordination and integration of care across different settings

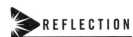 **REFLECTION**

How can the powerful data in this chapter about Spain as a BPSO Host be used to support the evidence-based practice movement in nursing, the BPSO Designation, and the global synergy in nursing through this work?

CONCLUSION

The Best Practice Spotlight Organization (BPSO) Designation in Spain is multicentered, covers different healthcare sectors (hospital, primary care, long-term care, and nursing homes), and addresses a wide range of healthcare problems. Key to the sustainment of the overall BPSO Designation, including the consolidation of the BPSO network and ongoing establishment of new cohorts, were: the alliances created on the micro and macro levels, continuous evaluation and feedback on implementation strategies, and the dissemination of results and development of related research.

The outcomes reported by our BPSOs and the overall BPSO Designation in Spain demonstrate that the RNAO BPG-implementation methodology can be replicated with success internationally. Strategies developed based on the local context contribute to the program's effectiveness, and, through a consolidated network, these strategies and the relevant BPG and implementation knowledge have been shared across healthcare settings to promote an evidence-based culture that reaches a wide spectrum of health professionals and patients.

KEY MESSAGES

■ Scaling up in the BPSO Host Model is influenced by nursing leadership, strategic planning, interprofessional team collaboration, and partnerships, which strengthen dissemination of good practices, reduce unreasonable variability in care, and increase quality.

■ Full engagement of nurses in the provision of evidence-based practice and monitoring its impact motivates passion for better performance and advancing people-centered healthcare.

■ The BPSO Host Model is a successful approach to spread evidence-based practice and inspire inter-organizational collaboration.

■ Evaluation of BPG impact is most effective if it addresses structure, process, and outcomes indicators measured in a consistent way.

■ The BPSO Host Model has demonstrated its powerful potential to impact client health outcomes at the local and regional levels, as well as outcomes for nurses, the profession, other healthcare providers, and healthcare organizations.

■ RNAO's overall BPSO Designation and implementation methodology, as demonstrated in Spain, can be replicated with success internationally.

REFERENCES

Albornos-Muñoz, L., González-María, E., & Moreno-Casbas, T. (2015). Implantación de guías de buenas prácticas en España. Programa de Centros comprometidos con la excelencia en cuidados. *MedUNAB, 17*(3), 163–169.

Comet-Cortés, P., Escobar-Aguilar, G., González-Gil, T., de Ormijana-Sáenz Hernández, A., Rich-Ruiz, M., & Vidal-Thomas, C. (2010). Establecimiento de prioridades de investigación en enfermería en España: estudio Delphi. *Enfermeria Clinica, 20*, 88–96.

González-María, E. (2014). Centros Comprometidos con la Excelencia en Cuidados o BPSO España. *NURE, 71.*

Grinspun, D. (2011). Guias de practica clinica y entorno laboral basados en la evidencia elaborados por la Registered Nurses' Association of Ontario (RNAO) (Evidence-based clinical practice and work environment guidelines prepared by the Registered Nurses' Association of Ontario). *Enfermeria Clinica (Clinical Nursing), 21*(1), 1–2.

Ministerio de Sanidad, Política Social e Igualdad. (2010). *Plan de Calidad para el Sistema Nacional de Salud.* Retrieved from http://www.mspsi.es/organizacion/sns/planCalidadSNS/pdf/pncalidad/PlanCalidad2010.pdf

Registered Nurses' Association of Ontario (RNAO). (2003). *Breastfeeding Best Practice Guidelines for nurses.* Toronto, ON: Registered Nurses' Association of Ontario.

Registered Nurses' Association of Ontario (RNAO). (2009). *Ostomy care and management.* Toronto, ON: Registered Nurses' Association of Ontario.

Registered Nurses' Association of Ontario (RNAO). (2011). *Prevention of falls and fall injuries in the older adult* [Supplement]. Toronto, ON: Registered Nurses' Association of Ontario.

Registered Nurses' Association of Ontario (RNAO). (2012). *Toolkit: Implementation of Best Practice Guidelines* (2nd ed.). Toronto, ON: Registered Nurses' Association of Ontario.

Registered Nurses' Association of Ontario (RNAO). (2013). *Assessment and management of pain* (3rd ed.). Toronto, ON: Registered Nurses' Association of Ontario.

Ruzafa-Martínez, M., González-María, E., Moreno-Casbas, T., del Río Faes, C., Albornos-Muñoz, L., & Escandell-García, C. (2011). Proyecto de Implantación de Guías de Buenas Prácticas en España 2011–2016. *Enf Clin, 21*(5), 275–283.

World Health Organization (WHO). (2015). *Nurses and midwifes: A vital resource for health. European compendium of good practices in nursing and midwifery towards Health 2020 goals.* Retrieved from http://www.euro.who.int/en/health-topics/Health-systems/nursing-and-midwifery/publications/2015/nurses-and-midwives-a-vital-resource-for-health.-european-compendium-of-good-practices-in-nursing-and-midwifery-towards-health-2020-goals

14

OVERCOMING CONTEXT AND LANGUAGE DIFFERENCES: BPSO TRAILBLAZERS IN CHINA

Hao Yufang, PhD
Guo Hailing, RN
Yan Lijiao, MS, RN
Tian Runxi, MSN, RN
Zhao Junqiang, BScN, RN

LEARNING OBJECTIVES

After reading this chapter, you will be able to:

- Understand the strategies for overcoming the contextual differences when implementing Best Practice Guidelines in a different culture

- Describe the facilitators and barriers within the Chinese context in implementing Best Practice Guidelines

- Develop an action plan related to implementing Best Practice Guidelines, building on the facilitators to tackle the identified barriers

- Discuss similarities and differences in the BPSO experience in an academic and a service setting

- Appreciate the impact of the BPSO Designation on patients, students, faculty, nursing staff, and organizations

INTRODUCTION

This chapter is about the groundbreaking partnership between the Registered Nurses' Association of Ontario (RNAO) and organizations in China to establish Best Practice Spotlight Organizations (BPSO). The experiences of a service BPSO and an academic BPSO are shared, alongside the tremendous success and spread resulting in several additional BPSOs in China. The chapter highlights the themes of capacity building, knowledge transfer, scope of practice changes, and the role of the BPSO lead in ensuring successful BPG implementation. In addition, the integration of traditional Chinese medicine and traditional Chinese nursing within the Chinese BPSO model is profiled as part of this specific context.

THE BACKGROUND OF INTRODUCING BPSOS IN CHINA

China represents approximately one-fifth of the world's population (Deloitte Touche Tohmatsu Limited, 2014). It is a nation with a severe nursing shortage. To accommodate the growing demands for quality and accessible healthcare, China is undertaking significant healthcare reforms (Zhu, Rodgers, & Melia, 2014), which have driven major changes in nursing education, practice, and research. Still, many challenges remain. First, in nursing education, the curriculum and teaching content cannot keep up with the rapid updates in knowledge. Second, monotonous teaching methods are not effectively engaging students, thus rendering them passive receptors of knowledge who lack innovation, creativity, and the ability to obtain knowledge. Third, there is a big gap in nursing between evidence and practice (Zhang, 2003). Most nurses prefer to use their own experiences as a reference for practice because of their many years of practice. At times, the practice delivered by nurses in China is based on textbooks, which are outdated. Moreover, many of the protocols developed for guiding nursing practice are based on expert consensus instead of more rigorous evidence (Jin et al., 2016). Even though some nurses are becoming familiar with the use of evidence-based practice, they rarely assess the feasibility and appropriateness of evidence for their own utilization.

With every challenge comes opportunity. Evidence-based nursing (EBN) provides a scientific framework that is based on nursing research and offers guides to clinical nursing practice and education. It is an effective approach to solve the dilemmas faced by nurses in China.

ESTABLISHING ACADEMIC AND SERVICE BPSOS IN CHINA

In 2015, the DongZhiMen Hospital and Beijing University of Chinese Medicine (BUCM) School of Nursing became the first two BPSOs in China. The goal for joining as BPSOs was and remains the urgent need to promote a culture of evidence-based nursing practice and management decision-making, and to optimize nursing care, education, and research through the systematic introduction of evidence-based nursing.

BUILDING UP THE BPSO TEAM

A structured and well-organized BPSO team is the prerequisite to implementing BPGs successfully. In China we set several priorities. First, the BPSO director acts as the scientific and administrative leader of an entity and oversees its general performance. Second, the BPSO leader is responsible for all BPG implementation. Third, BPG implementation involves various stakeholders. As an academic BPSO, BUCM School of Nursing aimed to ensure successful integration of BPGs into the curriculum by using the following strategies:

- Having an experienced faculty member instruct other faculty members in evidence-based practice, especially if they did not have experience in this area

- Selecting faculty directors as BPG leaders to be in charge of the BPG implementation in specific nursing courses

- Having BPG leaders discuss the BPSO Program with faculty, including strategies for implementation, because those faculty members will be central to integrating the selected BPGs into nursing curricula

- Engaging faculty in the planning process helps them adapt to the changes brought by the BPSO Program, and also to adjust their own teaching syllabus and methodology to embed the BPGs into their course

- Involving the students and identifying their preferred ways of gaining knowledge

The process of integration at the DongZhiMen Hospital has been similar, albeit more complex, because clinical nurses have to apply the BPGs recommendations in their day-to-day practice with their patients. Thus, their BPSO team composition needs to be more comprehensive, with much emphasis on training, data collection, and audit and feedback. Figure 14.1 shows an example of the infrastructure setup in DongZhiMen Hospital, which includes an overall steering committee as well as subcommittees for each of the three BPGs implemented.

SELECTING AND TRANSLATING BPGS

Selecting and translating BPGs and adapting them to the local culture are key steps to understanding the BPG development process and specific guideline content prior to implementation. Our BPSOs selected specific guidelines based on the following criteria:

- What are the prioritized nursing issues that need to be addressed in current nursing education and clinical practice?

- Can solutions be found in the BPGs?

- How does the knowledge from the BPGs fit with the current priorities and settings?

After selecting the guidelines, the translation process may commence. This step required careful planning and partnership with RNAO to ensure an accurate translation. At the BUCM School of Nursing, the translation team included a leader from the university who specializes in the topic, several master of science in nursing (MSN) candidates, and one or more specialized clinical staff. After translation, a careful review by RNAO is conducted to ensure that it is clear and accurate. The translated BPGs, with full acknowledgement of the contributors, are finally published on the RNAO website, providing free access for users.

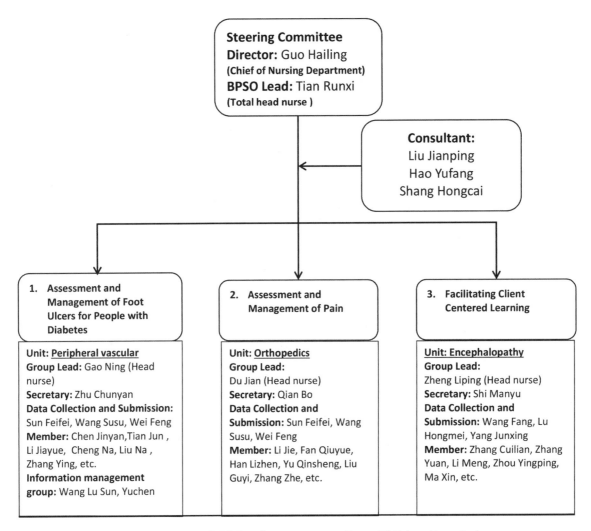

FIGURE 14.1 BPSO infrastructure at DongZhiMen Hospital.
Used with permission.

INTEGRATING BPGS INTO NURSING EDUCATION: THE BUCM EXPERIENCE

Integrating BPGs into the curriculum is a comprehensive process that gets embedded throughout the program. It engages all partners including nursing and other faculty, students, and clinical partners. Next we discuss the myriad of approaches we used to ensure we actively involved all partners in transforming our curriculum—in theory and teaching methodologies—into an evidence-based one.

IN THE CLASSROOM

After selecting the specific BPGs to be implemented, the BPG leader needs to study the content together with faculty who will incorporate it into their courses. In the case of the BPG *Assessment and Management of Foot Ulcers for People with Diabetes* (RNAO, 2013a), the content is often taught in medical and surgical nursing courses. When reviewing the content, the faculty responsible for those courses discussed the following questions:

- How is the BPG developed and organized?

- What are the recommendations of this BPG?

- What are the differences between current clinical practice and the BPG recommendations?

- In the past, only some key points on foot ulcer care for diabetic patients were taught in those courses within 1 hour of lecture. How can a significant amount of new knowledge be integrated into the same timeframe?

- What strategies can be used to embed the recommendations in the class and engage students' interest?

This discussion is an effective way to not only enhance and update educators' own knowledge in this specific topic, but also to understand the gap between recommendations and clinical practice. Based on such analysis, educators can then adjust the teaching syllabus to incorporate the evidence-based concepts and recommendations into the learning objectives. For example, the current objectives in a *Medical Nursing* course (You, 2012) directed at diabetic patient care are:

- Gain basic knowledge on evidence-based nursing and understand the differences between the course textbook and the RNAO Best Practice Guideline

- Understand key recommendations from the RNAO (2013a) BPG, *Assessment and Management of Foot Ulcers for People with Diabetes*

- Describe how to apply those recommendations in day-to-day clinical practice

Prior to each class, nursing educators provide reading materials, including parts of the BPG and additional references, for students to review in advance. During class, educators expand on the foundation of evidence-based nursing and key recommendations from the BPG and share specific examples of embedding evidence-based concepts into clinical practice. Various teaching methods are adopted to make the learning experience more interactive, such as peer teaching, role-playing, problem-based learning, team-based learning, and a flipped classroom. Since entering the BPSO Program, our own teaching methodologies have become more dynamic and engaging, enriched with techniques that we learned during our training sessions with RNAO.

To assess the impact of implementing BPGs in the curriculum, the course evaluation system required changes. First, questions on evidence-based nursing and BPG recommendations were added to the tests and final exam of the course. This change emphasized the significance of the new content and directed students' attention when reviewing. Second, the formative assessment was enhanced with metrics for evaluating students' performance in peer teaching, role-playing, and other exercises that promote dynamic learning.

INTRODUCING FACILITATING CLIENT-CENTRED LEARNING (RNAO, 2012) INTO A COURSE ON NURSING PRACTICE AT BUCM

Educators adopted the content of the *Facilitating Client-Centred Learning* (2012a) BPG in their lectures and also implemented some of the recommendations from the BPG as they applied to the student-educator situation in the classroom. The recommendations adopted included those listed below, with specific adaptations for the student learning situation identified following:

I. Educators can follow the six segments of the LEARNS Model (RNAO, 2012a, pp. 19–20) from the BPG:

- **L**istening to student needs—How can I encourage students to deliver their opinions and advice?

- **E**stablishing partnerships—How do I engage and build a trusting partnership with students?

- **A**dopting an approach to learning—How do I shift to a more formal, structured, and interactive approach to facilitating learning?

- **R**einforcing competency in nursing practice—How do I foster nursing knowledge and improve the nursing practice of students?

- **N**aming new knowledge—In what ways can I check for understanding amongst students?

- **S**trengthening self-learning—How can I promote or strengthen students' capacity for self-learning (e.g., after-school exercises, case study presentations, and using school resources)?

II. Based on the BPG recommendations 1, 2, 3, 4 and 8 (RNAO, 2012a, pp. 6–7), related to creating a safe environment to assess learning, assessing the learning needs, tailoring the approach by collaborating with students and colleagues, and assessing learning, we have designed the teaching methodology so students can engage in nurse/patient role-playing situations simulating appropriate teaching dialogues. If the topic is a specific disease or a nursing diagnosis, the "nurse" should try their best to explain it in plain language to the "client" and assess whether the "client" understands it. At the same time, the nurse should also think from the client's perspective and recognize the client's feelings. In this way, students may experience a relatively realistic clinical scenario and gain certain abilities in facilitating client-centred learning in future clinical practice.

III. Recommendation 6 is using plain language to promote health literacy (RNAO, 2012a, p. 6). We support students to become expert in this by asking them to give a short presentation at the beginning of each class, demonstrating how they would teach a client. The topic provided to the student can be a specific disease or a clinical nursing issue. For example, students can give a presentation on a cancer patient's diet. They can choose the content and presentation methods (oral presentation, PowerPoint, role-play, etc.) to make the knowledge understandable and memorable. After their presentation, the class would discuss the optimal way to provide health education to patients.

IV. Recommendation 7 is assessing the effectiveness of the education strategy (RNAO, 2012a, p. 6); educators use this in the curriculum by asking students questions about key lessons from previous classes where different teaching methods were employed. Through this, they can ascertain which methods were more conducive to knowledge uptake and explore a variety of approaches to making the class more engaging.

Evaluation of Students' Performance

Students are evaluated comprehensively through presentations, answering questions, group discussions, nursing situational conversation, and written exams. Presentations can provide students with chances to improve their confidence and oral communication skills. Through answering questions, teachers can test whether students have gained the specific knowledge. Case discussion in groups can help group members improve communication skills and cultivate a sense of teamwork. Situational conversation is an effective way to expose students to relatively real clinical contexts and emphasize the importance of listening and thinking from the patient's perspective. The written exam is still a necessary component for assessing whether students have fully absorbed the course material.

Outside the Classroom

Given the time constraints of in-class education, nurse educators devised additional methods for students to grasp evidence-based nursing. The following approaches were applied at the Beijing University of Chinese Medicine.

Second Classroom

Sophomore nursing students were asked to form teams and become familiarized with the RNAO (2012a) BPG, *Facilitating Client-Centred Learning*, during their winter break. In their teams, they discussed the BPG's contents, gaps between the BPG and current clinical practice, and changes in their knowledge and attitude toward health teaching in clinical practice after studying the BPG. At the beginning of the next semester, students were required to give presentations based on their discussions, using PowerPoint or other audio-visuals.

Summer Class

Students are provided with opportunities to attend classes during the summer break, and one class features lectures from evidence-based nursing experts. Their lectures are systematically arranged to cover the aspects of: asking clinical questions, searching for research evidence, appraising research evidence, and applying evidence to practice. From those lectures, students can gain in-depth understanding of evidence-based nursing concepts and practice.

Students' Association of Evidence-Based Nursing

The Students' Association of Evidence-Based Nursing is operated by graduate students who are BPG Champions. Its membership includes nursing undergraduate students from BUCM as well as students from other schools interested in evidence-based nursing. The main responsibilities of the association are to provide EBN training for undergraduate students, translate BPGs, and review BPGs with undergraduate students, with guidance from faculty. This is an effective approach for spreading the BPSO knowledge and preparing more BPG Champions in the organization.

IMPLEMENTING BPGS INTO CLINICAL NURSING PRACTICE: THE DONGZHIMEN HOSPITAL EXPERIENCE

The process of introducing a clinical guideline in the practice setting is similar to that used in the academic setting. RNAO's Toolkit (2012b) is a critical resource that provides detailed guidance on implementing BPGs in clinical practice. The general process is as follows:

1. Identify gaps between BPG and clinical practice. For non-English speakers, the first issue that needs to be tackled prior to BPG implementation is the thorough understanding of BPG content.

2. The next step is to hold a multidisciplinary team meeting to identify the gaps between BPG recommendations and clinical practice. In this meeting, each recommendation is reviewed and rated. The following questions are used for consideration:

    ■   What are the recommendations that have already been implemented?

    ■   Are there any recommendations that have only been partially implemented?

    ■   What are the gaps between current clinical practice and the recommended practice, and to what extent do they exist?

    ■   Are there any recommendations that can be implemented quickly?

    ■   What will be the barriers to implementing those recommendations, such as budget, staff skills, workload, etc.?

The meeting concludes with a final decision on which recommendations will be implemented. An example of the review process of a specific BPG is provided in Table 14.1.

TABLE 14.1   EXAMPLE OF GAPS IDENTIFIED AT DONGZHIMEN HOSPITAL

RNAO BPG *ASSESSMENT AND MANAGEMENT OF PAIN* (RNAO, 2013b)

GUIDELINE RECOMMENDATION	MET	PARTIALLY MET	UNMET	COMMENTS
1.1 Screen for the presence, or risk of, any type of pain: ■ On admission or visit with a healthcare professional ■ After a change in medical status ■ Prior to, during, and after a procedure	✓			Admission assessment sheet and the TCM nursing care guideline

GUIDELINE RECOMMENDATION	MET	PARTIALLY MET	UNMET	COMMENTS
1.2 Perform a comprehensive pain assessment on persons screened having the presence, or risk of, any type of pain using a systematic approach and appropriate, validated tools.	✓			Visual Analogue Scale/Score (VAS)
1.3 Perform a comprehensive pain assessment on persons unable to self-report using a validated tool.			✓	Patients in this unit are all able to self-report
1.4 Explore the person's beliefs, knowledge, and level of understanding about pain and pain management.	✓			Admission assessment sheet
1.5 Document the person's pain characteristics.	✓			Admission assessment sheet
2.1 Collaborate with the person to identify his/her goals for pain management and suitable strategies to ensure a comprehensive approach to the plan of care.		✓		Lack opinions from patients
2.2 Establish a comprehensive plan of care that incorporates the goals of the person and the interprofessional team and addresses: ■ Assessment findings ■ The person's beliefs and knowledge and level of understanding ■ The person's attributes and pain characteristics		✓		Lack opinions from patients
3.1 Implement the pain management plan using principles that maximize efficacy and minimize the adverse effects of pharmacological interventions including: ■ Multimodal analgesic approach ■ Changing of opioids (dose or routes) when necessary ■ Prevention, assessment, and management of adverse effects during the administration of opioid analgesics ■ Prevention, assessment, and management of opioid risk		✓		It's not suitable in China's context. Nurses are not allowed to do so.
3.2 Evaluate any nonpharmacological (physical and psychological) interventions for effectiveness and the potential for interactions with pharmacological interventions.	✓			

continues

TABLE 14.1 EXAMPLE OF GAPS IDENTIFIED AT DONGZHIMEN HOSPITAL (CONTINUED)

GUIDELINE RECOMMENDATION	MET	PARTIALLY MET	UNMET	COMMENTS
3.3 Teach the person, his/her family, and caregivers about the pain management strategies in their plan of care and address known concerns and misconceptions.		✓		Health education brochures, could involve patients more
4.1 Reassess the person's response to the pain management interventions consistently using the same re-evaluation tool. The frequency of reassessments will be determined by: ■ Presence of pain ■ Pain intensity ■ Stability of the person's medical condition ■ Type of pain, e.g., acute versus persistent ■ Practice setting	✓			
4.2 Communicate and document the person's responses to the pain management plan.	✓			Nursing record sheet
5.1 Educational institutions should incorporate this guideline, *Assessment and Management of Pain* (3rd ed.), into basic and interprofessional curricula for registered nurses, registered practical nurses, and doctor of medicine programs to promote evidence-based practice.			✓	Not suitable in clinical context, however suitable in academic BPSO
5.2 Incorporate content on knowledge translation strategies into education programs for healthcare providers to move evidence related to the assessment and management of pain into practice.			✓	Not suitable in clinical context, however suitable in academic BPSO
5.3 Promote interprofessional education and collaboration related to the assessment and management of pain in academic institutions.			✓	Not suitable in clinical context, however suitable in academic BPSO
5.4 Healthcare professionals should participate in continuing education opportunities to enhance specific knowledge and skills to competently assess and manage pain, based on this guideline, *Assessment and Management of Pain* (3rd ed.).		✓		There's training in this area, however, not as a special training program
6.1 Establish pain assessment and management as a strategic clinical priority.	✓			Supported by the nursing department

GUIDELINE RECOMMENDATION	MET	PARTIALLY MET	UNMET	COMMENTS
6.2 Establish a model of care to support interprofessional collaboration for the effective assessment and management of pain.	✓			There's a pain management group currently in our hospital
6.3 Use the knowledge translation process and multifaceted strategies within organizations to assist healthcare providers to use the best evidence on assessing and managing pain in practice.	✓			Support from academia, especially BUCM, BPSO
6.4 Use a systematic, organization-wide approach to implement *Assessment and Management of Pain* (3rd ed.) Best Practice Guideline and provide resources and organizational and administrative supports to facilitate uptake.			✓	BPSO work will help us with this over time, as we expand this BPG

The results of the gap analysis guided the BPG implementation work and led to greater involvement of patients in their care; enhanced client-centred teaching about pain; increased independence for nurses in carrying out pain assessment, interventions, monitoring, and evaluation; and a more consistent approach to pain management hospital-wide.

ASSESSING FACILITATORS AND BARRIERS TO BPG IMPLEMENTATION

The identification of facilitators can enable the BPSO team to maximize support for BPG implementation, and the identification of barriers allows the team to develop effective strategies for overcoming or mediating them early in the implementation process. This process can be augmented by interviewing identified stakeholders. An example of the facilitators and barriers identified in relation to implementing the *Assessment and Management of Foot Ulcers for People with Diabetes* (RNAO, 2013a) at DongZhiMen Hospital is provided in Table 14.2.

TABLE 14.2 FACILITATORS AND BARRIERS IDENTIFIED IN BPG IMPLEMENTATION AT DONGZHIMEN HOSPITAL

RNAO BPG: *ASSESSMENT AND MANAGEMENT OF FOOT ULCERS FOR PEOPLE WITH DIABETES (2013A)*		
Facilitators	Policy support	The national nursing development programs 2010–2015 and 2016–2020 have both made it clear that scientific methods shall be utilized to standardize clinical nursing practice.
	Leadership support	The program is highly supported by the directors of nursing department, medical department, and head nurses.
	Adequate source of patient data	The peripheral vascular disease in this department is authorized as the national key discipline, and the treatment of diabetic foot is its specialty. Annually, hundreds of patients with diabetic foot come to this department for treatment.
	Staff nurses' great interest and positive attitude	Even though staff nurses' professional knowledge of evidence-based nursing is generally inadequate, they have great interest in BPGs and are willing to learn more.
	Support from academia	The academic center provides training to staff nurses on the basic knowledge of evidence-based nursing and provides instructions on evidence utilization in practice.
Barriers	Human resources	Nursing shortages have become a critical issue throughout China, as well as the peripheral vascular department.
	Lack of knowledge and skills	Although many staff nurses have heard of evidence-based nursing, they seldom accept relevant training and do not have a clear and deep understanding of EBN.
	Scope of nursing practice	The scope of nursing practice varies greatly in different countries. Some recommendations are beyond nurses' scope of practice and are not quite suitable in China's clinical context (e.g., the recommendation to assess foot ulcer(s) for infection using clinical assessment techniques, based on signs and symptoms, and facilitate appropriate diagnostic testing, if indicated).
	Financial problem	BPG implementation not only implies a heavier workload in the short term, but also involves more costs for the unit. Additions such as new health-education brochures, new nursing record sheets, and training programs all require more funding and financial support.

DEVELOPING IMPLEMENTATION STRATEGIES

Guidelines developed by professional associations are sometimes quite general and not agency-specific, while protocols endorsed by a hospital are based on the specific hospital context, which provide detailed instructions and parameters for nursing practice. Thus it is necessary to translate the BPGs into evidence-based clinical nursing protocols. Within such protocols, the rationale of each chosen recommendation, the implementation method, and audit method are listed. An example of the pain management protocol developed by DongZhiMen Hospital is provided in Table 14.3.

TABLE 14.3   EXAMPLE OF PAIN MANAGEMENT PROTOCOL DEVELOPED BY DONGZHIMEN HOSPITAL

RNAO BPG ASSESSMENT AND MANAGEMENT OF PAIN (RNAO, 2013b)

RECOMMENDATIONS CHOSEN TO BE IMPLEMENTED	CLINICAL NURSING PRACTICE STANDARDS	AUDIT CRITERIA
1.1 Screen for the presence, or risk of, any type of pain: ■ On admission or visit with a healthcare professional ■ After a change in medical status ■ Prior to, during, and after a procedure	1. Perform pain screening on hospitalized and operated patients.	Admission assessment sheet and nursing record sheets
1.2 Perform a comprehensive pain assessment on persons screened having the presence, or risk of, any type of pain using a systematic approach and appropriate, validated tools.	2. Use an effective assessment tool to comprehensively assess the screened pain positive patients.	
1.4 Explore the person's beliefs, knowledge, and level of understanding about pain and pain management.	3. The assessment should include patient knowledge, comprehension of pain, and so on.	
1.5 Document the person's pain characteristics.	4. Document the person's pain characteristics.	
2.1 Collaborate with the person to identify his/her goals for pain management and suitable strategies to ensure a comprehensive approach to the plan of care.	5. The pain management plan should incorporate patient preference.	Patient interview or questionnaire

continues

TABLE 14.3 EXAMPLE OF PAIN MANAGEMENT PROTOCOL DEVELOPED BY DONGZHIMEN HOSPITAL (CONTINUED)

RECOMMENDATIONS CHOSEN TO BE IMPLEMENTED	CLINICAL NURSING PRACTICE STANDARDS	AUDIT CRITERIA
2.2 Establish a comprehensive plan of care that incorporates the goals of the person and the multi-professional team and addresses: ■ Assessment findings ■ The person's beliefs and knowledge and level of understanding ■ The person's attributes and pain characteristics	6. The pain management program requires collaboration between the patient and the professional team. It should include assessment findings, patient knowledge, and pain characteristics.	Nursing record sheets including nursing care plans and assessments
3.1 Implement the pain management plan using principles that maximize efficacy and minimize the adverse effects of pharmacological interventions including: ■ Multimodal analgesic approach ■ Changing of opioids (dose or routes) when necessary ■ Prevention, assessment, and management of adverse effects during the administration of opioid analgesics ■ Prevention, assessment, and management of opioid risk	7. Multimodal analgesic approach should be used. 8. Grasp the side effects and risks of opiates.	Nursing record sheets; survey for nurses
3.2 Evaluate any nonpharmacological (physical and psychological) interventions for effectiveness and the potential for interactions with pharmacological interventions.	9. Rational use of nonpharmacological therapy for patients.	Patient interview or questionnaire
3.3 Teach the person, their family, and caregivers about the pain management strategies in their plan of care and address known concerns and misconceptions.	10. Incorporate pain management strategies into patient education.	
4.1 Reassess the person's response to the pain management interventions consistently using the same re-evaluation tool. The frequency of reassessments will be determined by: ■ Presence of pain ■ Pain intensity ■ Stability of the person's medical condition ■ Type of pain (e.g., acute versus persistent) ■ Practice setting	11. Use a consistent tool for pain evaluation.	Nursing record sheets
4.2 Communicate and document the person's responses to the pain management plan.	12. Communicate and document the person's responses to the pain management plan.	

RECOMMENDATIONS CHOSEN TO BE IMPLEMENTED	CLINICAL NURSING PRACTICE STANDARDS	AUDIT CRITERIA
5.4 Healthcare professionals should participate in continuing education opportunities to enhance specific knowledge and skills to competently assess and manage pain, based on this guideline, *Assessment and Management of Pain* (3rd ed.).	13. Use the BPG in continuing education.	Continuing education material in nursing department

Based on the established protocol, the BPSO team developed new procedures and nursing record sheets where necessary. For example, recommendation 1.0 in the BPG *Assessment and Management of Foot Ulcers for People with Diabetes* (RNAO, 2013a, p. 18) is to "Obtain a comprehensive health history and perform physical examination of affected limb(s)." The team at DongZhiMen Hospital developed a table with a specific checklist of items mentioned in the BPG, including the history of presenting illness (initiating event, duration of ulceration, treatment undertaken, and outcome of the treatments), past medical history, glycemic control, nutritional status, and allergies. In relation to the BPG *Assessment and Management of Pain* (RNAO, 2013b), prior to its implementation, the admission assessment sheet only included one question: Do you feel pain? During the implementation process, the Dong-ZhiMen Hospital team developed a single pain assessment sheet, which requires patients to describe the pain experience at length. On top of adding new items to the existing nursing record sheets, other resources, such as health-education brochures for patients, needed to be enhanced.

CHAMPION DEVELOPMENT

In DongZhiMen Hospital, nurses and physicians participating in the BPG implementation process are regarded as BPG Champions. They are given BPG Champion badges and receive priority in attending relevant training programs. The BPSO Orientation Program is based on RNAO's toolkit and materials, including the PowerPoint presentations—all of which are provided to us as part of the agreement at no cost. The content of these materials includes theories of evidence-based curriculum and practice, as well as teaching methods.

The specialist nurses' training program focuses on the scope of nursing practice, which is one of the main obstacles to implementation of the BPG recommendations encountered at DongZhiMen Hospital. Indeed, we credit the BPSO Program with progressive changes in the scope of practice for nurses. For example, before implementing the BPG *Assessment and Management of Foot Ulcers for People with Diabetes* (RNAO, 2013a), the dressing change for patients with diabetic foot was often done by physicians. To shift the practice scope, the specialist nurses' training program was developed for wound care. After obtaining the approval of physicians in the peripheral vascular department, and after nurses earned qualifications on wound care, they are now able to conduct the dressing change for patients with physicians' full support.

INTERDISCIPLINARY COOPERATION

Interdisciplinary team cooperation is essential for effective BPG implementation. For patients with diabetic foot ulcers at DongZhiMen Hospital, a vascular surgeon, endocrinologist, nutritionist, and diabetes specialist nurse work closely with each other to develop the optimal treatment and care.

Similarly, another interdisciplinary team develops pharmaceutical and nonpharmaceutical therapies for patients suffering from pain.

OBTAINING ADDITIONAL RESOURCES THROUGH RESEARCH FUNDS

Another main barrier to BPG implementation is financial support. The BPSO team at DongZhiMen Hospital found the solution by applying for research funds both from the hospital and the Beijing government. We were successful in this endeavour thanks to our increased research capacity from the BPSO training and program work.

MONITORING BPG USE AND EVALUATING OUTCOMES

Evaluation and monitoring is a key pillar of the BPG Program and a critical aspect of the BPSO requirements for both service and academic BPSOs. All BPSOs participate in NQuIRE, RNAO's robust comprehensive database system, on an ongoing basis, and as well are expected to engage in other evaluation processes.

NQUIRE DATABASE

Each BPG implementation site is required to submit data monthly to the RNAO NQuIRE database. Based on the NQuIRE data reports, the DongZhiMen Hospital BPSO gains insight into BPG utilization outcomes. BUCM BPSO is working with RNAO to help determine appropriate education indicators that can become part of NQuIRE.

RNAO AUDIT

RNAO conducts an annual audit of the BPG implementation sites, and it provides constructive feedback on the structures and processes used by the BPSOs and BPG implementation, in practice and integration into the curriculum as well as sustained use/integration of evidence-based practice.

QUESTIONNAIRE ON PATIENT SATISFACTION

The DongZhiMen Hospital develops and administers questionnaires on patient satisfaction related to their pain control to evaluate the overall effect of implementing the RNAO (2013b) BPG, *Assessment and Management of Pain*. Results have shown increased patient satisfaction with pain management (see Figure 14.2).

Other indicators for evaluating outcomes include the length of hospital stay, patients' medical costs, and questionnaires on nurses' knowledge of BPGs, all of which have shown substantive improvements (see Figure 14.2).

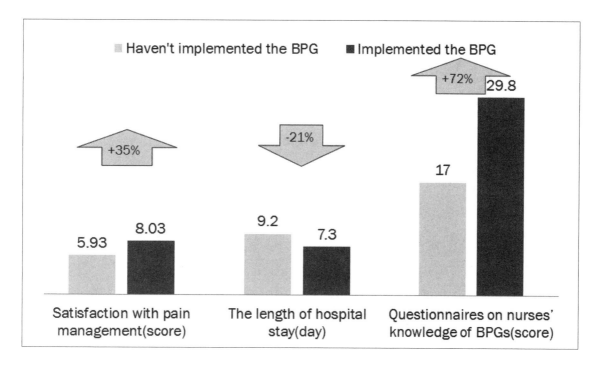

FIGURE 14.2 The effects of implementing the RNAO BPG *Assessment and Management of Pain* (2013b) using three indicators measured pre- and post-implementation.
Used with permission from DongZhiMen Hospital.

SUSTAINING BPG USE

Sustaining practice change related to implementation of BPGs is an important and vital activity for academic and service BPSOs. Key to success in this area is the use of a variety of sustainability strategies, many of which are discussed next.

DEVELOPING AN ANNUAL WORK PLAN

For planning and sustaining BPG implementation, an annual plan was developed to set goals and coordinate activities. Both the DongZhiMen Hospital and the BUCM School of Nursing use their annual plan as a framework for reporting to RNAO on a biannual basis, as a way to review strengths and areas for improvement.

MONTHLY REVIEW MEETINGS

The BPSO teams have monthly meetings to track the status of BPG implementation work.

MAINTAINING AND ENHANCING CHAMPION TRAINING

Since the launch of the BPSO Designation at DongZhiMen Hospital and the BUCM School of Nursing, BPSO Champions have made significant strides in nursing education, practice, and research. Using a train-the-trainer approach, RNAO has effectively transferred the knowledge and skills of BPG implementation to local Champions, who not only maintain but also augment the outcomes of the BPSO Designation.

ACHIEVEMENTS OF THE BPSO DESIGNATION IN CHINA

The BPSO Designation in China has resulted in a number of key changes in educational and clinical practices, scope of practice, and interprofessional work. Most importantly, it has already delivered positive results in education for both faculty and students, as well as improved patient and organizational outcomes. An added bonus is the enthusiastic attention that both the university and the hospital have received, which has translated into funding gains and high-level recognition of its leadership and staff. This section of the chapter discusses top achievements in these academic and service BPSOs.

ACHIEVEMENTS BY THE ACADEMIC BPSO

For students at the Beijing University of Chinese Medicine (BUCM), the introduction to evidence-based nursing through the RNAO BPSO Program enriched their knowledge of best practices and also cultivated their critical thinking. What's more, master's students gained a broader perspective on research topics related to guideline adoption, implementation, and synthesis. Some dissertations have already been developed on *Identification and Management of Dysphagia After Stroke: An Evidence-Based Nursing Practice* (Gao, 2015); *The Analysis of Application Situation for Colostomy Care Clinical Practice Guideline Recommendations* (Xue, 2017); and *Development of Evidence-Based Practice Protocols for High Risk of Diabetic Foot Ulcers* (Jiang, 2017).

STUDENT COMMENTS

Student A: "The guideline can not only help us to adjust our ways of thinking, but also help us to study knowledge of the practice of nursing and nursing skills. In addition, in the process of learning a guideline, we can also develop a collaborative academic atmosphere amongst the students, learning and cooperating together as a team."

Student B: "According to this BPG, if we as nurses want to succeed in facilitating client-centred learning, we should work hard to build a professional, therapeutic partnership relationship with our clients. In the academic setting the client is the student, whereas in the clinical setting the client is the patient. Lack of a partnership relationship is the main obstacle to the success of client-centred learning."

Nurse educators also gained new insights from the experience of implementing BPGs in an academic setting. Many educators at BUCM are now able to develop new teaching methods and learning resources that have enriched their teaching practices as well as student engagement. In particular, they have gained in-depth knowledge of student-centred teaching, which has brought a higher degree of innovation and interaction into their classroom.

TEACHER COMMENTS

Teacher A: "I finally found a way from the *Facilitating Client-Centred Learning* BPG to encourage students to ask questions to improve their understanding of what we taught."

Teacher B: "Students always enjoy our class and are more satisfied with teachers teaching skill and contents based on the guidelines."

Teacher C: "Sometimes the students find it difficult to understand some sentences or words in the BPGs, so I organize them to discuss those questions together. I think it is a good way to cultivate their critical-thinking ability."

Teacher D: "Since the *Ostomy Care and Management* guideline includes much new knowledge, such as ostomy assessment tools, new nursing skills, and so on, which we can hardly find in our textbook, we introduce the BPG as supplemental knowledge when teaching students how to provide better care for ostomy patients. In addition, we plan to design the colorectal cancer care lesson plans according to the content of this guideline in order to help students master the knowledge better."

Teacher E: "Before we incorporated the BPG into our curriculum, we gave lectures on pain assessment mainly based on the textbook. However, in the textbook, only a limited number of traditional pain assessment scales for general population were available. Students felt that it was difficult to apply these pain assessment tools in clinical practice.

Now we introduce the specific, operable pain assessment procedure and validated tools to our students from this BPG. Students come to understand how to perform a comprehensive pain assessment with a validated tool in special populations, especially those unable to self-report, such as newborn infants, older adults, and patients in critical condition. We also design the role-play to let the student complete a pain assessment for a patient in pain by following the BPG, and to find the barriers for pain assessment in real clinical practice."

At an organizational level, the BPSO Program has provided many new ideas for educational and teaching reform at the Beijing University of Chinese Medicine. These include student-centred learning and how to promote and sustain the application of knowledge to practice in a variety of clinical learning environments. The program has also led to increased research capacity and achievements. In 2015, several evidence-based nursing research projects were approved by the University; BUCM became the chief editor, compiling these projects into a graduate student textbook in 2016, *Evidence-Based Nursing*. Moreover, two influential journals in China established special columns for the BUCM School of Nursing to publish a series of articles on evidence-based nursing, including its BPSO-related work, in 2016.

With such achievements, and as a result of the heightened profile of BUCM in China and other countries, the BPSO team was invited to give EBN lectures at national conferences, universities, and hospitals. In 2016, the BPSO director at BUCM School of Nursing was invited to an international conference in Liaoning province and gave an oral presentation on "Implementation of BPGs in Nursing Practice." She was also invited to the 2016 national nursing Deans Summit in Guangxi province for an oral presentation on "Implementing BPGs in Nursing Education." She was also invited to give lectures on EBN at Peking Hospital, Shandong University, Third Medical University, and others.

ACHIEVEMENTS BY THE SERVICE BPSO

There have been many changes and successes achieved in nursing practice since the inception of the BPSO Program at DongZhiMen Hospital. Evidence-based practice has become the focus of global healthcare; however, the transformation of high-quality evidence into clinical practice is a challenge to nursing staff in many institutions.

At DongZhiMen Hospital, the BPSO team learned that BPG implementation is, first, an effective method to improve the quality of clinical care, and second, a catalyst for research and professional advancement. Many nurses have conducted research on BPG implementation and published a number of articles on their findings. In 2015 and 2016, nurses from the DongZhiMen Hospital won the first prize and top ten individual awards at the Beijing Municipal Administration of Traditional Chinese Medicine Competition. In addition, the hospital is gaining numerous external accolades. As well, the increased competency of nurses implies better pay and more opportunities for advancement. By improving their practice and research ability, nurses report feeling more confident and enthusiastic about their work. Nurses have also gained more trust and support from doctors and patients. Inter-professional collaboration has increased, as doctors are now more likely to collaborate with nurses in responding to patients' needs.

> *"It offered me a chance to grow professionally and improve my ability to be an effective leader and manager. I gained skills of communication, good judgment, and logical thinking ability. In my work, I started to develop more awareness of and improvement in my ability to solve problems and find solutions."*
>
> —Gao Ning, BPG implementation leader of *Assessment and Management of Foot Ulcers for People with Diabetes* (RNAO, 2013a)

Amongst the achievements at DongZhiMen Hospital BPSO is higher patient satisfaction with its nursing care because of nurses' attention to providing better patient care, and the greater respect they have for patients' perspectives, needs, and values. Before the introduction of the BPG *Assessment and Management of Foot Ulcers for People with Diabetes* (RNAO, 2013a), there were no stoma nurses at the hospital. Following the BPG recommendations, stoma specialist nurses were recruited, and a new dressing clinic was opened. Patients who were previously hospitalized for dressing change can now receive the service in the clinic, which shortens the time of hospitalization of patients and reduces their expenses. Furthermore, through the implementation of *Facilitating Client-Centred Learning* (RNAO, 2012a), nurses are showing a higher degree of attention to patients' needs and their perspective.

Like the BUCM School of Nursing, the nursing department at DongZhiMen Hospital experienced a similar boost in support and a higher research profile. It received more financial, policy, technical, and intellectual support from the hospital, as well as support from BUCM in the form of expert consultation and scientific research guidance. These valuable resources enabled the nursing department to experience an unprecedented surge in nursing research, where it has developed 17 approved research projects in 2016 and received research funds nearing 578,500 RMB. One project, entitled

"Implementation Scheme and Application of TCM Nursing in Diabetic Foot Ulcer," is a Beijing TCM (Traditional Chinese Medicine) bureau-level project and is related to the BPSO-led application of that BPG. In addition, the nursing department obtained two nursing patents and published four conference papers and several articles in journals. Nursing workflow has also been optimized; the integration of the diabetic foot ulcer assessment tool (PUSH scale) into clinical practice is one example.

CHALLENGES AND SOLUTIONS TO BPSO IMPLEMENTATION

There have been and will continue to be challenges to address and overcome in implementing EBP, including BPGs, in China. Overcoming these requires continuous leadership and strategic thinking and acting. Keeping in mind the end goal of improved nursing education and clinical practice for better patient, organizational, and health system outcomes, as well as perseverance to get to the finish line, are paramount to realize these goals. Both of our organizations are fully committed and invested in our work as BPSOs. Independently and together we are building creative solutions to sustain our work in our own BPSOs and spread the BPSO Designation and BPG uptake to other organizations and academic settings in China. The key challenges are discussed next.

HEAVY WORKLOAD

Heavy workload was identified as a major obstacle for nurses and educators, which may deter or hinder participation in the BPSO Program. The DongZhiMen Hospital is a tertiary hospital characterized by, and renowned for, its Traditional Chinese Medicine (TCM) treatment and nursing care. As such, nurses must conduct TCM nursing techniques as well as Western nursing practices, which gives them a much heavier workload in comparison with other hospitals. Seventeen nurses in the peripheral vascular department are responsible for 40 beds and implementing the BPG *Assessment and Management of Foot Ulcers for People with Diabetes* (RNAO, 2013a); 10 nurses in the orthopaedics department are responsible for 26 beds and implementing the BPG *Assessment and Management of Pain* (RNAO, 2013b); and 34 nurses in the encephalopathy department are responsible for 75 beds and implementing the BPG *Facilitating Client-Centred Learning* (RNAO, 2012a). The BPG implementation work has, to some extent, added to their current workload, which may impede the implementation process and quality.

Creating an incentive is one solution that the BPSOs offered to encourage educators and nurses to participate in BPSO activities. For example, they added indicators related to BPSO participation to the BUCM faculty's annual Key Performance Indicator System, which includes BPG translation, BPG implementation, and BPG leadership. With that, faculty are becoming more active in BPSO involvement. Using a more direct approach, the director of the nursing department at the hospital and at the BUCM School of Nursing spoke with BPSO leaders who volunteered for the position about the importance of BPG implementation and their role in its impact. As a result, the BPSO leaders felt highly favoured and more motivated to do the work well.

CULTURAL DIFFERENCES

Given the many differences in knowledge, attitudes, and practices, it is understandable that culture may form a barrier to understanding, and thus implementing, best practices. In particular, the BPG *Facilitating Client-Centred Learning* (RNAO, 2012a, p. 6) presented a challenge to Chinese BPSOs in its recommendation to "Engage in more structured and intentional approaches when facilitating client centred learning." The BPSO teams did not understand the meaning of "structured" approaches and thus felt unable to implement the recommendation correctly.

In order to effectively implement the BPGs and overall BPSO Program, both Chinese BPSOs have organized BPSO symposiums and other forums for reviewing and discussing the BPGs. Translation of the BPGs and regular meetings with the RNAO BPSO Host have also enhanced local capacity to develop an evidence-based culture. Professional training programs in English oral and writing skills have further cultivated an English learning environment for better uptake of the BPGs and implementation resources.

ATTITUDES, KNOWLEDGE, AND PRACTICES IN EVIDENCE-BASED NURSING

DongZhiMen Hospital and BUCM School of Nursing have encountered a range of attitudes toward evidence-based nursing. Despite a majority of positive views, some educators did not realize that nursing education needs to be evidence-based, while some nurses demonstrated reluctance or struggled with implementing evidence-based practice. In the early days of our work, some of the comments we heard are reflected in the voices from educators and nurses:

EDUCATOR AND NURSE COMMENTS

Teacher B: "I don't understand why they ask us to use BPGs in our course, I don't think it is so necessary."

Nurse A: "It's hard for us to implement BPGs in our practice."

Attitude plays a principal role in guiding human behaviour toward achieving goals (Ajzen & Fishbein, 2005). In order to increase positive beliefs and attitudes regarding the integration of BPGs into curriculum and to improve nurses' EBP knowledge and skills, several training programs were offered, and RNAO faculty were invited to give lectures on BPG development, implementation, and evaluation. In addition, a BPG Discussion WeChat group was created on a mobile platform for communication and sharing knowledge about BPGs. Using this, BPG Champions can readily engage in discussion or provide suggestions around BPG implementation, thereby enhancing their knowledge and enriching the overall evidence-based culture.

FUTURE PROSPECTS OF CHINA BPSOS

The current BPSOs in China recognize the tremendous potential of this EBP knowledge transfer strategy to transform nursing and nursing education in China. The future prospects for China BPSOs are very strong and discussed in the next section.

BUILDING AN EBN CULTURE

The work embarked upon by BUCM School of Nursing and DongZhiMen Hospital is almost unprecedented in academia and healthcare in China, as we assumed a leading role in integrating best practices into nursing education and clinical nursing practice. BPG implementation at the BUCM School of Nursing has caused a paradigm shift in multiple ways. Nursing educators have shifted to a student-centred approach and an evidence-based curriculum, both of which foster critical thinking amongst students. We will continue to revise and refine curricula to fully incorporate evidence-based nursing concepts into nursing education. Educators are also developing a comprehensive and long-term evaluation system to better assess whether the updated knowledge and evidence-based concepts are applied to nursing graduates' future clinical practice.

BPG implementation in the clinical setting has enhanced nurses' professional knowledge and research capacity and is cultivating an evidence-based culture in the nursing department and beyond. The BPSO team at DongZhiMen Hospital will continue with the rigorous implementation of the selected BPGs and strive for further innovation. By combining evidence-based practice, research, and quality improvement together, we aim to build a solid evidence-based nursing team with more nursing leaders and staff nurses involved. The overarching goal is to advance the evidence-based culture throughout the whole hospital.

INTRODUCTION OF EBN INTO TCM NURSING

With the advantages of simplicity, convenience, effectiveness, and low cost, Traditional Chinese Medicine (TCM) nursing techniques are well accepted and readily adopted in China and increasingly internationally. The main drawback is that most TCM nursing techniques lack standardization.

Although the Chinese government has promulgated TCM nursing handbooks and guidelines, these resources are developed based on experience, without support from scientific and rigorous research findings. With the assistance of the evidence-based nursing methodology we have gained from our BPSO experience, it may be possible to standardize TCM nursing techniques, thereby reducing the variability in their implementation and enabling their dissemination throughout the world.

BPSO DESIGNATION EXPANSION

With the great efforts made in disseminating BPSO-related work, an increasing number of hospitals and nursing schools are becoming interested in evidence-based nursing and joining this powerful movement. Once we achieve our BPSO Designation in April 2018, the BUCM School of Nursing and affiliated DongZhiMen Hospital plan to refine our program methodology and apply to RNAO to become a BPSO Host, the first in China. Our overall aim is to impact student learning, faculty development, clinical nursing excellence, and ultimately to improve the health of the population in China.

CONCLUSION

In China, the combination of healthcare reform, the early trending amongst some nursing leaders to embrace evidence-based practice, and the emergence of the BPSO Designation has resulted in groundbreaking accomplishments in nursing education and clinical practice that are transforming nursing. As pioneer BPSOs in academia and service in China, we have experienced much success based on focused activities to change education and clinical practices for better learning and health outcomes. We have also been purposeful in spreading this knowledge and sharing our experiences through numerous nursing and healthcare networks across China and abroad.

Lessons learned related to the use of a comprehensive planned methodology based on implementation science and knowledge transfer have spurred powerful changes in scope of practice, interprofessional care, and the status of nurses in the eyes of patients and other healthcare professionals, particularly medical doctors. The BPSO Designation in China has reflected the local context and supported adaptations as necessary to enable the integration of traditional Chinese medicine and traditional Chinese nursing. Finally, as true innovators, our two founding BPSOs are linking with new BPSOs as mentors to maximize the benefits of evidence-based education and clinical practice to advance outcomes for all, especially our patients.

KEY MESSAGES

- Changing the way we do things can be a challenging experience and process. Successful BPSO leaders strongly believe that change in academia and clinical practice based on evidence is the best way for improvement.

- Leadership is a key factor for the success of developing a culture of evidence-based practice and education in China.

- There's no one-size-fits-all method for BPG implementation. The specific cultural and organizational context needs to be considered.

- BPGs augment TCM with strong mainstream evidence to the benefit of students and patients in China.

- The BPSO Designation is a robust program that brings EBP to the classroom and the bedside pragmatically and effectively.

REFERENCES

Ajzen, I., & Fishbein, M. (2005). The influence of attitudes on behavior. In D. Albarracín, M. P. Zanna, & B. T. Johnson (Eds.), *The handbook of attitudes* (pp. 3–19). New York, NY: Lawrence Erlbaum Associates.

Deloitte Touche Tohmatsu Limited. (2014). 2014 global health care outlook: Shared challenges, shared opportunities. Retrieved from https://www2.deloitte.com/au/en/pages/life-sciences-and-healthcare/articles/2014-global-health-care-outlook.html

Gao, S. (2015). *Identification and management of dysphagia after stroke: An evidence-based nursing practice* (Research thesis). Beijing University of Chinese Medicine, Beijing.

Jiang, Y. T. (2017). *Development of evidence-based practice protocols for high risk of diabetic foot ulcers* (Thesis). Beijing University of Chinese Medicine, Beijing.

Jin, Y., Wang, Y., Zhang, Y., Ma, Y., Li, Y., Lu, C., . . . Shang, H. (2016). Nursing practice guidelines in China do need reform: A critical appraisal using the AGREE II instrument. *Worldviews on Evidence-Based Nursing, 13*(2), 124–138.

Registered Nurses' Association of Ontario (RNAO). (2012a). *Facilitating client-centred learning.* Toronto, ON: RNAO. Retrieved from http://rnao.ca/bpg/guidelines/facilitating-client-centred-learning

Registered Nurses' Association of Ontario (RNAO). (2012b). *Toolkit: Implementation of Best Practice Guidelines* (2nd ed.). Toronto, ON: RNAO. Retrieved from http://rnao.ca/bpg/resources/toolkit-implementation-best-practice-guidelines-second-edition

Registered Nurses' Association of Ontario (RNAO). (2013a). *Assessment and management of foot ulcers for people with diabetes* (2nd ed.). Toronto, ON: RNAO. Retrieved from http://rnao.ca/bpg/guidelines/assessment-and-management-foot-ulcers-people-diabetes-second-edition

Registered Nurses' Association of Ontario (RNAO). (2013b). *Assessment and management of pain* (3rd ed.). Toronto, ON: RNAO. Retrieved from http://rnao.ca/bpg/guidelines/assessment-and-management-pain

Xue, D. Q. (2017). *The analysis of application situation for colostomy care clinical practice guideline recommendations.* (Thesis). Beijing University of Chinese Medicine, Beijing.

You, L. M. (2012). *Medical nursing.* People's Medical Publishing House. (in Chinese).

Zhang, L. Y. (2003). Factors influencing and measures of the development of evidence-based nursing. *Chinese Journal of Nursing, 38*(1), 57–58. (in Chinese).

Zhu, J., Rodgers, S., & Melia, K. M. (2014). The impact of safety and quality of health care on Chinese nursing career decision-making. *Journal of Nursing Management, 22*(4), 423–432.

15

THE LATIN-AMERICAN BPSO EXPERIENCE: A CONSORTIUM MODEL

Aracelly Serna Restrepo, BScN
Maribel Esparza-Bohórquez, MSc, BScN, RN
Sonia Abad Vasquez, MA, BScN, RN
Olga L. Cortés, PhD, MSc, CCN, RN
Lina Maria Granados Oliveros, MSc, RN
Alejandra Belmar Valdebenito, BScN
Josephine Mo, BA (hon)
Doris Grinspun, PhD, MSN, BScN, RN, LLD(hon), Dr(hc), O.ONT

LEARNING OBJECTIVES

After reading this chapter, you will be able to:

- Gain an appreciation for the impact of the RNAO BPSO Designation in Latin America

- Understand processes used to adapt the BPSO Designation to fit local contexts, generating engagement and leading to sustainment

- Explain how key strategies of change such as awareness raising, alignment with organizational values, use of a Champions model, and attention to monitoring and evaluation have facilitated creation of evidence-based practice cultures and collective identity in Latin American BPSOs

- Describe the value of a BPSO consortium approach in BPSO spread, BPG uptake, resource management, innovation, sustainability, and outcomes

- Identify how RNAO has managed fidelity processes of the BPSO Orientation Program and the audit and feedback, along with a train-the-trainer approach, to bolster resources and acknowledge local leadership strengths

INTRODUCTION

In July 2012, the Registered Nurses' Association of Ontario's (RNAO) Best Practice Guidelines made its formal debut in Latin America when RNAO signed agreements with two facilities in Chile and two in Colombia to become Best Practice Spotlight Organizations (BPSO) Direct. These pioneers are the Universidad de Chile, Escuela de Enfermería, and Clínica las Condes in Chile; and two hospitals—Cardioinfantil Foundation of Cardiology Institute (FCI-IC) and Fundación Oftalmológica de Santander (FOSCAL) in Colombia. They formed the Latin America BPSO Consortium and received together their orientation and Champions training. They committed to a 3-year BPSO qualifying experience, wherein they would focus on enhancing their evidence-based nursing practice and decision-making cultures, with the mandate to implement and evaluate multiple clinical practice guidelines. The Chilean and Colombian organizations chose the guidelines they deemed most beneficial to their patients and students, including those focused on treating pressure ulcers, establishing therapeutic relationships, providing end-of-life care, preventing falls in older people, assessing and managing pain, and developing and sustaining nursing leadership.

The BPSO Direct program is a partnership between RNAO, who acts as BPSO Host, and an academic or health service organization, which assumes responsibility for all deliverables and costs associated with achieving the BPSO Designation. With oversight and support from RNAO, the BPSO Direct builds capacity through training of BPSO Champions; develops and delivers specific implementation activities; engages in regular knowledge exchange, monitoring, planning, and evaluation sessions with RNAO staff; participates in RNAO's NQuIRE database; and utilizes a variety of dissemination methods to share learnings, resources, and achievements with the wider healthcare community.

RNAO's role as BPSO Host is to launch the program with a 5-day orientation based on a systematic implementation and evaluation framework (RNAO, 2012b). Through a train-the-trainer approach, RNAO imparts the knowledge and skills to the BPSO Lead(s) and staff or faculty at the organization, who then train additional Champions and develop a network to support and enhance BPG implementation. The BPSO journey in Latin America started with the formal signing of agreements in July 2012, followed by the Orientation Program, which was delivered in Spanish at CLC to the full consortium (RNAO, 2012a).

Knowledge exchange is key to the success of the BPSO Designation, not only for peer learning and mentorship, but also for cultivating a spirit of individual and collective improvement. Virtual meetings prove to be very effective for RNAO to connect with international BPSOs and support their ongoing activities. The Hispanic consortium has been strengthened by regular virtual meetings every 2 months between the RNAO BPSO mentor to the consortium, CEO Dr. Doris Grinspun; RNAO BPSO Coordinator for Latin America, Josephine Mo; and the BPSO Leads in each country alongside their executive and/or full implementation teams.

The consortium holds annual BPSO research conferences organized by one of the BPSOs on an alternating basis. These conferences serve as another valuable mode of knowledge exchange, included as a deliverable of the program, which brings together all BPSOs in this particular region to present and discuss their strategies and outcomes. Engagement of the media at these events, as well as officials from government and the broader health community, heightens the profile of both the participating organizations and the BPSO Designation, while promoting the value of evidence-based nursing practice (EBP) and the robust contribution nurses are making to patients and organizational- and health-system outcomes.

RNAO also conducts a yearly audit of the BPSOs in Chile and Colombia to ensure program fidelity and progress with implementation of BPGs. The audit is composed of visits to the implementation sites, as well as review of materials related to the structure, process, and outcomes of the program. In addition to dynamic progress with the program, the audits also show a shared and very strong BPSO collective identity and pride. At each of the four institutions there is high visibility of the BPSO logo in units and the availability of BPSO-branded resources everywhere. These act as symbols of inspiration and motivation for nurses and also spark the interest of patients and their families who receive care and education based on BPGs. With its added presence on the organizations' websites and Intranet, the BPSO Designation has attained even greater profile and reach.

The case studies in this chapter explore the perspectives of three BPSOs: Clínica las Condes, Cardioinfantil Foundation of Cardiology Institute (FCI-IC), and Fundación Oftalmológica de Santander (FOSCAL).

CASE STUDY

THE EXPERIENCE OF FCI-IC IN IMPLEMENTING RNAO EVIDENCE-BASED GUIDELINES

Clinical practice guidelines (CPGs) are a type of knowledge synthesis at the highest level of the literature, with a selection of care recommendations based on the best existing evidence (Dearholt & Dang, 2012). Given the advanced information they contain, they are instrumental in the decision-making of health professionals about specific care situations (Dearholt & Dang, 2012). Clinical practice guidelines review, evaluate, and combine evidence related to problems, while incorporating all relevant aspects and values that determine a clinical decision, such as risk, prognosis, costs, patient values, and institutional achievements (DiCenso et al., 2002). CPGs need to be implemented in real practice situations by caregivers and thus be able to reduce adverse events (e.g., falls) and increase positive indicators (e.g., education) in the target population. This requires professionals with critical thinking and leadership skills who can transform routine care into scientific-based nursing care (Grinspun & Aninyam, 2014).

In order to achieve excellence in care, nurse leaders of the Nursing Department of the Cardioinfantil Foundation of Cardiology Institute—FCI-IC, located in Bogotá, Colombia—entered the Best Practice Spotlight Organization (BPSO) partnership with RNAO through a formal agreement which was signed in 2012. FCI-IC is a private, nonprofit hospital. It has a total of nine hospitalization services for adults and a total of three hospitalization services for children; 90 intensive care beds, of which 19 are neonates, 20 are paediatric, and 51 are adult; and a total capacity of 340 beds.

The overall purpose of joining the RNAO BPSO Designation was to implement and evaluate three RNAO Best Practice Guidelines (BPG) in selected adult-care services at FCI-IC. Our organization also sought to adapt the RNAO leadership model in the implementation process and evaluate the results in patients under our care. This collaboration included the commitment to submit data on each BPG to NQuIRE, RNAO's global BPG-related indicator data system. This international data set would provide a general reference on the impact of BPG implementation worldwide. Lastly, FCI-IC aimed to promote the progress resulting from BPG implementation in order to demonstrate the importance of evidence-based practice and the advances in terms of quality and patient safety, particularly in a care institution for patients with cardiovascular diseases and risk factors.

Taking into account that nursing care and its effectiveness based on the use of BPGs is not a common practice in Colombia, we were cognizant of how our experience might encourage the understanding of other colleagues about this process. Our case study thus includes a brief description of the implementation methodology, our outcomes during the BPSO predesignation period

(2012–2015), sustainability, leadership, research, and future development.

SELECTION OF BEST PRACTICE GUIDELINES

The implementation planning process began in mid-2012, after the BPSO Agreement was signed. Training Champions was the first step of processes related to BPG uptake and implementation. Over 10 years of evaluation data at our institution allowed us to have an understanding of the problems related to the incidence of events such as falls, skin pressure ulcers, and foot ulcers in diabetic patients. In order to select the most appropriate BPGs, we needed to identify the priority healthcare problems that we could overcome with the implementation of those guidelines. We performed a baseline diagnostic evaluation through a survey, which identified a number of existing problems. These included issues in the use of diagnostic tools for risk assessment for both falls and pressure ulcers; an underreporting of events in the electronic medical record; a prevalence of falls with injuries; use of bed railings for all patients, with no consideration of patient risks; and a prevalence of grade III and grade IV pressure ulcers. Based on this evaluation, three BPGs were selected: two focused on preventive care, *Prevention of Falls and Fall Injuries in the Older Adult* (RNAO, 2011a) and *Risk Assessment and Prevention of Pressure Ulcers* (RNAO, 2011b), and the third on *Assessment and Management of Foot Ulcers for People with Diabetes* (RNAO, 2013a). The selection phase lasted 6 months.

SETTINGS FOR IMPLEMENTATION AND POPULATION

The next phase involved the identification of hospital services for implementing the selected BPGs, including services that provided care for adults (≥ 18 years) and those with a high prevalence of events such as falls, pressure ulcers, and foot ulcers. For the implementation of *Prevention of Falls and Fall Injuries in the Older Adult* (RNAO, 2011a), two services were selected: internal medicine-general surgery and cardiology. For the

implementation of *Risk Assessment and Prevention of Pressure Ulcers* (RNAO, 2011b), we selected two intensive care units (ICU): medical and surgical. Finally, for the implementation of *Assessment and Management of Foot Ulcers for People with Diabetes* (RNAO, 2013a), we chose to include all adult hospitalization services (eight services in total).

STUDY AND CRITICAL ANALYSIS OF SELECTED RNAO GUIDELINES

The objective of this phase was to identify the strength of the evidence in each BPG and to select the recommendations with high or medium level of evidence for implementation. We also identified common interventions used routinely in our institution that should not be modified, as well as interventions currently in place that were not based on evidence.

We performed an analysis of the interventions and their levels of evidence (Ia, Ib, IIa, IIb, III, IV) (Scottish Intercollegiate Guidelines Network [SIGN], 2008) and reviewed the recommendations in each of the BPGs. We selected those recommendations that had the best level of evidence, were most needed for services, and could be implemented with our existing hospital resources (material, personal, and administrative). An example of recommendations selected for one BPG is presented in Table 15.1.

Current practice patterns and use of risk scales were evaluated. The instruments for risk assessment were selected for each guideline. They included the STRATIFY Falls Risk Assessment Tool, the Braden Scale for pressure ulcers, and the University of Texas Diabetic Wound Classification. We also obtained the necessary instruments for monitoring and documentation (Fundación Cardio-Infantil IC, 2012). The selected interventions were integrated into our practice and were illustrated in flow charts and diagrams and were part of comprehensive care processes for patients at risk. We needed to learn or to unlearn certain interventions in the change process, such as unlearning the use of guardrails for all hospitalized patients.

TABLE 15.1   RECOMMENDATIONS SELECTED FROM THE RISK ASSESSMENT AND PREVENTION OF PRESSURE ULCERS BPG

	RECOMMENDATIONS THAT WERE SELECTED FROM *RISK ASSESSMENT AND PREVENTION OF PRESSURE ULCERS* (RNAO, 2011B) BPG AND IMPLEMENTED	LEVEL OF THE EVIDENCE
Assessment	Perform an initial assessment of the state of the skin from head to toe and subsequently every day for those patients at risk of deterioration of skin integrity.	IV
	The risk of pressure ulcers is determined by combining clinical criteria and the use of a reliable risk assessment tool (e.g., Braden Risk Scale).	IV
	If patients are in bed or seated for long periods or following surgery, pressure, friction, and shear forces should be controlled in all positions. All pressure ulcers are identified and classified according to the NPUAP criteria *. Assessment and management of pressure ulcers in stages I to IV. All data are documented at the time of initial assessment and continuously on a regular basis thereafter.	IV
Planning	A personalized care plan is based on assessment data, risk factors, and goals in order to meet the patient needs. The plan should include the patient, family, and health personnel.	IV
Interventions	Programming of position changes. (For example, with clock use.) Use appropriate techniques during position changes (do not pull the patient across the sheets; position change must be done with the help of other professionals). Assess the pain and take into account the impact.	IV
	Lubricate the skin while avoiding massage and/or friction on bony prominences.	IIb
	Patients at risk of pressure ulcers should not remain on conventional mattresses. A low-pressure high-density foam mattress is used. In the case of high-risk patients undergoing surgical intervention, it is advisable to use pressure relief mechanisms.	Ia
	Establish interventions for patients with bed rest or sitting. Protect and promote the integrity of the skin. Protect the skin from excessive moisture and incontinence. Conduct a nutritional assessment if nutritional deficiencies are suspected.	IV

continues

TABLE 15.1 RECOMMENDATIONS SELECTED FROM THE RISK ASSESSMENT AND PREVENTION OF PRESSURE ULCERS BPG (CONTINUED)	
RECOMMENDATIONS THAT WERE SELECTED FROM *RISK ASSESSMENT AND PREVENTION OF PRESSURE ULCERS* **(RNAO, 2011B) BPG AND IMPLEMENTED**	**LEVEL OF THE EVIDENCE**
Educational program for the prevention of pressure ulcers.	III
Best Practice Guidelines in nursing can be successfully implemented if resources, planning, and administrative and institutional support exist.	IV

*NPUAP: National Pressure Ulcer Advisory Panel. www.npuap.org

SELECTION OF OUTCOMES (INDICATORS)

In this phase, the outcomes of each BPG were analyzed, and we carried out structural changes in order to ensure the valid documentation of the information (events and nursing care plans) into the electronic chart. In addition, communication systems (visual or by notes) were structured in the same electronic clinical history in order to convey the risk of each patient (for falls or pressure ulcers) to the medical staff and the interdisciplinary team.

The indicators selected for *Risk Assessment and Prevention of Pressure Ulcers* (RNAO, 2011b) were:

- The percentage of admitted patients diagnosed with the risk scale selected (Braden Scale)

- The percentage of patients newly evaluated at 24 hours with the same scale

- Patients at risk for pressure ulcer (%)

- The incidence of grade II to grade IV pressure ulcer (number of patients with new pressure ulcer/clients at risk of pressure ulcer) in a given period of time

The evaluation indicators for the *Assessment and Management of Foot Ulcers for People with Diabetes* (RNAO, 2013a) included:

- The percentage of those patients assessed who received leg assessment

- Percentage of those patients who had a foot ulcer assessment at the time of admission

- Percentage of those patients and families that received education

- Reduction of wound size (ulcer), at least 50% standing

Finally, the indicators for the *Prevention of Falls and Fall Injuries in the Older Adult* (RNAO, 2011a) included:

- The percentage of patients diagnosed with risk for falls at the time of admission, using the falls risk scale

- The total number of individuals who entered the fall prevention program

- The percentage of use of guardrails

- The rate of falls (number falls/days/patient) and post-fall injuries

IMPLEMENTATION AND MONITORING

In order to ensure the successful implementation of the BPGs, we selected spontaneous leaders or leaders with outstanding knowledge of each hospital service. Shift leaders (morning, afternoon, and evening) received training and were motivated with knowledge of the aims and content of BPGs, and also of the assessment of indicators and education strategies, in order to disseminate each BPG. This procedure took into account the RNAO (2013c) BPG, *Developing and Sustaining Nursing Leadership*, and the use of other general educational organizational strategies.

Educational material was developed in order to carry out dissemination sessions in three ways: peer-to-peer, in small groups, and in large groups (see Figure 15.1a and Figure 15.1b). The dissemination sessions included reading meetings, critical case analyses, lectures, and

direct monitoring with staff. Nursing staff (professional, auxiliary, and coordination) and hospital directors were made aware of BPGs and their relevant contents at every opportunity.

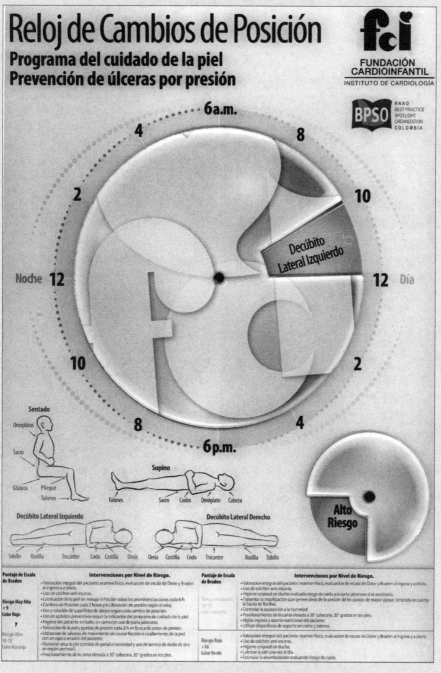

FIGURE 15.1A   BPSO educational materials developed by FCI-IC.
Used with permission.

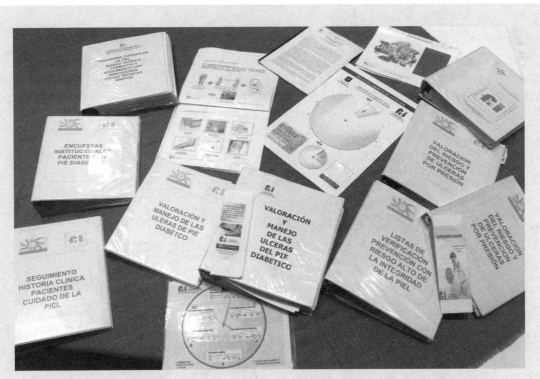

FIGURE 15.1B   BPSO educational material developed by FCI-IC.
Used with permission.

In order to monitor adherence to evidence-based recommendations, adverse events data, and patient outcomes in each of the services, we built formats to collect information related to the screening of patients in the selected services, to identify total population admitted, total population at risk (for falls or for pressure ulcers), in addition to information on the indicators for each BPG. Nursing coordinators of the morning, afternoon, and evening shifts initially collected this information with supervision from the implementation leaders of the falls prevention and pressure ulcer prevention in particular. This information was validated through the use of institutional databases and confirmed in the medical records. Indicator information was recorded in the RNAO database NQuIRE on a quarterly basis.

The entire staff was involved in both the presentations of the BPSO Designation and in the educational sessions related to each BPG. In general, a total of eight institutional BPSO Designation sessions and 10 BPG-specific tutorial sessions were conducted throughout the implementation process. The training of 800 professionals was carried out in six sessions in large groups, and six sessions were organized for only the leaders of the selected services with a dedication of 30 hours per leader. Interprofessional groups were organized to monitor the adherence to the BPGs, including physicians and other health professionals.

RESULTS OF BPG IMPLEMENTATION

An evaluation and validation of the BPGs selected and implemented by FCI-IC were conducted for the period between January 1, 2014 and December 31, 2015. The results were obtained from data reported to the NQuIRE database. For the evaluation of the *Prevention of Falls and Fall Injuries in the Older Adult* BPG (RNAO, 2011a), we analyzed 2,208 patients admitted to the cardiology and cardiac surgery services and 4,154 patients in the internal medicine-surgery services up to December 2015. Amongst the most outstanding results of the implementation was the adherence of nursing staff to the use of the Falls STRATIFY risk scale for the assessment of 100% of newly admitted patients. There was also a significant reduction, approximately 80%, in nursing staff's use of handrails with patients at risk for falls (see Figure 15.2).

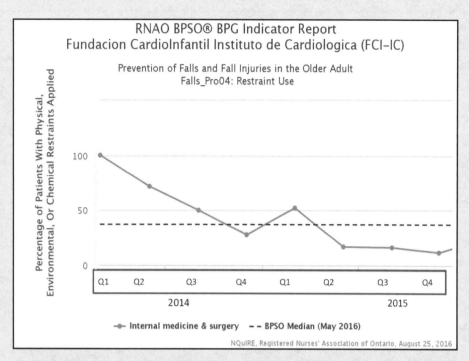

FIGURE 15.2   NQuIRE reporting on reduction of the use of railings in beds (physical restraints), FCI-IC.
Used with permission.

Two intensive care units (one healthcare unit and one surgical care unit) were included in the evaluation of the *Risk Assessment and Prevention of Pressure Ulcers* BPG (RNAO, 2011b), with a total of 5,952 patients admitted. The adherence of the nursing staff was 100% in the use of the Braden Scale with patients at the time of admission and with patients at 24 hours post-admission. One hundred percent of patients had access to "anti-bedsore" mattresses, as part of institutional policy.

Finally, the results of the evaluation of the *Assessment and Management of Foot Ulcers for People with Diabetes*

BPG (RNAO, 2013a) showed a 100% increase in care activities for diabetic patients, such as assessments in lower limbs, assessment of feet and ulcers (University of Texas Classification), and an increase in education given to the patient and their family based on the medical history report (see Figures 15.3a and 15.3b). The assessment of size reduction in a diabetic foot ulcer was 30%. Amputations have limited observation of healing in the short and medium term.

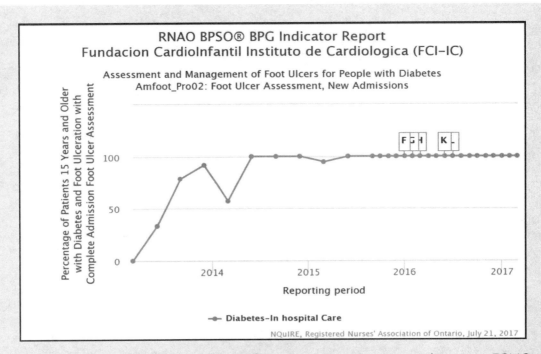

FIGURE 15.3A NQuIRE reporting on foot ulcer assessment, new admissions, FCI-IC.
Note: The letters F, G, H, and K indicate cases where patients received amputations during hospitalization.
Used with permission.

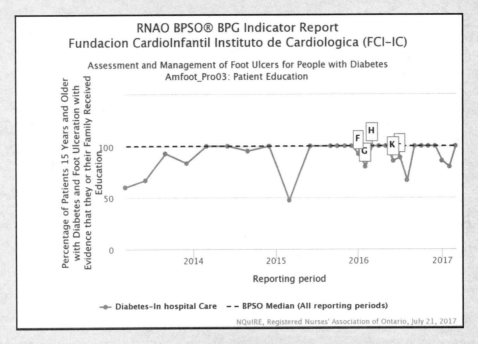

FIGURE 15.3B NQuIRE reporting on education to patients with foot ulcers and their families.
Note: The letters F, G, H, and K indicate cases where patients received amputations during hospitalization.
Used with permission.

POSITIVE STRATEGIES FOR SUSTAINING THE IMPLEMENTED BPGS

The sustainability of implementation has been planned as part of knowledge transfer (KT). First of all, there are budget-oriented measures to maintain the training of nurses, such as the Champions. Secondly, all education strategies are aimed at new staff and continue to target basic nursing staff in order to maintain the effectiveness of the interventions of each BPG. Finally, there is a solid relationship between the nursing department and the direct-care services that are implementing BPGs, which is strengthened through projects, research, and improvement plans to reduce adverse events.

Strengthening nursing leadership through continuing education, ongoing feedback, and specific education makes it possible to reduce the variability of care. Working teams set goals and prioritize the focus of their care based on continuous improvement using the BPG indicators. This cycle helps sustain the integration of best practices into nursing, thus ensuring improvements in the health experience of patients and their families.

The increased focus on research in this area is promoting scientific development in evidence-based nursing care. One prominent example is the PENFUP study, which focuses the use of skin protectors to prevent pressure ulcers, based on a randomized controlled trial. This study received a grant from the Institute of Science and Technology Colombia (COLCIENCIAS), which was submitted in partnership with RNAO and FOSCAL (BPSO Direct in Colombia). The participation of nursing and health professionals in this project has further promoted evidence-based practice in the prevention of pressure ulcers. We anticipate that final outcomes of the study will augment the evidence in future editions of the *Risk Assessment and Prevention of Pressure Ulcers* BPG (RNAO, 2011b).

EFFECTING CHANGE THROUGH BPG IMPLEMENTATION: A PERSPECTIVE OF THE NURSING STAFF

In general, the implementation of RNAO BPGs, the ongoing connection with RNAO, and the BPSO and Champions networks have enabled FCI-IC to witness the tremendous

impact of the BPSO Designation on improving care and its outcomes for patients. The quarterly analysis of data from each service has enhanced the understanding of the value of evaluation by demonstrating the impact of interventions on care. The general enthusiasm and individual nurse ownership of this knowledge have contributed to the formation of implementation teams and the identification of new institutional leaders. The visibility of nursing has significantly increased in our hospital as a result of the evidence-based interventions we adopted and the impact of our advances. This has also been a motivation for other teams.

Our participation in the RNAO BPSO Program involves serious, coordinated, and structured work aimed at reducing adverse events in the population under our care. The decrease in the variability of care has allowed us to increase quality standards, in accordance with national and international accreditation assessments.

Likewise, this work has allowed us to strengthen the critical thinking of healthcare providers. The process of organizational implementation has led to improved documentation of events in electronic records and a stronger focus on evaluation and critical analysis of indicators in groups and by services, and has impacted the national and international accreditation assessments.

In terms of continuing education at FCI-IC, the teaching methodology was transformed by including pedagogical models to achieve learning objectives, from induction to specific training programs to maintain the sustainability of interventions. Electronic medical records were transformed by including some of the BPG recommendations on diagnosis, evaluation, and follow-up for individuals and their families. A large body of educational material has been established for staff and the community. This presents the opportunity for further evaluation of such elements and their impact on BPG implementation.

Finally, the collaborative work between FCI-IC and RNAO has triggered several organizational improvements for nurses and nursing care. First, BPGs are now built into institutional policies and have served to enrich our human resource allocation to guarantee the daily physical and emotional well-being of the people under our care. In addition, there is now nursing representation and participation in the decisions related to new acquisitions and changes in infrastructure. The BPGs, policies, and the achievement of better patient and family outcomes now form part of the strategic objectives and performance of the FCI-IC Department of Nursing (Lucía Cortés et al., 2016).

Finally, the implementation process, as a result of the RNAO guidelines, has guided our nursing practice toward care that is based on the use of best evidence, from assessment of risk, to prevention of adverse events, to interventions leading to better outcomes. As for next steps, we aim to strengthen our nursing research capacity, as well as the evidence behind BPG recommendations, through further research studies.

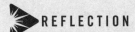

REFLECTION

What were the key drivers in the success of the BPSO Designation in FCI-IC? What key barriers were overcome and how?

THE EXPERIENCE OF FOSCAL IN IMPLEMENTING RNAO EVIDENCE-BASED GUIDELINES

The Ophthalmological Foundation of Santander (FOSCAL) is a tertiary and quaternary care institution, located strategically in the northeast region of Colombia. It has a capacity of 256 hospital beds (229 adults, 19 paediatrics, and 8 obstetrics), 46 beds in the intensive care unit (34 for adults and 12 for paediatric), 18 operating rooms, emergency service, and a parturition center (maternal and child center). On average it handles a volume of 1,584 monthly visits, an average stay of 5.8 days, and a 93% bed occupancy rate, a situation that allows for the presence of risks in the different services and care processes carried out in the institution.

As an institution of this level of complexity, with a serious interest in improving the quality of care, it was necessary to generate a change in nursing care processes. Such a change would require knowledge of different aspects: organizational size and culture, type of care, characterization of the population, problems or weaknesses detected, and, more importantly, the health human resources. The transformation of knowledge within organizations is what generates this change, but where and how do you start toward this goal?

We believed this change could be achieved with the implementation of the evidence-based RNAO Best Practice Guidelines (BPG). In FOSCAL's application to the RNAO Best Practice Spotlight Organizations (BPSO) Designation, these goals were outlined, and an implementation plan was developed.

PREPARATION PHASE

This phase consists of a number of the steps required in the BPSO application process, which are highlighted here.

1. **Raising awareness about the RNAO BPGs and BPSO Designation**—The first step in the change process is to share and promote information about the internationally renowned RNAO program, which disseminates evidence-based guidelines to health-care organizations around the world and supports their uptake and implementation. The rollercoaster of change model is a helpful illustration to guide the change process in nursing practice (Haines, 2005).

2. **Establishing a positive approach**—Commitment and enthusiasm from the outset are key factors in the success of the process. The leadership of the organization initiates the process by preparing a letter of intent that outlines their mentoring role to staff and stakeholders and shows keenness to receive the expertise and resources of RNAO.

3. **Commitment**—The letter of intent elaborates on the organization's goal to participate in the BPSO Program and attain BPSO Designation.

4. **Coordination**—The organization appoints a BPSO leader who will receive BPSO orientation and training in leadership and capacity-building methodology.

5. **Selection of guidelines to be implemented**— Knowledge of critical nursing issues during the care process assists in the review of RNAO BPGs to identify the priorities to be addressed through this methodology. Criteria used for BPG selection include the impact within the care process on nursing, the patient, family, institution, and also the resources available or necessary for implementation. FOSCAL selected the BPGs on *Prevention of Falls and Fall Injuries in the Older Adult* (RNAO, 2011a) and *Risk Assessment and Prevention of Pressure Ulcers* (RNAO, 2011b) for their preventative benefits for patients and the institution. The BPG *Assessment and Management of Pain* (RNAO, 2013b) was selected for its systematic approach to care, and quality interventions to provide comfort to patients. The overarching objective was to improve the care of patients.

VALIDATION OF THE GUIDELINES WITH AGREE II AND AGLI METHODOLOGY

The RNAO guidelines were evaluated with the AGREE II methodology in order to assess their methodological rigor and transparency, and the AGLI methodology to determine the recommendations to be implemented (see Table 15.2).

TABLE 15.2   EVALUATION OF BPGS WITH AGREE II AND AGLI

BPG	AGREE II	AGLI
Assessment and Management of Pain	91.3%	Of 18 recommendations, 17 are implementable and 1 is implementable with conditions
Prevention of Falls and Fall Injuries in the Older Adult	89.3%	Of 13 recommendations, 9 are implementable, 2 are implementable with conditions, and 2 are nonimplementable
Risk Assessment and Prevention of Pressure Ulcers	81.5%	Of 31 recommendations, 23 are implementable, 2 are implementable with conditions, and 6 are nonimplementable

SELECTION OF SERVICES

This phase focuses on locating and prioritizing the issues within healthcare services for the start of the implementation process. Services were selected by performing an environmental analysis and evaluating the prevalence of related events. For skin lesions, pilot implementation of recommendations from *Risk Assessment and Prevention of Pressure Ulcers* (RNAO, 2011b) was aimed at internal medicine, neurosurgery, and the adult intensive care unit. The delivery room and oncology were selected to implement the *Assessment and Management of Pain* guideline (RNAO, 2013b). For the *Prevention of Falls and Fall Injuries in the Older Adult* (RNAO, 2011a), consistent with the BPSO requirements, hospital-wide implementation was planned, beginning with two internal medicine services.

SELECTION OF CHAMPIONS

Following the selection of services, key people (BPG Champions) are identified to lead BPG implementation activities and monitoring of adherence to the process. Each of the guidelines has a leader responsible for the transfer of knowledge to the service staff. Champions receive specially designed BPSO pins that recognize their role.

ORGANIZATION OF EDUCATION FOR CHAMPIONS

This stage involves preparing the themes; identifying demands on faculty, availability of human resources to participate, and logistics of training; and the act of institutional recognition.

BPSO AGREEMENT

The BPSO Agreement between FOSCAL and RNAO was signed in 2012 for a period of 3 years and includes stipulations related to BPG selection, development of a BPSO infrastructure, capacity building, implementation, dissemination, and evaluation activities. Part of the dissemination requirement of the agreement is the publication of a scientific article on the implementation experience. To meet this deliverable, FOSCAL published an article in the *MedUNAB* journal (Esparza-Bohórquez, Granados Oliveros, & Joya-Guevara, 2016) entitled "Implementation of Best Practice Guidelines: Risk Assessment and Prevention of Pressure Ulcers: Experience of the Ophthalmological Foundation of Santander (FOSCAL)." Other parts of the BPSO Agreement include organizing an annual international research congress, submitting quarterly reports, participating in the NQuIRE database, undergoing an annual BPSO audit, and motivating other institutions to partake in this methodology.

ELABORATION AND UPDATE OF PROCEDURES

The existing recommendations in each guideline implemented were reviewed, and the impact; viability; and human, administrative, and economic resource requirements were assessed based on the evidence. The resulting protocols developed are being updated every 2 years, incorporating relevant new evidence from RNAO's new editions of these BPGs. A logo was designed to identify the services where BPGs were being implemented. These were seen as BPSO Units. See Figure 15.4.

STAFF TRAINING

The nursing division of FOSCAL and RNAO both conducted training for the BPG implementation teams.

STAKEHOLDER IDENTIFICATION

Stakeholders were identified by brainstorming who could influence our processes and who would be influenced by them. Then given the role and influence of these staff members and others in the implementation process, it is important to obtain their support for the methodology and identify the actions that various staff groups must carry out.

SELECTION OF TOOLS

The tools selected to assess the risk of patients for conditions as identified in the different guidelines are shown in Table 15.3.

FIGURE 15.4 BPSO plaque developed at FOSCAL.
Used with permission.

TABLE 15.3 TOOLS TO ASSESS PATIENT RISK

TOOLS	
BPG	Scales
Risk Assessment and Prevention of Pressure Ulcers	Braden
Prevention of Falls and Fall Injuries in the Older Adult	Morse
Assessment and Management of Pain	Old Cart—Campbell

These scales are systematized in the electronic medical record, which establishes the risk according to the score and aids in providing users with multifactorial intervention plans, based on the assessment data. These plans are designed using the recommendations and related evidence for each guideline and are included in the training program for nursing personnel.

INDICATORS

Analysis of the indicators of each BPG is necessary for selecting the ones to implement in each procedure and an instrumental part of monitoring in each service. The technical data sheets were designed with the purpose of systematically collecting indicator data for each BPG. The indicators selected for the guidelines are shown in Table 15.4.

TABLE 15.4   INDICATORS SELECTED FOR BPGS

BPG	SELECTED INDICATORS
Risk Assessment and Prevention of Pressure Ulcers	■ Risk assessment ■ Risk reassessment ■ Intervention ■ Classification of pressure ulcers
Prevention of Falls and Fall Injuries in the Older Adult	■ Risk assessment ■ Posterior post-fall reassessment ■ Multifactorial plan ■ Immobilized patients ■ Falls rate ■ Falls injury
Assessment and Management of Pain	■ Pain detection ■ Pain assessment ■ Pain management ■ Customer satisfaction with pain control

IMPLEMENTATION PHASE

An orientation day was designed and delivered to staff of the pilot services and to stakeholders. The BPGs and implementation methodology were also incorporated into the training program for new staff. Within the annual training program, 1 month is assigned to providing updates on guidelines and tips on implementation. For the training of staff and families, educational material is developed to convey the BPG recommendations in a practical way, during the hospital stay and at discharge.

Data collection was initiated at the pilot services, starting with registration in the NQuIRE data system and proceeding to analysis of results and elaboration of quality-improvement plans.

AUDIT AND MONITORING PHASE

For the audit and monitoring process, BPG rounds were conducted as follows:

■ **Protecting the FOSCAL skin**—The implementation of the selected strategic interventions is evaluated using a checklist that measures staff adherence to BPG recommendations, and the data required for NQuIRE submission are collected.

■ **Days without falls**—The institutional billboard of each service shows daily updates with information on days without falls. The service is recognized for this achievement. Families' understanding of the education provided on preventing skin lesions and falls is evaluated using a knowledge questionnaire.

■ **Humanization rounds**—These rounds were created to provide staff support and acknowledgement to the services by verifying the assessment and management of pain and reinforcing the adherence of staff to the activities of prevention and identification of pain in patients.

EVALUATION

NQuIRE is a database of quality indicators designed for BPSOs to systematically monitor progress and evaluate the results of implementing BPGs. It is the first international quality-improvement initiative of its kind, and involves the development and measurement of structure, process, and outcome indicators related to each BPG. The FOSCAL nursing division performs follow-up every month when reviewing the data on each indicator for the implemented guidelines. For this process, it is necessary to appoint a general administrator for the organization, and involve the implementation team leaders in collecting data on and monitoring each guideline, analyzing the behaviour for informed decision-making, and correcting any deviations. The most important indicators of each guideline are presented below, reflecting the first 3 years of implementation.

Results on the indicators of *Prevention of Falls and Fall Injuries in the Older Adult* are displayed in Figures 15.5a, 15.5b, and 15.5c.

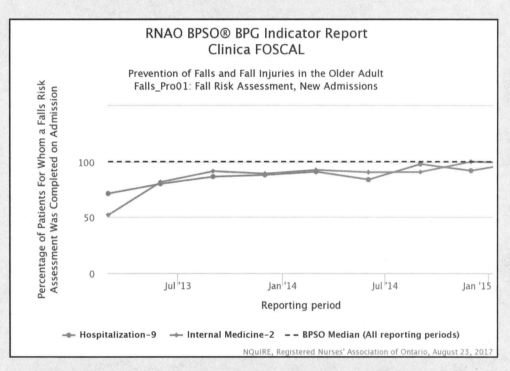

FIGURE 15.5A   NQuIRE reporting on fall risk assessment, new admission, FOSCAL. Used with permission.

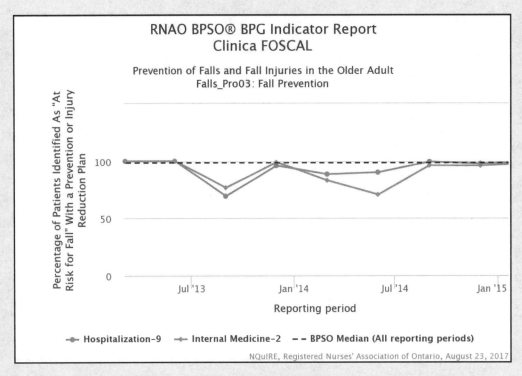

FIGURE 15.5B NQuIRE reporting on fall prevention, FOSCAL.
Used with permission.

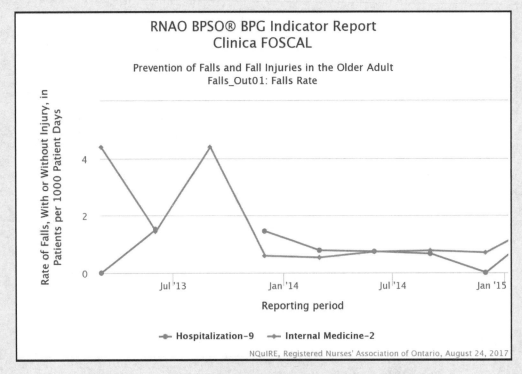

FIGURE 15.5C NQuIRE reporting on falls rate, FOSCAL.
Used with permission.

The results on the indicators of *Risk Assessment and Prevention of Pressure Ulcers* are displayed in Figures 15.6a, 15.6b, and 15.6c.

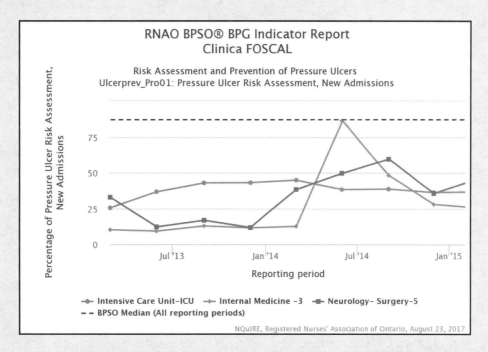

FIGURE 15.6A   NQuIRE reporting on pressure ulcer risk assessment, new admissions, FOSCAL. Used with permission.

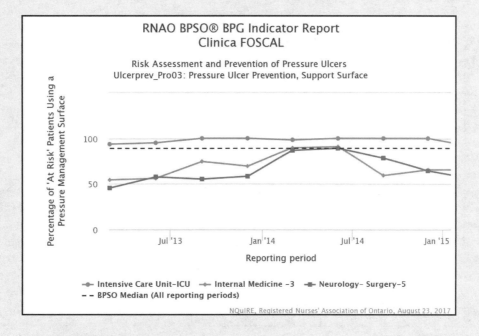

FIGURE 15.6B   NQuIRE reporting on pressure ulcer prevention, FOSCAL. Used with permission.

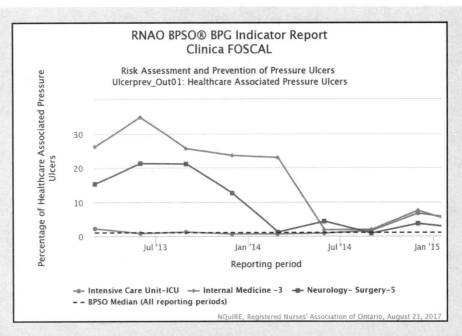

FIGURE 15.6C NQuIRE reporting on healthcare-associated pressure ulcers, FOSCAL.
Used with permission.

Results on the indicators of *Assessment and Management of Pain* are displayed in Figures 15.7a and 15.7b.

FIGURE 15.7A NQuIRE reporting on pain screening, FOSCAL.

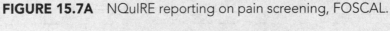

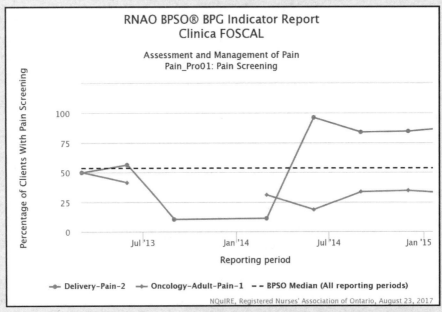

Used with permission.

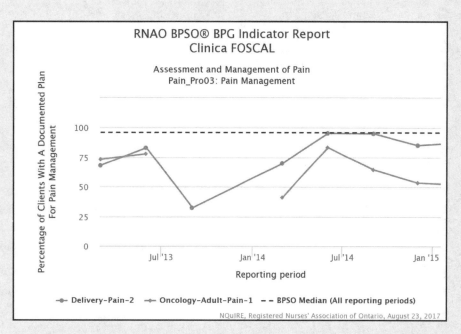

FIGURE 15.7B   NQuIRE reporting on pain management, FOSCAL.
Used with permission.

LEADERSHIP

Nursing leadership is a process that promotes the improvement of health and well-being of the population. It includes the attainment of nursing care objectives and the achievement of goals set for health services. Therefore, it is a process that favours social, professional, and organizational development.

The achievements with the implementation of evidence-based guidelines have been recognized at the institutional, local, and national level, drawing attention to improvements in the care process and elevating the profile of nursing (Grinspun, 2011, 2015). This is the result of several years of work and commitment of all professionals, with the sole purpose of providing quality care to the patient and significantly reducing the indicators that negatively impact on their health and well-being.

The development of knowledge, strengthening of professional decision-making, standardization, and resolution of issues in nursing practice culminate in improved care and health outcomes. Based on its results in preventing falls and fall injuries in older adults, the institution has been identified as a leader in best practices and as an exemplar in decreasing the incidence of falls using evidence-based interventions and monitoring outcomes.

FOSCAL's leadership serves as a reference for the Ministry of Health and Social Protection in strengthening the process in different institutions around the country.

OUTCOMES AND ACHIEVEMENTS

FOSCAL successfully attained its BPSO Designation in April 2015, at the RNAO Designation ceremony in Toronto, Canada (RNAO, 2015). Prior to that, in 2014, FOSCAL participated in the IV International Congress of Nursing, hosted by fellow BPSO Hospital Cardio-Infantil (FCI-IC) in Bogotá, Colombia. There, FOSCAL presented two posters and participated in a forum on the experience of implementing evidence-based guidelines. Furthermore, FOSCAL's accomplishments as part of the BPSO Program have been recognized through:

- An invitation to participate in the XIV Pan-American Nursing Research Colloquium

- Being featured in a video by the Ministry of Health and Social Protection as an exemplary institution at the national level, in best practices

- Earning second place in the Oral Mode of the Leadership Prize in Prevention of Skin Damage

■ Presentation at the National Nursing Days of Alicante, Spain, on FOSCAL's experience with local success and international leadership related to implementing RNAO's clinical guidelines

■ Publication of an article in the *MedUNAB* journal titled "Implementation of Best Practice Guidelines: Experience at the Ophthalmological Foundation of Santander (FOSCAL)" (Esparza-Bohórquez et al., 2016)

CONCLUSION

As a group of nurses at FOSCAL, we have become leaders in Colombia in the implementation of evidence-based guidelines, and we demonstrate a tangible impact on the outcomes and quality of care, which we provide to patients with a high level of warmth. Evidence-based knowledge has enabled FOSCAL to exercise nursing leadership in achieving change and motivating other organizations to participate in this important process—this is the best part of our experience. Our gains are further reflected in the decrease of adverse events; increase in the satisfaction of patients and work teams during the care process; updating of care processes; participation in academic events, and national and international publications; and sharing their experiences in the process of transferring knowledge to practice and advancing nursing.

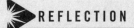

REFLECTION

What were the key drivers in the success of the BPSO Designation in FOSCAL? What key barriers were overcome and how?

CASE STUDY

THE EXPERIENCE OF CLÍNICA LAS CONDES IN IMPLEMENTING RNAO EVIDENCE-BASED GUIDELINES

Clinical practice in current health systems is undergoing an important paradigm shift. Since the 1980s, the Evidence-Based Medicine (EBM) movement has endorsed the need to have trained professionals at the forefront of knowledge, so that we can ensure safe, quality care for our patients. It is widely accepted that professional practice based on evidence or results from research and its use contributes to improving the health of the population. However, according to some studies published in this regard, at least 40% of patients do not receive care consistent with the results of the research and, consequently, between 20% and 25% of care may be unnecessary and even potentially harmful (Grinspun, Melnyk, & Fineout-Overholt, 2010; Moreno-Casbas, Fuentelsaz-Gallego, Gonza, Rey, & Carlos, 2016).

In addition to this, there are several barriers to research use in nursing: lack of time, lack of motivation, lack of support from management, structures of organizations, lack of support from coworkers, lack of funding, scarce staffing, and insufficient methodological knowledge (Moreno-Casbas et al., 2016). These factors result in low interest in and adherence to evidence-based work—a reality that Clínica las Condes faced and grappled with.

It is in this context that, at the beginning of 2010, the nursing management at Clínica las Condes (CLC) wanted to expand its field of action and decided to partner with the Registered Nurses' Association of Ontario (RNAO) through its international BPSO Designation, which not only allowed the institution to learn the best practices in nursing care based on scientific evidence, but also enabled its implementation, evaluation, and subsequent maintenance. This has undoubtedly become an incentive for nursing staff, who strive daily to provide quality, safe, and efficient care to their patients based on the best scientific advice available.

Today, CLC's collaborators have a sustainable and firm theoretical framework that allows them to shape the decisions they make with their patients with the support of evidence-based documents (clinical guidelines and recommendations) prepared by the RNAO BPG Program. This in turn empowers the nursing role and positions nurses solidly as knowledge professionals providing quality care in our institution. The purpose of this case study is to describe the experience of CLC in the implementation of clinical practice guidelines in nursing.

THE BEGINNING

In 2010, the nursing management at CLC initiated the first steps of their BPSO journey, which began with outreach by the chief nurse at the time to RNAO and their beginning conversations about the BPSO partnership. Once this was set in motion, CLC formed working groups that were led by the chief nurses of each clinical unit. They discussed the scope of the program and identified the BPGs for implementation: *Risk Assessment and Prevention of Pressure Ulcers* (RNAO, 2011b) and *Assessment and Management of Stage I to IV Pressure Ulcers* (RNAO, 2007a).

Despite the striking initiative and keenness shown by the heads of nursing, they were met with challenges to internalize the BPSO Designation and comply with all of the deliverables requested by RNAO. CLC's nurses went ahead and added the two above BPGs to their already scheduled work, without necessarily being trained or prepared for other aspects of the program. The situation was compounded by changes in nursing leadership during the period between 2010 and 2012. Thus, in order to stabilize the conditions for the BPSO Designation, the BPSO Lead was appointed and responsible for facilitating the program, raising awareness, and motivating nurses and other health professionals to participate and collaborate. Working groups were also solidified in a way that each member assumed a function of supporting implementation of a particular guideline (see Figure 15.8).

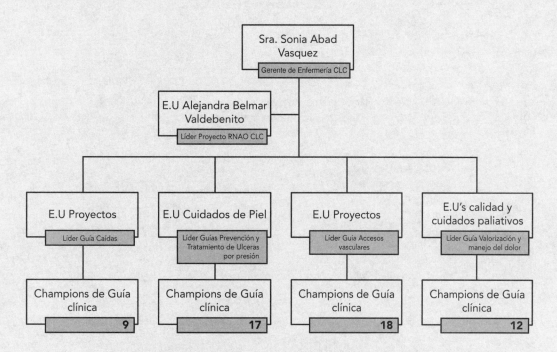

FIGURE 15.8 BPSO team structure at CLC, 2017.

These working groups are primarily composed of a nurse educator, palliative care nurse, wound nurse, ostomy nurse, quality nurse in surgical pavilions and project nurse, and teaching and research nurses. They began work in 2013 on implementing the *Risk Assessment and Prevention of Pressure Ulcers BPG* (RNAO, 2011b) and adapting the institutional policy according to the BPG's recommendations. This work was complemented by the development of two specific institutional policies: one for hospitalized patients and the second for patients treated in surgical rooms. At the same time, there was work on developing BPSO badges and educational brochures for patients and families, which promoted BPG dissemination (see Figures 15.9a and 15.9b).

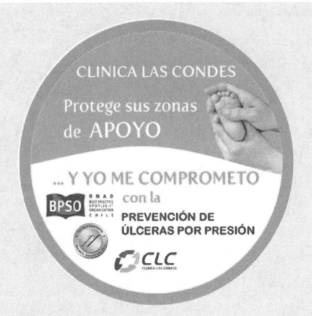

FIGURE 15.9A   BPSO badge developed by Clínica las Condes.
Used with permission.

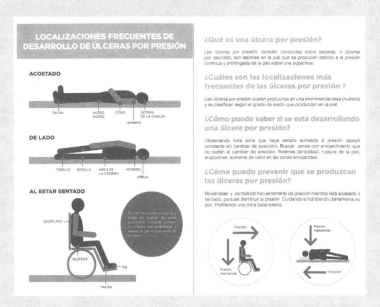

FIGURE 15.9B   BPSO educational brochure developed by Clínica las Condes.
Used with permission.

As the program's infrastructure and activity became established and functional, it gradually earned recognition by the heads of nursing in each clinical unit.

By the end of 2013, the team began the creation of eLearning training for the prevention of pressure ulcers, based on the RNAO BPG, aimed at nurses and nursing technicians. The goal was to facilitate improved uptake of knowledge through distance learning, leading to improved clinical outcomes. More details on the eLearning program will be shared later in this case study.

With time, the BPSO Program gained stability and took shape. One of the key actions was to set the ideal composition of the working group, which should include nurses in the areas of quality of care, wound care, pain management, and project management. As a whole, this would ensure that a specific guideline is fully implemented, along with capacity-building and other related objectives. Figure 15.8 summarizes the organization of the team for the year 2017 and demonstrates the BPSO leadership and the BPG Leader and Champion team for each BPG being implemented.

CHAMPIONS

The development of BPG Champions began in 2011 with the adoption of the guideline on *Risk Assessment and Prevention of Pressure Ulcers* (RNAO, 2011b). From the outset, participation in the BPSO Program was entirely voluntary, which fosters greater commitment and

endurance of the participants. Today, CLC counts amongst its staff a total of 64 Champions for the different BPGs implemented (see Figure 15.10). The Champions' main functions include the following:

- Carefully review clinical guidelines for their work group

- Actively review action guides and protocols of Clínica las Condes that correspond to the guideline of their RNAO working group

- Motivate colleagues to follow nursing best practices within their clinical services

- Present on the BPG recommendations and results on a semi-annual basis through participatory meetings in their respective clinical services

- Present on the results and themes to the RNAO group on an annual basis

- Ensure compliance with the guidelines implemented in each clinical service

It is also important to note that, although the program started by recruiting only nurses as Champions, there are already other health professionals who have joined the BPG implementation process on a continuous basis, as detailed in Figure 15.10. The chart provides a more global and interdisciplinary view of the Champions program at CLC.

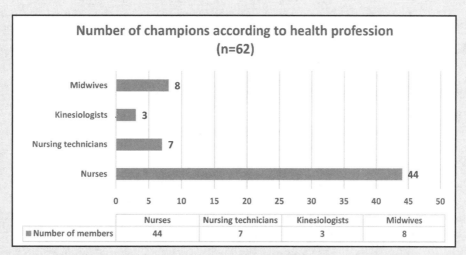

Number of champions according to health profession (n=62)

	Nurses	Nursing technicians	Kinesiologists	Midwives
■ Number of members	44	7	3	8

Midwives — 8
Kinesiologists — 3
Nursing technicians — 7
Nurses — 44

FIGURE 15.10   Number of Champions by profession, CLC.
Used with permission.

This is how, almost 6 years after the start of Champions training, some of them have referred to the program through the following testimonials:

"Being part of the BPG Champion Network has been very gratifying, since you can contribute to the overall approach to nursing care and give quality care to patients. Being a member of a group of nurses and other health professionals who belong to different services, I got to know other realities that we face day to day. Thus together across disciplines and services, we seek the best way to solve problems with best evidence. We all work for the same purpose, giving better care to our patients."

—Paulina Sanhueza, Nurse, Surgical Services

"I volunteered to be a Champion almost a year ago. It has been a time full of challenges, a lot of dedication and teamwork. Seeing how the BPSO has emerged has been super rewarding for me on a personal and professional level. In internalizing the existence of the RNAO BPGs, I realized that it not only provides us with an evidence-based framework for our professional work, but also helps us to generate more evidence. In relation to CLC, our strong commitment to evidence-based practice and our results have given us an international profile of excellence in care."

—Barbara Silva, Nurse, Paediatric Services

"It has been interesting because working with people from other disciplines is good. As a kinesiologist, being in the fall prevention group has contributed positively to my work and has been very enriching for me. I am now much more aware of falls and fall prevention, and we have taken precautions to strengthen patient safety."

—Giancarlo Calcagno, Kinesiology

MILESTONES

One of the most important milestones in the implementation of RNAO's Best Practice Guidelines took place in 2014, with the launch of eLearning training for the prevention of pressure ulcers. This educational program was born from the need to maintain nursing skills without demanding the time of collaborators to attend in-person classes. Furthermore, the use of information and communication technologies made it possible to facilitate knowledge transfer on a much more efficient level compared to traditional face-to-face methodology. In this way, a total of approximately 941 nurses and nursing technicians were trained through eLearning technology (see Figure 15.11).

Since 2005, CLC has adopted this system of learning, which its staff has rated as excellent, given the possibility to complete training from home or another location, based on their schedule. On top of this, further advantages of distance learning have been identified as follows (Villaverde, 2013):

- Exceeds the limits of the classroom

- Adapts to the pace of the individual learner

- Allows flexible use of time

- Employs a variety of means and resources

- Does not detach people from their work or family environment

- Promotes the autonomy of the participants

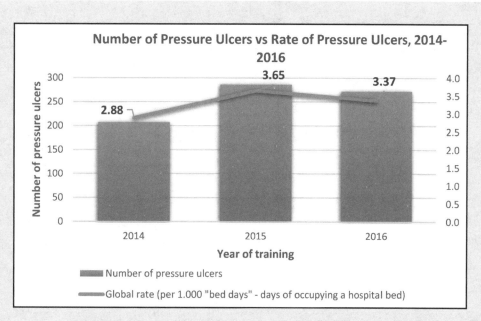

FIGURE 15.11   Number of staff trained by eLearning, CLC.
Used with permission.

The benefits of using educational software in teaching and learning are as follows (Barrios Araya, Masalán Apip, & Cook, 2011):

- It is a medium that offers students information visually through the laptop or computer.

- It has a great capacity for motivating students.

- Communication can be bidirectional, establishing continuous feedback with the student.

- The work can be adapted to the work and style of learning of each student individually, which corroborates the principle of individualization advocated by the new education system.

- Correction and evaluation of exercises can be immediate if there is interactivity.

- It is a means capable of showing and simulating reality almost perfectly.

The value of this learning methodology in building the knowledge base of nurses in relation to wound prevention and care was reflected in the patient wound outcome data. CLC opened its new hospital building in 2014, with double its previous bed capacity and almost double the number of existing staff. In spite of these factors, the rate of pressure ulcers reported at the institutional level did not suffer great variations (see Figure 15.12). On the contrary, the rate decreased in 2015, a fact that affirms the effectiveness of evidence-based care and its diffusion through eLearning methodology.

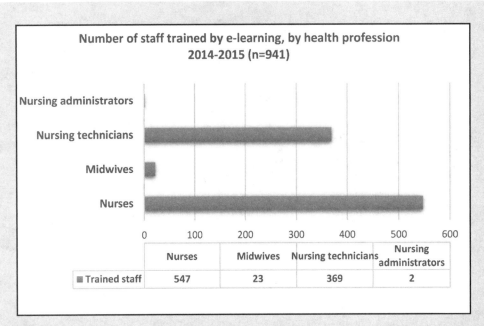

FIGURE 15.12 Number of pressure ulcers in CLC vs. global rate of pressure ulcers, 2014-2016, CLC.
Used with permission.

PROGRESS AND RESULTS TO DATE

CLC has been an innovator and become a leader amongst the country's hospitals through engagement in the BPSO Designation and promoting staff learning and their adherence to BPG implementation.

At present, RNAO's BPGs and their implementation have become indispensable to the care of our patients. Following the implementation of evidence-based guidelines, four institutional protocols have been modified to date in all areas of CLC, which were approved by the Nursing Manager and Medical Director. These mandate the compliance of all health professionals involved in patient care. In addition, the search for the best scientific evidence to integrate in care has been included in the plans for continuous improvement of clinical units, in all institutional training, and in all orientation processes for nurses and nursing technicians. This is slowly generating a cultural change that, on top of providing knowledge, empowers clinical staff to make the best-informed decisions in the care of their patients.

The formation of BPG Champions has been fundamental to the BPSO success at CLC. Their commitment is reflected in the low turnover (2 people out of 66), which can be linked to their voluntary application to the program and their high degree of participation in the improvement measures proposed for the detected issues. Furthermore, being prepared to lead a theme and guide their colleagues toward continuous improvement based on best practices induces a greater motivation in the Champions to always be up-to-date in knowledge and to transmit it in a timely manner. Peer recognition fuels the further success of Champions, as there is better receptiveness, and in turn learning, that takes place amongst peers.

Another factor that has contributed to the motivation of Champions is the recognition and continuous positive reinforcement by the CLC Chief Nurse, the nursing managers, and BPSO team at CLC. Activities such as the certification of Champions, held in December 2016 with RNAO CEO Dr. Doris Grinspun, acknowledge teamwork and commitment, as well as encourage staff to play a greater role in clinical practice. Through this they are empowered and motivated to provide optimal care to patients.

NEXT STEPS

CLC is currently working on the implementation of two new guidelines: the BPG for the *Subcutaneous Administration of Insulin in Adults with Type 2 Diabetes* (RNAO, 2009) and *Integrating Smoking Cessation into Daily Nursing Practice* (RNAO, 2007b). These guidelines have been revised with the purpose of being implemented in centers for prevention and treatment of these pathologies, which extends CLC's services to ambulatory patients and their families. At the same time, both centers (diabetes center and cancer clinical center) are drafting the institutional policy, based on the RNAO BPG recommendations, to ensure full and sustained adoption following its launch. The full process is expected to take place at the end of 2017.

The BPSO team is also working on new strategies to motivate existing Champions to take on new challenges, offering them greater visibility and accountability to their colleagues. A clear example of this is Champions' participation in the recording of the new version of the eLearning on prevention of pressure ulcers. Also part of the portfolio of upcoming projects is the development of vascular care access equipment in accordance with the RNAO BPG *Assessment and Device Selection for Vascular Access* (RNAO, 2008), massive campaigns for prevention for falls, and beginning of supervision of the implementation of *Assessment and Management of Pain* BPG (RNAO, 2013b). For the latter, CLC Champions, supported by members of the BPSO team, will supervise compliance with the BPG recommendations and guide their colleagues toward the correct filling of pain rating scales.

Finally, Clínica las Condes is promoting programs to recognize Champions. The objective is to highlight the involvement of participants in the BPSO Designation, to maintain their motivation, and to empower them and help them empower their colleagues as knowledge professionals. Through this, their positive performance is acknowledged and reinforced, which in turn will motivate more health professionals to join the BPSO journey.

CONCLUSION

The implementation of clinical practice guidelines allows us to have clear guidance for changes and improvements that must be made in our daily actions, in favour of the standardization of care based on evidence and the reduction of clinical variability.

The use of innovative strategies, empowerment of professionals, and ongoing motivation methods have enabled us to maintain and scale out BPG implementation to more areas of the institution, as well as to more health professionals. The Nursing Manager of CLC, Mrs. Sonia Abad Vasquez, also emphasizes the spread of evidence-based practice at every opportunity, such as during her address at the 2017 Nursing Day:

"Managing care in a timely, safe, and satisfactory manner implies responding to our patients with the best evidence available to make the best decisions about caring for people. Evidence-based nursing is thus emerging as a valid instrument to sustain nursing practice and improve quality of care."

Adding to this is her opinion on the next challenges for CLC in that direction:

"The challenge of nursing at Clínica las Condes is to continue in this way, strengthening our profession based on knowledge and contributing to the health team in such a way to achieve the best results for our patients."

Undoubtedly, Clínica las Condes has changed its paradigm of patient care over the last several years. Today, quality and safety of care are basic pillars guiding our standards, and it is within this framework that evidence-based nursing, embracing RNAO's Best Practice Guidelines, plays a fundamental role in fulfilling these pillars. In addition, the development of Champions has allowed us to bring out the best in our collaborators and enable and empower them to participate in the improvement plans for better care.

Finally, one of the greatest challenges for a health organization is to not only maintain, but to advance methodological rigor in our implementation, measurement of results, and creation of improvement plans in each area. We continue to strive for this, as well as motivating health professionals to use the best evidence available with patients, thereby always ensuring that we improve our quality of service.

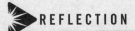

REFLECTION

What were the key drivers in the success of the BPSO Designation in CLC? What key barriers were overcome and how?

THE LATIN AMERICA BPSO CONSORTIUM: FROM STRENGTH TO GREATER STRENGTH

Much has been said about RNAO's BPSO Designation, its comprehensiveness and overall success (Grinspun, 2015, 2017). The Latin America BPSO Consortium is a lived example of the BPSO Designation's success in the Latin American context. The BPSOs in the consortium derive tremendous strength individually and as a group. Together they have developed a unique bond and strong collective identity, which is continuously expressed in their visual symbols, as well as their mutual support and desire to work as partners. This cognitive, social, and emotional sharing of knowledge and experiences, successes, and failures has served them well in advancing BPG uptake and sustainability, as well as BPSO Program fidelity. It has also become a source of strength and inspiration for new BPSOs in the region and elsewhere.

In 2014, the *Programa de Enfermería at Universidad Autónoma de Bucaramanga (UNAB)*, in Bucaramanga, Colombia, joined as a BPSO Direct-Academia. In 2017, the consortium gained three new BPSO Hosts—two of these in Chile and one in Peru—which together bring 20 new service and academic organizations. Evolving from a modest consortium of 4 hospitals and 1 university in 2012 to a sizable 25 organizations in 2017, the Latin America BPSO Consortium has moved to be the third largest partner in the RNAO BPSO Program following Canada and Spain. What's more important is the nature of the three BPSO Hosts that have recently joined and the capacity they have to catapult the Latin America BPSO Consortium to new heights of collaboration, achievements, and the furthering of the RNAO BPSO Program's collective identity flavoured by its unique cultural context.

The first BPSO Host is Universidad de Chile, which applied and was approved to move from being a BPSO Direct to a BPSO Host and will take five Chilean universities as its direct academic BPSOs. The second BPSO Host is the Ministerio de Salud de Chile, known as MINSAL, where the agreement was signed in a formal televised ceremony by their national Minister of Health and RNAO'S CEO, marking the highest level international agreement signed to the program. The MINSAL agreement began with seven BPSO Direct-Service hospitals in various Chilean regions and will quickly expand to additional public hospitals and primary care organizations in that country (El America, 2017; RNAO, 2017). The third BPSO Host, the Colegio de Enfermeros del Peru, began its journey leading with six BPSO Direct-Service hospitals and two BPSO Direct-Academia universities (The Trujillo Com, 2017; Panamericana TV, 2017; RNAO, 2017).

From the onset, all these BPSOs gained tremendous support from the consortium founding members and the robust infrastructure that RNAO has in place. The Orientation Program for each of these new BPSOs was co-led by RNAO's CEO and one of the founding regional BPSO leaders, knowing that the newcomers would benefit from RNAO's expertise and also the experience and local knowledge context of an existing academic and/or service BPSO leader in the region.

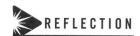

REFLECTION

Compare and contrast the BPSOs from perspectives of success factors, approaches to engagement, management of barriers, a unique focus, and results.

All new BPSOs have joined the regular knowledge-exchange bimonthly meetings, where they learn from the strategies and successes of other BPSOs and receive mentoring for any challenges encountered. For example, UNAB was introduced to the innovative eTraining modules developed by Clínica las Condes, which through its in-kind obligations with RNAO provides access to these and other resources it created as part of its solid educational repository. All the new BPSO leads have benefited from attending the BPSO annual regional conference, which rotates between countries. In addition, some have joined a working group of academic BPSOs that is developing NQuIRE indicators particular to the integration of BPGs into curricula.

CONCLUSION

The Latin America BPSO Consortium is a success story at many levels. First, the partners' incredible enthusiasm, unwavering commitment, and extraordinary leadership is inspiring to all and an exemplar to the RNAO BPSO Designation overall, fuelling success, sustainability, and fidelity. Second, their capacity to share, support, and propel one another within and between countries is limitless. This rich exchange takes place on a continuous basis both formally through the consortium's meetings with RNAO and informally amongst themselves via emails, phone calls, and onsite visits. Thirdly, this consortium lives in their narratives and in their actions the collective identity that characterizes the social movement of educational and clinical practice changes that the BPSO Designation has created. Fourth and last, it was the Latin America Consortium that propelled RNAO to create its train the trainer models. With its rapid expansion in a region that uses Spanish, it was imperative for RNAO to create solutions that are both responsive and cost effective.

The Latin America Consortium was amongst the first to experience the benefits of RNAO's capacity building programs of Certified BPSO Orientation Trainers and Auditors. These programs are detailed in Chapter 12, *RNAO's Global Spread of BPGs: The BPSO Designation Sustainability and Fidelity.* Their use with the Latin America BPSO Consortium at UNAB, MINSAL and its 7 BPSO Directs, as well as the Colegio de Enfermeros del Peru and its 7 BPSO Directs, exemplifies RNAO's maturity and ability to continuously innovate its BPG Program infrastructure and BPSO delivery models. By building capacity in its established processes for training and onsite audits, RNAO enables continued growth and sustainability of a widespread BPSO Designation. In the case of Latin America, this is proving to be beneficial because the certification of BPSO Leads as trainers and auditors in the region is resulting in less travel, cost-effectiveness for BPSOs, greater ease of communication, and recognition of regional expertise.

KEY MESSAGES

- The BPSO Designation is adaptable to different contexts with outstanding results.

- Energized leadership locally and regionally is critical in spreading the BPSO Designation across different cultures and contexts.

- Organizational and staff readiness in conjunction with a clear, meaningful, and comprehensive organizational-level BPG implementation strategy, such as the BPSO Designation, can lead to a sustained cultural shift.

- Key BPSO deliverables related to creating an infrastructure, capacity building, comprehensive implementation plans, attention to evaluation, dissemination of results, and adherence to RNAO monitoring requirements all impact success as a BPSO.

- Peer support amongst BPSOs is a strong lever in successful uptake of BPGs and their sustained use.

- RNAO's NQuIRE is a robust tool to position the impact of excellence in nursing practice in organizations.

- BPSOs have proven to be a powerful mechanism to sustain and spread the use of RNAO's BPGs, as well as maintain the Program's fidelity.

- The BPSO Training of Trainers Model has contributed to rapid expansion of BPSOs in the Latin American region, impacting costs, communication, development, and recognition of local and regional leaders.

- The Latin America BPSO Consortium showcases a strong collective identity developed over time through common experiences and emotional investment, which fosters sustained BPG use in practice and education, resulting in positive outcomes for patients and organizations.

REFERENCES

Barrios Araya, S., Masalán Apip, M. zP., & Cook, M. P. (2011). Health education: In search of innovative methodologies. *Science and Nursing, 17*(1), 57–69. https://dx.doi.org/10.4067/S0717-95532011000100007

Dearholt, S., & Dang, D. (2012). *Johns Hopkins nursing evidence-based practice: Model and guidelines* (2nd ed.). Indianapolis, IN: Sigma Theta Tau International.

DiCenso, A., Virani, T., Bajnok, I., Borycki, E., Davies, B., Graham, I., . . . Scott, J. (2002). A toolkit to facilitate the implementation of clinical practice guidelines in healthcare settings. *Hospital Quarterly, 5*(3), 55–60.

El América. (2017). http://elamerica.cl/2017/12/13/chile-y-canada-celebran-convenio-de-acuerdo-para-la-implementacion-de-guias-de-practica-clinica-basadas-en-evidencia/ Diciembre 13, 2017

Esparza-Bohórquez, M., Granados Oliveros, L. M., & Joya-Guevara, K. (2016). Implementación de la guía de buenas prácticas: Valoración del riesgo y prevención de úlceras por presión: Experiencia en la Fundación Oftalmológica de Santander (FOSCAL). *MedUNAB, 19*(2), 115–123.

Fundación Cardio-Infantil IC. (2012, October 17). *Informe anual de gestión. Fundación Cardio-Infantil IC. Bogotá, 2009–2012.* [PowerPoint slides]. Retrieved from http://www.slideshare.net/pasante/1caso-de-xito-fundacin-cardioinfantil-turismo-de-salud

Grinspun, D. (2007). Healthy workplaces: The case for shared clinical decision making and increased full-Time employment. *Healthcare Papers* (Special Issue), 7, 69–75.

Grinspun, D. (2011). Guías de práctica clínica y entorno laboral basados en la evidencia elaboradas por la Registered Nurses' Association of Ontario (RNAO). *Enfermeria Clinica, 21*(1), 1–2.

Grinspun, D. (2015). Transforming nursing practice through evidence. Revista *MedUNAB, 17*(3), 133–134.

Grinspun, D. (2017). Leading evidence-based nursing care through systematized processes (Editorial). Revista *MedUNAB*, *19*(2), 83–84. Retrieved from http://revistas.unab.edu.co/index.php?journal=medunab&page=article&op=view&path%5B%5D=2615

Grinspun, D., & Aninyam, C. (2014). Leadership. In S. Coffey & C. Anyinam (Eds.), *Interprofessional health care practice* (1st ed.), (131–158). Toronto, Canada: Pearson Canada Inc.

Grinspun, D., Melnyk, B. M., & Fineout-Overholt, E. (2014). Advancing optimal care with rigorously developed clinical practice guidelines and evidence-based recommendations. In B. M. Melynk & E. Fineout-Overholt (Eds.), *Evidence-based practice in nursing & healthcare. A guide to best practice* (3rd ed.), (182–201). Philadelphia, PA: Lippincott, Williams & Wilkins.

Haines, S. (2005). *Leading strategic change.* San Diego, CA: Systems Thinking Press.

Lucía Cortés, O., Serna-Restrepo, A., Salazar-Beltrán, L. D., Rojas-Castañeda, Y. A., Cabrera-González, S., & Arévalo-Sandoval, I. (2016). Implementación de guías de práctica clínica de la Asociación de Enfermeras de Ontario-RNAO: Una experiencia de enfermería en un hospital colombiano. *MedUNAB, 19*(2), 103–114.

Moreno-Casbas, T., Fuentelsaz-Gallego, C., González-María, E., & Gil de Miguel, A. (2010 May-June). Barreras para la utilización de la investigación. Estudio descriptivo en profesionales de enfermería de la práctica clínica y en investigadores activos. *Enfermeria Clinica. 20*(3), 153–164. doi.org/10.1016/j.enfcli.2010.01.005

Panamericana TV. (2017). https://panamericana.pe/24horas/salud/237180-enfermeros-peru-canada-firman-importante-acuerdo-internacional

Registered Nurses' Association of Ontario (RNAO). (2007a). *Assessment and management of stage I to IV pressure ulcers.* Toronto, ON: Registered Nurses' Association of Ontario.

Registered Nurses' Association of Ontario (RNAO). (2007b). *Integrating smoking cessation into daily nursing practice.* Toronto, ON: Registered Nurses' Association of Ontario.

Registered Nurses' Association of Ontario (RNAO). (2008). *Assessment and device selection for vascular access.* Toronto, ON: Registered Nurses' Association of Ontario.

Registered Nurses' Association of Ontario (RNAO). (2009). *Best Practice Guideline for the subcutaneous administration of insulin in adults with type 2 diabetes.* Toronto, ON: Registered Nurses' Association of Ontario.

Registered Nurses' Association of Ontario (RNAO). (2011a). *Prevention of falls and fall injuries in the older adult.* Toronto, ON: Registered Nurses' Association of Ontario.

Registered Nurses' Association of Ontario (RNAO). (2011b). *Risk assessment and prevention of pressure ulcers.* Toronto, ON: Registered Nurses' Association of Ontario.

Registered Nurses' Association of Ontario (RNAO). (2012a, July 9). *RNAO's clinical Best Practice Guidelines debut in Chile and Colombia.* Toronto, ON: Registered Nurses' Association of Ontario.

Registered Nurses' Association of Ontario (RNAO). (2012b). *Toolkit: Implementation of Best Practice Guidelines* (2nd ed.). Toronto, ON: Registered Nurses' Association of Ontario.

Registered Nurses' Association of Ontario (RNAO). (2013a). *Assessment and management of foot ulcers for people with diabetes* (2nd ed.). Toronto, ON: Registered Nurses' Association of Ontario.

Registered Nurses' Association of Ontario (RNAO). (2013b). *Assessment and management of pain.* Toronto, ON: Registered Nurses' Association of Ontario.

Registered Nurses' Association of Ontario (RNAO). (2013c). *Developing and sustaining nursing leadership.* Toronto, ON: Registered Nurses' Association of Ontario.

Registered Nurses' Association of Ontario (RNAO). (2015, April 9). *RNAO celebrates milestone anniversary with international flare.* Retrieved from http://rnao.ca/news/media-releases/2015/04/09/rnao-celebrates-milestone-anniversary-international-flare

Scottish Intercollegiate Guidelines Network (SIGN). (2008). *SIGN 50: A guideline developer's handbook.* Retrieved from http://www.sign.ac.uk/guidelines/fulltext/50/

The Trujillo Com. (Enero 4, 2018). https://detrujillo.com/colegio-de-enfermeros-del-peru-firma-convenio-con-canada-para-implementar-modelo-de-buenas-practicas-clinicas/

Villaverde, M. F. (2013). Distance education and its relation with the new technologies of the information and the communications. *MediSur, 11*(3), 280–295. Retrieved from http://scielo.sld.cu/scielo.php?script=sci_arttext-t&pid=S1727-897X2013000300006&lng=en&tlng=en

EVALUATING OUTCOMES, PROVING RESULTS: THIRD PILLAR FOR SUCCESS

16

EVALUATING BPG IMPACT: DEVELOPMENT AND REFINEMENT OF NQUIRE

Valerie Grdisa, PhD, MS, BScN, RN
Doris Grinspun, PhD, MSN, BScN, RN, LLD(hon), Dr(hc), O.ONT
Gurjit Kaur Toor, MPH, BScN, RN
Yaw O. Owusu, PhD, MS, MSc, BSc
Shanoja Naik, PhD, MPhil, MSc, BEd, BSc
Kyle Smith, BSc

L E A R N I N G   O B J E C T I V E S

After reading this chapter, you will be able to:

- Understand the background, history, and purpose of the NQuIRE data system

- Understand the Donabedian Model and how it applies to the NQuIRE indicators

- Describe the stages of the NQuIRE indicator development process and the safeguards for NQuIRE security and privacy

- Describe the NQuIRE Data Quality framework and how it contributes to a robust data system

- Describe how health information data are critical for healthcare service provision and used for many secondary purposes including quality improvement, accountability, and research

- Be inspired by the impact of BPG implementation within BPSOs based on NQuIRE outcomes analysis

- Describe the RNAO evaluation methodologies that demonstrate the value and outcomes of BPG implementation in BPSOs and long-term care homes

This chapter focuses on RNAO's evaluation of its Best Practice Guidelines (BPG) impact. In particular it zeroes in and traces the history of NQuIRE, Nursing Quality Indicators for Reporting and Evaluation, from its conception stage through to the early beginning as a data system. The chapter highlights the current state of NQuIRE poised to produce comparative reports, the Nursing Trends Report, and to be a robust source of data for practitioners, administrators, educators, researchers, and policymakers. We describe NQuIRE's history, purpose, and infrastructure. Examples of structure, process, and outcome indicators are shared alongside the impact of BPGs around the world. We also discuss key supports for BPSOs, including capacity building to use NQuIRE and ensuring data quality.

INTRODUCTION

Evidence-based clinical guidelines aim to improve the quality of care and optimize health outcomes, organizational performance, and health system results. However, many efforts to implement programs designed to improve the quality and outcomes of clinical care have not always delivered on their promise.

While single studies and a few systematic reviews exist on the value proposition of clinical guidelines, a comprehensive and longitudinal approach is hard to find. Lugtenberg, Burgers, and Westert (2009) conducted a systematic review of studies evaluating the effects of Dutch evidence-based guidelines on both the process and structure of care and patient outcomes. A total of 20 studies were included, and 17 showed significant improvements in the process and structure of care. The effects of guidelines on patient health outcomes were studied far less. This is the reason behind the birth of NQuIRE, an international data system developed by the Registered Nurses' Association of Ontario (RNAO) in Canada (Grinspun, Lloyd, Xiao, & Bajnok, 2015).

RNAO's BPGs are being implemented in 550 Best Practice Spotlight Organizations (BPSO) worldwide, located on four continents. There is mounting evidence that shows that BPG implementation contributes to better outcomes at the client, nurse, team, organizational, and health system levels, and at a lower cost—thus achieving better value. Local evaluations report substantive improvements in patients' clinical outcomes and financial performance for BPSOs. Chapter 17, *Value for Money: Measuring the Economic Impact of BPSOs in Australia*, details such an impact in Australia.

As described in Chapter 1, *Transforming Nursing Through Knowledge: The Conceptual and Programmatic Underpinnings of RNAO's BPG Program*, the program is composed of three main pillars: development, implementation, and evaluation. This chapter focuses on the latter, and Figure 16.1 depicts the four areas of focus within the evaluation and monitoring pillar of the BPG Program. The BPSOs have created a platform for innovative evaluation methodologies for RNAO to measure the impact of evidence-based nursing care for both quality improvement and future research. NQuIRE consists of a database with an online data entry system; data dictionaries, including a set of organization-level structural indicators, as well as a set of process and outcome indicators for each clinical BPG; and data collection and reporting processes.

Through NQuIRE, RNAO collects, analyzes, and reports quality indicator data submitted by all of RNAO's BPSOs. The system is designed to support BPSOs in monitoring and evaluating the impact of

BPG implementation in their organizations, enabling them to track progress, do intra-organizational comparisons, and in the future, perform inter-BPSO comparative analysis. It sharpens the capacity of BPSOs to make effective practice improvements by identifying areas for intervention and/or areas for further investment to optimize clinical, organizational, and health system outcomes.

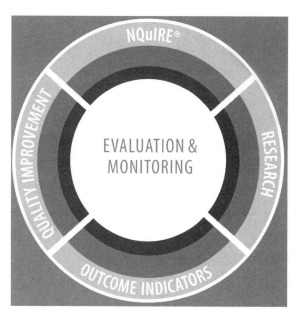

FIGURE 16.1   Evaluation & Monitoring pillar of RNAO BPG Program.

"We see that we need to move to looking at NQuIRE being the first step and not the eighth step in the BPG implementation process. Understanding the data dictionaries was a learning curve for us, but a very helpful step in benchmarking against ourselves and similar BPSOs."

–Karen Cziraki
PhD student, MSc, BScN, RN
BPSO Lead Cambridge Memorial Hospital BPSO Direct

The nursing workforce forms the backbone of the health system, and it is essential to quantify nursing care and nurse-led quality-improvement initiatives that are informed by unit-level benchmarks and local, national, or international peer averages (VanDeVelde-Coke et al., 2012). Standardized measurement of nursing-sensitive indicators and outcome evaluation is essential to evaluate nursing interventions and implement quality-improvement initiatives (Doran, Mildon, & Clarke, 2011). RNAO's NQuIRE is the first international quality-improvement initiative of its kind, consisting of a data system of quality indicators derived from evidence-based guideline recommendations.

By monitoring, evaluating, and reporting quality improvements in nursing care across the globe, NQuIRE is producing BPSO-validated and -endorsed quality indicators that will contribute to sustainability and enhance understanding of the full impact of evidence-based nursing practice on healthcare quality and health outcomes. The RNAO BPSO Designation has created a platform for innovative evaluation methodologies to measure the impact of evidence-based nursing care (Lloyd,

Xiao, Albornos-Munoz, González-María, & Joyce, 2013), and NQuIRE is
the data system to achieve it.

As the global population grows, migrates, and ages, health systems need to
boldly transform to better meet population health needs. Governments and
planning authorities are eager to spread, scale up, and scale out proven
quality-improvement strategies such as RNAO's evidenced-based Best
Practice Guidelines (BPG) and the Best Practice Spotlight Organization
(BPSO) model.

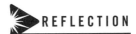

*Why is it important to
have measures that
demonstrate the impact
of evidence-based
nursing practice?*

HISTORY AND PURPOSE OF NQUIRE

NQuIRE, RNAO's groundbreaking international data system, was launched in August 2012 for
BPSOs to monitor performance of RNAO BPG implementation and evaluate their impact on nursing
practice, clients, organizations, and health system outcomes. Evidence shows that BPGs reduce variation in care, transfer research evidence into practice, help identify knowledge gaps, assist in clinical
decision-making, redesign organizational processes, improve organizational and system performance,
and reduce the cost of care. NQuIRE has a web-based user interface and database storage system that
serves to collect, analyze, and report back to BPSOs comparative data on indicators reflecting the
structure, process, and outcomes of care resulting from BPG implementation. From 2012 to 2014,
NQuIRE was a voluntary option for BPSOs to join. In 2014, NQuIRE became a mandatory BPSO
requirement to promote evaluation of nursing quality improvement and advance nursing knowledge
through BPG implementation.

NQuIRE indicators have been developed for clinical BPGs based on the
practice, education, and organization/policy recommendations to demonstrate how evidence-based nursing practice improves health outcomes and
transforms healthcare. When the BPSO chooses the BPG for implementation, they also choose the specific indicators for each BPG. The BPSOs
embrace the importance of evaluating the uptake and impact of their
evidence-based implementation efforts and demonstrating the value of
the nursing practice changes and improved outcomes. As the data system
expands, NQuIRE will continue to impact practice, management and policy
decisions, education, and health system research.

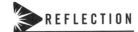

*Are you familiar with
other data repositories
that demonstrate the
impact and value of
evidence-based nursing
care, such as NQuIRE?*

THE DONABEDIAN MODEL OF STRUCTURE, PROCESS, AND OUTCOMES AND NQUIRE INDICATORS

The evaluation of nurses' contribution to improved health and healthcare using RNAO's evidence-based BPGs is based on a well-established theoretical evaluation framework. NQuIRE's architecture is based on the Donabedian Model, which categorizes the structural attributes of the settings
in which care occurs, processes of care, and desired outcomes (Donabedian, 1966, 1988, 2005). The
three dimensions include: structure (e.g., organizational structures, human resources, and material

resources), process (e.g., assessment, interventions, and education), and outcomes (e.g., patient, client or resident; healthcare provider; organization). The structure-process-outcome (SPO) model has been used to evaluate a diverse range of quality improvement initiatives, including the development and classification of nursing-sensitive indicators. Nursing-sensitive indicators are "based on nurses' scope and domain of practice, and for which there is empirical evidence linking nursing inputs and interventions to the outcome" (Doran, 2003, p. vii). The SPO model can be applied to a diverse range of quality improvement projects, such as:

- Introducing enhanced recovery pathways for elective colorectal surgery (Moonesinghe et al., 2017)

- Demonstrating the value of nurse-led teams in emergency departments designed to address the needs of frail older persons living in the community and residential aged care facilities (Marsden et al., 2017)

- Demonstrating the value of advanced practice nursing interventions in Switzerland (Bryant-Lukosius et al., 2016)

- Implementing evidence-based nursing interventions in a neonatal intensive care unit in China (Chen et al., 2016)

- Improving surgical procedures (Ingraham, Richards, Hall, & Ko, 2010)

- Improving the structures and processes of trauma care (Moore, Lavoie, Bourgeois, & Lapointe, 2015)

Kelley and Hurst (2006) use the SPO dimensions in a conceptual framework for the Organisation for Economic Co-operation and Development's (OECD) Health Care Quality Indicator Project. The OECD recently demonstrated the economic impact of the success or failure of patient-safety interventions within a patient-safety improvement context (Slawomirski, Auraaen, & Klazinga, 2017). With 5 decades of literature demonstrating the applicability of the SPO model, it has been an effective organizing framework for the NQuIRE data system to help BPSOs evaluate their structural inputs and impact of their implementation efforts on outcomes.

TAXONOMY OF QUALITY MEASURES

The NQuIRE data system collects structural indicators, as well as nursing-sensitive process and outcome indicators derived from the practice recommendations in RNAO's BPGs. Data dictionaries have been developed for 20 clinical BPGs of the 53 RNAO BPGs. Each data dictionary consists of the links to specific BPG practice recommendations, rationale for creating the indicator, operational definition, numerators and denominators, the target population, data collection frequency, and a list of comparable data sources. Each data dictionary has four to eight process and outcome indicators on average, for a total of 140 NQuIRE indicators.

STRUCTURAL INDICATORS

Within NQuIRE, the structural indicators represent organizational measures that are not BPG specific. Structural indicators capture staffing and other human resource characteristics of the BPSO implementation site. The six NQuIRE measures include: the number of nursing hours per patient day or patient visit, nursing skill mix including hours worked and agency/purchased hours worked, nurse absenteeism and nurse turnover rates (as studied by Nantsupawat et al., 2017), type of education received, and the model of care delivery.

PROCESS INDICATORS

Process indicators capture nursing care provided to patients or clients, such as the assessments and interventions recommended in a specific BPG. The coding of process indicators for the NQuIRE data system generally follows the steps of the nursing process: assessment, planning, implementation/intervention, and evaluation. A numerical order (pro01, pro02, etc.) usually follows the steps of the nursing process. For example, falls_pro01 is falls risk assessment for new admissions and falls_pro02 is a falls risk assessment following a fall.

OUTCOMES INDICATORS

Outcome indicators capture the effects of nursing care on the patient's health status or their level of satisfaction with their nursing care. Thus, it is critical to ensure that planned changes in the processes of care are "validated by demonstrating their relationship to desirable outcomes" (Mainz, 2003, p. 527). To fully understand outcomes as measures of quality improvement, one must account for structural indicators related to the organization and/or sector, as well as variables specific to the patient. In addition, matters of data quality must be addressed to ensure that what we measure is valid and reliable. NQuIRE's Data Quality framework is discussed later in this chapter.

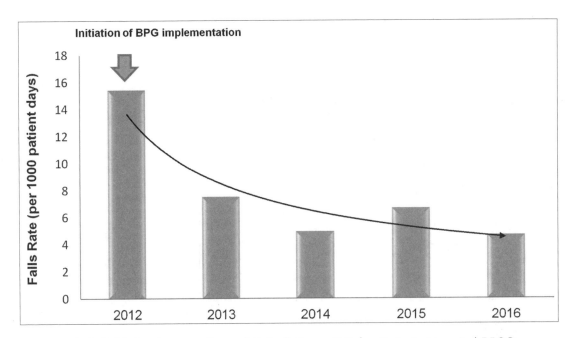

FIGURE 16.2 Average Rate of Falls (falls_out01) for Ontario Hospital BPSO.

Given that long periods of time elapse before the manifestation of a desired outcome in specific sectors such as public health, implementing evidence-based practice interventions that have demonstrated effect in the systematic review is essential. Outcome indicators are derived from the BPG practice recommendations and purpose statements that identify desired outcomes and also follow a numerical order. For example, falls_out01 is for average rate of falls and falls_out02 is injury rate following a fall.

Figure 16.2 demonstrates a 70% (15.4 to 4.7) decrease in the NQuIRE outcome indicator, falls rate per 1.000 patient days, following implementation of the RNAO BPG *Prevention of Falls and Fall Injuries in the Older Adult* (2011) in one hospital BPSO. The nursing processes of care were changed in 2012 based on the BPG recommendations, and the desired outcomes have been sustained for 4 years.

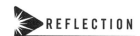
REFLECTION

Using the Donabedian Model of Structure, Process, and Outcomes, can you identify indicators that are being measured or should be measured within your clinical practice?

FREQUENCY OF DATA COLLECTION

BPSOs collect indicator data monthly, quarterly, or annually depending on the type of indicator and the level of indicator utilization and/or stability. For example, data on initial assessment of new pressure injury patients on admission are collected monthly, whereas the numbers of educational visits on childhood obesity prevention to a school by the public health nurse are collected quarterly, and data on nurse turnover rate (structural indicator) are collected annually. The next section provides an overview of the NQuIRE indicator development process and planned refinements to align with the BPG development process and respond to BPSO feedback based on their lived experiences using NQuIRE.

NQUIRE INDICATOR DEVELOPMENT PROCESS

RNAO's International Affairs and Best Practice Guideline (IABPG) Centre staff work together with BPSOs throughout all phases—including development, implementation, and evaluation—to develop indicators. In 2012, the indicator development process was established based on steps identified within a systematic review of 48 articles (Kotter, Blozik, & Scherer, 2012). As an international data system, approaches used for indicator development by leading national and international organizations were examined. The World Health Organization (WHO) incorporates an advisory committee and statistical tests of indicators during its testing phase to enhance inter-jurisdictional comparisons (von Schirnding, 2002). The Organisation for Economic Co-operation and Development (OECD) maintains and continuously reviews and refines indicators (Kelley & Hurst, 2006).

The Centers for Disease Control and Prevention (CDC) uniquely uses logic models to understand the relationship amongst program goals, activities, outputs, and intended outcomes, and an explanation of baseline data (CDC, 2007). The National Institute for Health and Care Excellence (NICE) integrates an advisory committee's prioritization results and tests the prioritized indicators in their process (NICE, 2014).

Amongst Canadian agencies, the inter-Resident Assessment Instrument (inter-RAI) integrates algorithms and clinical assessment protocols in the indicator development process (inter-RAI, 2017). The Public Health Agency of Canada (PHAC, 2012) uses focus groups and content analysis of data collected from survey participants. Health Quality Ontario (HQO), an advisory agency to the Government of Ontario, Canada, recently introduced a modified Delphi process into its process to build consensus on key indicators for public reporting (HQO, 2016). The RNAO uses a modified-Delphi process for building consensus on the BPG recommendation statements, and these findings lead to robust discussions amongst BPG Expert Panel members on potential evaluation measures.

The initial NQuIRE indicator development process (2012 to 2016) involved a five-step process which includes: 1) guideline selection; 2) extraction of recommendations; 3) quality indicator selection; 4) practice test/validation; and 5) implementation (see Figure 16.3). As previously indicated, 20 data dictionaries have been developed for 20 clinical BPGs for a total of 140 indicators. BPSOs receive education and training regarding the data dictionaries and engage in a discussion with the IABPG Centre team, including their BPSO coach, to select the NQuIRE indicators that would address the practice gaps and capture the impact of their implementation efforts for each BPG.

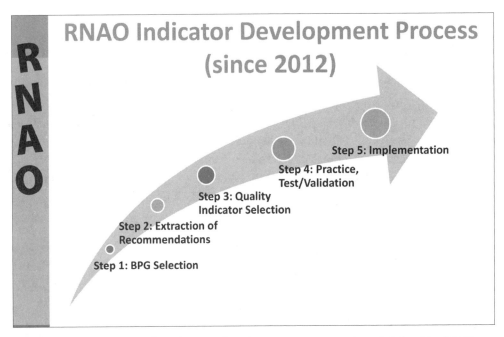

FIGURE 16.3   RNAO indicator development process (established in 2012).
© Registered Nurses' Association of Ontario. All rights reserved. Used with permission.

The RNAO indicator development process steps are summarized here:

1. **Guideline selection**—Indicators are developed for clinical BPGs that are focused on health system priorities, utilized most frequently, and/or requested by BPSOs.

2. **Extraction of recommendations**—Practice recommendations, potential measures identified in the BPG Evaluation and Monitoring chart, and RNAO Nursing Order Sets (if applicable) are reviewed to extract or identify potential measures for indicator development. The Nursing Order Sets are clear, concise, and actionable evidence-based intervention statements— derived from the BPG process recommendations—that can be readily embedded within an organization's electronic health information system (see Chapter 5, *Technology as an Enabler of Evidence-Based Practice*). Several criteria are considered when developing indicators, such as the strength of supporting evidence, impact on patient/client outcomes, or feasibility to measure and monitor. The practice recommendations that have significant policy implications and/or associated costs are also carefully considered.

3. **Quality indicator selection and development**—For new BPGs (new topics) or next edition BPGs (supplements with a literature review or subsequent editions with updated systematic reviews), indicators are identified using various established health information data libraries or repositories of quality measures, such as those from Accreditation Canada, Resident Assessment Instrument (RAI) Minimum Data Set, Canadian Institute of Health Information, Health Quality Ontario, and Joint Commission. For each next edition BPG with an updated systematic review, the previous NQuIRE indicators are reviewed for possible alignment with the updated and/or new practice recommendations. Most importantly, indicator definitions are aligned with available administrative data and existing performance measures wherever possible, adhering to a "collect once, use many times" principle. By complementing other established and emerging performance measurement systems, NQuIRE strives to leverage reliable and valid measures, minimize reporting burden, and align evaluation measures to enable comparative analyses.

4. **Practice test/validation**—Internal validation of face validity and content validity is conducted by the IABPG team, led by the Evaluation and Monitoring team. External validation of content validity and feasibility of data collection is conducted by the BPSOs. This process involves review of each draft data dictionary for new or next edition BPGs through a survey instrument. International BPSOs are included in the external validation to better understand the implications of the indicators in a global context. For example, our BPSO Host in Spain—Investén-isciii—which oversees about 80 service organizations and academic institutions across that country, conducted an expert review to select the NQuIRE indicators for the BPG, *Assessment and Management of Foot Ulcers for People with Diabetes*, 2nd Edition (RNAO, 2013).

As the majority of BPSOs represent the hospital care sector, and most nursing-sensitive indicators measure nursing care in hospitals (Heslop & Lu, 2014), the IABPG team makes a concerted effort to work closely with BPSOs from other sectors (e.g., home care, long-term care, public health, and primary care) to validate sector-specific NQuIRE indicators. For example, the indicators *falls_pro05* (rate of daily physical restraint) and *falls_out02* (injury rate following a fall) were both developed for the long-term care sector and align with the long-term care mandatory reporting requirements.

5. **Implementation**—The data dictionaries are published on the NQuIRE website. The RNAO Information Management and Technology department and the Evaluation and Monitoring team create NQuIRE web forms and data import Excel spreadsheets for data collection. BPSOs are informed about the new indicators within the new or revised data dictionaries. BPSOs provide ongoing feedback regarding validity, feasibility of data collection, utilization of the automated NQuIRE reports, and recommendations for any future refinements.

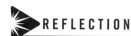**REFLECTION**

Think of a clinical topic you are passionate about, and using the NQuIRE indicator development process, identify three ideal process indicators that would capture nursing interventions.

PURPOSEFUL EVOLUTION OF NQUIRE

As described in Chapter 1, RNAO's BPG Program engages in purposeful evolution to continuously reflect current science and respond to the needs in the field.

BPGs are updated every 5 years, at which time NQuIRE indicators are also revised for the new or updated recommendation statements. Importantly, if a next edition BPG has a STOP recommendation, then any indicator related to that STOP recommendation will be removed or revised in NQuIRE and the data dictionary. During review of each next edition BPG, the decision to remove or revise existing NQuIRE indicators is based on the following criteria:

- Indicator is not well defined and it cannot be further defined or clarified based on the BPG recommendation statement.

- Indicator is no longer relevant to nursing practice or overall client outcomes.

- Indicator does not permit useful comparisons.

- Indicator is not supported by the systematic review and evidence summaries.

- Indicator is not relevant or coherent, based on sufficient feedback from BPSOs.

NQUIRE INDICATORS: REFINEMENT

As RNAO's guideline development methodology evolves to assess the strength of recommendations using GRADE (Grading of Recommendations, Assessment, Development, and Evaluation), the indicator development process is being refined accordingly. As discussed in Chapter 2, *The Anatomy of a Rigorous Best Practice Guideline Development Process*, GRADE involves a focus on outcomes identification prior to the systematic review, which informs the research questions and affects the indicator development process.

The refined NQuIRE indicator development process will maintain the established five main steps with the addition of a sixth step that focuses on conducting the data quality assessments and ongoing evaluation to create a continuous cycle (see Figure 16.4). Within the refined NQuIRE indicator development cycle, changes include:

- Identify evaluation measures from the evidence profiles based on the systematic review (conducted by the BPG development team)

- Apply schematic algorithms to aid decision-making regarding potential indicators

- Make concerted efforts to consistently align new or revised indicators with other publicly reported measures that align with the BPG purpose, scope, and/or recommendation statements

- Apply and test the new organizing framework to categorize core, novel, and sector-specific indicators (see Figure 16.5)

- Enrich the current participation of BPSOs in the testing phase through a formalized, structured, modified-Delphi process for consensus building during external validation

"If we ask people to do more work for data collection, we need to be strategic about what we ask and how we support them so that it gets done."

—Sara Leblond, M.Sc.N., RN, IIWCC
BPSO Co-Lead
Montfort Hospital, Ontario
BPSO Direct

- Introduce new statistical tests to measure the degree of consensus (or concordance) amongst the reviewers of draft indicators as well as other psychometric tests such as reliability (Chen et al., 2016)

- Conduct annual data quality assessments to inform indicator revisions and identify the frequency of indicator utilization by BPSOs and robustness of the indicator dataset

- Create a checklist for each indicator to standardize data collection for the data elements identified in the data dictionaries

- Evaluate the indicators by conducting regular tests by BPSOs post-implementation to compare to the baseline to determine if further modifications are necessary

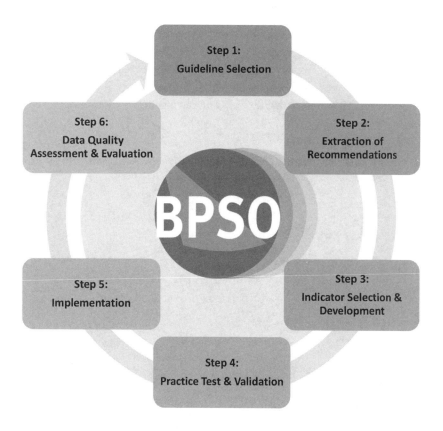

FIGURE 16.4 NQuIRE indicator development cycle (effective 2017).
© Registered Nurses' Association of Ontario. All rights reserved. Used with permission.

As RNAO evolves the NQuIRE indicator development process, the reporting burden is expected to lessen, and the core, new, or novel indicators are expected to be more specific to the practice setting and sector. Indicator definitions will be further aligned with available administrative data and mandatory performance measures from other data repositories wherever possible, to adhere to a "collect once, use many times" principle. BPSOs worldwide have access to NQuIRE's unique international data system to evaluate the uptake and impact of evidence-based clinical and Healthy Work Environment BPGs on nursing practice and health outcomes. This has been made possible through a collective sense of ownership of the BPSO Program and NQuIRE and an intense desire to make a difference that has led to a powerful collaboration of BPSOs globally. As described in Chapter 1, there is a collective identity about BPSOs and about NQuIRE; together we shape the program and share our outcomes with the world.

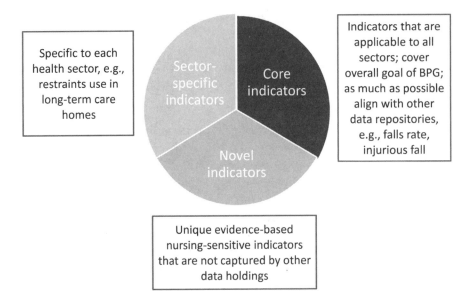

FIGURE 16.5 Categorization of NQuIRE indicators.

ACADEMIC INDICATORS

The field of academic indicators and their testing is in an early stage of development. RNAO and its academic BPSOs are trailblazers of discovery in this area. Together, we have pilot initiatives underway to develop and test academic indicators for participating academic BPSOs (see Chapter 9, *Enhancing the Evidence-Based Nursing Curriculum and Competence in Evidence-Based Practice*).

NQUIRE INTERNATIONAL ADVISORY COUNCIL

In 2013, RNAO established the NQuIRE International Advisory Council (IAC) to provide strategic advice on the theoretical framework underpinning the use of indicators in research and evaluation. The IAC advises on ongoing quality-control processes and strategic use of NQuIRE data to inform research initiatives and practice, education, management, and policy deliberations at local, national, and international levels. This advisory council also recommends strategies for information analysis, including benchmarking, comparative reporting, and data triangulation.

The council meets twice a year for open discussions as RNAO continues to make strides in the field of nursing to impact health outcomes. Part of the IAC's recommendations has been to align indicators with national and international publicly reported indicators to reduce the reporting burden of BPSOs while maintaining the overall desired outcomes of the BPG. The IAC has been a source of expert advice on high-level directions and on subject-specific matters such as the NQuIRE Data Quality framework, as discussed in the next section.

"I have watched the BPG Program from its inception and have seen the amazing impact of BPSOs worldwide. With NQuIRE we have a real opportunity to prove once and forever that evidence-based nursing practice serves to optimize results for patients and health organizations. As already shown in several chapters of this book, NQuIRE will increasingly allow us to make the necessary connections between evidence-based practice and evidence-based policy—an essential link to ensure nurses' full contribution to the health and healthcare of people."

—Judith Shamian, PhD, MPH, BA, RN, D.Sc(hon), LLD(hon), FAAN
NQuIRE Founding Chair
ICN Past President

NQUIRE SECURITY AND PRIVACY

The RNAO data governance requirements are operationalized through RNAO's data governance policy and the related committees representing all departments. The Privacy Impact Assessment (PIA) provides documentation of RNAO's legal obligations toward privacy legislation, which includes Ontario's *Personal Information Protection and Electronic Documents Act, 2000* and the *Personal Health Information Protection Act, 2004*. RNAO, through NQuIRE, collects only de-identified aggregated data from BPSOs at the unit level, and not personal health information. The threat risk assessment details RNAO's legal responsibilities to BPSOs in the event of a data breach and provides evidence that RNAO has secured the NQuIRE data system at multiple levels—data, host, application, and network—against such a breach (see Figure 16.6).

The innermost layer details the security of the NQuIRE data. The NQuIRE data system includes the web-based interface, where BPSOs submit data and access their reports, and the NQuIRE database, which houses the NQuIRE data submitted by BPSOs. All data is encrypted in our secure database, and the encryption key is outside the database and the web root directory. NQuIRE datasets are subsets of the data housed within the NQuIRE database (e.g., falls data for a specific BPSO).

The second layer outlines security for the NQuIRE application. The web-based data system has role-based access control. There are two roles for BPSO users: a BPSO Lead role and an Implementation Site role. These roles are assigned automatically, and assignment is dependent on the initial invitation to NQuIRE. The data are stored in the database with access limited by the application to specific RNAO staff with a unique username and password login. Access to the application is logged and tracked through IP addresses. Access to the server and site is limited to authorized RNAO Information Management and Technology (IMT) department staff and specific IABPG Centre staff.

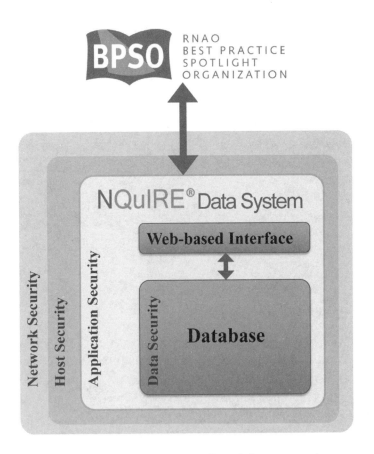

FIGURE 16.6 NQuIRE multilayer security.

The NQuIRE application is developed using open source software that enables many data integrity and security features for its database. The NQuIRE application encrypts user data submissions before storing them in the NQuIRE database. The third layer includes security of the host. All data are stored entirely on RNAO-controlled and owned servers. The host is housed within RNAO's home office, and physically the server is restricted to IMT staff. The RNAO building has electronic security access, and additional electronic swipe entry is required for IMT staff to access a locked server room at the RNAO home office.

The fourth and outermost layer outlines security for RNAO networks. The networks are regularly monitored by IMT staff ensuring no unauthorized access to the network or any host or application. This multilayer security ensures that the NQuIRE data is protected at each layer. The practices for privacy and security of NQuIRE data have been established through RNAO's IMT governance processes and NQuIRE-specific data governance (i.e., the NQuIRE Data Usage Agreement). This multilayer approach to data security and privacy, combined with the NQuIRE Data Quality framework described next, are fundamental to overall data management.

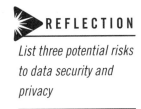

REFLECTION

List three potential risks to data security and privacy

NQUIRE DATA QUALITY FRAMEWORK

The NQuIRE Data Quality framework was developed to support comprehensive data quality assessments. This required an in-depth understanding of the data system, including what the data represent and their use. Data represent selected characteristics of a phenomenon (i.e., events, concepts, and objects) and their interpretation. Specifically, data elements must be interpreted within the context of their creation, which determines "fitness for use" (Sebastian-Coleman, 2012; Wang & Strong, 1996). For NQuIRE the context is RNAO, led by the IABPG Evaluation and Monitoring team, and the fitness for use is tested by the BPSOs during BPG implementation. Data constitute an organizational asset, and appreciation of its value provides direction to reduce risks associated with flawed data (Loshin, 2011). In essence, NQuIRE must embed approaches that support high-quality data to demonstrate the impact and value of BPG implementation.

In health systems around the globe, data quality is impacted by the state of documentation systems, ranging from paper-based documentation to hybrid systems to fully electronic documentation. Data quality begins with the source, making it paramount to identify and mitigate the risks for collecting flawed data (Strome, 2013). Lack of documentation standards, duplicate records within and between organizations, different staff collecting and entering data, and outdated data-collection tools are common factors that affect data quality. According to Loeb (2004), data collection is also hindered by:

- Organizations that are unwilling or unable to change existing data-collection processes

- Ambiguous data requirements and definitions

- Challenges with data availability

- No internal, external, or independent audits of the data

- Variation in data collection and management within and across organizations

- Lack of support for those collecting data from database developers

Despite these challenges, healthcare data are critical to service delivery and used for the three categories of performance measurement (Solberg, Mosser, & McDonald, 1997): quality improvement (e.g., identifying practice issues, evaluating practice changes), accountability (e.g., reporting requirements, accreditation), and research (e.g., observational studies, case studies).

Both learning health systems and comparative effectiveness research programs use secondary health data from health information systems to apply evidence (i.e., patient, practice, and population level outcomes) in healthcare decision-making and quality improvement and to generate new knowledge (Institute of Medicine [IOM], 2007; Lopez, Holve, Sarkar, & Segal, 2012; Safran et al., 2007). Both utilize existing administrative and health information systems within and across health organizations to gather individual or aggregated data. The RNAO and BPSOs are part of learning health systems using secondary aggregated data in NQuIRE to evaluate guideline implementation. As BPSOs transform care and improve outcomes, high-quality data is critical to demonstrating the impact and value of the BPG implementation efforts (IOM, 2013; Kahn et al., 2015). The NQuIRE Data Quality framework provides the blueprint for continuously enhancing the quality of data received from BPSOs provincially, nationally, and internationally. The next section summarizes how BPSO perspectives and clinical and health data repositories from other data quality frameworks informed the development of RNAO's Data Quality framework.

RESPONDING TO THE BPSOs TO ENHANCE DATA QUALITY

Consistent with all aspects of the BPG Program and its BPSOs, end user engagement is critical to ensure uptake, sustainability, and program fidelity. In the case of NQuIRE, BPSOs are the data creators, users, and data stewards. Thus, to enhance data quality, it is important for RNAO to fully understand and account for BPSOs' perceptions, needs, and experiences in using NQuIRE.

ENRICHING THE UNDERSTANDING OF BPSOS' PERCEPTIONS, NEEDS, AND EXPERIENCES WITH NQUIRE

A comprehensive and iterative approach was used to engage BPSOs' experiences using NQuIRE and to identify data quality challenges and potential solutions. It entailed a focus group, seven onsite visits, and two virtual visits. The focus group participants consisted of a sample of BPSO Leads (n=5) representing five different sectors (i.e., public health, long-term care, hospital, home care, and primary care) within Ontario. The five BPSO Leads reported into NQuIRE for more than 6 months and had comprehensive knowledge regarding all aspects of the BPSO Designation. A semi-structured questionnaire was used to guide the focus group discussion on NQuIRE and barriers to data quality within their respective organizations. Interpretive descriptive analysis was applied to identify preliminary themes based on the verbatim transcription of the BPSO focus group.

To further understand and validate the identified themes, seven onsite visits and two virtual visits were conducted with a different subset of BPSOs with the same inclusion criteria: represented one of five sectors, reported to NQuIRE for more than 6 months, and had comprehensive knowledge of the BPSO Program. The two virtual visits were conducted with international BPSOs from Europe and Asia to ensure transferability of findings in other countries.
For each visit, a structured questionnaire was used for data collection. To ensure credibility, three individual transcribers were present at each visit, and transcripts were compared and contrasted to assess consistency and reduce bias and gaps in information.

A secondary thematic analysis was conducted, and several themes were similar to the documentation and data-collection challenges previously summarized. The following were specific to NQuIRE data quality for RNAO BPGs:

- BPG purpose and scope may result in exceptions to NQuIRE indicators (e.g., BPG restricted to adults only is adapted for paediatric setting and indicator does not include paediatric population).

- NQuIRE indicators need to better represent sector-specific BPG implementation (e.g., falls intervention in public health is significantly different from hospital care).

"The client's chart is paper-based and kept at home and then only comes to office upon discharge at which point data is manually extracted for NQuIRE. This reporting burden may change once we complete transition to an electronic health record."

—Sandra M McKay, PhD
NQuIRE lead
VHA Home HealthCare, Ontario
BPSO Direct

- Data collection should start prior to BPG implementation to demonstrate effect.

- NQuIRE indicator data-collection cycle needs to be established to follow the implementation-to-sustainability cycle (e.g., pressure injury assessment indicator is collected months after steady state achieved and no data collection end date identified).

- Standardized training throughout predesignation period is required for specific topics: NQuIRE launch, data collection, data quality, data analysis, and indicator development.

- NQuIRE supporting documents such as the data dictionaries, training materials, and glossary should be more succinct and understandable for BPSO Leads to champion NQuIRE purpose and reporting.

- NQuIRE indicators should be better aligned with existing performance measures from other data repositories to decrease reporting burden.

COMPARATIVE REVIEW OF DATA QUALITY FRAMEWORKS

Data quality frameworks from other clinical and health data repositories were reviewed to develop the RNAO framework (see Table 16.1). The Canadian Institute for Health Information (CIHI) framework is based on three inputs: data quality literature, the principles of Continuous Quality Improvement (CQI), and methods and guidelines from Statistics Canada. CIHI's framework includes five data quality dimensions: accuracy, relevance, timeliness, comparability, and usability (CIHI, 2009). The New Zealand Ministry of Health (NZMH) developed a framework that includes the five CIHI dimensions and another dimension, security and privacy (Kerr, 2003; Kerr & Norris, 2004, 2007).

The Organisation for Economic Co-operation and Development (OECD), which houses international health and economic data, developed a framework that overlaps with three CIHI dimensions and has four additional dimensions—credibility, accessibility, interpretability, and coherence—and the factor of cost-efficiency (OECD, 2012). The Australia Capital Territory (ACT, 2013) Data Quality framework has seven dimensions, which include three dimensions common to all frameworks and overlaps with three of the OECD dimensions and introduces institutional environment.

Although there are differences in the dimensions between the four frameworks studied, there are many similarities and overlapping characteristics. The four frameworks informed the conceptualization and development of the NQuIRE Data Quality framework within the context of IABPG Centre initiatives and BPSO Designation goals and desired outcomes related to BPG implementation. With NQuIRE having a solid approach to security and privacy within the data system architecture, RNAO selected five similar dimensions: relevance, timeliness, interpretability, coherence, and institutional environment. It also introduced one new dimension, integrity.

TABLE 16.1   COMPARISON OF DATA QUALITY DIMENSIONS ACROSS FRAMEWORKS

DATA QUALITY DIMENSIONS	CIHI	NZMH	OECD	ACT	RNAO
Accuracy	✓	✓	✓	✓	
Relevance	✓	✓	✓	✓	✓
Timeliness	✓	✓	✓	✓	✓
Comparability	✓	✓			
Usability	✓	✓			
Security and Privacy		✓			
Credibility			✓		
Accessibility			✓	✓	
Interpretability			✓	✓	✓
Coherence			✓	✓	✓
Institutional Environment				✓	✓
Integrity					✓

THE DATA QUALITY FRAMEWORK

The NQuIRE Data Quality framework was developed to support comprehensive data quality assessments to ensure a robust data system that demonstrates the impact of BPG implementation within BPSOs.

FOUR COMPONENTS OF THE NQUIRE DATA QUALITY FRAMEWORK

The framework consists of four essential components (see Figure 16.7):

1. The BPSO is the data source where NQuIRE data is created and used (core).

2. The RNAO BPG cycle of guideline development, implementation, and evaluation impacts data quality during BPSO predesignation and designation phases (inner three circles).

3. The key features include culture of data quality, innovation and integration, and complexity and multiplicity to support high-quality data in NQuIRE (outer circle).

4. The six data quality dimensions of coherence, relevance, timeliness, institutional environment, integrity, and interpretability ensure NQuIRE data meet the goals and expectations of data users, producers, and stewards (outer pinwheel).

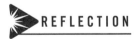

REFLECTION

Based on the data quality dimensions, which dimensions do you believe are most important to high quality data?

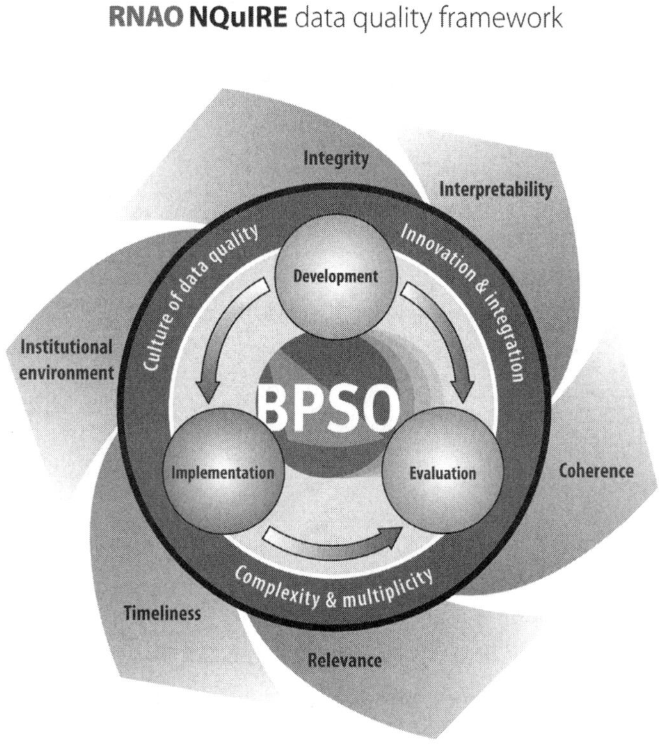

RNAO NQuIRE data quality framework

FIGURE 16.7   NQuIRE Data Quality framework.

The four framework components are described in more detail in the next section.

BPSO CONTEXT AND DATA QUALITY RECOMMENDATIONS

RNAO has collaborative relationships with local, national, and international BPSOs, as all work together for the common goal of speaking out for nurses and speaking out for health, and to demonstrate the impact of their BPG implementation efforts. BPSOs analyze gaps between current practice and BPG recommendations and identify desired goals and outcomes prior to selecting relevant NQuIRE indicators and determining data sources and data-collection processes. Within each sector (i.e., public health, primary care, hospital care, long-term care, and home care), BPSOs consider the best approaches to optimize the data from their existing health information systems. The two BPSO types (service and academic) and two BPSO models (Direct and Host) have implications for which data elements are collected and reported. By placing BPSOs in the center of this framework, the RNAO is committed to actively involve BPSOs throughout the BPG cycle—from development to implementation to evaluation—to support high-quality data in NQuIRE.

To engage BPSOs in data quality improvement, the IABPG Evaluation and Monitoring team organized six in-person NQuIRE Boot Camps (autumn 2016) with local BPSOs, and five virtual NQuIRE Boot Camps (winter 2017) with international BPSOs, to collectively identify strategies to strengthen BPSOs' participation in NQuIRE, including the needs of different practice settings. The main purpose of the Boot Camp was to provide a knowledge-exchange forum for BPSOs to develop a collective understanding of NQuIRE's value to the nursing profession and enhance the quality of data in the NQuIRE data system. BPSOs recommended the development and/or refinement of sector-specific indicators, as many of the NQuIRE indicators are focused on hospital care. This recommendation would address variation in nursing care and service delivery in different practice settings and enable "like sector" comparisons in the future. Currently, the absence of some sector-specific indicators results in exceptions and requests for customized indicators. The stratification of NQuIRE indicators by sector explains the need for this BPSO recommendation, as the data system has robust data for hospital care (60%) and long-term care (20%) and emerging data for home care (9%), public health (8%), and primary care (3%).

> *"Good job especially with international countries. The networking and knowledge exchange is great. It will be very interesting to compare the data between a Caribbean country and a Canadian site, similar in structure and size."*
>
> —Judy-Ann Henry, MScHA, CCRN, RN
> BPSO Lead
> University Hospital of the West Indies, Jamaica
> BPSO Direct

Boot Camp participant recommendations to improve data quality were also focused on institutional environment and timeliness of data collection, as monthly data collection was more challenging than quarterly data collection, which aligns with other mandatory reporting requirements. Participants recommended that NQuIRE indicators need more external validation and practice tests during the indicator development process to determine relevance and coherence with other data repositories. Participants highlighted the importance of using other data sources, both qualitative and quantitative, to improve the data quality and to champion robust evaluation that demonstrates the profound impacts of BPG implementation within BPSOs around the globe. Finally, participants highlighted the importance of defining the time period for data collection for process indicators that measure changes in the processes of care, and recommended ending data collection for specific indicators when a steady state has been sustained and targets have been achieved during the designation stage.

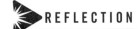 **REFLECTION**

Why do you believe it is important to establish a Data Quality framework for a large data system like NQuIRE? Have you been involved in such an initiative, and if yes, what did you learn?

BPG CYCLE AND ITS IMPACT ON DATA QUALITY

As described in Chapter 1, the BPG Program has three main pillars: development, implementation, and evaluation. As detailed in this section, each one of these pillars has a bearing on NQuIRE data quality.

BPG Development

During the BPG development phase, the purpose, scope, and inclusion and exclusion criteria form the basis for the research questions that guide the systematic review. The evidence summaries lead to the development of actionable and measurable practice recommendation statements. This initiates the early identification of NQuIRE indicators and comparison to other data repositories through the indicator development process. The practice recommendation statements lead to the identification of process indicators while the outcome indicators are derived from the purpose, scope, and desired outcomes of the BPGs. This phase of the BPG cycle is critical to setting the foundation for data quality.

The BPSOs recognize the importance of evaluating evidence-based nursing interventions and nurse-led quality improvement initiatives as demonstrated by the number of BPSOs registered in the NQuIRE data system. Eighty-four percent are submitting data into NQuIRE, and the remaining portion (16%) are not yet submitting data because they are part of a new cohort of: service BPSOs and are in the early phase of selecting indicators and collecting data; academic BPSOs (piloting new academic-specific NQuIRE indicators); or service BPSOs that need data quality follow-ups. This level of participation contributes significantly to data quality.

BPG Implementation

The BPSOs interpret and adapt the evidence to their clinical context or practice setting during the predesignation phase. The BPSO Agreement ensures continuous flow of consistent data into NQuIRE. BPSOs identify practice gaps prior to BPG implementation to focus their efforts on changes in nursing and/or interprofessional care. RNAO BPSO coaches support organizations during implementation and evaluation activities to meet requirements for BPSO Designation. The training, support, and tools provided during this phase impact how BPSOs select indicators, identify data sources, develop data-collection processes, and submit data to NQuIRE. Each of these activities is pertinent to building capacity to comprehensively evaluate BPG implementation. These implementation efforts impact NQuIRE utilization, inform indicator selection for other BPSOs, and improve data quality throughout the 3-year period.

BPG Evaluation

BPSOs use NQuIRE indicators, other data elements from other data repositories, and their BPSO qualitative reports to evaluate BPG implementation. The unit of observation for NQuIRE data is at the implementation site level. This means aggregated data is collected at the source of BPG implementation within an organization (e.g., mental health unit in a hospital, public health program within a public health unit, or long-term care home within a long-term corporation). BPSOs need to pre-emptively plan for evaluation during the proposal stage to ensure they have an evaluation infrastructure and understand the evaluation culture. Their planning continues into the pre-implementation stage, while they conduct the gap analysis to embed necessary structures that support NQuIRE utilization. During predesignate phase, through discussions with their RNAO Coaches or the BPSO report review meetings, BPSOs discuss opportunities to further strengthen performance audit and feedback processes using NQuIRE data. These combined activities impact the data quality housed in NQuIRE. In conclusion, the interrelationships of the BPG Program pillars— 1) guideline development; 2) dissemination, implementation, and sustainability; and 3) evaluation and monitoring—have a cascading effect on data quality.

Three key features were identified to support BPSOs and the IABPG team in ensuring high-quality data in NQuIRE:

1. Creating a culture of data quality is essential, because data quality is everyone's responsibility.

2. Innovation and integration throughout the BPG cycle supports high-quality data.

3. NQuIRE as a multipurpose international data system must proactively address the complexity and multiplicity of data quality needs within each BPSO.

CULTURE OF DATA QUALITY

A comprehensive and pervasive data quality culture is essential throughout the IABPG Program and all its components. This means that data quality is everyone's responsibility for all IABPG Program staff and BPSOs. Establishing data stewardship throughout the NQuIRE data lifecycle is essential and includes planning, creating, processing, analyzing, preserving, sharing, and reusing data (Faundeen et al., 2014). For NQuIRE, the data lifecycle starts with indicator development and data collection by BPSOs. The lifecycle ends with the NQuIRE reports and dashboard utilization by BPSOs to evaluate the impact of guidelines. This requires that NQuIRE data are governed and managed throughout the lifecycle with clear documentation; metadata; data quality; and data security, backup, and recovery procedures in place. Since its inception in 2012, NQuIRE's initial data architecture and design have evolved to meet the needs of BPSOs and the RNAO. These continuous data quality improvement efforts strengthen data quality.

INNOVATION AND INTEGRATION THROUGHOUT THE BPG CYCLE

Data-driven innovation is central to ensuring BPSOs have the right information to improve quality and make better decisions (Health Canada, 2015). As a high-quality data holding, NQuIRE generates automated reports and supports both real-time and retrospective decision-making regarding quality-improvement efforts. The nature of the relationship between RNAO and BPSOs, both collaborative and reporting, fosters innovation and a feedback loop that informs ongoing NQuIRE enhancements.

Integration of BPSO data submissions involves strategies to resolve the semantic conflicts between heterogeneous data sources from multiple BPSOs representing different sectors and jurisdictions (Streiner & Norman, 2008). As previously indicated, certain concepts and definitions in respective schemas such as "screening for pain upon admission" (*pain_pro01*) may have different meanings in different practice environments, organizations, sectors, and countries. RNAO works closely with the BPSOs in a continuous feedback loop to resolve such challenges throughout all phases of BPSO predesignation. The collaboration helps explicitly define or refine components of the indicators within the data dictionaries to resolve semantic conflicts and improve data quality. This enables the data sources to be directly comparable so they can be integrated even when the characteristics of the BPSOs are different.

COMPLEXITY AND MULTIPLICITY THAT IMPACT DATA QUALITY

BPSO participation in NQuIRE has implications on several levels (i.e., clinical, organizational, and health system), and the NQuIRE datasets for each BPG can be used for multiple purposes:

- Quality improvement for BPSOs to measure impact of BPG implementation
- Accountability as BPSOs submit and report on data to meet required deliverables
- Future research that will require the highest-quality data

The complexity and multiplicity of the NQuIRE data system and its multiple purposes impact data quality. The NQuIRE data system was primarily designed for clinical and organizational quality improvement. Measurement for quality improvement occurs when: 1) identifying the practice gap or problem; 2) gathering preimplementation data; and 3) collecting post-implementation data. Measurement of quality improvement includes a small subset of "easy to collect" measures for a defined period of time (usually shorter) for a specific setting or process using a small sample size and simple data-collection processes.

For accountability purposes, measurement characteristics are more complex, with data being collected for specific indicators over a long period of time using large samples. This is done to manage performance and to compare to benchmarks for peer organizations.

For research, many precise and valid measures are collected for long time periods with large sample sizes and complex data-collection processes (Solberg et al., 1997). In 2012, NQuIRE was launched as a nursing quality-improvement database, and over the past 5 years, NQuIRE reporting and monitoring by BPSOs have demonstrated the impact of BPG implementation at the organizational level. NQuIRE has evolved into a robust data system that can be used for comparative reports and the Nursing Trends Report.

In conclusion, data quality requirements for quality improvement are less rigorous when compared to the requirements for accountability or research. The decision to mandate NQuIRE in 2014 has significantly enhanced data quality, and the datasets for the most-utilized BPGs are robust. This mandatory requirement added complexity to the data quality needs of NQuIRE and drove changes to the data system architecture and design to support the participation of all BPSO types, models, sectors, and countries. In anticipation of data usage for future research, data quality improvement procedures based on the framework dimensions are currently being tested.

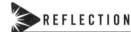

REFLECTION

Can you provide examples of how data have been used for the different purposes of quality improvement, accountability, and research?

DATA QUALITY DIMENSIONS

The data quality dimensions describe the fundamental components to ensure that high-quality data are inputted into NQuIRE. Each of these dimensions is integral, interrelated, and overlapping, which implies that failure in one dimension can result in failure in other dimensions. Six data quality dimensions were identified as crucial to NQuIRE and the BPG Program: integrity, relevance, interpretability, coherence, timeliness, and institutional environment. These dimensions are the core components of the Data Quality framework for continuous monitoring and data quality improvement implementation procedures. The characteristics of each data quality dimension are described here.

Integrity

This dimension determines accuracy of NQuIRE data in describing and representing the event, object, or concept they were intended to measure (e.g., goals for guideline implementation and impact on outcomes for target population). This includes the comprehensiveness of the BPG dataset for each BPSO and sensitivity to change to represent the impact of BPG implementation on nursing care and outcomes. Completeness of the NQuIRE dataset for each BPG by the BPSO is determined by the established data-collection processes. *Completeness* is defined by the proportion of data in the data system to the potential 100% complete data for any data element. The consistency of data reported within BPSOs and across BPSOs within a sector for specific data elements provides opportunity for comparability.

Potential data-collection and reporting errors are documented, and upon identification, corrections are made in a timely manner. Most BPSOs report one structural indicator, one process indicator, and one outcome indicator for each clinical BPG. RNAO conducts data quality assessments to improve data quality over time and identify inconsistencies in data submissions. Recently, a "missingness assessment," which involves identification and analysis of missing data, was conducted. It rank-orders valid data for each indicator based on the number of BPSOs submitting data for that particular indicator. The results of this missingness assessment supported improvements in the NQuIRE data system including the indicator development, indicator refinement, and data analysis to better demonstrate the impact and value of BPG implementation.

Relevance

This dimension refers to NQuIRE's ability to address the needs of users. For BPSOs, it refers to how well the data supports evaluation of BPG implementation (i.e., for the purpose of quality improvement). NQuIRE data dictionaries outline the operational definition of indicators with the target population. This includes inclusion and exclusion criteria to identify the relevance of the data to the user. A BPSO may implement a guideline organization-wide but only report data to NQuIRE for specific areas or settings within the organization. For example, a BPSO may report data on a single long-term care home when the BPG is being implemented across five long-term care homes. Finally, the NQuIRE reports and dashboard must meet the needs of the BPSOs.

Interpretability

This dimension differentiates whether BPSOs can correctly interpret their results and use their NQuIRE report and dashboard to support evaluation of their BPG implementation efforts. The data collected from BPSOs are de-identified and aggregated at the implementation site level, which is important to discern data quality challenges associated with analysis and interpretation. RNAO resources (e.g., data dictionaries, metadata, training materials, and other resources) provide BPSOs with information and context for analysis and interpretation of the NQuIRE reports and dashboard.

Coherence

This dimension ensures internal consistency and comparability of the NQuIRE data by the individual BPSO or with similar indicators from secondary data repositories (when applicable). Coherence should be apparent through standardized definitions, concepts, and data-collection processes over time. Coherence should also occur within a single NQuIRE dataset for each BPG by BPSO and across NQuIRE datasets for multiple BPSOs. Common definitions and concepts, with appropriate documentation, provide an opportunity for comparability of BPSO data. Coherent indicators within sectors and between countries are identified to allow for "like" BPSO-to-BPSO comparisons. Revisions to NQuIRE indicators may be required with new BPG editions, or data-collection practices change over time, resulting in restricted comparability of NQuIRE data to specific time periods, BPGs, and/or BPSO cohorts.

Timeliness

This dimension identifies the currency of the data (i.e., data is available when expected and needed). Acceptable differences in timing between guideline implementation and reporting data to NQuIRE need to be continuously examined and refined. The usefulness of the real-time and retrospective NQuIRE reports and dashboards at specific points in time (e.g., BPG launch, implementation, post-implementation phases) needs to be fully understood to further support implementation and sustainability efforts. The data collection stop date needs to be identified for relevant process indicators when steady state and/or desired outcomes are achieved (Mainz, 2003). The expected data collection frequency is clearly outlined, and adherence to monthly, quarterly, or annual submission is pertinent for this dimension.

Institutional Environment

This dimension identifies a BPSO's capacity to collect quality data for NQuIRE. Institutional factors such as adequacy of available resources and support (budget, human resources, time, equipment, processes, etc.) to collect data have a significant impact on BPSO data submission and NQuIRE data quality. Prior to participating in NQuIRE, the BPSO mandate to collect NQuIRE data is a key factor in ensuring BPSOs adhere to contractual requirements and submit data. The commitment of BPSO staff and support staff (e.g., information technology, decision support, clinical informatics, administration, etc.) to collect and report data with objectivity and transparency is fundamental.

INNOVATIVE DATA QUALITY ASSESSMENT APPROACHES TO IMPROVE DATA QUALITY

These six dimensions led to the development of subjective and objective metrics to conduct data quality assessments. *Subjectivity* considers the perception, needs, and experiences of data producers, consumers, and stewards. The BPSO focus group and visits (onsite and virtual) to develop the framework inform the subjective metrics. *Objectivity* includes measures to test whether the criteria and characteristics of each dimension are met. Objective data quality metrics can be developed within the context of data usage or independently. For the integrity dimension, considerable analysis for completeness and usability was completed.

The following metrics were developed: missing percentage, valid percentage, and weighted measure. The "missing percentage" is the proportion of missing data from the total data submissions by BPSOs. The "valid percentage" is the proportion of valid data from the total data submissions by BPSOs. Using the "valid percentage" and the number of BPSOs submitting data for a specific NQuIRE measure, a "weighted measure" was calculated. The "weighted measure" provides insight regarding the most reliable and frequently used BPG-specific indicators. Sector-specific analysis was also conducted to develop a better understanding of data quality by sector and inform areas for improvement. Data quality metrics for all dimensions are being developed to support comprehensive assessments to continuously monitor and improve NQuIRE data quality. By comparing the number of BPSOs using each indicator along with the valid data percentage, RNAO identified inconsistencies in data submission which have led to technological enhancements to the data system. Also, the weighted measure by NQuIRE indicator revealed the most robust datasets for 30 indicators that can be further examined to demonstrate the impact of BPG implementation within individual BPSOs (see Figures 16.8 and 16.9). This analysis also provides the foundation for choosing NQuIRE indicators that can be used in comparative reports and the Nursing Trends Report to demonstrate the value of the BPSO Designation.

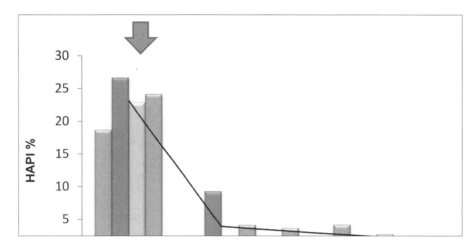

FIGURE 16.8   Quarterly average of HAPI for international hospital BPSO (ulcerprev_out01).
Used with permission.

Figure 16.8 demonstrates a 91% (23.08 to 2.09) decrease in the NQuIRE outcome indicator, health-care-acquired pressure injury (HAPI), following implementation of the RNAO BPG *Risk Assessment and Prevention of Pressure Ulcers* (2005) in an international hospital BPSO. The nursing processes of care were changed in 2013 based on the BPG recommendations, and the desired outcomes have been sustained for 3 years.

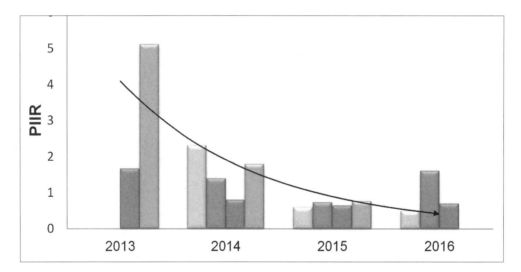

FIGURE 16.9   Quarterly average of pressure injury incidence rate for international hospital BPSO.
Used with permission.

Figure 16.9 demonstrates an 86% (5.1 to 0.7) decrease in the NQuIRE outcome indicator, pressure injury incidence rate (PIIR), following implementation of the RNAO BPG *Risk Assessment and Prevention of Pressure Ulcers* (2005) in a different international hospital BPSO than the previous example. The nursing processes of care were changed in 2013 based on the BPG recommendations, and the desired outcomes have been sustained for 3 years.

SUMMARY OF NQUIRE DATA QUALITY FRAMEWORK

The NQuIRE data system, a technology-enabled data profiling and reporting system for the evaluation of BPG implementation by BPSOs, is a first-in-its-class innovation by RNAO. The NQuIRE Data Quality framework highlights the key features and dimensions required for focused data quality improvement efforts. The six data quality dimensions are fundamental to assessing data quality and continuous data quality improvement. In comparison to existing frameworks, the NQuIRE Data Quality framework puts the BPSO at the center and integrates the BPG cycle. BPSOs, the main data producers from multiple sectors and diverse jurisdictions, have their own health information systems and data-collection processes, which leads to unique data quality challenges and opportunities for NQuIRE. This framework demonstrates the rigor behind the NQuIRE data system and increases BPSO confidence in the value of NQuIRE for quality improvement, accountability, and research.

FUTURE DIRECTIONS: EVIDENCE BOOSTERS AND BPSO-NQUIRE EVALUATION MODEL

Over the past 5 years, there has been a continuous feedback loop with BPSOs around the globe regarding their NQuIRE experience, insights, and advice. RNAO has formally and continuously engaged BPSOs for the NQuIRE indicator development process, NQuIRE orientation sessions, NQuIRE Boot Camps, and RNAO evaluation workshops. RNAO engages the NQuIRE IAC to receive strategic advice on the theoretical framework underpinnings, quality-control processes, as well as future directions and use for the data system. Our active participation in the Guidelines International Network (GIN) allows us to contribute learnings from our experience and glean insights from others on guideline development, implementation strategies, and performance measures.

RNAO regularly reviews the literature, assesses processes and frameworks of other jurisdictions, and consults its partners, such as Health Quality Ontario, Accreditation Canada, and Resident Assessment Instrument (RAI) Minimum Data Set. All of these efforts inform enhancements to the NQuIRE data system, the refined NQuIRE data indicator development process, and NQuIRE's Data Quality framework for ongoing BPSO Program evaluation and future research. With a robust BPG Program, active BPSO engagement, and a strong measurement system, RNAO is now confident in its ability to demonstrate value of the BPSO efforts. We discuss this next.

Value is defined as the relationship between outcomes and costs. Health systems worldwide are focusing on enhancing value by engaging in quality-improvement strategies in which:

- Outcomes remain stable, but costs are decreased

- Outcomes improve, but costs remain stable

- Outcomes improve *and* costs are decreased

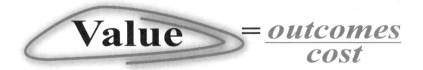

$$Value = \frac{outcomes}{cost}$$

ECONOMICS OF NURSING

Health systems are complex, and at any moment there are many ideas for ways to improve the system, but in order to achieve the health system goals and improve health system sustainability, no major initiatives should move forward without clearly addressing value enhancement. Value must become the backbone of global health transformation strategies. RNAO has developed two-page value proposition reports: RNAO Evidence Boosters (EBs). They demonstrate the value and impact of BPG implementation by BPSOs using NQuIRE indicators. The NQuIRE indicators chosen for the RNAO EBs have achieved high scores in the weighted measure of the data quality assessment. The Evidence Boosters are trending reports from BPG launch to implementation to sustainability and demonstrate the economic impact (see Figure 16.10).

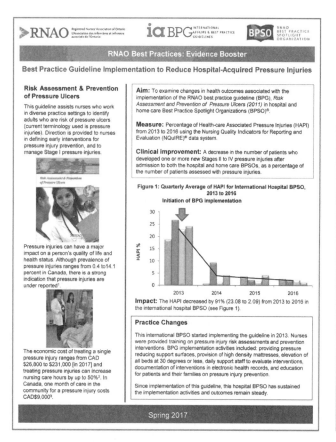

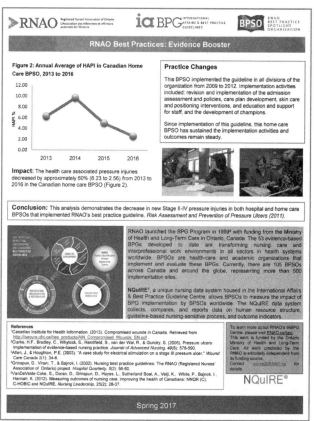

FIGURE 16.10 Examples of RNAO Evidence Boosters: Pressure injury incidence rate and hospital-acquired pressure injuries.

The Evidence Boosters (EB) depicted in Figure 16.10 showcase the BPG implementation results in a graphic and include a brief description of the BPG in the upper-left corner and the BPSO aim, measure, clinical improvement, and practice changes in the right column. In the bottom-left corner, the economic impacts are reported. For example, treating pressure injuries increases nursing care hours by up to 50% (Clarke et al., 2005), and 1 month of care in the community for a pressure injury costs approximately CAD $9,000 (Allen & Houghton, 2003). An 86% decrease in pressure injury incidence rate and a 91% decrease in hospital-acquired pressure injuries would result in significant cost savings to the patient, organization, and health system. See Appendix A at the end of this chapter for a full view of each EB.

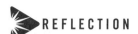

▶ REFLECTION

Is the impact and value of evidence-based nursing care depicted in your workplace? Would you benefit from using a data system such as NQuIRE to demonstrate the impact of nurse-led quality improvement? If yes, in which way would you benefit and how can you introduce it?

BPSO-NQUIRE EVALUATION MODEL: STRATEGIC FOCUS

The BPSO-NQuIRE Evaluation Model (see Figure 16.11) encompasses: 1) the NQuIRE Data Quality framework; 2) the rigorous indicator development and revision cycle for each clinical BPG; and 3) the BPSO reporting and data collection that occurs within NQuIRE and myBPSO, which is the online reporting system. The five pillars within the model represent RNAO's analytic approaches to robust evaluation to demonstrate the health impact and value of BPG implementation by BPSOs. These analytic approaches include:

1. Quantitative data analysis of the NQuIRE datasets

2. Qualitative data analysis based on case studies from myBPSO reports

3. Data mapping and secondary data analysis of other health system data repositories (e.g., inter-RAI and CIHI) to complement NQuIRE and myBPSO data analysis

4. Data analysis focused on implementation science indicators that complement the Donabedian Model (see Chapter 4, *Forging the Way with Implementation Science*)

5. Inter-BPSO comparative analysis for publication of NQuIRE comparative reports and Nursing Trends Report

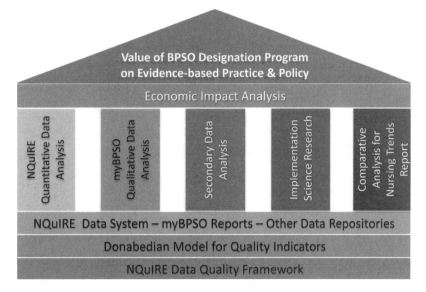

FIGURE 16.11 BPSO-NQuIRE Evaluation Model.

As shown in Figure 16.11, RNAO's multimethod approach supports BPSOs to demonstrate the value of their implementation efforts and ultimately the value of the RNAO BPGs to BPSOs and health systems.

CONCLUSION

Health systems need to fully embrace evidence to boldly transform and meet population health needs. As discussed in Chapters 1 and 12, scaling up, scaling out, and scaling deep programs that have demonstrated results are urgently needed to meet this challenge. RNAO's BPG Program is revolutionizing nursing's contribution to patients', organizational, and health system outcomes worldwide. The NQuIRE data system will increasingly make this contribution visible by quantifying processes of nursing care and its value locally, nationally, and internationally. The RNAO BPSO Designation has created a platform for robust evaluation methodologies to measure the impact of evidence-based nursing care, as well as the impact of evidence and structural indicators such as staffing on patients' outcomes. RNAO has developed rigorous approaches to development of NQuIRE indicators, establishment of the NQuIRE Data Quality framework, and completion of data quality assessment using innovative statistical techniques. With the current state of NQuIRE and the BPSO Evaluation Model, RNAO is poised to produce comparative reports, the Nursing Trends Report, and be a source of data for practitioners, administrators, educators, researchers, and policymakers, now and into the future.

KEY MESSAGES

- Quantifying the impact of evidence-based nursing practice on patient, organizational, and health system outcomes enables us to showcase nurses' full contributions.

- The Donabedian Model is an effective framework to build structure, process, and outcome indicators to evaluate the impact of BPG implementation.

- A robust indicator development process that is evidence-based and informed by RNAO's BPG development methodology, BPSOs, other data repositories, end users, and other RNAO partners is foundational to evaluate the uptake of, and impact of, RNAO BPGs.

- Security and privacy safeguards, as well as ensuring data quality, are central features of a robust data system.

- The NQuIRE Data Quality framework puts the BPSO at the center, demonstrates the rigor behind the NQuIRE data system, and increases BPSO confidence in the value of NQuIRE for quality improvement, accountability, and research.

- Purposeful evolution of NQuIRE indicator development with a programed refinement cycle is critical to ensuring that the BPG evaluation measures remain abreast with new BPG editions and current research.

- Access to data in daily practice is critical in understanding gaps in care, measuring improvement, and demonstrating impact of evidence-based practice on outcomes.

REFERENCES

Allen, J., & Houghton, P. E. (2003). A case study for electrical stimulation on a stage III pressure ulcer. *Wound Care Canada*, *2*(1), 34–36.

Australian Capital Territory (ACT) Health. (2013). *ACT health Data Quality framework*. Retrieved from http://health.act. gov.au/sites/default/files/Policy_and_Plan/Data%20Quality%20Framework.pdf

Bryant-Lukosius, D., Spichiger, E., Martin, J., Stoll, H., Kellerhals, S. D., Fliedner, M., . . . De Geest, S. (2016). Framework for evaluating the impact of advanced practice nursing roles. *Journal of Nursing Scholarship*, *48*(2), 201–209.

Canadian Institute for Health Information (CIHI). (2009). *The CIHI Data Quality framework*. Retrieved from https://www. cihi.ca/en/data_quality_framework_2009_en.pdf

Centers for Disease Control and Prevention (CDC). (2007). *Developing evaluation indicators*. Retrieved from https://www. cdc.gov/std/Program/pupestd/Developing%20Evaluation%20Indicators.pdf

Chen, L., Huang, L.-H., Xing, M.-Y., Feng, Z.-X., Shao, L.-W., Zhang, M.-Y., & Shao, R.-Y. (2016). Using the Delphi method to develop nursing-sensitive quality indicators for the NICU. *Journal of Clinical Nursing*, *26*, 502–513. doi: 10.1111/jocn.13474

Clarke, H. F., Bradley, C., Whytock, S., Handfield, S., van der Wal, R., & Gundry, S. (2005). Pressure ulcers: Implementation of evidence-based nursing practice. *Journal of Advanced Nursing*, *49*(6), 578–590.

Donabedian, A. (1966). Evaluating the quality of medical care. *Millbank Memorial Fund Quarterly*, *44*(Suppl.), 166–206.

Donabedian, A. (1988). The quality of care: How can it be assessed? *Journal of American Medical Association*, *260*, 1743–1748.

Donabedian, A. (2005). Evaluating the quality of medical care. *Milbank Quarterly*, *83*, 691–729.

Doran, D. M. (2003). Preface. In D. M. Doran (Ed.), *Nursing-sensitive outcomes: State of the science* (2nd ed.) (pp. vii–ix). Sudbury, MA: Jones and Bartlett.

Doran, D., Mildon, B., & Clarke, S. (2011). Towards a national report card in nursing: A knowledge synthesis. *Canadian Journal of Nursing Leadership*, *24*(2), 38–57.

Faundeen, J. L., Burley, T. E., Carlino, J. A., Govoni, D. L., Henkel, H. S., Holl, S. L., . . . Zolly, L. S. (2014). *The United States geological survey science data lifecycle model: U.S. geological survey open-file report 2013–1265*. Retrieved from https:// pubs.usgs.gov/of/2013/1265/

Grinspun, D., Lloyd, M., Xiao, S., & Bajnok, I. (2015). Measuring the quality of evidence-based nursing care: NQuIRE – Nursing Quality Indicators for Reporting and Evaluation Data-System. *Revista MedUNAB*, *17*(3), 170–175.

Health Canada. (2015, July). *Unleashing innovation: Excellent healthcare for Canada*. Report of the Advisory Panel on Healthcare Innovation. Retrieved from https://www.canada.ca/en/health-canada/services/publications/health-system-services/report-advisory-panel-healthcare-innovation.html

Health Quality Ontario (HQO). (2016, October). *Quality standards: Process and methods guide*. Retrieved from http://www. hqontario.ca/portals/0/documents/evidence/quality-standards/qs-process-guide-1610-en.pdf

Heslop, L., & Lu, S. (2014). Nursing-sensitive indicators: A concept analysis. *Journal of Advanced Nursing*, *70*(11), 2469–2482.

Ingraham, A. M., Richards, K. E., Hall, B. L., & Ko, C. Y. (2010). Quality improvement in surgery: The American College of Surgeons National Surgical Quality Improvement Program approach. *Advances in Surgery*, *44*(1), 251–267.

Institute of Medicine (IOM). (2007). *The learning healthcare system: Workshop summary*. Retrieved from https://www.ncbi. nlm.nih.gov/books/NBK53481/

Institute of Medicine (IOM). (2013, 26 March). *Digital data improvement priorities for continuous learning in health and health care: Workshop summary*. Retrieved from https://www.ncbi.nlm.nih.gov/books/NBK207329/

inter-RAI. (2017). Instruments: An overview of the inter-RAI suite. Retrieved from http://www.interrai.org/instruments/

Kahn, M. G., Brown, J. S., Chun, A. T., Davidson, B. N., Meeker, D., Ryan, P. B., . . . Zozus, M. N. (2015). Transparent reporting of data quality in distributed data networks. *eGEMs*, *3*(1), 1052.

Kelley, E., & Hurst, J. (2006, March 9). *Health care quality indicators project conceptual framework paper. Organisation for Economic Co-operation and Development* (OECD), *Health Working Paper No. 23*. Retrieved from http://www.oecd.org/els/health-systems/36262363.pdf

Kerr, K. (2003). *The development of a Data Quality framework and strategy for the New Zealand ministry of health*. Department of Information Systems and Operations Management, University of Auckland, New Zealand. Retrieved from http:// mitiq.mit.edu/Documents/IQ_Projects/Nov%202003/HINZ%20DQ%20Strategy%20paper.pdf

Kerr, K., & Norris, T. (2004). *The development of a healthcare Data Quality framework and strategy*. Proceedings of the ninth international conference on information quality (ICQ-04). Retrieved from http://mitiq.mit.edu/ICIQ/Documents/IQ%20Conference%202004/Papers/TheDevelofaHealthcareDQFramework.pdf

Kerr, K., & Norris, T. (2007). The development of a health Data Quality programme. In L. Al-Hakim (Ed.), *Information quality management: Theory and applications* (pp. 94–118). Hershey, PA: Idea Group Publishing.

Kotter, T., Blozik, E., & Scherer, M. (2012). Methods for the guideline-based development of quality indicators—A systematic review. *Implementation Science, 7*(21), 1–22.

Lloyd, M., Xiao, S., Albornos-Munoz, L., González-María, E., & Joyce, A. (2013). Measuring the process and outcomes of foot ulcer care with guideline-based nursing quality indicators. *Diabetic Foot Canada, 1*(2), 15–19.

Loeb, J. M. (2004). The current state of performance measurement in health care. *International Journal for Quality in Health Care, 16*(Suppl.), i5–i9.

Lopez, M. H., Holve, E., Sarkar, I. N., & Segal, C. (2012). Building the informatics infrastructure for comparative effectiveness research (CER): A review of the literature. *Medical Care, 50*(Suppl.), 38–48.

Loshin, D. (2011). *The practitioner's guide to data quality improvement.* Burlington, MA: Elsevier.

Lugtenberg, M., Burgers, J. S., & Westert, G. P. (2009). Effects of evidence-based clinical practice guidelines on quality of care: A systematic review. *BMJ Quality & Safety, 18*(5), 385–392.

Mainz, J. (2003). Methodology matters: Defining and classifying clinical indicators for quality improvement. *International Journal for Quality in Health Care, 15*(6), 523–530.

Marsden, E., Taylor, A., Wallis, M., Craswell, A., Broadbent, M., Barnett, A., . . . Glenwright, A. (2017). A structure, process and outcome evaluation of the Geriatric Emergency Department Intervention model of care: A study protocol. *BMC Geriatrics, 17,* 76.

Millar, A., Simeone, R. S., & Carnevale, J. T. (2001). Logic models: A systems tool for performance management. *Evaluation and Program Planning, 24,* 73–81.

Moonesinghe, S. R., Grocott, M. P. W., Bennett-Guerrero, E., Bergamaschi, R., Gottumukkala, V., Hopkins, T. J., . . . The Perioperative Quality Initiative (POQI) I Workgroup. (2017). American Society for Enhanced Recovery (ASER) and Perioperative Quality Initiative (POQI) joint consensus statement on measurement to maintain and improve quality of enhanced recovery pathways for elective colorectal surgery. *Perioperative Medicine, 6,* 6.

Moore, L., Lavoie, A., Bourgeois, G., & Lapointe, J. (2015). Donabedian's structure-process-outcome quality of care model: Validation in an integrated trauma system. *The Journal of Trauma and Acute Care Surgery, 78*(6), 1168–1175.

Nantsupawat, A., Kunaviktikul, W., Nantsupawat, R., Wichaikhum, O.-A., Thienthong, H., & Poghosyan, L. (2017). Effects of nurse work environment on job dissatisfaction, burnout, intention to leave. *International Nursing Review, 64,* 91–98.

National Institute for Health and Care Excellence (NICE). (2014, April). *Health and social care directorate indicators process guide.* Retrieved from https://www.nice.org.uk/media/default/Standards-and-indicators/Quality-standards/Quality-standards-process-guide-April-2014.pdf

Organisation for Economic Co-operation and Development (OECD). (2012, 17 January). *Quality framework and guidelines for OECD statistical activities version 2011/1.* Retrieved from http://www.oecd.org/officialdocuments/publicdisplaydocumentpdf/?cote=std/qfs(2011)1&doclanguage=en

Personal Health Information and Protection Act, 2004, S.O. 2004, c. 3, Sched. A. Retrieved from the Ontario Laws website: https://www.ontario.ca/laws/statute/04p03

Personal Information Protection and Electronic Documents Act, S.C. 2000, c. 5. Retrieved from the Government of Canada Justice Laws website: http://laws-lois.justice.gc.ca/eng/acts/P-8.6/index.html

Public Health Agency of Canada (PHAC). (2012). *Canadian sexual health indicators survey—Pilot test and validation phase.* Retrieved from http://publications.gc.ca/site/eng/415217/publication.html

Registered Nurses' Association of Ontario (RNAO) (2005). *Risk assessment and prevention of pressure ulcers.* (Revision Supplement 2011). Toronto, ON: Registered Nurses' Association of Ontario.

Registered Nurses' Association of Ontario (RNAO). (2011). *Prevention of falls and fall injuries in the older adult.* Toronto, ON: Registered Nurses' Association of Ontario.

Registered Nurses' Association of Ontario (RNAO). (2013). *Assessment and management of foot ulcers for people with diabetes* (2nd ed.). Toronto, ON: Registered Nurses' Association of Ontario.

Safran, C., Bloomrosen, M., Hammond, W. E., Labkoff, S., Markel-Fox, S., Tang, P. C., & Detmer, D. E. (2007). Toward a national framework for the secondary use of health data: An American Medical Informatics Association white paper. *Journal of American Medical Informatics Association, 14*(1), 1–9.

Sebastian-Coleman, L. (2012). *Measuring data quality for ongoing improvement: A Data Quality assessment framework.* Waltham, MA: Morgan Kaufmann.

Slawomirski, L., Auraaen, A., & Klazinga, N. (2017, 26 June). *The economics of patient safety: Strengthening a value-based approach to reducing patient harm at national level.* OECD Health Working Papers, No. 96., OECD Publishing, Paris. Retrieved from https://www.bundesgesundheitsministerium.de/fileadmin/Dateien/3_Downloads/P/Patientensicherheit/The_Economics_of_patient_safety_Web.pdf

Solberg, L. I., Mosser, G., & McDonald, S. (1997). The three faces of performance measurement: Improvement, accountability, and research. *Journal of Quality Improvement, 23*(3), 135–147.

Streiner, D., & Norman, G. (2008). *Health measurement scales: A practical guide to their development and use* (4th ed.). New York, NY: Oxford University Press Inc.

Strome, T. (2013). *Healthcare analytics for quality and performance improvement.* Hoboken, NJ: John Wiley & Sons.

VanDeVelde-Coke, S., Doran, D., Grinspun, D., Hayes, L., Sutherland Boal, A., Velji, K., . . . Hannah, K. (2012). Measuring outcomes of nursing care, improving the health of Canadians: NNQR (C), C-HOBIC and NQuIRE. *Nursing Leadership, 25*(2), 26–37.

von Schirnding, Y. (2002). *Health in sustainable development planning: The role of indicators.* Geneva, CH: World Health Organization. Retrieved from http://www.who.int/wssd/resources/indicators/en/

Wang, R., & Strong, D. M. (1996). Beyond accuracy: What data quality means to data consumers. *Journal of Management Information Systems, 12*(4), 5–33.

APPENDIX A: EVIDENCE BOOSTERS DEMONSTRATING BPG IMPACT IN BPSO

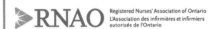 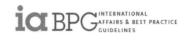 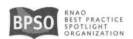

RNAO Best Practices: Evidence Booster

Best Practice Guideline Implementation to Reduce Hospital-Acquired Pressure Injuries

Risk Assessment & Prevention of Pressure Ulcers

This guideline assists nurses who work in diverse practice settings to identify adults who are risk of pressure ulcers (current terminology used is pressure injuries). Direction is provided to nurses in defining early interventions for pressure injury prevention, and to manage Stage I pressure injuries.

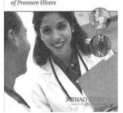

Pressure injuries can have a major impact on a person's quality of life and health status. Although prevalence of pressure injuries ranges from 0.4 to14.1 percent in Canada, there is a strong indication that pressure injuries are under reported[1].

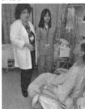

The economic cost of treating a single pressure injury ranges from CAD $26,800 to $231,000 [in 2017] and treating pressure injuries can increase nursing care hours by up to 50%[2]. In Canada, one month of care in the community for a pressure injury costs CAD$9,000[3].

Aim: To examine changes in health outcomes associated with the implementation of the RNAO best practice guideline (BPG), *Risk Assessment and Prevention of Pressure Ulcers (2011)* in hospital and home care Best Practice Spotlight Organizations (BPSO)®.

Measure: Percentage of Health-care Associated Pressure Injuries (HAPI) from 2013 to 2016 using the Nursing Quality Indicators for Reporting and Evaluation (NQuIRE)® data system.

Clinical improvement: A decrease in the number of patients who developed one or more new Stages II to IV pressure injuries after admission to both the hospital and home care BPSOs, as a percentage of the number of patients assessed with pressure injuries.

Figure 1: Quarterly Average of HAPI for International Hospital BPSO, 2013 to 2016

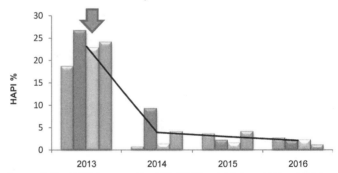

Impact: The HAPI decreased by 91% (23.08 to 2.09) from 2013 to 2016 in the international hospital BPSO (see Figure 1).

Practice Changes

This international BPSO started implementing the guideline in 2013. Nurses were provided training on pressure injury risk assessments and prevention interventions. BPG implementation activities included: providing pressure reducing support surfaces, provision of high density mattresses, elevation of all beds at 30 degrees or less, daily support staff to evaluate interventions, documentation of interventions in electronic health records, and education for patients and their families on pressure injury prevention.

Since implementation of this guideline, this hospital BPSO has sustained the implementation activities and outcomes remain steady.

Spring 2017

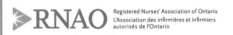
RNAO Registered Nurses' Association of Ontario
L'Association des infirmières et infirmiers
autorisés de l'Ontario

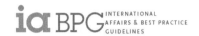
ia BPG INTERNATIONAL AFFAIRS & BEST PRACTICE GUIDELINES

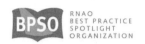
BPSO RNAO BEST PRACTICE SPOTLIGHT ORGANIZATION

RNAO Best Practices: Evidence Booster

Figure 2: Annual Average of HAPI in Canadian Home Care BPSO, 2013 to 2016

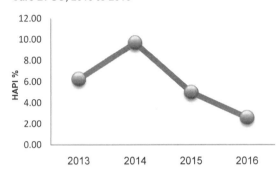

Impact: The health care associated pressure injuries decreased by approximately 60% (6.23 to 2.56) from 2013 to 2016 in the Canadian home care BPSO (Figure 2).

Practice Changes

This BPSO implemented the guideline in all divisions of the organization from 2009 to 2012. Implementation activities included: revision and implementation of the admission assessment and policies, care plan development, skin care and positioning interventions, and education and support for staff, and the development of champions.

Since implementation of this guideline, this home care BPSO has sustained the implementation activities and outcomes remain steady.

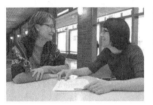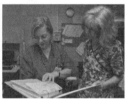

Conclusion: This analysis demonstrates the decrease in new Stage II-IV pressure injuries in both hospital and home care BPSOs that implemented RNAO's best practice guideline, *Risk Assessment and Prevention of Pressure Ulcers (2011)*.

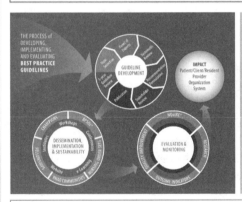

RNAO launched the BPG Program in 1999[4] with funding from the Ministry of Health and Long-Term Care in Ontario, Canada. The 53 evidence-based BPGs developed to date are transforming nursing care and interprofessional work environments in all sectors in health systems worldwide. BPSOs are health-care and academic organizations that implement and evaluate these BPGs. Currently, there are 105 BPSOs across Canada and around the globe, representing more than 500 implementation sites.

NQuIRE[5], a unique nursing data system housed in the International Affairs & Best Practice Guideline Centre, allows BPSOs to measure the impact of BPG implementation by BPSOs worldwide. The NQuIRE data system collects, compares, and reports data on human resource structure, guideline-based nursing-sensitive process, and outcome indicators.

References

[1]Canadian Institute for Health Information. (2013). Compromised wounds in Canada. Retrieved from http:///secure.cihi.ca/free_products/AiN_Compromised_Wounds_EN.pdf .

[2]Clarke, H.F., Bradley, C., Whytock, S., Handfield, S., van der Wal, R., & Gundry, S. (2005). Pressure ulcers: Implementation of evidence-based nursing practice. *Journal of Advanced Nursing, 49*(6): 578-590.

[3]Allen, J., & Houghton, P.E. (2003). "A case study for electrical stimulation on a stage III pressure ulcer." *Wound Care Canada 2*(1): 34-6.

[4]Grinspun, D., Virani, T., & Bajnok, I. (2002). Nursing best practice guidelines: The RNAO (Registered Nurses' Association of Ontario) project. *Hospital Quarterly, 5*(2): 56-60.

[5]VanDeVelde-Coke, S., Doran, D., Grinspun, D., Hayes, L., Sutherland Boal, A., Velji, K., White, P., Bajnok, I., Hannah, K. (2012). Measuring outcomes of nursing care, improving the health of Canadians: NNQR (C), C-HOBIC and NQuIRE. *Nursing Leadership, 25*(2): 26-37.

To learn more about RNAO's IABPG Centre, please visit RNAO.ca/bpg. This work is funded by the Ontario Ministry of Health and Long-Term Care. All work produced by the RNAO is editorially independent from its funding source. Contact nquire@RNAO.ca for details.

NQuIRE®

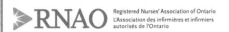 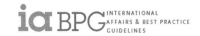 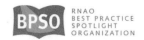

RNAO Best Practices: Evidence Booster

Best Practice Guideline Implementation to Reduce Pressure Injuries Incidence Rate

Risk Assessment & Prevention of Pressure Ulcers

This guideline assists nurses who work in diverse practice settings to identify adults who are at risk of pressure ulcers (current terminology used is pressure injuries). Direction is provided to nurses in defining early interventions for pressure injury prevention and to manage Stage I pressure injuries.

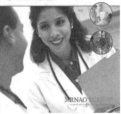

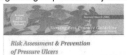

Pressure injuries can have a major impact on a person's quality of life and health status. Although prevalence of pressure injuries range from 0.4 to14.1 percent in Canada, there is a strong indication that pressure injuries are under reported[1].

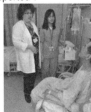

The economic cost of treating a single pressure injury ranges from CAD $26,800 to $231,000 [in 2017] and treating pressure injuries can increase nursing care hours by up to 50%[2]. In Canada, one month of care in the community for a pressure injury costs CAD$9,000[3].

Aim: To examine changes in health outcomes associated with the implementation of the RNAO best practice guideline (BPG), *Risk Assessment and Prevention of Pressure Ulcers (2011)*, in two hospital-based Best Practice Spotlight Organizations (BPSO)®.

Measure: Incidence rate of pressure injuries from 2013 to 2016 based on Nursing Quality Indicators for Reporting and Evaluation (NQuIRE)® data system.

Clinical improvement: A decrease in number of patients who developed one or more new Stages II to IV pressure injuries after admission to hospital BPSOs, as a percentage of the number of patients assessed with pressure injuries.

Figure 1: Quarterly Average of Pressure Injury Incidence Rate (PIIR) for International Hospital BPSO-I, 2013 to 2016

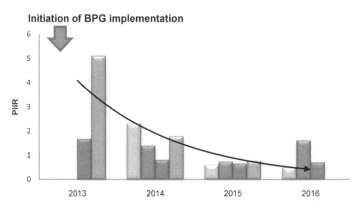

Impact: The pressure injury incidence rate decreased by 86% (5.1 to 0.7) from 2013 to 2016 in the international hospital BPSO-I (see Figure 1).

Practice Changes

This hospital BPSO-I implemented the guideline between 2012 to 2015. Implementation activities included: policies and procedures aligned with the guideline recommendations; standardized orientation and workshops for staff with learning materials; consistent changes in practices across the organization for admissions, transfers and discharges; and hourly rounding.

Since implementation of this guideline, BPSO-I has sustained the implementation activities and outcomes remain steady.

Spring 2017

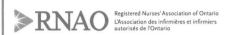 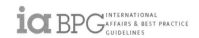 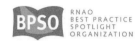

Registered Nurses' Association of Ontario
L'Association des infirmières et infirmiers autorisés de l'Ontario

ia BPG INTERNATIONAL AFFAIRS & BEST PRACTICE GUIDELINES

BPSO RNAO BEST PRACTICE SPOTLIGHT ORGANIZATION

RNAO Best Practices: Evidence Boosters

Figure 2: Pressure Injury Incidence Rate (PIIR) in Canadian Hospital BPSO-II, 2013 to 2016

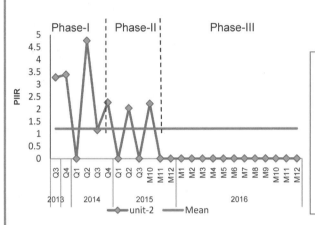

Impact: In Phase-I, the PIIR decreased by 63% (3.28 to 1.21) and had the highest variation in data. In Phase-II, the PIIR had consistent variations in data. By Phase-III, the PIIR decreased by 100% (3.28 to 0) between 2013 to 2016 and has remained at zero pressure injuries (see Figure 2).

Practice Changes

This hospital BPSO-II implemented the guideline from 2012 to 2015. Implementation activities included: standardized assessment tools, education and related materials for staff and patients, documentation changes, and standard therapeutic surfaces to reduce pressure for all patients.

Since implementation of this guideline, BPSO-II has sustained the implementation activities and outcomes remain at zero.

Conclusion: This analysis demonstrates a decrease in new Stage II-IV pressure injuries in two BPSOs (Canadian and International) that implemented RNAO's best practice guideline, *Risk Assessment and Prevention of Pressure Ulcers (2011)*.

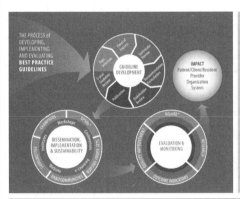

RNAO launched the BPG Program in 1999[4] with funding from the Ministry of Health and Long-Term Care in Ontario, Canada. The 53 evidence-based BPGs developed are transforming nursing care and interprofessional work environments in all sectors in health systems worldwide. BPSOs are health-care and academic organizations that implement and evaluate these BPGs. Currently, there are 105 BPSOs across Canada and around the globe, representing more than 500 implementation sites.

NQuIRE[5], a unique nursing data system housed in the International Affairs & Best Practice Guideline Centre, allows BPSOs to measure the impact of BPG implementation by BPSOs worldwide. The NQuIRE data system collects, compares, and reports data on human resource structure, guideline-based nursing-sensitive process, and outcome indicators.

References

[1]Canadian Institute for Health Information. (2013). Compromised wounds in Canada. Retrieved from http://secure.cihi.ca/free_products/AiN_Compromised_Wounds_EN.pdf .

[2]Clarke, H.F., Bradley, C., Whytock, S., Handfield, S., van der Wal, R., & Gundry, S. (2005). Pressure ulcers: Implementation of evidence-based nursing practice . Journal of Advanced Nursing, 49(6): 578-590.

[3]Allen, Jill, and Pamela E. Houghton. "A case study for electrical stimulation on a stage III pressure ulcer." Wound Care Canada 2.1 (2003): 34-6.

[4]Grinspun, D., Virani, T., & Bajnok, I. (2002). Nursing best practice guidelines: The RNAO (Registered Nurses' Association of Ontario) project. Hospital Quarterly, 5(2): 56-60.

[5]VanDeVelde-Coke, S., Doran, D., Grinspun, D., Hayes, L., Sutherland Boal, A., Velji, K., White, P., Bajnok, I., Hannah, K. (2012). Measuring outcomes of nursing care, improving the health of Canadians: NNQR (C), C-HOBIC and NQuIRE. Nursing Leadership, 25(2): 26-37.

To learn more about RNAO's IABPG Centre, please visit RNAO.ca/bpg. This work is funded by the Ontario Ministry of Health and Long-Term Care. All work produced by the RNAO is editorially independent from its funding source. Contact nquire@RNAO.ca for details.

NQuIRE®

Spring 2017

17

VALUE FOR MONEY: MEASURING THE ECONOMIC IMPACT OF BPSOS IN AUSTRALIA

Rob Bonner
Jennifer Hurley, MHSM, RN, RM
Edith Ho, GradDipBus(AdminMgmt), BNg, RN
Elizabeth Dabars, AM

LEARNING OBJECTIVES

After reading this chapter, you will be able to:

- Understand the process and impact of the BPSO Host and BPSO Direct Designations in Australia

- Describe the responsibilities, benefits, and excitement of becoming a BPSO Host

- Gain awareness of the client, provider, organizational, and system outcomes of the BPSO Designation in Australia, in particular those related to economic impacts

INTRODUCTION

Every day in their practice, nurses around the globe have to share good news and bad with their patients. They have to provide the information in a way that is accessible to their patients, not sending mixed signals or unclear information, but sharing it in a way that meets the needs of the individual patient and their loved ones.

Our journey in measuring the economic analysis and outcomes of evidence-based practice began in order that we could make accessible the results of our work with patients and the public, health system funders, governments, and health bureaucrats. We cannot expect people who are not clinicians or from a clinical background to share the nursing culture based on achieving great results for our patients. Great results that cost more may not find favour in health systems that are increasingly cost-constrained. However there is growing acceptance that more effective care can also save money. Avoiding misadventure, readmission to hospital, or acquisition of secondary illnesses or complications are accepted as objectives that should be sought for both quality and cost outcomes.

So why embark on exploring the financial outcomes of our own Best Practice Spotlight Organization journeys? First, as we have described already, our healthcare system is increasingly dominated by managerialists. Clinicians have lost control and influence of the health and hospital systems with decision-making increasingly influenced by budgets, financial performance, and data analysis. Medical dominance, which has traditionally challenged nursing as a professional discipline, has been replaced by these managers. However, this new domination comes with a loss of the shared focus and experience of working directly with patients and clients, which at least gave nurses and doctors a common language and a set of client-centred goals.

This new domination is reflected in the political landscape, with policy debate increasingly focused on economic and fiscal performance. The economic debate has become an end in itself rather than an instrument to sustain and support wider societal well-being and improvement. Increasingly in Australia, governments and healthcare executives are using system reforms and innovation in practice to disguise or become the vehicle for budget cuts to the system. Whether it be case mix as a classification system, consumer-directed models of care (disability and aged care), or even the intended application of internationally benchmarked clinical standards (Transforming Health, South Australia), all have been used as or were the vehicles for budget-savings measures to be achieved.

This is not of itself necessarily a bad thing. If savings can be made by the adoption of evidence-based clinical standards, then so be it. However, our argument is that the adoption of the standards and their implementation should come first. If that results in savings along with the expectation of improved care, then that would be optimal. In Australia, too often the budget savings measures have actually been seen to drive the adoption of standards to give a cloak of clinical propriety to the measures. In fact, what it is doing is creating mistrust by clinicians and in the general community over the language of best practice and standards-based approaches, which is the reverse of what we should be seeking to achieve.

Nurses have historically attempted to describe the outcomes of their care using qualitative statements or measures. Improvement in the quality of outcomes and patient benefit and satisfaction have been central, with a number of well-known studies confirming the impact of nursing care on the morbidity and mortality of the client population (Aiken, Rafferty & Sermeus, 2014; Aiken et al., 2017; Barton, Johnson, & Price, 2009; Cheung, Aiken, Clarke, & Sloane, 2008; Twigg, Duffield, Thompson, & Rapley,

2010). Conversion of the learning to the economic impact that nurses make is less developed, although in some cases obvious. Measures that reduce the length of stay in hospitals through interventions, such as those that reduced the incidence of pressure ulcers, urinary tract infections, and falls, are well reported (Garrard, Boyle, Simon, Dunton, & Gajewski, 2014; Lloyd, Xiao, Albornos-Muñoz, González-María, & Joyce, 2013; Mitchell, Ferguson, Anderson, Sear & Barnett, 2016; VanDeVelde-Coke et al., 2012). The fact that there is a reduction in the length of stay clearly impacts cost of care but is rarely quantified in the reports.

Our experience is that we cannot assume health bureaucrats and politicians will understand and accept that such savings flow from these improved nursing-driven clinical outcomes. Instead, we should explicitly seek to quantify and state these savings where they exist, in order to make them understood by and able to influence decision-makers. This does not reduce the need to apply qualitative approaches. Rather, in this chapter we argue and demonstrate that it adds to the picture and allows a new way of entering the discussion on quality and value of nursing interventions with people of influence, whose primary interest and language is economic rather than clinical.

This chapter discusses the role, work, and journey of the Australian Nursing and Midwifery Federation (SA Branch) (referred to as ANMF [SA Branch]) as the Best Practice Spotlight Organization Designation (BPSO) Host in Australia, working in partnership with the Registered Nurses' Association of Ontario (RNAO) and the South Australian government, to establish, develop, implement, and evaluate the impact and value of evidence-based practice. We highlight the challenges and opportunities of the initial stages of our journey, including gaining government support and attracting health services to engage, invest, and participate to become accredited as BPSOs.

We then discuss the first phase of the BPSO Designation, the establishment at two South Australian public local health networks (across multiple sites and specialties), and how the RNAO Nursing Quality Indicators for Reporting and Evaluation (NQuIRE) database contributes to the evaluation of the patient/client, provider, and organization outcomes. To that end, pilot programs were submitted for analysis of hospital performance indicators and national quality care indicators, including average length of stay, falls, pressure injuries, use of mechanical restraints, urinary tract infections, and other indicators known to be sensitive to nursing practice and interventions.

We acknowledge that there is a wealth of qualitative statements and measures that describe health outcomes and benefits of nursing care. However, converting these measures to quantifiable savings that support the economic value of nursing and evidence-based practice appears to be a gap in the research. In order to provide an argument for sustained funding of the Australian BPSO Designation and demonstrate the economic benefits of the program, the ANMF (SA Branch), as the national BPSO Host, has worked to establish, quantify, and calculate the financial gains made from sound evidence-based practice and improved patient outcomes.

The evaluation demonstrates very significant improvements, not only with patient and nurse satisfaction, but at a system level with evidence of enhanced efficiencies and financial performance. These demonstrations convinced funding authorities of the program's value, resulting in expansion of the BPSO Designation. The economic evaluation of the Australian BPSO Designation and its outcomes provides a model for the measurement of financial impacts of nursing care, which is increasingly important within a financially constrained system.

BACKGROUND OF THE ANMF

The ANMF (SA Branch) is the largest professional and industrial organization representing nurses, midwives, and assistants in nursing in South Australia. We cultivate and promote knowledge-based nursing and midwifery practices and promote quality of work life and excellence in professional development. The organization has an important role advocating, influencing, and promoting the nursing and midwifery profession, practice, and healthcare policy.

In South Australia, the ANMF (SA Branch) has continuously lobbied for improved patient care and safety and is committed to promoting the integration of evidence-based practice and the provision of healthy work environments across all sectors of healthcare. Through the course of the organization's networking to improve evidence-based practice in South Australia, the ANMF (SA Branch) engaged with the RNAO and was attracted to the BPSO Designation. On March 2, 2012, the ANMF (SA Branch) signed an agreement with the RNAO to become a BPSO Host and lead the development and implementation of the BPSO Designation in Australia. In April 2012, the ANMF (SA Branch) finalized a contract with the Department of Health and Ageing (SA) to provide funding for the program as well as grant permission to use two of its sites to facilitate uptake of the program in South Australia.

ANMF (SA BRANCH): THE AUSTRALIAN BPSO HOST

Once the agreement with the RNAO was signed, the ANMF (SA Branch) became the second international host of the RNAO BPSO Designation (with the government of Spain being the first). This enabled the ANMF (SA Branch) to adapt the program to the Australian context. In our role of designated host, we lead and are responsible for BPSOs within Australia, in addition to directly working with RNAO and its network of international BPSO partners.

As the Australian BPSO Host, we select, coach, and support healthcare organizations to achieve BPSO Designation by implementing, disseminating, and evaluating the RNAO Best Practice Guidelines (BPG). Furthermore, we facilitate the establishment and development of a network of BPSO Leads for the purposes of knowledge transfer and exchange. Through regular meetings, reporting, and knowledge exchange forums, we monitor and provide reports to the RNAO with updates from the BPSOs as well as an overview of successes, challenges, questions, and issues of the BPSO Designation in Australia. As part of our participation in RNAO's Nursing Quality Indicators for Reporting and Evaluation (NQuIRE), we facilitate quarterly input of structural, process, and outcome indicator data by providing user education sessions, mentoring, and partnership with the RNAO and BPSOs to ensure data integrity, accuracy, and agreement on common definitions.

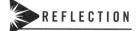

REFLECTION

Consider the early processes used in developing the Australia BPSO Host Model and identify what factors related to implementation science principles contributed to its success.

In return, the RNAO provides free-of-charge expert mentorship and consultation on guideline dissemination, implementation, uptake, sustainability, and evaluation. This includes all materials related to call for proposals, scoring of applications, and training materials, which enables full consistency of this internationally renowned program.

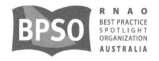

One of our key learnings is the importance of being able to actively engage with and become part of the implementation team. We are involved in leading the BPSO Designation institutes and workshops at the local level and providing continuing support for the Steering Committee, BPSO Lead, and nurses and midwives at the front line.

THE AUSTRALIAN BPSO MODEL

Since 2012, the Australian BPSO Designation has expanded. We now have four public health network sites participating in the Program: two designated BPSOs—Central Adelaide Rehabilitation Services (CARS, also referred to as Hampstead Rehabilitation Centre [HRC]) and Northern Adelaide Local Health Network (NALHN); and two predesignate BPSOs—Central Adelaide Local Health Network Mental Health Directorate (MHD) and Women's and Children's Health Network (WCHN). The adapted Australian BPSO Model in Figure 17.1 depicts the structures that have been established to support and enable the implementation of the BPSO Designation and BPGs, with an Executive Sponsor and ownership at the local level.

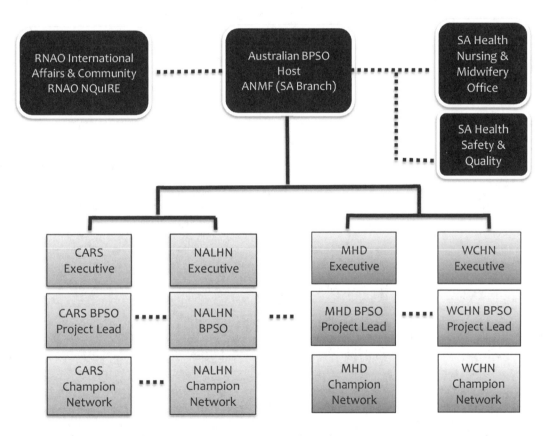

FIGURE 17.1 Australian BPSO governance and implementation structure as of June 2017. Copyright ANMF (SA Branch), 2017. Used with permission.

THE BEGINNINGS OF THE BPSO HOST MODEL

In April 2012, the BPSO Project Steering Committee was established to provide overarching leadership and governance. The Steering Committee is responsible for the appointment of the BPSO Program Manager and the selection of the BPSO candidate sites. The BPSO Steering Committee monitors and evaluates the BPSO sites' progress to ensure compliance with contractual obligations and ensure that candidate and designate key deliverables are met, key milestones are achieved, and strategies to mitigate potential risks are implemented.

In Australia, the designated BPSO Program Manager works collaboratively with the SA Government, Local Health Networks, Executive Directors, Directors of Nursing/Midwifery, and the BPSO Leads. This BPSO Program Manager's leadership role, vital to the success of the program, includes:

- Consultation with the pilot sites to select the appropriate and relevant guidelines to be implemented

- Delivery of education and training to the BPSO Leads and Practice Champions

- Program management and coordination

- Provision of support and advice for the duration of the project

- Establishment of the Australian BPSO knowledge exchange forums

- Establishment of regular consultation meetings with the RNAO to support and provide advice on the project

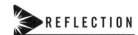

REFLECTION

How do you think these key activities of the BPSO Host Lead impacted the success of the first phase of the BPSO Designation in Australia and helped it spread? How could you modify these activities to be part of a role description for BPSO Lead in your setting?

AUSTRALIAN BPSO PROJECT ADVISORY COMMITTEE

In February 2013, the BPSO Project Advisory Committee was established to provide guidance and advice to the Program Manager on the BPSO evaluation framework and learnings. Reporting to the BPSO Steering Committee, the Project Advisory Committee is composed of representatives from SA Health Nursing and Midwifery Office, Safety and Quality Unit, and Nursing/Midwifery executives, as well as representatives from South Australian universities, BPSO project sites, and the ANMF (SA Branch).

RNAO BPSO DESIGNATION ADAPTATION TO THE AUSTRALIAN CONTEXT

Adapting the RNAO BPSO Model to the Australian context required communication on how this internationally successful model was indeed different from previous change models. Using the RNAO's philosophy enabled the establishment of meaningful dialogue and engagement with potential sites across the five local health networks in South Australia.

As part of the BPSO 3-year candidacy period, BPSO sites are required to implement a minimum of three clinical Best Practice Guidelines (BPG) and to successfully complete all activities mandated by RNAO and ANMF (SA Branch) to qualify for BPSO Designate status. This includes the establishment of the Best Practice Champion Network: training and engaging a minimum of 15% of the total nursing/midwifery workforce in the acute sector to become Champions for each BPG across the sites. In addition to the three clinical BPGs selected at each site, the ANMF (SA Branch) supported the implementation of the BPSO Designation with the complementary RNAO Healthy Work Environment BPGS to promote direct-care leadership at the bedside. Each of the selected RNAO BPGs and education materials was contextualized to reflect the South Australian legislation, population, practice, and healthcare system.

It is important to note the RNAO BPGs were mapped against the Australian National Safety and Quality Health Service Standards to ensure the initiatives were aligned to state and local health network priorities and goals and the national quality standards that improve health outcomes, system efficiencies, and effectiveness. This provided measures for evaluating the BPSO Designation in Australia.

PHASE 1: BPSO PILOT PROGRAM, 2012–2015

The BPSO Designation pilot extended for a 3-year period. It was structured to fit the Australian context and provide data to our government funders to demonstrate its impact. What follows is a description of the specific activities carried out during the first phase.

Selection of the Australian BPSOs

Interested local health networks submitted proposals to participate in the BPSO Designation, and two sites were eventually selected to commence their 3-year BPSO candidacy. The two candidates were Central Adelaide Rehabilitation Services (CARS) and Northern Adelaide Local Health Network (NALHN).

Establishment of the Local Australian BPSO Designation Governance and Leadership Structure

Similar to the Australian BPSO structure, the two sites established local leadership and governance structures. The Local Health Network BPSO Steering Committees provided executive leadership and drove the establishment, implementation, and evaluation of the BPSO Designation. Both sites worked collaboratively with the BPSO Program Manager and local health network executives.

During Phase 1, BPSO candidate sites selected the appropriate RNAO Best Practice Guidelines based on a number of factors, including the South Australian Government's and Local Health Network's strategic priorities and goals. Organization-wide audits identified gaps in practice knowledge and procedures, which determined the three priority areas for the inaugural BPSO Designation. Engagement of the Consumer Advisory Council resulted in advocacy for the BPSO Designation, as it promoted the partnership and value of consumers in healthcare. The established National Safety and Quality Health Service Standards Working Parties at the local health networks supported the incorporation and inclusion of the BPSO Designation and the three selected clinical BPGs, resulting in standardization of assessment, documentation, procedures, processes, practices, and policies.

Australian BPSO Leads

BPSO Leads were recruited at both sites to lead the implementation of the program. Working collaboratively with the BPSO Program Manager, the BPSO Lead also worked closely with the existing working parties, committees within the hospital, local health network, and government throughout the project. Together with the executives, both BPSO Leads participated in the Australian BPSO Learning Institute to enhance knowledge, skills, and expertise in the linkages between research, education, evidence-based practice and quality patient/resident/person care. A key element of the learning institute is the knowledge-transfer-change management model, and tools and resources for creating, innovating, and sustaining change to facilitate the implementation and uptake of the program.

Each site developed and enacted a 3-year project plan that identified the strategies, actions, resources, deliverables, and key milestones to support the implementation and sustainability of the BPSO Designation.

Australian BPSO Best Practice Champions

Critical to implementing the BPSO Designation as stated in the formal contract is the role of best practice Champions. To become Champions, nurses and other healthcare professionals participate in orientation workshops designed to provide them with strategies to champion Best Practice Guidelines in their organization and join the Best Practice Champions Network. The Champions model is well established in the RNAO literature as an effective model of knowledge transfer to incorporate evidence into practice (Garrard et al., 2014; Hewitt-Taylor, 2013; VanDeVelde-Coke et al., 2012). Through monthly meetings, the Champions share their learnings and experience, explore new opportunities, and support knowledge dissemination and local practice and cultural changes that are based on the highest level of evidence.

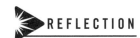

REFLECTION

Consider how the relationship of the BPG Champion Network and point of care leadership affect BPG uptake and quality of care.

PHASE 2: BPSO DESIGNATION, 2015–2018

The achievements from Phase 1 of the BPSO Designation, utilizing the BPSO Best Practice Champion model, have supported the bottom-up approach to change and facilitated evidence-based knowledge transfer. It has enabled nurses and midwives at the front line to lead, influence, and embed practice changes at the local level. The economic analysis has also enabled the BPSO project evaluation to quantify the benefits in dollar value, which will be discussed later in this chapter.

In January 2016, in Phase 2 of our BPSO Host activities, Central Adelaide Local Health Network Mental Health Directorate and Women's and Children's Health Network commenced their BPSO journey.

Site 3: Central Adelaide Local Health Network Mental Health Directorate (MHD)

The MHD offers a range of inpatient, outpatient, emergency, and community mental health services, including acute, recovery, and specialist mental healthcare services for people in the Adelaide region. It contains 100 acute inpatient beds and 16 beds for older people with mental health conditions, located across three different campuses. The three selected BPGs for implementation by MHD are:

- *Promoting Safety: Alterative Approaches to the Use of Restraints* (RNAO, 2012a)

- *Assessment and Care of Adults at Risk for Suicidal Ideation and Behaviour* (RNAO, 2009)

- *Person- and Family-Centred Care* (RNAO, 2015)

Site 4: Women's and Children's Health Network (WCHN)

The WCHN provides a range of trauma, emergency, inpatient, outpatient, and specialist obstetric and maternity services for women, babies, paediatrics, and adolescents. It contains 295 acute inpatient beds, mental health services, and family community services. The three selected BPGs for implementation by WCHN are:

- *Person- and Family-Centred Care* (RNAO, 2015)

- *Woman Abuse: Screening, Identification, and Initial Response* (RNAO, 2012c)

- *Care Transitions* (RNAO, 2014)

BPSO AND BPG IMPLEMENTATION

The process of implementing the BPGs across the organizational, educational, and practice levels is guided and outlined by the RNAO (2012b) *Toolkit: Implementation of Best Practice Guidelines*. The Toolkit is a comprehensive resource manual for teams who are responsible for implementing BPGs at their organization. It is grounded in theory, research, and experience, and is focused for use at the organizational or departmental level through a systematic process. The Toolkit was used at both sites as the guiding document for change and BPG implementation.

PHASE 1 PILOT SITE 1: CENTRAL ADELAIDE REHABILITATION SERVICE (CARS)

CARS provides state-wide specialized rehabilitation services for people who are severely affected by acquired brain injury, major burns, spinal cord injury and multitrauma, stroke, orthopaedic conditions, amputations, and medical deconditioning. CARS has inpatient, outpatient, and community-based services, and is composed of 124 inpatient rehabilitation beds, a rehabilitation in-home program, and outpatient and community rehabilitation programs. The model of care aims to maximize an individual's level of function and independence through physical and nonphysical therapy with a multidisciplinary team approach. The multidisciplinary team works to develop and coordinate a set of goals based on the individual's psychosocial, health, education, recreational, and vocational needs.

The three selected and successfully implemented RNAO Best Practice Guidelines are:

- *Client Centred Care* (RNAO, 2006a)

- *Promoting Safety: Alternative Approaches to the Use of Restraints* (RNAO, 2012a)

- *Supporting and Strengthening Families Through Expected and Unexpected Life Events* (RNAO, 2006b)

PHASE 1 PILOT SITE 2: NORTHERN ADELAIDE LOCAL HEALTH NETWORK (NALHN)

NALHN provides a diverse range of health services for people living in the northern metropolitan area of Adelaide. NALHN encompasses the:

- Lyell McEwin Hospital and Modbury Hospital

- Primary health, subacute, and transitional care services

- Aboriginal healthcare services

- Northern Mental Health service

The Lyell McEwin Hospital is a 336-bed, specialist referral public teaching hospital that provides a full range of high-quality intensive, coronary, medical, surgical, maternity, paediatrics, mental health, diagnostic, emergency, and support services. Modbury Hospital is a 174-bed, acute care teaching hospital that provides inpatient, outpatient, and emergency services.

NALHN's model of care focuses on the patient journey, safe environments, clinical teaching and research, sustainability, and fostering innovation and best practice.

The three RNAO BPGs selected by NALHN are:

- *Client Centred Care* (RNAO, 2006a)

- *Prevention of Falls and Fall Injuries in the Older Adult* (RNAO, 2011a)

- *Risk Assessment and Prevention of Pressure Ulcers* (RNAO, 2011b)

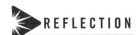

REFLECTION

How do you feel that ownership of practice change by nurses leads to positive engagement and the ability to impact positive outcomes?

BPSO PHASE 1 EVALUATION

The Australian BPSO Designation has been evaluated broadly in terms of the overall impact on the organization and the effects of embedding evidence-based practice and cultures. It has also been evaluated in terms of BPG recommendations and how they improve patient care and enrich professional practices of nurses and midwives. RNAO's NQuIRE comprehensive database system was used extensively in our evaluation processes.

MEASURING CLIENT, PROVIDER, AND ORGANIZATIONAL OUTCOMES USING NQUIRE

Aiming to monitor and assess the impact of the Australian BPSO Phase 1 Program, the evaluation was conducted in consultation with the South Australian Government and the South Australian Local Health Networks, Safety and Quality Units. The hospital data performance measures; safety and quality nurse-sensitive indicators; and NQuIRE structural, process, and outcome indicators were used to analyze and evaluate practice changes.

NQuIRE has been developed by the RNAO to enable BPSOs to systematically monitor and evaluate their progress and outcomes and measure and compare structural, process, and outcome indicators for "like" organisations at the individual ward/unit level for each of the BPGs. The NQuIRE indicators have facilitated the development and contextualization of the Australian BPSO Evaluation Model. In recognition of the capability and future development of the RNAO's NQuIRE database, ethics approval (HREC-14-SAH-21) was obtained through the SA Health Human Research Ethics Committee, which enabled international comparison and contribution to evidence-based practice research.

AUSTRALIAN BPSO EVALUATION FRAMEWORK, MODEL, AND TOOLS

In constructing the framework, the Australian BPSO Host, Local Health Networks, and BPSOs reviewed the international, national, and state indicators influencing patient and nursing outcomes. This led to the development of the Person-Organisation-Practice (POP) framework, shown in Table 17.1, which incorporates qualitative and quantitative measurements that are aligned to the SA Health policy, safety, and quality and reform agendas.

TABLE 17.1 PERSON-ORGANIZATION-PRACTICE (POP) FRAMEWORK

PERSON DATA	ORGANISATIONAL DATA	PRACTICE
Client-centred care specific patient discharge surveys	Structural indicators OBDs N/MHPPD Skill Mix	Percent of nursing/midwifery workforce trained in a specific BPG area such as CCC, Alternatives to Restraints, etc.
Patient testimonials and suggestions	SA Health safety and quality data	BPG-specific surveys that benchmark staff perspectives
Partnership with Consumer Advisory Groups and volunteers		Stakeholder consultations (ongoing Steering and Advisory Committee feedback)

Copyright ANMF (SA Branch), 2017. Used with permission.

The Australian BPSO Designation evaluation was designed to examine the following questions and the relationships between them (see Figure 17.2):

- Has the implementation of the BPG changed staff's attitudes, beliefs, and knowledge?
- Has the practice changed?
- Has it achieved the intended outcomes?

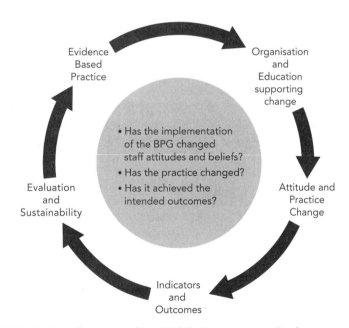

FIGURE 17.2 The Australian BPSO Designation Evaluation Model.
Copyright ANMF (SA Branch), 2017. Used with permission.

Quantitative Tools

As guided by the Evaluation Model, and in order to capture data to answer questions related to person, organization, and practice, a number of quantitative tools were developed and administered, as described in the following sections.

Tool 1: BPSO Practice Champion Survey

Literature reviews on the role of Practice Champions in a change-management context were conducted and identified that the attitudes and beliefs of nurses and midwives are integral to the successful implementation of the BPG (Price, 2015; RNAO, 2015; VanDeVelde-Coke et al., 2012). Nurses and midwives' confidence in working in a new way affects their acceptance of the proposed changes. Therefore, "considering how people will perceive and be affected by an innovation" is critical for change to be successful (Hewitt-Taylor, 2013, p. 35). Furthermore, the literature indicated that the level of support offered to change agents is essential to sustainment of attitude changes (Maben et al., 2012).

In summary, without these proven strategies and organizational support, the literature clearly states that innovations or new ways of working will often fail if the strong attitudinal barriers in nursing and midwifery are overlooked or unaddressed. In the absence of relevant tools to measure the attitudinal impact of each BPG, Practice Champion surveys were developed and validated to support the evaluation. The aim of the Practice Champion survey was to determine an individual's attitude and level of knowledge prior to and following BPSO workshops on each selected BPG. In order to enable this comparison and measure the impact of the specific Practice Champion workshop, two surveys were administered pre- and post-workshop. The surveys were composed of a series of attitudinal statements, and participants were asked to rate their level of agreement with those statements, ranging from 0 to signify that they strongly disagree, to 10, strongly agree.

Tool 2: Consumer Experience Survey

In order to assess interactions and satisfaction levels between the nursing and midwifery workforce and consumers, as well as to meet the NQuIRE requirements, the Consumer Experience Survey tool was developed. The survey investigated the patient's experience of care across the recognized NQuIRE domains and how their experience relates to the implementation of the *Client Centred Care* BPG recommendations (RNAO, 2006a). The survey was provided to patients (or their nominated person) on discharge with a prepaid envelope.

Tool 3: Nurse Staff Survey: Alternative to Restraints

The literature review on the use of alternatives to restraints showed that knowledge, in addition to understanding of how and when to apply restraint alternatives, is critical in establishing and sustaining a restraint-free practice environment (Barton, Johnson, & Price, 2009; Fariña-López et al., 2014; RNAO, 2012a). For this reason, as part of the evaluation process, a survey was developed to measure staff's knowledge, attitude, and confidence in when and how to apply alternatives to restraints. A subgroup analysis was conducted to assess the effectiveness of the BPSO Practice Champions workshop. This survey was administered to all nursing staff across the health unit, with a 47% response rate.

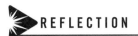

Qualitative Measures

Again, in keeping with the Evaluation Model and to answer the evaluation questions fully, focus groups and interviews were used to collect qualitative data, as described in the following sections.

Measure 1: Australian BPSO Focus Group

The BPSO focus group captured the experience of Practice Champions and assisted in facilitating knowledge transfer between peers. The focus group was held in July 2014 with the aim of evaluating how Practice Champions viewed the BPSO Designation and their journey in the BPG implementation process.

REFLECTION

What in your view are the benefits of conducting BPG implementation evaluation using structure, process, and outcome level indicators? How extensively was this carried out in the Australian experience?

Measure 2: BPSO Interviews

RNAO strongly emphasizes the importance of leadership throughout the BPG implementation processes. By *leadership*, the RNAO refers to leaders at all levels, including consumers, nurses, and executive management (Edwards & Grinspun, 2011; RNAO, 2004; RNAO, 2013). RNAO recommends that Practice Champions and the network should be established and supported by the leadership team to facilitate and role-model cultural change at the bedside. This further suggests that the leadership culture in a practice environment serves as a vital linkage between clinical practice at the bedside and senior management (RNAO, 2012b). Qualitative video interviews were conducted with all of the BPSO Executives, Leads, Consumer Advisory Council, and Working Parties.

BPSO PHASE 1: EVALUATION RESULTS AND FINDINGS

For the purpose of this section, we will focus on the evaluation of the Australian BPSO Designation at CARS—the inaugural site that has successfully implemented the RNAO clinical and Healthy Work Environment BPGs and attained designate status.

HAS THE IMPLEMENTATION OF THE BPG CHANGED STAFF'S ATTITUDES, BELIEFS, AND KNOWLEDGE?

Next we discuss the results of qualitative and quantitative measures administered in order to address this question.

CCC Practice Champion survey (Tool 1)

The Client-Centred Care Practice Champion surveys were conducted over an 8-month period. Their key results are shown in Figure 17.3.

The positive impact of the Client-Centred Care Practice Champions workshops is clearly illustrated by the survey results. The analysis found that overall, the workshops improved Practice Champions' knowledge and understanding of client-centred care; significantly impacted their confidence and belief in the implementation of evidence-based practice; and increased their belief that the active engagement of patients and their family results in safe patient care and better outcomes.

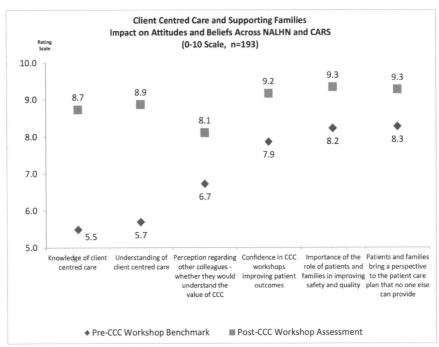

FIGURE 17.3 Results of the Client-Centred Care Practice Champion surveys: May–December, 2014. Copyright ANMF (SA Branch), 2017. Used with permission.

Improved knowledge, understanding, and perception of client-centred care:

- The Practice Champions' knowledge of client-centred care improved from a mean score of 5.5 out of 10 preworkshop to 8.7 postworkshop. This represents statistically significant improvements (p <0.001).

- The Practice Champions' understanding of client-centred care also improved from 5.7 out of 10 preworkshop to 8.9 postworkshop. This represents statistically significant improvements (p <0.001).

- The Practice Champions' perception of client-centred care improved as well from 6.7 out of 10 preworkshop to 8.1 postworkshop. This represents statistically significant improvements (p <0.001).

Increased confidence in client-centred care improving patient outcomes:

- The Practice Champions' confidence that client-centred care improves patient outcomes increased from 7.9 out of 10 preworkshop to 9.2 postworkshop (p <0.001).

Enhanced knowledge of the need to engage and involve patients and families in all aspects of care:

- The Practice Champions' belief that involving patients and their family members will improve patient safety and quality of care increased from 8.2 out of 10 preworkshop to 9.3 postworkshop.

- The Practice Champions' attitude toward engaging patients and families as active participants in care increased from 8.3 out of 10 preworkshop to 9.3 postworkshop.

Promoting Safety: Alternative to Restraints Practice Champion Survey (Tool 1).

This survey sought to measure the effect of workshops related to the BPG *Promoting Safety: Alternative Approaches to the Use of Restraints* (RNAO, 2012a), conducted ahead of BPG implementation. The results are illustrated by Figures 17.4a and 17.4b. The analysis has found that the workshops have improved Practice Champions' knowledge and understanding of promoting safety and the use of restraints; their ability to identify alternatives; their understanding that restraints are high-risk interventions; and their belief that engagement with patients and their family is important in the use of restraints. In summary, the noticeable changes in knowledge, understanding, and attitude are essential to successful implementation of the guideline recommendations.

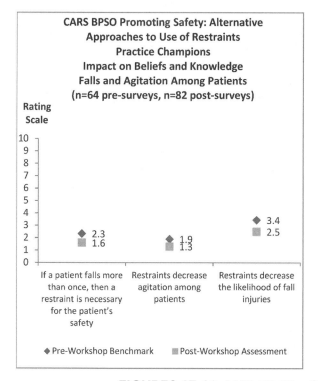
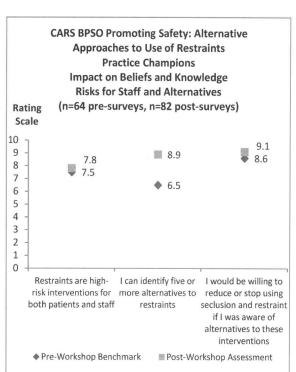

FIGURES 17.4A AND 17.4B CARS Practice Champion surveys
Copyright ANMF (SA Branch), 2017. Used with permission.

BPSO Focus Group (Measure 1)

A semi-structured BPSO Champions focus group was moderated by the BPSO Leads and the BPSO Program Manager (see Figure 17.5). Focus group participants were asked the following questions:

- What have you experienced throughout your BPSO journey?

- What do you think is the difference of the BPSO Project?

- What does BPSO mean to you?

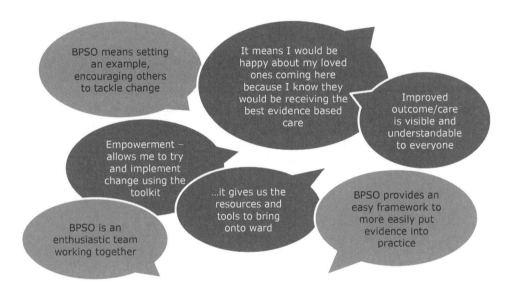

FIGURE 17.5 BPSO focus group responses.
Copyright ANMF (SA Branch), 2017. Used with permission.

The key themes that emerged from the focus group are:

- The BPSO Designation has empowered Practice Champions to lead and innovate practice change using the latest research and evidence.

- Practice Champions commonly referred to their reflective journey throughout the BPG implementation process as an avenue that encouraged them to learn, think, and act collectively.

- The BPSO Designation has been pivotal in improving Practice Champions' clinical practice by increasing their knowledge and confidence in implementing BPG recommendations.

- The most common perspective related to the practicality of the program, because it revolves around easy-to-use and easy-to-adapt tools.

Nurse Staff Survey—Alternatives to Restraints (Tool 3)

Out of the 114 responses, 38 nurses attended the BPSO Promoting Safety and Alternatives to Restraints Workshop, and at the time of the survey, 76 nurses had not attended the workshop. The findings of the survey are shown in Figures 17.6a, 17.6b, and 17.6c.

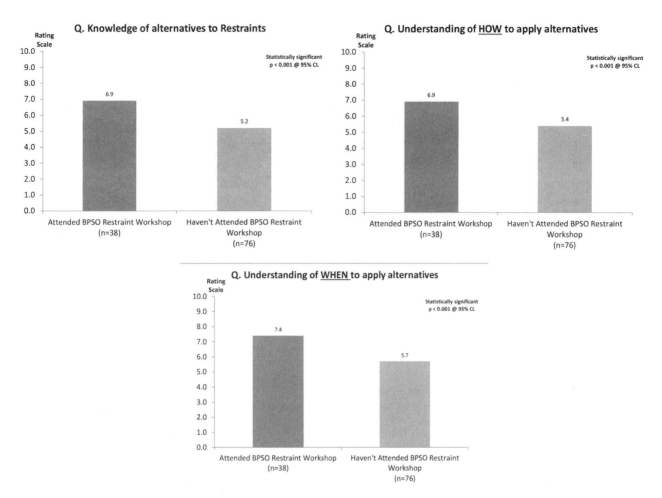

FIGURES 17.6A, 17.6B, 17.6C Staff survey results reflecting changes in knowledge and understanding: Alternatives to least restraints.
Copyright ANMF (SA Branch), 2017. Used with permission.

The responses confirm significant improvements amongst workshop attendees in their knowledge and understanding of how and when to apply alternatives to restraints. To sum up, the BPSO workshop on *Promoting Safety: Alternative Approaches to the Use of Restraints* (RNAO, 2012a) has resulted in enhanced knowledge in this area of practice, which is critical to improving patient outcomes, minimizing risks, and engaging patients and families at the centre of care.

HAS THE PRACTICE CHANGED?

To measure the practice change, clinical audits were undertaken. Below are two sample audits that were conducted during the BPSO Designation at CARS, in relation to the selected BPGs that were implemented and the evidence on how the practice changes have been embedded.

Clinical Practice Audit

The BPSO Designation and the Practice Champion workshops have contributed to the positive cultural and attitudinal change within CARS. This clinical practice change is evident in the CARS (HRC) Hourly Rounding Audit. Clinical Rounding was introduced to ensure patient safety and care needs were met each hour.

The audit has shown significant improvements in client-centred practice (see Figure 17.7). Improvements have occurred in all audited areas when compared to the September 2013 audit results. The high average compliance rate in the January 2015 audit has also indicated that HRC is achieving positive practice changes.

ARE THE FOLLOWING CHECKS OF PATIENT SAFETY AND CARE COMPLETED AT HOURLY ROUNDING?		AUDIT JAN 2015	AUDIT SEPT 2013
1	Comfort & safety	96%	52%
2	Call bell is in reach	96%	44%
3	Client status (sleeping, absent, therapy, in common areas)	96%	52%
4	Pain	96%	52%
5	Pressure injury prevention	96%	52%
6	Hydration	96%	52%
7	Continence	96%	48%
8	Handover—Client present	96%	0%
	Staff initials	96%	40%
	Average Total	96%	44%

Data Source: HRC Audit Reports

FIGURE 17.7 CARS–Hampstead Rehabilitation Centre audit report. Audit: Hourly rounding audit collation results. Auditor: R Pearl. Wards: All wards (1C, 1D, 2A, 2B, 2CD).
Copyright ANMF (SA Branch), 2017. Used with permission.

CARS Practice Audits: Bed Rails Audit

HRC's positive achievement has also been reflected in the bed rails audits. As part of the implementation process, bed rails/cot-sides were removed, and a matrix was developed to guide the clinical decision. Figure 17.8 displays the results from two audits, conducted in October 2014 and January 2015. The initial audit was designed to look at the compliance rate after the initial introduction of the bed/cot-side matrix.

The October 2014 audit identified areas that needed improvements, including the need to:

- Improve documentation on risk assessment on admission (Q.2)

- Follow the recommendations from the risk assessment (Q.3)

- Improve documentation on clinical reasoning (Q.4)

- Improve documentation on Bed Rail needs reassessment (Q.7)

In comparing the results of the two bed rail audits, it is evident that such improvements have indeed been achieved. The practice of removing bed rails has been embedded, leading to a 100% score in the latest audit, which indicated that, "no bed rails were required to be removed." This practice change followed the recommendations from admission assessments, as seen in an increase from 15% in 2014 to 95% in 2015. In cases where recommendations were not followed, there was an increase in documentation on clinical reasoning.

	Section A	Audit Jan-2015			Audit Oct-2014			Comments
		Yes	No	n/a	Yes	No	n/a	
1	Are Bed Rails insitu on bed?	40%	60%	0%	45%	55%	0%	Decrease in Bed Rails in situ on bed
2	Is there documented evidence that a risk assessment has been completed on admission or within first 24 hrs?	95%	5%	0%	20%	80%	0%	Increase in document evidence
3	Have recommendations been followed?	95%	0%	5%	15%	70%	15%	Increase – recommendations have been followed
4	If not, have staff documented clinical reasoning for not following the recommendations in the clinical records?	5%	0%	95%	0%	65%	35%	Improvement in documentation clinical reasoning
5	Have the Bed Rails been removed from the bed if not recommended? (identify in n/a section if client has requested)	20%	0%	80%	55%	25%	20%	Increase in n/a due to no bed rails being on the bed already or the client has requested to keep them
6	Have the Bed Rails been removed from the bed once client is discharged?	0%	0%	100%	65%	25%	10%	100% n/a (no bed rails are required to be removed)
7	Is there documented evidence that the need for Bed Rails has been reviewed?	25%	60%	15%	0%	95%	5%	Increase in document evidence

Data source: HRC audit reports

FIGURE 17.8 Hampstead Rehabilitation Centre practice audit report, January 2015 vs. October 2014.
Audit: Bed Rails
Auditor: S McCormack
Wards: 1C, 1D, 2A, 2B

Documentations on risk assessment and admission also improved. In summary, the challenging behaviour/restraint data and the bed rails audit have confirmed that HRC has achieved a positive cultural shift and evidence-based practice change.

HAS THE BPG IMPLEMENTATION ACHIEVED THE INTENDED OUTCOMES?

This section discusses the impact of BPG implementation on consumer experience.

CARS Consumer Experience Survey (Tool 2)

The implementation of the HRC Consumer Experience Survey commenced in July 2013, with small sample sizes for analysis. In analyzing the nurse-patient interactions, patients reported improvements in always being treated by nurses with courtesy and respect; nurses always explaining things in a way they could understand; and nurses always listening to them carefully. The patient discharge surveys were collated and analyzed in quarterly periods for comparison purposes.

The charts in Figures 17.9a, 17.9b, and 17.9c provide a summary of the findings.

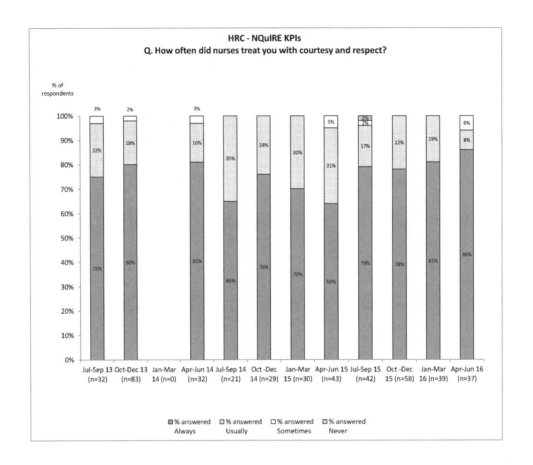

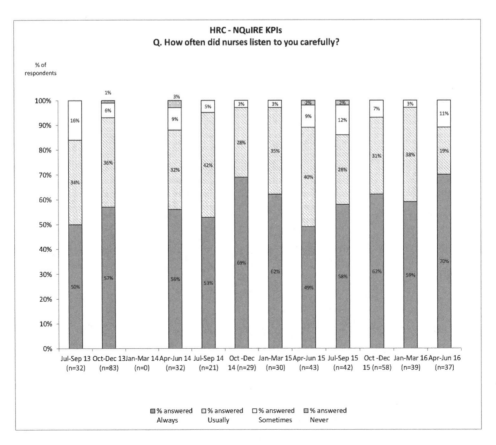

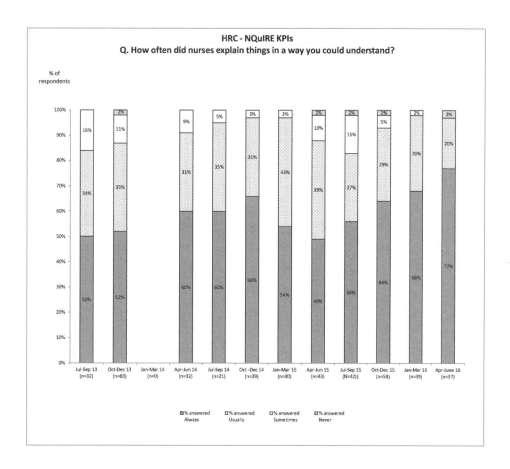

HRC – NQuIRE KPIs
Q. How often did nurses explain things in a way you could understand?

FIGURES 17.9A, 17.9B, AND 17.9C HRC Consumer Experience Surveys between July 2013 and June 2016.
Data Source: HRC Consumer Experience Survey, July 2013—June 2016
Note: Period January 2014—March 2014: No surveys were received.
Copyright ANMF (SA Branch), 2017. Used with permission.

The analysis of consumers' experiences has been an enabler of practice and process improvements. It is noted that the proportion of respondents who mentioned "always" in the three survey questions fluctuated across reporting periods. During the same periods, the South Australian Government made the major announcement that the HRC would be closed, with over 100 rehabilitation beds being realigned to other local health networks. This clearly had a significant impact on rehabilitation nurses and the workplace environment.

SA HEALTH SAFETY AND QUALITY INDICATORS

Evidence-based nursing and midwifery interventions, and systematic collection, analysis, and reporting of nursing-sensitive indicators, have supported the BPG implementation and outcome evaluation with the end goal of improving patient outcomes and quality of care. Nursing-sensitive quality indicators and structural indicators are important in establishing, monitoring, and evaluating evidence-based practice guidelines. It is internationally accepted and recognized that the link between the number of nurses/midwives, education levels, and skill mix directly influence patient outcomes (Aiken et al., 2002; Aiken et al., 2014; Aiken et al., 2017).

PATIENT SAFETY INDICATORS

In order to evaluate the BPSO pilot and how it complemented other safety and quality agenda and organizational priorities, the internationally recognized nursing-sensitive indicators, such as incidence of falls and pressure ulcers, have been analyzed based on their relation to the implementation of the BPG recommendations. Assessment and evaluation were based on the data currently being captured by the systems within the organization.

All (SAC 1 and SAC 2) Incidents—Serious Incidents—Mandatory Reporting Requirement

SAC, Safety Assessment Code, is a numerical score that rates incidents affecting a patient. The score is based on the consequence of that incident and the likelihood of its recurrence, using a risk type matrix. The scale is from 1 to 4, with SAC 1 (extreme) indicating a major incident with significant harm or death, and 4 (insignificant) being a near miss or no harm. The SAC is mandated by SA Health and is used by all public hospitals across South Australia (Government of South Australia—SA Health, 2016). Reporting on the total number of all SAC 1 and SAC 2 incidents at CARS since FY 2012/13 (see Figure 17.10) demonstrates a decrease in both categories that is consistent with the SA Health trend.

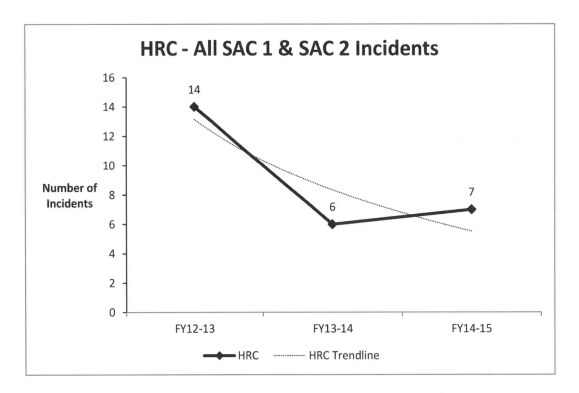

FIGURE 17.10   CARS (HRC) all SAC 1 and SAC 2 incidents, FY 2012/13 to FY 2014/15. Copyright ANMF (SA Branch), 2017. Used with permission.

All (SAC 1 and SAC 2) Falls Incidents—(With Harm and Injury)

From the findings on falls-related incidents with harm and injury, there has evidently been a reduction at HRC (from 11 in FY 2012/13, to 4 in FY 2013/14, and 5 in 2014/15). Moreover, for comparison purposes, there was a 64% reduction of SAC 1 and SAC 2 falls incidents during the 2012/13 period at HRC, compared to an 18.6% reduction in SA Health (across all local health networks). See Figure 17.11.

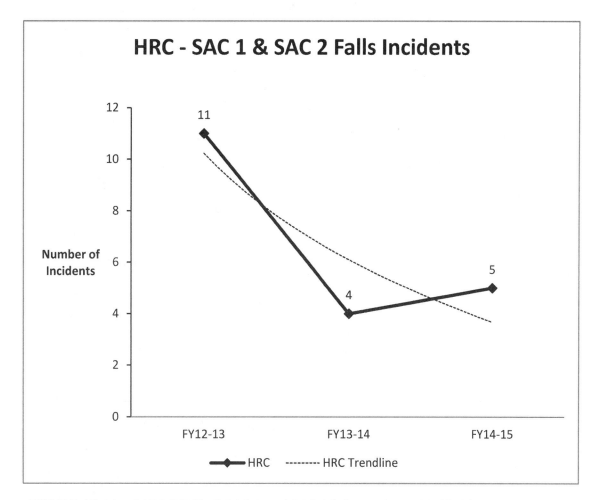

FIGURE 17.11   CARS (HRC) all SAC 1 and SAC 2 falls incidents, FY 2012/13 to FY 2014/15.
Copyright ANMF (SA Branch), 2017. Used with permission.

CARS Hospital Acquired Pressure Injury Incidents

At HRC, there has been a reduction (50%) in hospital-acquired pressure injury incidents from 78 in FY 2012/13 to 39 in FY 2014/15 (see Figure 17.12).

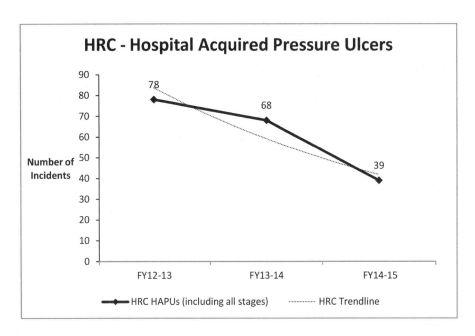

FIGURE 17.12   CARS (HRC) hospital-acquired pressure injury incidents, FY 2012/13 to FY 2014/15. Copyright ANMF (SA Branch), 2017. Used with permission.

Reduction in Restraint

HRC showed an increase in number of reported challenging behaviour incidents and a decrease in the number of patients being restrained (see Figure 17.13). These trends indicate more success in de-escalation, thus reflecting the success of BPG implementation.

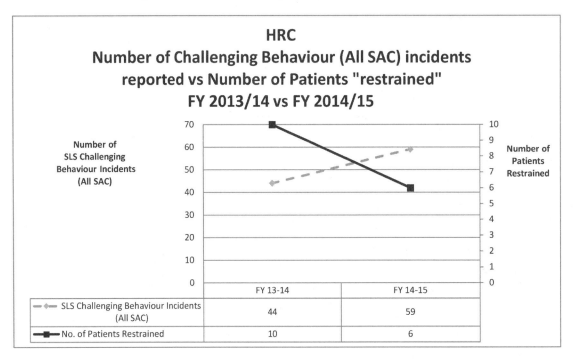

FIGURE 17.13   CARS (HRC) challenging behaviour and restraint incidents, FY 2013/14 to FY 2014/15. Copyright ANMF (SA Branch), 2017. Used with permission.

SUMMARY

The adaptation and application of the RNAO BPSO Designation to the Australian context has proven to be successful. Overall, staff and consumer surveys, clinical practice audits and indicator data showed:

- Nurses are better informed and have improved knowledge, understanding, and attitudes toward implementing and embedding evidence-based practice.

- Patients'/clients' hospital experience and nurses/midwives interactions with patients/clients improved.

- There has been a reduction of all incidents (SAC1 and SAC2).

- There has been a reduced incidence of patient/client falls (SAC1 and SAC2).

- There has been a reduced incidence of hospital-acquired pressure ulcers.

- There has been a reduced use of restraints in the environment.

MEASURING ECONOMIC OUTCOMES OF THE AUSTRALIAN BPSO DESIGNATION

To strengthen the case for value of the BPSO Designation for South Australia, it was necessary to consider the cost effectiveness of evidence-based practice in nursing and how the clinical improvements can be translated to an economic argument in terms of "savings" to the health system. There are four main types of economic evaluation in healthcare:

1. Cost minimization, where the consequences are assumed to be the same so only the costs are compared

2. Cost effectiveness, where a ratio of the differences in costs and outcomes is calculated—that is, an incremental cost effectiveness ratio (ICER)

3. Cost utility, where the ICER is based on cost per quality adjusted life years (QALY)

4. Cost benefit, where both costs and outcomes are valued in monetary terms (Gray, Clarke, Wolstenholme, & Wordsworth, 2012; Simoens, 2009)

ECONOMIC IMPACT OF BPG IMPLEMENTATION SHOWN THROUGH COST BENEFIT ANALYSIS

To measure the economic impact of the Australian BPSO Designation, we selected the fourth option: the cost benefit of the program to the South Australian health system, which is illustrated in Table 17.2.

TABLE 17.2 COST-BENEFIT ANALYSIS RELATED TO IMPLEMENTATION OF FALLS AND PRESSURE INJURY BPGS

Australian BPSO Designation Evaluation Indicator	Nurse-Sensitive Indicator Change	Number of Changes in Incidences	$/Incident* (Based on RNAO Financial Estimates)	Total Savings/ Costs
Reduced incidence of patient/client falls (SAC1 and SAC2)	From total of 11 incidences in 2012/13 to 5 incidences in 2014/15	6	$35,000 per fall	$210,000
Reduced incidence of hospital acquired pressure ulcers	From total of 78 incidences in 2012/13 to 39 incidences in 2014/15	39	$9,000 per pressure injury	$351,000
Total Savings				$561,000
Less Investment	($50,000 per annum to site BPSO Lead)			$100,000
Cost Benefit (Net Saving)				$461,000

Copyright ANMF (SA Branch), 2017. Used with permission.

OTHER SAVINGS THAT ARE RELATED TO REDUCTION IN RESTRAINT

The systematic cost of restraint is difficult to quantify. There is limited information in the literature on the economic evaluation that demonstrates the link between cost savings and prevention of restraints.

It has been established by RNAO, as part of the literature reviews, that a relationship does exist between restraint and patient/client falls. However, there is a large degree of variability based on the outcome or injury of the patient fall—serious/life threatening to no physical harm. In the Australian BPSO economic evaluation, we have explored and considered multiple factors, such as staffing (hours per patient day), reductions in length of stay, and range of interventions. Therefore, we are exploring a model that could provide to the base for the economic measurement of the benefits of reduction in restraints. The potential financial savings and implications associated to each of the restraint episodes are depicted elements of the model in Figure 17.14.

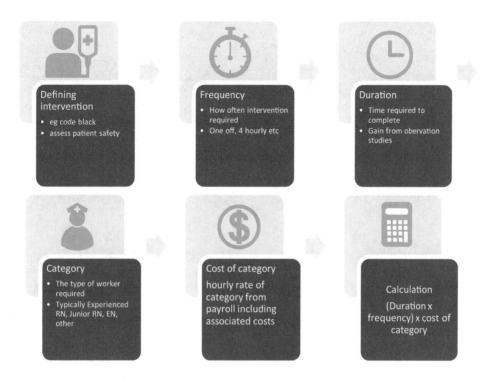

FIGURE 17.14 Financial implications and potential savings model.
Copyright ANMF (SA Branch), 2017. Used with permission.

CALCULATION METHODOLOGY

The calculation methodology was based on:

- Defining the intervention eliminated or reduced (actions related to restraint such as code black team attendance, evaluation of impact on skin integrity, safety, etc.)

- Identifying the frequency of the interventions that would have been required

- Identifying the duration of the intervention (time required)

- Identifying the person(s) who would be required to undertake the intervention (by staff category)

The calculation is performed in two parts. First, the total amount of nursing time is calculated based on the intervention frequency and duration. Then the total nursing time is multiplied by the cost of relevant staff, which equals the costs saved.

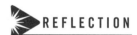

REFLECTION

How do these evaluation results relate to your own experiences and, in your view, have they been effectively captured? Consider how you would explain the value-add of BPG implementation using these results.

CONCLUSION

The adapted RNAO BPSO Designation has contributed significantly to the growing body of knowledge and understanding of how to successfully bridge the gap between evidence, knowledge, and practice in Australia. Following the success of Phase 1, the Australian BPSO Designation has been extended to Phase 2. The coaching, mentoring, and support for three (out of four) metropolitan local health networks in South Australia has led them to fulfill their goal of becoming the "change that they wanted to see." The systemic approach used in the BPSO Designation, and specifically with BPG implementation, has resulted in a shift to an evidence-based practice culture in which decision-making about healthcare and service delivery is based on the best evidence possible; hospital policies and procedures are standardised; and care variation is reduced, thus ensuring consistent, quality, safe care.

We have successfully advocated for and attained funding for the Australian BPSO Designation within a financially constrained system. Our comprehensive evaluation was able to demonstrate significant improvements, not only with patient and nurse satisfaction, but at a system level with evidence of enhanced efficiencies and financial performance. Based on data and testimony, the value for money proposition further reinforces that nurses and midwives using evidenced-based practice within a healthy work environment do make a difference at all levels.

KEY MESSAGES

- Implementing evidence-based practice guidelines requires a systematic, organizational-level approach.

- Nursing practice based on evidence produces positive clinical outcomes for patients.

- Nursing practice based on evidence saves money for the system.

- The BPSO Designation and its impact on client, provider, organization, and system outcomes has led to increased respect from government for nurses as knowledge professionals and for the nursing association's work.

REFERENCES

Aiken, L., Clarke, S. P., Sloane, D. M., Sochalski, J., & Silber, J. H. (2002). Hospital nurse staffing and patient mortality, nurse burnout, and job dissatisfaction. *JAMA, 288*(16), 1987–1993.

Aiken, L., Rafferty, A. M., & Sermeus, W. (2014, April 30). Caring nurses hit by a quality storm. *Nursing Standard, 28, 35*, pp. 22–25.

Aiken, L. H., Sloane, D., Griffiths, P., Rafferty, A. M., Bruyneel, L., McHugh, M., . . . Sermeus, W. For the RN4CAST Consortium. (2017). Nursing skill mix in European hospitals: Cross-sectional study of the association with mortality, patient ratings, and quality of care. *BMJ Quality & Safety, 26*, 559–568.

Barton, S. A., Johnson, M. R., & Price, L. V. (2009). Achieving restraint-free on an inpatient behavioural health unit. *Journal of Psychosocial Nursing & Mental Health Services, 47*(1), 34–40.

Cheung, R. B., Aiken L. H., Clarke, S. P., & Sloane, D. M. (2008). Nursing care and patient outcomes: International evidence. *Enfermeria Clinica, 18*(1), 35–40.

Edwards, N., & Grinspun, D. (2011). *Understanding whole systems change in healthcare: The case of emerging evidence-informed nursing service delivery models*. Retrieved from http://www.cfhi-fcass.ca/SearchResultsNews/11-10-07/7eccd93b-a091-4d01-b625-3cd8279afbc2.aspx

Fariña-López E. L., Estévez-Guerra G. J., Gandoy-Crego, M., Polo-Luque, L. M., Gómez-Cantorna, C., & Capezuti, E. A. (2014). Perception of Spanish nursing staff on the use of physical restraints. *Journal of Nursing Scholarship*, *46*(5), 322–330.

Garrard, L., Boyle, D. K., Simon, M., Dunton N., & Gajewski B. (2014). Reliability and validity of the NDNQI Injury Falls Measure. *Western Journal of Nursing Research*, *38*(1), 111–123. doi: 10.1177/0193945914542851

Government of South Australia—SA Health. (2016, August). *Patient Incident Management TOOL 2: Safety assessment code matrix*. Retrieved from http://www.sahealth.sa.gov.au/wps/wcm/connect/29f2ff004e2bd4aca30cfbc09343dd7f/TOOL+2+Code+Matrix+WEB.pdf?MOD=AJPERES&CACHEID=29f2ff004e2bd4aca30cfbc09343dd7f%20%0d%0d-cheers,%20Deb%0d

Gray, A. M., Clarke, P. M., Wolstenholme, J. L., & Wordsworth, S. (2012). *Applied methods of cost-effectiveness analysis in health care*. Oxford, UK: Oxford University Press.

Hewitt-Taylor, J. (2013). Planning successful change incorporating processes and people. *Nursing Standard*, *27*(38), 35–40.

Lloyd, M., Xiao, S., Albornos-Muñoz, L., González-María, E., & Joyce, A. (2013). Measuring the process and outcomes of foot ulcer care with guideline-based nursing quality indicators. *Diabetic Foot Canada*, *1*(1), 15–19.

Maben, J., Peccei, R., Adams, M., Robert, G., Richardson, A., Murrells, T., & Morrow, E. (2012). *Exploring the relationship between patients' experiences of care and the influence of staff motivation, affect and wellbeing*. Final report. NIHR Service Delivery and Organisation Programme. Retrieved from http://www.netscc.ac.uk/hsdr/files/project/SDO_FR_08-1819-213_V01.pdf

Mitchell, B. G., Ferguson J. K., Anderson. M., Sear. J., & Barnett. A (2016). Length of stay and mortality associated with healthcare-associated urinary tract infections: A multi-state model. *Journal of Hospital Infection*, *93*(1), 92–99. doi: 10.1016/j.jhin.2016.01.012

Price, B. (2015). Understanding attitudes and their effects on nursing practice. *Nursing Standard*, *30*(15), 50–57. doi: 10.7748/ns.30.15.50.s51

Registered Nurses' Association of Ontario (RNAO). (2004). *A phenomenal journey: The dissemination and uptake of the nursing Best Practice Guidelines across Canada—Final report*. Retrieved from http://rnao.ca/bpg/guidelines/links/phenomenal-journey

Registered Nurses' Association of Ontario (RNAO). (2006a). *Client centred care*. Toronto, ON: Registered Nurses' Association of Ontario.

Registered Nurses' Association of Ontario (RNAO). (2006b). *Supporting and strengthening families through expected and unexpected life events*. Toronto, ON: Registered Nurses' Association of Ontario.

Registered Nurses' Association of Ontario (RNAO). (2009). *Assessment and care of adults at risk for suicidal ideation and behaviour*. Toronto, ON: Registered Nurses' Association of Ontario.

Registered Nurses' Association of Ontario (RNAO). (2011a). *Prevention of falls and fall injuries in the Older Adult*. Toronto, ON: Registered Nurses' Association of Ontario.

Registered Nurses' Association of Ontario (RNAO). (2011b). *Risk assessment and prevention of pressure ulcers*. Toronto, ON: Registered Nurses' Association of Ontario.

Registered Nurses' Association of Ontario (RNAO). (2012a). *Promoting safety: Alterative approaches to the use of restraints*. Toronto, ON: Registered Nurses' Association of Ontario.

Registered Nurses' Association of Ontario (RNAO). (2012b). *Toolkit: Implementation of Best Practice Guidelines* (2nd ed.). Toronto, ON: Registered Nurses' Association of Ontario.

Registered Nurses' Association of Ontario (RNAO). (2012c). *Woman abuse: Screening, identification, and initial response*. Toronto, ON: Registered Nurses' Association of Ontario.

Registered Nurses' Association of Ontario (RNAO). (2013). *Developing and sustaining nursing leadership Best Practice Guideline* (2nd ed.). Toronto, ON: Registered Nurses' Association of Ontario.

Registered Nurses' Association of Ontario (RNAO). (2014). *Care transitions*. Toronto, ON: Registered Nurses' Association of Ontario.

Registered Nurses' Association of Ontario (RNAO). (2015). *Person- and family centred care*. Toronto, ON: Registered Nurses' Association of Ontario.

Simoens, S. (2009). Health economic assessment: A methodological primer. *International Journal of Environmental Research and Public Health*, *6*(12), 2950–2966. doi: 10.3390/ijerph6122950

Twigg, D. E., Duffield, C., Thompson, P. L., & Rapley, P. (2010). The impact of nurses on patient morbidity and mortality—The need for a policy change in response to the nursing shortage. *Australian Health Review*, *34*(3), 312–316. doi: 10.1071/AH08668

VanDeVelde-Coke, S., Doran, D., Grinspun, D., Hayes, L., Sutherland Boal, A., Velji, K., . . . Hannah, K. (2012). Measuring outcomes of nursing care, improving the health of Canadians: NNQR (C), C-HOBIC and NQuIRE. *Nursing Leadership*, *25*(2), 26–37.

NEXT STEPS:
FROM PRACTICE TO POLICY

18

SCALING DEEP TO IMPROVE PEOPLE'S HEALTH: FROM EVIDENCE-BASED PRACTICE TO EVIDENCE-BASED POLICY

Doris Grinspun, PhD, MSN, BScN, RN, LLD(hon), Dr(hc), O.ONT
Mariam Botros, DCh, IIWCC, CDE, Wounds Care Fellowship University of Toronto
Lynn Anne Mulrooney, PhD, MPH, RN
Josephine Mo, BA(hon)
Ronald Gary Sibbald, MD, BSc, FRCPC(Med, Derm), MACP, FAAD, MEd, FAPWCA, DSc(hon)
Tasha Penney, MN, RN

LEARNING OBJECTIVES

After reading this chapter, you will be able to:

- Understand how nursing can become a body politic and why this is important to advance healthy public policy

- Grasp the central role of professional and labor associations in taking political leadership to ensure the public has the highest-quality health system

- Describe how nurses make a contribution at the micro, meso, and macro levels and why nursing involvement at all levels is vital to a healthy society

- Outline the pillars and stages of the Framework for Advancing Healthy Public Policy and describe how each is necessary to shape the health policy agenda and achieve change

- Discuss how RNAO's BPGs and evidence-based clinical recommendations can be used to influence policy improvements at the macro systems level

- Discuss the concept of social movements and how it applies to successful advocacy

- Identify the components of a successful advocacy campaign and the role of nurses and of the professional association in such a campaign

INTRODUCTION

"We must create a public opinion which must drive the government, instead of the government having to drive us—an enlightened public opinion, wise in principles, wise in details."

—Florence Nightingale, 1892

This book, of which this is the last chapter, is primarily about using evidence, in particular clinical evidence and evidence relating to healthy work environments, with the aim to improve people's health. The book's focus so far has been mainly on strengthening nurses' clinical practice through the systematic application of evidence drawing from the leadership and experience of the Registered Nurses' Association of Ontario (RNAO). Health policy has not been salient, except for a peripheral focus in some of the chapters, particularly Chapters 10, 12, and 17.

Realizing nursing as a body politic is central to advancing healthy public policy and ensuring that the public—in any and all countries and communities around the world—fully benefit from nursing and nurses' contribution as evidence-based experts. As this book shows, nurses must and do impact the micro systems of patient care, the meso systems of health organizations, and the macro health systems (Grinspun, 2006a, 2006b, 2013, 2015). This chapter argues it is the impact to health systems that nurses must continue to conquer.

In reality, it is seldom the case that policy changes can be achieved only with the persuasion of clinical evidence—a point we emphasize below. Furthermore, many changes required to improve health outcomes fall outside the realm of clinical evidence. This is especially true for social and environmental determinants of health, health system design, and nursing human resources. Thus, given RNAO's broad scope of policy interventions, our need to continue to shape clinical practice through evidence goes hand-in-hand with our need to shape healthy public policy through evidence. This is why, 20 years ago, we endeavoured to learn systematically how to impact the political and policy sphere. What we uncovered follows.

This chapter focuses specifically on the link between evidence-based practice and evidence-based policy and how to move from one to the other and leverage both to achieve healthy public policy. How do you shift from making a difference for a patient or a health organization, in the case of bedside or street-side nursing, or for a community, in the case of public health, to influencing systemic change in the provision of health services across an entire jurisdiction?

NURSING AS BODY POLITIC

This chapter also tells a larger story about how a nursing organization can become a transformative social force and an effective policy advocacy machine that is respected and influential in a key jurisdiction—the province of Ontario, Canada's largest—as well as in Canada and internationally. It is the story of how a group of nurses, who 2 decades ago sat many times on the sidelines as spectators and watched policy processes unfold, is now a leading contributor and formulator of policy. This is a success story that is worth telling because it has lessons for nursing organizations that want to become policy and politically relevant, anywhere. It shows how one can link the clinical work that nurses do with the policy frameworks and social contexts that enable or hinder their day-to-day work. It shows, with concrete examples, how nurses' evidence-based work impacts patient health outcomes and how nurses can leverage evidence and advocacy to affect health system policy changes that ultimately feed back into practice.

If one were to measure RNAO's current stage of political development using Cohen's four stages of political development framework (Cohen et al., 1996), it would be categorized as stage 4, where nursing "leads the way." This is a stage in which the profession is envisioned as providing proactive political leadership on broader policy issues that speak to the public's interests. Here the profession is leading agenda-setting for a broad range of health and social policy issues, introducing terms that reorder the debate, and initiating coalitions with nursing and non-nursing stakeholders for broad policy concerns. At this stage, many nurses are sought to fill nursing and health policy positions because of the value of nursing expertise and knowledge. The authors argue that the further the profession is able to move into this stage, the more the public will benefit from nursing's expertise and the advocacy on behalf of the public (Cohen et al., 1996). Indeed, the sophistication of RNAO and its members—both in evidence-based practice through our Best Practice Guidelines (BPG) Program and in evidence-based policy activation as described in this chapter—is well recognized in Canada and abroad (Amela, 2012; Factor Hispano, 2006; Gardner, 2010; Jordan, 2005; Marti, 2014; Pantaleoni, 2014).

Ellenbecker and colleagues (2017) propose a staged approach to nursing education in health policy at each level of nursing education, very much in following with Cohen's four stages of political development in nursing. The focus of health policy content these scholars propose is to progress from the organizational level to local, state, and finally national level health policies. While we fully concur with such an approach to nursing education, we urge a parallel fast-tracked approach by all nursing associations, nursing labour organizations, and others to embrace policy and politics as much as we have embraced evidence-based clinical practice if we are to reach our full potential for influence and impact at the organizational and governmental levels—locally, nationally, and internationally (Grinspun, 2016c). We hope the experience of RNAO inspires others to mobilize their expertise to shape policy and galvanize their power to conquer politics.

THE NECESSITY BUT INSUFFICIENCY OF AN EVIDENCE-BASED APPROACH

For nurses embedded in an evidence-based practice approach, the shift to health policy raises a striking realization: Evidence—even the best and most robust evidence—is a necessary but for the most part insufficient tool to shape healthy public policy. Policy advocates over the years have learned to accept that evidence alone does not influence whether a policy change will occur, nor how it occurs or when; it is but one factor in a seemingly disorderly array of influences, vested interests, and scarce resources. Years ago, a highly esteemed Canadian researcher approached some of us for comments on a polished, evidence-based paper on a policy change that had just taken hold in Ontario. As we read it, we smiled, as the paper was as exquisite as everything else this scholar had written. The paper, however, was naive and inaccurate in its thinking that evidence alone had moved forward the government's policy decision. Indeed, how nice it would be if that were the case, and how sad to recognize that it seldom is that way.

This reality—of policy driven by small politics and entrenched interests rather than evidence on how to advance the right values and services—was the fuel that propelled RNAO to fast track our own journey into the arena of political and policy engagement. Indeed, the key purpose of RNAO is to advance healthy public policy to affect people's health, healthcare, and nursing services. Undaunted, like most nurses, we decided to tackle the challenge as problem solvers. And, like most nurses, we never gave up (Grinspun, 2017). Instead, we set ourselves to observe and articulate what truly moves policy forward and came up with a basic operational framework that has guided RNAO's advocacy work and has delivered profound changes.

This evolution started with the vision of a professional association that would influence policies pertaining to the practice of the nursing profession, as well as the healthcare system and the broader set of public policies that affect health and well-being—namely, social and environmental determinants of health. This vision embodied a different kind of professional association, a high-profile one that is an agenda setter in public policy. No other nursing association in Canada, and only a handful in the world, has dared to adopt—in depth—such a broad and ambitious mandate.

What follows is a glimpse into this transformation that we hope will whet the appetite of others to learn more. First, we introduce the conceptual framework that has guided this work (Grinspun, 2006b; 2007a). Next, with two lived-experience case studies we provide a flavour of the actual work and accomplishments that have followed. The first case study focuses on supervised injection services as part of a comprehensive harm-reducing strategy. The second case study relates to improving access to health services, in particular universal access to offloading devices for persons with diabetes and foot ulcers. Following the case studies, we draw a conclusion and explore what will come next.

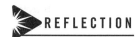

REFLECTION

Think about a healthcare policy that has been implemented in your jurisdiction; does it surprise you that evidence may not have been the primary motivator in the adoption of it? Why or why not?

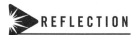

REFLECTION

Do you think the description provided here about the political advocacy ability of nurses in Ontario, Canada mirrors nursing in your jurisdiction? Around the world? If so, in what ways?

FOUNDATIONAL IDEAS AND CONCEPTUAL FRAMEWORK FOR ADVOCACY

In considering how advancing public policy becomes a reality, does robust evidence suffice? In this section we address the unsettling recognition that the answer to this question is "no." In fact, there is hardly any historical experience where this has been the case. Policy change requires, in addition to solid evidence, the mustering of political will through concerted and informed advocacy. The following discussion presents foundational ideas related to advancing public policy and how they have been conceptualized as a framework built on two key pillars of evidence and advocacy to realize evidence-based policy and practice.

THE TWO PILLARS FOR ADVANCING HEALTHY PUBLIC POLICY

The fundamental recognition that evidence is necessary but not sufficient is at the root of our framework for advancing healthy public policy. Thus, the two pillars to RNAO's framework for advancing healthy public policy are robust evidence and robust advocacy. The first is the design of robust evidence-based policies—we refer to this as the "evidence" pillar. The second is engaging advocacy action with nurses, the media, and the public to create the political will to make them a reality—we refer to this as the "political action" or "advocacy action" pillar. Both of these pillars provide support to the five stages of policy advancement.

Table 18.1 provides a template of RNAO's Framework for Advancing Healthy Public Policy (adapted from Grinspun 2007b), useful for drafting a plan to advance healthy public policy on a specific agenda. The table presents the two pillars of the framework in the left column, and the stages required to successfully advance the policy goal in the upper row. The resulting matrix when completed with data relevant to the policy issue creates an evidence-based plan of action.

TABLE 18.1   RNAO'S FRAMEWORK FOR ADVANCING HEALTHY PUBLIC POLICY PLANNING TEMPLATE
© REGISTERED NURSES' ASSOCIATION OF ONTARIO. ALL RIGHTS RESERVED.

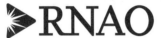

RNAO
Registered Nurses' Association of Ontario
L'Association des infirmières et infirmiers autorisés de l'Ontario

Speaking out for nursing. Speaking out for health.

PILLARS	STAGES/ DOMAINS OF ACTION	FRAMING (POSITIONING THE ISSUE)	PROMOTING AWARENESS (BUY-IN)	ENSURING UPTAKE (INFLUENCE)	SUSTAINING CHANGE (IMPACT)	EVALUATION (MEASURING OUTCOMES)
Evidence	Statistics					
	Policy papers					
	BPGs					
Advocacy	Knowledge mobilization					
	Communication and grassroots mobilization					
	Coalition building					
	Mass media and social media					
	Direct advocacy with politicians and civil servants					

Adapted from Grinspun, 2007b.
Used with permission.

THE FIRST PILLAR: AN EVIDENCE-BASED APPROACH

A foundational aspect of RNAO's approach to policy is that it should be evidence based. This is the reason for the first pillar, which starts from the belief that policy should rest on careful analysis and research—this is what we refer to as "evidence-based policy." The nature of the evidence varies depending on the subject matter or the desired policy outcome. On matters of social determinants of health, statistics and a plethora of interdisciplinary social policy evidence become relevant. Similarly, on environmental determinants, the evidence arises from the natural social and epidemiological sciences. On nursing and health policy issues, the relevant literature applies. We use a variety of "knowledge tools" that are deployed to the specific policy imperative, including the use of statistics and available data that are essential no matter what policy topic we are pursuing. On clinical issues that are the focus of this book, we rely on the best clinical evidence, and for RNAO the BPGs are central to related policymaking.

RNAO's evidence-based approach to policy also requires disregarding positions based on narrow concepts of self-interest and insists that core values—such as human dignity, people's well-being, health for all, and the public interest—should guide policy. The intent is that policy design harnesses the best available evidence on how to advance those values. That's why RNAO has produced some of the best and most detailed policy documents from health professionals in North America and arguably in the world. Many of these policy documents and policy proposals, especially in areas of nursing and health policy, are directly linked to our work on BPGs; and that is also the case in both case studies in this chapter.

Using evidence encompasses a number of forms: a mindset for statistics, accessing the most robust literature on the topic, and approaching the best experts in the field for their knowledge and insights. The end goal is to present rock-solid policy proposals that are fully backed by evidence.

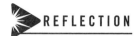

REFLECTION

How could you see yourself using this Framework for Advancing Healthy Public Policy? Would it also be a helpful tool to use in analyzing a policy initiative from the perspective of evidence and advocacy as well as the five stages of policy advancement? In what ways? See the list of RNAO policy initiatives in this chapter for consideration.

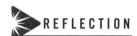

REFLECTION

If there are so many factors influencing the creation of public policy, why do you think it is so important to have the best evidence to back political advocacy work?

THE SECOND PILLAR: PURSUING A STRATEGIC ADVOCACY CAMPAIGN

The second pillar involves a political and advocacy campaign to create the political will for change. This is a multipronged, adaptive, and nimble approach that entails the use of a variety of tools and tactics that are individually important and collectively powerful. It includes knowledge mobilization; communication and grassroots mobilization of members; coalition building; intensive use of mass social and alternative media; as well as direct engagement with politicians, bureaucrats, and opinion leaders. Each one of these tactics is based on long traditions of work and theoretical insights about their effectiveness in advancing policy change (Stachowiak, 2013).

The analysis of policy change processes helps us understand the myriad of factors that influence successful policy mobilization and the need to intervene at multiple levels to secure policy uptake (Edwards, Rowan, Marck, & Grinspun, 2011). In designing an advocacy campaign, one must determine the potential for moving evidence into policy adoption; this requires understanding the factors that influence the uptake of new policies and the mechanisms that come into play that either accelerate or hinder adoption (Edwards et al., 2011; Grinspun, 2012, 2015).

The necessity of this second pillar arose early on with the realization that little is achieved if outstanding policy proposals end up lying dormant on someone's desk. That's why we set out to transform and galvanize RNAO's membership into becoming a highly informed, courageous, mobilized, and politically involved group of health professionals. RNs, NPs, and nursing students in Ontario have given massive support for such an activist approach. Moreover, this also has resulted in substantive increases in membership numbers that in turn strengthen our collective voice. RNAO's successes have made us keenly aware of the power of nursing as a body politic to advance collective good.

The second pillar entails the strategic use of five key advocacy domains (Grinspun, 2006b, 2007a). Each domain, in turn, applies a number of tactics and tools according to the circumstances and needs. These five domains of advocacy reflect the collective experience of others and have been adapted and perfected through repeated use in multiple RNAO policy campaigns:

- **Knowledge mobilization**—Knowledge mobilization encompasses activities relating to the production and use of research results, including knowledge synthesis, dissemination, transfer, and exchange. In particular, it informs public debate, policies, and practices in a particular area (Social Sciences and Humanities Research Council [SSHRC], 2017). For RNAO, advocacy action on a particular issue starts with making evidence-based knowledge available to RNAO members, other health professionals as appropriate, researchers, policymakers, stakeholders, and civil servants. It happens through various means including conferences, seminars, webinars, background papers, summary sheets, slide presentations, newsletter items, poster campaigns, as well as the President and CEO columns in RNAO's *Registered Nurse Journal (RNJ)* (Grinspun, 2014).

- **Communication with members and grassroots mobilization**—RNAO's work builds on a long tradition of grassroots movements, which believes groups can gain power by engaging in collective action for change (Alinsky, 1989). As discussed below, grassroots mobilization of its members is central to RNAO's policy successes, including those in the two case studies that follow. This has entailed keeping members well informed through a monthly "In the Loop" e-newsletter; building a grassroots organization for all members supported by RNAO's staff, board of directors, assembly, local chapters, and interest groups; a culture of political action; nurturing of a collective identity; and the refining of tools such as action alerts, nursing week campaigns, and the various topics we tackle in the *RNJ*.

- **Coalition building**—An advocacy coalition is an effective tool to advance changes in public policy; it involves seeking out allies with similar core beliefs and coordinating actions with them. Thus, advocacy coalitions include participants that both share similar policy core beliefs and engage in nontrivial degree of coordination (Weible & Sabatier, 2006, p. 128). RNAO has not only been effective in seeking powerful coalition allies, but also often plays a leading role, as exemplified in the case studies in this chapter.

■ **Mass social and alternative media**—RNAO is keenly aware of the agenda-setting role of mass media and its power to shape public opinion and influence how we picture public affairs (McCombs, 2014). From the outset, RNAO's advocacy role required connections with journalists and a concerted effort to have its voice amplified through mass media: op-eds, letters to the editor, interviews, etc. RNAO also sought a variety of other venues to bring forward its message. As stated above, RNAO's *RNJ* has played an important role as each issue highlights key policy interventions RNAO and its members are making, and RNAO's CEO and President's columns are carefully dedicated to difficult policy areas we are collectively tackling (Burkoski, 2015; McNeil, 2012). Other venues can include, for example, nursing week posters in public transportation (RNAO, 2010). We have made concerted investments in talent development and, with much success, on expanding the use of social media (Twitter, Facebook, Instagram) and RNAO's influence within the alternative media such as blogs, websites, online media, etc. (Grinspun 2015). Media presence in all its forms is captured and evaluated.

■ **Direct engagement with politicians, bureaucrats, and other opinion leaders**—RNAO recognizes the reality of concentrated power and influence and the power of key people to effect change. RNAO's planning of a policy campaign includes a detailed understanding of the distribution of power and decision-making on the subject matter. Thus, advocacy efforts focus on influencing key individuals, organizations, and political levers. In the case of RNAO, this has entailed a close working relationship with, and advocacy campaign toward, the Government of Ontario. The quality of the engagement matters substantively; for example, RNAO's strictly nonpartisan and issue-focused approach to policy engagement has earned it the respect of all political parties in Ontario and the ability to work with governments of any stripe. The engagement itself is done through the wise use of formal and informal meetings, calls, letters, participation in public consultations, Twitter, email, and phone call campaigns targeting particular individuals (such as with RNAO's Action Alerts).

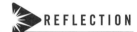 **REFLECTION**

What are the characteristics of a professional association that make it most suitable as an advocacy body? Are there any characteristics that may have a negative impact on advocacy activities?

ADVANCING HEALTHY PUBLIC POLICY INITIATIVES

RNAO success stories in the province of Ontario, Canada (Grinspun, 2012, 2015, 2016a, 2017):

■ **Nurse practitioner legislation and funding (1998)**—The Ontario government issues legislation and funding for NPs after ongoing advocacy by RNAO to promote their integral contributions and to widen their scope of practice.

■ **Baccalaureate entry to practice (2000)**—Provincial government passes legislation making a baccalaureate degree mandatory for RN practice in Ontario.

■ **New graduate employment guarantee (2007)**—Provincial government establishes a full-time employment guarantee for Ontario's new nursing graduates.

■ **Ontario's Nurse Practitioner-Led Clinics (2007)**—Canada's first NP-Led Clinic opens in Sudbury, Ontario. The following year, the provincial government promises to open 25 clinics in communities across Ontario.

■ **Ontario's Poverty Reduction Strategy (2008)**—The Ontario government announces this strategy, signalling a new vision for a fairer society.

- **Provincial prohibition of pesticides for cosmetic use (2008)**—Bill 64, provincial legislation to ban the use and sale of pesticides for cosmetic purposes, is passed.

- **Expanded scope of practice of NPs (2010)**—Important changes to the NP role are made, granting NPs the authority to work autonomously, prescribe without "a list," and to admit, treat, transfer, and discharge patients in hospital. Ontario becomes the first jurisdiction in North America, and Canada one of only three countries in the world, to enjoy the expanded scope of practice for NPs.

- **Empowering leadership positions in nursing (2011)**—The Ontario government operationalizes the 2011 *Excellent Care for All Act* (Bill 46) and amends regulations to mandate that chief nursing executives (CNE) are appointed as permanent members of hospital boards and quality committees, and the same for chief nursing officers (CNO) in public health units. Bill 46 also demands a focus on evidence-based practice for health organizations.

- **Closing of coal plants (2011)**—Ontario's Minister of Energy announces the permanent closure of two additional coal-fired generators, in partial response to an RNAO, Canadian Association of Physicians for the Environment, and Ontario Clean Air Alliance campaign to close coal plants immediately.

- **70% full-time employment in nursing (2012)**—RNAO's "70% solution" is implemented province wide, whereby at least 70% of the RNs in each work setting are permanent full-time (RNAO, 2003, 2005). As a result, in Ontario, 68.6% of RNs had full-time employment in 2012, while in Canada the corresponding rate was 54% (RNAO, 2014).

- **Banning medical tourism (2014)**—Ontario Health Minister issues a directive to all Ontario hospitals to not market to, solicit, or treat international patients, except in cases related to existing contracts. He also asks hospitals not to enter into new international contracts that include treating foreign nationals in Ontario (Glauser, 2014).

- **Protecting refugee health (2015)**—Provincial government listens to the outcry from RNAO and other healthcare providers against cuts to the Interim Federal Health Program (IFHP), a national health insurance program covering refugees and refugee claimants until they are eligible for provincial and territorial health plans. They also vow to make IFHP more comprehensive than it was before the cuts.

- **Adoption of RNAO's ECCO model for community care (2016): Bill 210**—Patients First Act is introduced, with the release of a discussion paper by the Ontario Health Minister, which proposes that Local Health Integration Networks (LHINs) assume responsibility for whole system planning and performance accountability. In addition, it proposes that major sectors of the health system be aligned under one umbrella: LHINs. The report credits RNAO's work and cites its groundbreaking report *Enhancing Community Care for Ontarians* (ECCO) (RNAO, 2012, 2014) by name.

- **Adoption of $15 minimum wage (2017)**—The Ontario government raises minimum wage to $15 per hour, the largest increase in the province's history.

- **Public inquiry into the safety and security of residents in long-term care (2017)**—Ontario appoints a judge to lead an independent public inquiry into the policies, procedures, and oversight of long-term care homes, which may have contributed to the assault and death of eight residents who were under the care of convicted serial killer and former registered nurse, Elizabeth Wettlaufer.

Building a Grassroots Movement

A crucial element in the second pillar has been RNAO's ability to mobilize its members—currently counting over 41,000—around public policy issues. In effect, this has been a strategy to build a grassroots movement, ready to mobilize in a concerted fashion and apply maximum pressure at all levels, from the "bottom" and from "above."

It all starts with genuine, purposeful, and continuous capacity-building of members, utilizing policy backgrounders, webinars, political action workshops, and more. It also entails supporting members through ongoing mentorship and equipping them with the tools they need to uptake political action and deploy their individual and collective power (RNAO, 2015c). Members receive training, and often these meetings (in person or virtually through webinars) happen with much personal connectedness, commitment, and passion. Members also link through RNAO's network of regional chapters and interest groups, thus creating local and specialty contingents of committed members ready to mobilize on particular policy matters of interest (e.g., fetal alcohol syndrome disorder) or bring voice to collective concerns and solutions (e.g., RN replacement) to the local level. Getting to know local politicians and other local stakeholders has earned members respect in their local setting and expanded the scope of influence of RNAO collectively. Members are also encouraged and supported to participate in public forums, attend chapter and interest group meetings, and express views through the media, "action alerts," and letters to the editor.

The RNAO board of directors and the RNAO staff have inculcated a sense of empowerment in members by demonstrating that being a member of RNAO means being in the loop, being part of the bigger picture, and being able to gain influence and have a positive impact. Not surprisingly, RNAO's presence, influence, and impact have escalated over the past decade, in Ontario, across Canada, and abroad. The growth in membership has meant a scaling up of mobilization. The outcome has been a remarkable policy and advocacy effort that has engaged Ontario governments of different political stripes to effect positive change in the nursing profession and the healthcare system.

An important example is RNAO's assembly of representatives—the association's formal leadership—composed of about 140 RNs, nurse practitioners, and nursing students, including the leaders of all 35 local RNAO chapters and 31 interest groups across the province of Ontario. Recognizing the paramount importance of political activism, RNAO has invested time and resources to advance capacity-building amongst these leaders.

For the past 20 years, the assembly has been formally trained and continuously supported by RNAO staff in each of the five advocacy domains. This includes providing them with materials and guidance on how to use the evidence that is relevant to the policy imperative the association is advocating for; coordinating and providing them with backgrounders to actively engage with members of the provincial parliament and/or of the federal parliament; and leveraging media and communications through the stages of our policy advocacy. As you will read in the first case study, RNAO also issues evidence-based action alerts focused on topic-specific areas that are sent to all parties' political leaders.

Direct Advocacy with Politicians and Civil Servants

As part of a rich array of advocacy tactics that have been built over 2 decades, RNAO conducts three formal yearly policy activation events, with one leading to the next.

Take Your MPP to Work: Created in 2001, this initiative takes place every year during nursing week and targets the three main political parties. RNs, NPs, and nursing students invite an MPP (member of the provincial parliament) to see firsthand the expertise needed to provide high-quality healthcare to Ontarians every day. The site visits also allow the politicians to better understand the breadth and depth of nursing practice across Ontario (Canada's largest jurisdiction), and the opportunities and challenges associated with providing care in different settings. Since its inception, *Take Your MPP to Work* has grown into a popular signature event for nurses and MPPs alike. Our members have taken premiers, cabinet ministers, opposition leaders, and backbench MPPs to work in primary care settings, NP-led clinics, street nursing programs, public health units, schools, hospitals, rehabilitation centers, long-term care homes, and more. Every year about 60 to 70 MPPs enjoy the unique experience of seeing RNs, NPs, and nursing students deliver health services in every type of practice setting across Ontario (RNAO, n.d.-c).

Queen's Park on the Road (QPOR): This initiative takes place from September to December. QPOR was originally proposed in 2013 as an event to replace RNAO's Queen's Park Day (discussed next) because the legislature in that year had been prorogued and elections had been called. The event was so successful that members told us they wanted to meet with MPPs in their riding offices every year. Since then, every year, RNs, NPs, and nursing students—members of RNAO—meet with MPPs from all political parties in the MPPs' offices and urge them to adopt specific recommendations. In these meetings, members focus on increasing access to nursing services, improving healthcare, and enhancing social and environmental determinants of health. Nurses come to the meeting well prepared with a comprehensive evidence-based policy package (titled "backgrounders"), prepared by RNAO's expert policy department and communications' staff. Queen's Park on the Road (QPOR) is an effective political engagement activity for members. The opportunity to meet with MPPs to discuss priority nursing and health issues empowers nurses and demonstrates that they can make an impact on public policy and influence healthy change for all (RNAO, n.d.-b).

Queen's Park Day is a dynamic and very meaningful event for both RNAO and the political leaders. It occurs in February when the legislature is in session, which allows RNAO's board of directors and the assembly leaders (composed of 140 representatives) to visit and meet with members of the provincial parliament (MPPs) for a full day at the legislature. It begins with a breakfast with MPPs, followed by seating at Question Period where many of the nurses and nursing student leaders are individually recognized by their local MPPs, and then a full hour to have dialogue and ask questions with Ontario's Premier and the Minister of Health, as well as an hour with each of the opposition party leaders and their health critics (RNAO, 2017d).

Ontario has 107 MPPs. In total, 98 to 104 MPPs participate in at least one of the events throughout the year, every year. Over 60 participate in two, and up to 45 in all three events.

RNAO evaluates each of these events to ensure our continued effectiveness in impacting healthy public policy. What is most important is that these political activation initiatives are anchored in deep-seated values at RNAO aimed at achieving health for all. Fuelled by sound, evidence-based intellectual work, and a good dose of courage, this extensive membership advocacy

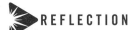

REFLECTION

How do these three advocacy tactics influence the political process? Can you give an example of how an initiative incubated at such an event could develop to become part of a broader policy agenda?

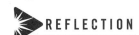

REFLECTION

Can you identify similar advocacy tactics used by your professional association and reflect on their outcomes?

work empowers RNAO and its members to persuade politicians to muster the will to do what's right for the public (Grinspun, 2017). The case studies below exemplify this critical point.

STAGES OF POLICY ADVOCACY

As indicated in the upper row of Table 18.1, the framework for advancing healthy public policy delineates five stages in the advocacy campaign to advance a particular policy issue. Successfully advancing from one stage to the next requires the strategic engagement of both pillars of action—harnessing evidence and pursuing an effective advocacy campaign involving a number of action domains. The strategic challenge of a campaign is to select the "which," "how," and "when" of the domains and specific actions within each domain to be engaged at each turn singularly or collectively. The five stages are:

1. **Framing (positioning of the issue)**—According to linguist George Lakoff (2004), *frames* are mental structures that shape the way we see the world. Frames shape the goals we seek, the way we act, and what counts as good or bad. In politics, our frames shape social policies, what we support, and what we reject. To change our frames is to change all this; thus, reframing represents social change (Lakoff, 2004, p. xv). RNAO's advocacy work starts by framing the issue at hand for our members, the public, and the opinion leaders. We want to frame the issue in a way that makes people care, that speaks to their values and interests, and that makes it clear why change must happen. In the first case study, why should we care if people die in the streets as a result of drug overdoses? In the second case, why should we care if two thousand amputations happen every year?

2. **Promoting awareness (buy-in)**—This is the stage when decision-makers decide they must act. This could be the result of effective framing of the issue amongst important sectors of the public through a successful awareness campaign. Or it could be the result of an efficacious advocacy campaign with substantial political impacts for decision-makers and the recognition that the only way to stop the campaign is by acting on the demands. No matter how the buy-in of policymakers happens, this is the stage where a policy direction is adopted or promised. It represents an important milestone in the advocacy campaign, but by no means the end. This is a progression stage that as you will see in the case studies is vulnerable, as promises do not always get us to the finish line.

3. **Ensuring uptake (influence)**—As stated above, in an ideal world, once decision-makers have decided to act and have announced their plans, all is settled. In reality, the struggle around the adoption of new policies continues throughout its implementation. At this stage, advocacy focuses on making sure the right changes and effective policies are enacted. With entrenched interests surely affected by the proposed policies, the fight will be on the terms, timing, and depth of the new policies. So this is all about making sure that what was promised actually happens. It is a process, with setbacks and successes that can be prolonged and uneven. When it comes to successful fruition, the policy changes have been implemented and institutionalized. Again, we will see evidence of this stage in both case studies.

4. **Sustaining change (ensuring impact)**—This is the stage where policy changes are implemented. Advocacy focuses on sustaining the change—making sure that political, financial, or other resources, such as education, policy uptake by stakeholders, and monitoring progress, are there to sustain change. At this stage, it is critical to continue being vigilant about particular

interests that may continue to try to derail or dilute change or distort its implementation. This is a stage of accompaniment of the expected changes, which may entail active support for implementation or "low-key" advocacy action.

5.   **Evaluation (measuring impact)**—This is a longer-term stage where the actual impacts of the policy change are evaluated and measured. Were the results of the policy those that were expected when the policy was envisioned? Or were the results different and unexpected? This is a stage of extracting lessons and analyzing results. In most cases, this evaluation is complex given the challenge of isolating the impacts of one particular policy change from many other changes in the policy environment.

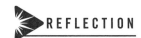

REFLECTION

As you read the case studies presented next, consider using the Framework for Advancing Healthy Public Policy to help guide your assessment of how this framework directed the process.

We turn now to the presentation of the two case studies. The next section presents a case study on supervised injection services, and the following one, a case study of access to services for persons with diabetes.

CASE STUDY

LINKING EVIDENCE AND ADVOCACY FOR SUPERVISED INJECTION SERVICES IN ONTARIO

Comprehensive harm-reduction programs are critical to save lives and help people with substance use, minimize stigma, and build healthier communities. RNAO has developed two well-recognized Best Practice Guidelines (BPG) on the topic. The first is *Supporting Clients on Methadone Maintenance Treatment* (MMT) released in 2009. The second is *Engaging Clients Who Use Substances* (RNAO, 2015a).

Supervised injection services (SIS) are an important component of a comprehensive harm-reduction program. SIS have generated much debate, scrutiny, and calls to shape policy with evidence. The issue came to the forefront in 2011, when Insite, North America's first legal SIS facility (Vancouver, British Columbia [BC]), was threatened with closure by a federal government that refused to heed the evidence and took the matter to the Supreme Court of Canada.

RNAO is a staunch supporter of Insite as an evidence-based public health service that demonstrates harm-reduction benefits to individuals and communities (Grinspun, 2016b). In 2007, RNAO's resolution in support of nursing advocacy to ensure Insite's long-term sustainability was passed at the Annual General Meeting of the Canadian Nurses Association. RNAO formed a coalition of nursing organizations to seek intervener status and present arguments before the Supreme Court of Canada. We secured intervener status and spread the word through the media (RNAO, 2011c), and communications to members (RNAO, 2011b). Ultimately, the evidence and public interventions contributed to the ruling that allowed Insite to keep its doors open. Insite's victory laid the groundwork for bringing SIS to Canadians in other provinces, including Ontario.

This case study examines the integral role of evidence in advocating for and informing change and how RNAO mobilized the profession, media, and public to move evidence into policy. We highlight the multipronged approach RNAO played in the association's pivotal role to land the approval of three proposed SIS sites throughout Toronto. We end the case study with a return to evidence-based practice as RNAO launches the development of a BPG centered on the nursing care of persons at SIS.

MOBILIZING CHANGE WITH EVIDENCE

According to 2012 Statistics Canada data, about six million people (about 21.6% of Canadians) met the criteria for a substance use disorder during their lifetime (Pearson, Janz, & Ali 2013). While tobacco and alcohol are responsible for more deaths and hospitalizations than illicit drugs (Single, Rehm, Robson, & Truong, 2000), dramatic increases in sudden deaths due to opioid overdoses prompted British Columbia's Minister of Health to call for recognition of a "national public health emergency" (Woo, 2017). Jane Philpott, Canada's then Minister of Health, acknowledged that the escalating number of overdoses deaths may be "the greatest public health crisis we face in Canada" (Woo, 2017, para. 2).

Preliminary federal estimates for 2016 are that there were 2,458 opioid-related deaths in Canada, which is an average of almost seven people per day (Public Health Agency of Canada, 2017). These numbers are sure to increase as the data do not include Quebec and use Ontario data from 2015. The annual rate of opioid-related deaths in Ontario has increased 285% from 1991 (144 deaths) to 2015 (734 deaths) (Gomes et al., 2017). In 2015, on average two people died in Ontario every day of opioid-related causes (Gomes et al., 2017). The crisis continues to escalate. Ontario announced there were 412 opioid-related deaths during the first 6 months of 2016, which is an 11% increase compared with the same time period in 2015 (MOHLTC 2017). In addition to deaths from prescribed opioids, the introduction of fentanyl and carfentanil into substances purchased illicitly greatly increases the chances of fatal overdoses (Howlett, 2016; Howlett, Giovannetti, Vanderklippe, & Perreaux, 2017).

MOBILIZING CHANGE WITH POWER: SPEAKING OUT FOR INSITE

Insite opened in 2003 as the first legal supervised injection site in North America. It is an integrated part of Vancouver Coastal Health's continuum of care, where people with problematic substance use can inject preobtained drugs and connect with healthcare and addiction services (RNAO, 2011a). It operates on the premise of harm reduction, which aims to decrease the adverse health, social, and economic effects of drug use without requiring abstinence from using drugs (RNAO, 2011a). Having opened under the leadership of the federal Liberal government, Insite faced a number of attempts to shut its doors since the Conservatives came to power in 2006. Despite two court decisions in BC in favour of its continued operation, the Supreme Court of Canada agreed in June 2010 to hear the federal government's appeal of those rulings. Recognizing the threat to Insite as well as its clients, nurses, other employees, and overall impact of harm reduction, RNAO invited the Canadian Nurses Association (CNA) and the Association of Registered Nurses of British Columbia (ARNBC) to form a "nursing coalition" to counter politics with evidence (RNAO, n.d.-a, 2011a).

The nursing coalition spoke out about the effectiveness of Insite, based on ample evidence and research. For instance, Insite received an average of 702 daily visits in 2009 and saw an average of 491 supervised injections (RNAO, 2011b). Nearly 500 overdose interventions were performed with no fatalities, and more than 6,200 people were referred to detox and addiction treatment at other service agencies (RNAO, 2011b). More than 30 peer-reviewed studies yielded findings of Insite's benefits to clients and the greater community, ranging from reduced public injecting, to lower levels of HIV risk behaviours and an increase in the pursuit of addiction treatment (RNAO, 2011b). Anecdotal accounts, such as RNAO's (2011b) *RNJ* feature on two RNs working in harm reduction, further supplement the data to demonstrate that Insite is run by knowledgeable professionals and powered by evidence to make a difference in people's lives. The nursing coalition drew on the strong evidence and the collective force of nursing to earn intervener status before the Supreme Court of Canada at the hearing in May 2011 (RNAO, 2011d). Later that year, the coalition celebrated the high court's unanimous ruling to keep Insite open (RNAO, 2011c).

The victory for Insite represented progress in more than one direction. It affirmed the life-saving and life-changing effect of supervised injection services as integral to harm reduction for clients who need help and support. It highlighted the contribution of nurses, both to their clients' well-being and to the decisions that affect nurses and the public we serve. The victory that was attained through collective action reflected the power of combining evidence, policy expertise, media, and communications. It is the same elements of this framework that would guide RNAO's efforts in the next phase of bringing supervised injection services to Ontario.

AMPLIFYING THE CALL FOR SIS IN ONTARIO

Although the 2011 ruling in favour of Insite was an encouraging sign for the harm-reduction movement, another barrier arose in 2013 when the federal government introduced Bill C-65 (RNAO, 2013c). The new bill posed onerous requirements designed to prevent SIS implementation. This regressive move contrasted with the research evidence that recommended the integration of SIS into existing health services in Toronto and Ottawa (Bayoumi et al., 2012). In order to respond to the documented need for SIS sites, the Toronto Drug Strategy Implementation Panel struck a working group (of which RNAO was a member) to look at SIS implementation and challenges. With the release of the working group's *Supervised Injection Services Toolkit* (2013) and staff recommendations from Toronto Public Health, the Board of Health was urged to advocate for provincial funding to integrate SIS into existing clinical health services and to oppose Bill C-65.

RNAO showed support for SIS implementation in Toronto by providing a quote in a media release by Toronto Public Health (2013). CEO Dr. Doris Grinspun represented RNAO as the first speaker to the Toronto Board of Health with a clear message: "Implementing SIS is a pragmatic, evidence-based policy that will improve health outcomes, prevent needless deaths, and contribute to safer communities" (RNAO, 2013a, para. 2). CEO Grinspun pointed out that strong leadership from Toronto was "critical not only for the people of Toronto but also for vulnerable people across Ontario and Canada" (RNAO, 2013a, para. 7).

At the same time, RNAO submitted an open letter to then-Minister of Health and Long-Term Care (MOHLTC) Deb Matthews, copied to the Premier and provincial opposition party leaders, which urged the Ontario government to speak out against Bill C-65 and fund the integration of SIS into existing clinical health services (RNAO, 2013b). In the spirit of combined action, RNAO cited its support for the latter alongside the Canadian Nurses Association, Canadian Medical Association, Canadian Public Health Association, Community and Hospital Infection Control Association-Canada, Public Health Physicians of Canada, and Urban Public Health Network (RNAO, 2013b).

RNAO also solicited further support with an action alert. RNAO *action alerts* mobilize nurses, other health professionals, and members of the community to be part of a movement by joining, and thus amplifying, the voice for change. Members are equipped with the necessary background on the issue as well as modes of action. In this case, they could sign the action alert to reinforce the asks in RNAO's open letter, which would also reach the Health Minister, Premier, and provincial party leaders (RNAO, 2013c). As a result, 1,038 people sent a strong message to the Minister and Premier. This action alert is featured in Figure 18.1, while the sidebar shows a later action alert (RNAO, 2017a), asking the provincial government to provide immediate funding for SIS.

ASK QUEEN'S PARK TO PROVIDE IMMEDIATE FUNDING FOR SUPERVISED INJECTION SERVICES (SIS)

Thank you to the more than 750 people who have signed RNAO's action alert urging Premier Wynne to announce funding for SIS in Toronto and Ottawa. We are getting traction and that is why we ask those of you who haven't yet signed to please take a minute to add your voice to urge immediate funding for renovations at four prospective sites so that Health Canada's SIS approval process can move forward.

Every 13 hours, an opioid-related death occurs in Ontario. As in British Columbia, many of these deaths are from accidental overdoses linked to fentanyl. Supervised injection services (SIS) can prevent overdose deaths, but these services are not currently available in Ontario.

The evidence is conclusive: Access to SIS will save lives.

The Ontario government must immediately announce funding for SIS in Ottawa and Toronto to complement existing health services and save lives.

Copies will be sent to:

- Premier Kathleen Wynne
- Patrick Brown, PC Leader
- Andrea Horwath, NDP Leader
- John Fraser, Parliamentary Assistant to Minister of Health and Long-Term Care
- Jeff Yurek, PC Health Critic
- France Gélinas, NDP Health Critic

RNAO (2017a) Action Alert: Ask Queen's Park to Provide Immediate Funding for Supervised Injection Services (SIS). Used with permission.

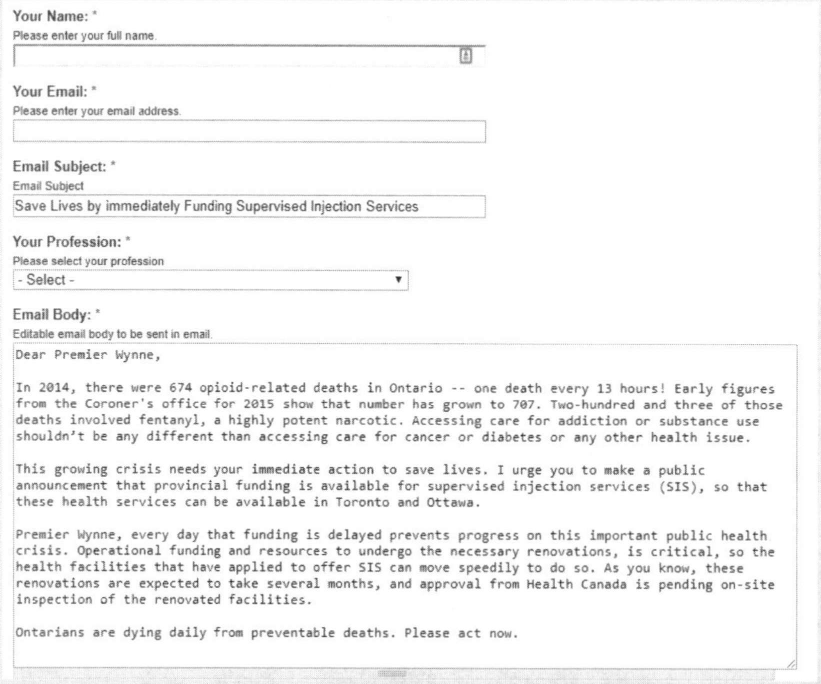

Your Name: *
Please enter your full name.

Your Email: *
Please enter your email address.

Email Subject: *
Email Subject
Save Lives by immediately Funding Supervised Injection Services

Your Profession: *
Please select your profession
- Select -

Email Body: *
Editable email body to be sent in email.

Dear Premier Wynne,

In 2014, there were 674 opioid-related deaths in Ontario -- one death every 13 hours! Early figures from the Coroner's office for 2015 show that number has grown to 707. Two-hundred and three of those deaths involved fentanyl, a highly potent narcotic. Accessing care for addiction or substance use shouldn't be any different than accessing care for cancer or diabetes or any other health issue.

This growing crisis needs your immediate action to save lives. I urge you to make a public announcement that provincial funding is available for supervised injection services (SIS), so that these health services can be available in Toronto and Ottawa.

Premier Wynne, every day that funding is delayed prevents progress on this important public health crisis. Operational funding and resources to undergo the necessary renovations, is critical, so the health facilities that have applied to offer SIS can move speedily to do so. As you know, these renovations are expected to take several months, and approval from Health Canada is pending on-site inspection of the renovated facilities.

Ontarians are dying daily from preventable deaths. Please act now.

FIGURE 18.1 RNAO action alert: Save lives by immediately funding supervised injection services (RNAO, 2017c).
Used with permission.

URGING EVIDENCE-BASED DECISION-MAKING

Although support for SIS was endorsed by the Toronto health board, more work and pressure were needed for it to materialize. Such pressure came in September 2015, when the Toronto Public Health Unit's Medical Officer of Health Dr. David McKeown presented a report to the board on trends, prevention, and response for overdose in Toronto. The report underlined concerns about the rise in drug-induced deaths in Toronto over the last decade. MOHLTC called a meeting that RNAO attended, and the focus was on the use and misuse of narcotics in Ontario (RNAO, 2015b). Following that, RNAO issued a letter to the Premier with recommendations on ways that the province could prevent premature deaths and improve health outcomes related to drugs (2015b). Of these, SIS was a key recommendation for government to prevent deaths from overdose (RNAO, 2015b).

The next window of opportunity came in March 2016, when the Toronto Board of Health considered the proposal for three health services in Toronto to add small-scale SIS to their existing clinical services. RNAO (2016c) again secured a deputation, and in addition to using robust evidence, it echoed the voices of lived experience that gave weight to the decision at hand. Just ahead of RNAO's deputation, a mother who had lost her daughter to a drug overdose, Donna May, made a heart-wrenching deputation. For RNAO's CEO, it was clear. The remarks she had brought, so well prepared and filled with evidence, were no longer sufficient. Grinspun's deputation was spontaneous, unapologetically sharp, and harsh.

The proposal was unanimously approved and moved to Toronto City Council.

MOBILIZING CHANGE WITH EVIDENCE, COMMUNICATIONS, AND MEDIA

To increase momentum, RNAO called on members and the media to give legs to the SIS movement. In a matter of days, RNAO issued two letters to the editor (*National Post*, 2016; *Toronto Star, 2016*), and CEO Dr. Doris Grinspun was quoted and counted in "Toronto VIPs [who] give support to safe injection sites" (Davidson, 2016). By injecting evidence into each media response, RNAO positioned itself and the issue firmly for serious consideration.

RNAO also harnessed the power of narrative, such as in the sad instance of Brad Chapman, who collapsed on a downtown Toronto street from a drug overdose (Chapman & Grinspun, 2016). Brad is the brother of Leigh Chapman, a registered nurse and member of RNAO. Leigh became an advocate, speaking with insight from her brother's experience, for evidence-based public policies including supervised injection services to prevent further tragedies.

"What else do you need to make a unanimous decision in favour of SIS," Grinspun asked the councillors. *"How many more mothers who have lost their children do you need to hear? How many more fathers, husbands, or sisters do you need to see suffering to say—unanimously—that the time for SIS is now? Nurses urge you to act swiftly,"* she added.

CHAPMAN: LEARNING FROM THE TRAGIC DEATH OF A BROTHER

Brad Chapman was found collapsed on a downtown Toronto street from a drug overdose in August 2015 and died eight days later in hospital. When not in jail, Brad lived on the streets for the last 20 years. He died at 43, but his mental health and addiction challenges took him away long before then.

Over the past few months, Brad's sister, Leigh, and mother, Cori, have had the privilege of meeting several people who shared memories of Brad. They learned that Brad could still play the guitar, liked to rollerblade, and brightened the lives of others with a kind word and a smile. It consoled them to know that Brad is missed—not just as a son, brother, father, grandfather, and uncle, but also as a friend and a member of the community.

But even with this consolation, Leigh Chapman, a registered nurse, knows there are evidence-based public policies that could have helped save Brad.

A supervised injection service is a health service that provides a safe and hygienic space where people can inject preobtained drugs under the supervision of nurses. There are more than 90 SIS sites world-wide, including those in Australia, Germany, Luxembourg, Netherlands, Norway, Spain, Switzerland, and two in Vancouver. Two decades of research on SIS show they reduce deaths from overdoses, reduce transmission of infectious diseases, increase use of detox and other addiction treatment services, and improve community safety.

Brad felt safe at a nearby harm reduction program where he could exchange used needles for clean ones, access safer crack kits, and engage with nonjudgmental public health staff. He would regularly call home from this facility, which offered Brad a sense of belonging and way of checking in with those who loved him.

But a needle exchange is different from SIS. Brad got his needles but then shot up alone, unsupervised, in an alley, which is where he was found by police after overdosing.

What if, instead, Brad had been able to access SIS within a harm reduction program where he felt welcome? Would he still be with us today?

There is also naloxone, a short-acting drug used to reverse a suspected narcotic overdose. Health Canada has determined naloxone's ability to quickly respond to an overdose far outweighs its minimal risks. Ottawa Public Health has successfully trained at least 150 people to provide naloxone, and about 50 local overdoses have been reversed. Because of the increasing number of deaths associated with prescription and nonprescription narcotics, some jurisdictions in the United States are training those most likely to arrive first at a scene (fire and police personnel) to recognize overdoses and administer naloxone. What if the first responders who arrived on the scene had been able to immediately give Brad naloxone and start CPR?

This is why the Registered Nurses' Association of Ontario has spoken out for SIS and called for easier access to naloxone. Nurses were at the forefront of creating Insite, the safe injection site in Vancouver, and RNAO fought then-prime minister Stephen Harper to keep it open.

The City of Toronto is moving forward with plans for SIS. Isn't it time other municipalities such as Ottawa—where overdoses took the lives of 40 people in 2014—took similar steps to avert tragedies? We have the evidence; we just need the political will. And with federal Health Minister Jane Philpott expressing her support for Insite, nurses are hopeful we can prevent others like Brad from dying.

Leigh Chapman *is a registered nurse and the sister of Brad Chapman.* Doris Grinspun *is a registered nurse and the chief executive officer of the Registered Nurses' Association of Ontario (RNAO).*

From http://ottawacitizen.com/opinion/columnists/chapman-learning-from-the-tragic-death-of-a-brother.

RNAO (2016g) wove evidence, narrative, and media into another powerful action alert for its members and the public to voice their support for SIS. It provided an update on developments since the deputation, including a vote by the Ottawa Board of Health in favour of proposals to set up SIS at community health centers, and studies underway in London and Thunder Bay on the need and feasibility of SIS in their communities (RNAO, 2016g). It also provided a letter template for members to write to their city councillor, in advance of the SIS motion proceeding to the Toronto City Council.

GAINS, LESSONS, AND NEXT STEPS FOR SIS IN ONTARIO

Advocates for SIS saw the fruits of their labour in July 2016, when Toronto City Council approved 36-3 the proposal to support integration of three supervised injection services into existing health facilities throughout the city (RNAO, 2016b). To celebrate the milestone, RNAO (2016f) added its own announcement of a new Best Practice Guideline (BPG) on SIS. Using a systematic review and guided by a panel of experts in the field, RNAO's BPG will provide recommendations to guide this critical harm-reduction initiative.

The cochairs supporting the guideline include Toronto's former Medical Officer of Health, Dr. David McKeown, who helped make SIS a reality in Toronto under his leadership; and Marjory Ditmars, a registered nurse with 5 years of practical and leadership experience at Insite.

IMPLEMENTING SUPERVISED INJECTION SERVICES: A HEALTH EQUITY BPG

In November of 2016, RNAO convened the SIS guideline development panel consisting of individuals with expertise in harm reduction and substance use. The panel includes individuals holding clinical, administrative, and academic positions, as well as those with lived experience. These experts work either directly with people who inject drugs (PWID) in a variety of health settings (e.g., supervised injection services, community health centers, harm-reduction programs, and primary healthcare), or indirectly in other types of organizations, such as associations and academic institutions.

To determine the purpose and scope of the guideline, the RNAO BPG Development Team conducted a gap analysis of existing guidelines, 12 key informant interviews, and two focus groups with experts in the field. These experts included direct-care staff, administrators, researchers, and individuals with lived experience, representing various Canadian organizations in Toronto, Vancouver, Edmonton, and Ottawa. It became apparent that a guideline was required for nurses and other health workers in SIS to provide recommendations on the most effective way to deliver service to PWID that would: 1) improve client engagement and inclusion; 2) support positive health outcomes; and 3) reduce harms associated with injection drug use. The main focus of the guideline was to ensure equity-oriented services for PWID though harm-reduction, trauma-informed, and culturally safe approaches.

Specifically, the practice recommendations provide guidance on how to engage PWID in SIS through establishing trusting relationships; practicing critical inquiry (i.e., reflective practice); and promoting and engaging in shared decision-making. The education recommendations provide direction on the structure and format of educational programs shown to be effective at increasing knowledge, skill, and confidence of individuals working with PWID. The policy recommendations provide guidance to organizations and the health system on how to build SIS that promote high-quality, equitable care for PWID. This includes: the integration of peers and comprehensive services into SIS operations, as well as the integration of SIS into existing health settings (e.g., hospitals); access considerations for rural environments and for vulnerable PWID; considerations related to facility size and hours of operation; and implementation of regulations and operational procedures that support people who require assisted injections and youth who inject drugs.

The latest achievement for SIS is the commitment by the Ontario government to fund renovations and operating costs at three SIS facilities in Toronto and one in Ottawa (RNAO, 2017c). This was announced as part of the 2017 provincial budget, which RNAO was pleased to see following its letter to political leaders urging provincial support and funding for SIS (RNAO, 2016d), and its earlier recommendation in a prebudget submission (RNAO, 2017b).

Through this strategic and planned advocacy initiative, RNAO and its coalition partners leveraged different avenues for shaping policy, all of which were rooted in evidence. Submissions and letters to the government form the starting point, first setting out the concerns and asks in relation to the issue at hand, as well as recommendations for action. Mobilizing a collective voice made up of nurses, healthcare professionals, and community members is the next step in amplifying the call to action. The media serves as another powerful platform for strengthening the call, and one supported by evidence gives substance and credibility to both the association and the media agency. The landmark achievements for SIS in BC and Ontario set a precedent not only for harm reduction, but on a broader scale, for linking evidence with advocacy and policy, to effect real change.

In a time of a global opioid crisis, RNAO publicly promoted the research evidence demonstrating that SIS saves lives and, armed with evidence, advocated politically for SIS as a necessary harm-reduction strategy. This advocacy work and subsequent development of a SIS BPG is one example of how a nursing professional association can effectively link evidence-based practice and evidence-based policy to advance healthy public policy and the health and well-being of people. See Figure 18.2.

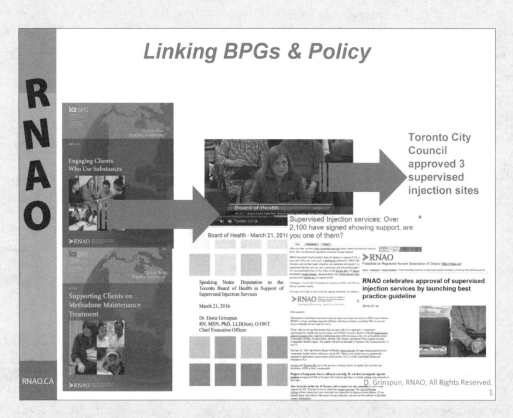

FIGURE 18.2   Linking BPGs and policy—supervised injection services.

LINKING EVIDENCE AND ADVOCACY FOR FUNDING OFFLOADING DEVICES IN ONTARIO

Diabetes is a serious metabolic condition that affects people of all age groups, worldwide (Canadian Diabetes Association Clinical Practice Guidelines Expert Committee, 2013). The International Diabetes Federation (IDF) estimates that the global prevalence of diabetes in 2012 was 8.3% (approximately 371 million people) (International Diabetes Federation, 2012). Moreover, 4 out of 5 people living with diabetes reside in low- and middle-income countries. Indigenous and South East Asian populations, both in Canada and abroad, are especially vulnerable to the disease (Davis, 2011).

People with diabetes are at high risk of developing long-term complications, including foot ulcers and amputations. Diabetes-related foot problems, ulcerations, and amputations significantly impact the person and the community in which patients live. Foot ulceration precedes 84% of nontraumatic lower extremity amputations in those with diabetes. The risk of death is 2.4-fold greater than for patients without ulcerations (Singh, Armstrong, & Lipsky, 2005). The treatment of diabetes-related foot ulcers is an expensive, lengthy, and time-consuming process when ulcers are not detected and managed early. In fact, it accounts for an estimated 15% of total healthcare resources dedicated to diabetes in high-income countries and as much as 40% in low- and middle-income countries (International Diabetes Federation, 2017). The International Diabetes Federation indicates that comprehensive diabetic foot assessments and foot care, based on prevention, education, and a multidisciplinary team approach, may reduce foot complications and amputations by up to 85% (International Diabetes Federation & International Working Group on the Diabetic Foot, 2005).

As alarming as this evidence is, evidence is not always enough to create change. Next in this chapter we discuss a successful case study leveraging three necessary factors—evidence, political pressure, and opportunity—to secure a policy change regarding universal funding for patients with diabetes living with foot complications to prevent amputation (Elliott, 2015). We will explore practical principles of government advocacy to empower our readers to help achieve positive policy change that can improve patient outcomes.

COMING TOGETHER

In 2012, Canada's Council of the Federation endorsed the Registered Nurses' Association of Ontario (RNAO)'s *Best Practice Guideline Assessment and Management of Foot Ulcers for People with Diabetes* for national implementation (The Council of the Federation Health Care Innovation Working Group, 2012). Provincial governments across Canada have publicly declared that foot care for people with diabetes is a significant health challenge and one of their top priorities for care. RNAO was committed to supporting the dissemination, adoption, and uptake of their guidelines at a national level (see Figure 18.3).

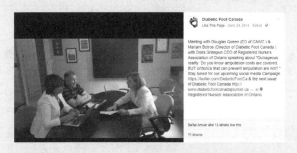

FIGURE 18.3 Meeting between Wounds Canada and RNAO.
Used with permission.

For 2 decades, Wounds Canada (formerly the Canadian Association of Wound Care) has been leading the charge in wound treatment and prevention across Canada. Wounds Canada worked with both Public Health Canada and Diabetes Canada (formerly the Canadian Diabetes Association) from 2009 to 2012 to raise awareness of diabetes-related foot complications and of prevention and management strategies. In 2012, Wounds Canada established a new division, Diabetic Foot Canada (DFC), to focus solely on foot disease in those living with diabetes, with a strong tie-in to the important etiological issues surrounding diabetes. Diabetic Foot Canada was designed to be the national go-to program for online information and education for clinicians and patients in support of effective self-monitoring, early detection, prevention, and treatment.

In 2013, Wounds Canada and RNAO identified this area of healthcare as a priority that affects both quality of life and healthcare costs. Thus, they joined forces to produce the *Diabetic Foot Canada Journal* (DFCJ), an online publication targeted at multidisciplinary healthcare professionals, to provide education, disseminate best evidence and educational tools, and raise awareness of the importance of preventing diabetes-related foot complications and amputations.

Wounds Canada and RNAO also recognized that, historically, the Canadian diabetic foot care community has struggled to fully leverage the power of our collective voices. Thus, they formed a coalition with each other, along with Diabetes Canada and the Canadian Association for Enterostomal Therapy (CAET), to jointly engage the government. One of the key alliance goals of this coalition is to prevent diabetes-related foot complications, including preventable lower limb amputations, through evidence-based Clinical Practice Guidelines (CPGs) and timely management of abnormalities.

JOINT LETTER TO MINISTRY OF HEALTH AND LONG-TERM CARE (MOHLTC)

On December 9, 2014, Wounds Canada, RNAO, and nearly 50 other supporters delivered a letter on care for diabetes-related foot ulcers to the top levels of the Government of Ontario. This letter is one of the most powerful and unified messages that has ever been delivered to a Canadian government on the issue of diabetes-related foot care.

In the letter, the Coalition highlighted to the ministry the importance of a coordinated and integrated system of care to improve patient outcomes, while providing the healthcare system with substantial cost savings. Currently, most Ontarians with diabetes-related foot complications have to pay out of pocket for the care they need, which includes preventative shoes, socks,

offloading devices, and chiropody, podiatry, or nursing treatment. As a result, many of the people most in need of the devices and care are least able to afford it. The letter presented a number of key suggestions the ministry could implement to drastically improve the diabetes-related foot care situation in the province, including:

- Providing universal access to preventative foot care services, including supplying preventative shoes, socks, and offloading devices to those in need, free at the point-of-care, for all Ontarians living with diabetes

- Developing policies that enable every Ontarian with diabetes to have appropriate foot assessments as outlined by the International Diabetes Federation 2017 guideline document (an annual exam for all persons with diabetes, with higher-risk individuals having assessments more frequently)

- Adopting an Ontario-wide interprofessional approach to diabetics-related foot care, with at least one interprofessional diabetes foot-care team, with a well-defined referral pattern, in each Local Health Integration Network (LHIN)

- Publishing, on an annual basis, reliable data on diabetes-related foot care, using internationally recognized metrics, to assist ongoing quality-improvement efforts

Chief amongst these gaps is the fact that most Ontarians with diabetes-related foot complications have to pay out of pocket for the care they need, which includes preventative shoes, socks, offloading devices, and chiropody, podiatry, or nursing treatment.

The coalition believes that universal access to preventative foot care for people living with diabetes will decrease the number of ulcers and amputations in the same way that retinopathy screening and treatment has decreased diabetes-related blindness. In addition, it will also decrease overall provincial spending (see Figure 18.4).

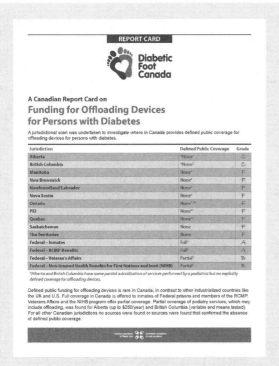

FIGURE 18.4 A Canadian report card on funding for offloading devices for persons with diabetes.
Used with permission.

The letter and subsequent meetings have focused on increasing policymakers' awareness by outlining cost-effective methods for improving foot care for people with diabetes and, ultimately, reducing the number of preventable amputations in the province. A jurisdictional report on offloading funding was also created and submitted. However, these meetings were not followed up with specific commitments from the MOHLTC.

INCREASING AWARENESS

Following the delivery of the letter, meetings and other events were held to increase the awareness of policymakers about these issues. The organizations and individuals of the coalition continued to work together and separately to improve the provincial politicians' awareness about the issue in general and advocate for universal public funding of offloading devices in particular.

To reinforce the message, the coalition highlighted cost-effective methods for improving foot care for people with diabetes and, ultimately, reducing the number of preventable amputations in the province. For example, in early 2015, Diabetes Canada developed an economic analysis and accompanying report revealing that diabetic foot ulcers currently cost the government of Ontario between $320 million and $400 million a year, whereas the public funding of offloading devices could produce a net savings of between $48 million and $75 million (Somerville & Nagpal, 2015).

Later that year, Diabetes Canada and its volunteers held an information session with MPPs at Queen's Park to advocate for amputation-prevention supports and public funding for offloading devices. An embargoed copy of Diabetes Canada's economic analysis and report was provided to the Health Minister's Office, which was in turn shared with the Treasury Board and Finance Minister's Office.

In April 2016, RNAO and Wounds Canada hosted a successful reception with 28 members of the Ontario legislature, partnering associations, clinicians, and patients to lobby the ministry to fund offloading devices. Materials had been developed as part of the legislators' information packages. These materials were designed to help them assess the problem and impact of not changing policies. The event itself included an overview of the problem through presentations from clinical and policy experts and the sharing of patient stories by patients and family members. Representatives from each political party delivered a response to the information they had received and their plans for addressing the issues. What is interesting is that many of the attendees, including many in key policy and decision-making positions, were surprised to learn that something as seemingly minor as a foot ulcer could lead to amputation and increased mortality (see Figure 18.5).

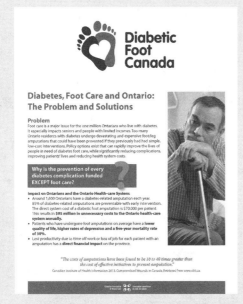

FIGURE 18.5 Diabetes, foot care and Ontario: The problem and solutions. Used with permission.

The problem is that "evidence is often not presented in a language that governments speak." (Elliott, 2015, pg. 9)

MEDIA AND OPPOSITION

Following the April event, a media release outlining the problem and stating the recommendations of the coalition was used by several news outlets to develop stories about the issue, many of which included interviews with representatives of coalition organizations (Artuso, 2016; RNAO, 2016a).

Over the next many months, the coalition continued to work collectively to increase political pressure and engage all political parties, including the opposition.

LEVERAGING OPPOSITION

On World Diabetes Day, November 14, 2016, the Ontario Minister of Health was challenged during Question Period on the issue of offloading devices by Ontario Progressive Conservative Health Critic Jeff Yurek, prompted by Diabetes Canada.

FORMALIZING THE PROCESS

The coalition was invited to submit a formal Ontario Health Technology Advisory Committee (OHTAC) request outlining the evidence supporting removable cast walkers (RCW) and RCWs rendered irremovable (ITCC) in May 2016. OHTAC is composed of a group of evidence-based experts from across the province who review health technology assessments and make recommendations on which healthcare services and devices should be publicly funded.

SUCCESS AT LAST: THE HEALTH MINISTER'S COMMITMENT

In February of 2017 at RNAO'S Queen's Park event, the Minister of Health committed to public funding for offloading devices and to accepting OHTAC's recommendations to publicly fund total contact casts (TCC), RCWs, and ITCC for diabetic neuropathic foot ulcers.

After this long process of providing information, recommendations, and follow-up, the coalition recognized that decision-makers were finally beginning to understand the impact of diabetes on the health of Canadians. However, comprehension is only the first step. It is important to acknowledge that the "what" is only part of the equation. The "how" is also necessary for successful implementation of the recommendations. Therefore, the coalition has continued to advise the ministry on successful options for safe and effective rollout of this initiative.

Part of the coalition strategy was the creation for the ministry of a document comparing three implementation methods for ensuring direct-care patient access to offloading devices for people with diabetes and foot ulcers. These are:

- Offloading devices added to formularies and accessed at point-of-care

- An Assistive Devices Program (ADP) funding model accessed by the organization where offloading devices are obtained by patients at the point-of-care

- A direct-to-patient ADP funding model

The implementation method recommended by the coalition is #1: offloading devices added to formularies and accessed at point-of-care.

Specific recommendations to support this option include:

- Immediate point-of-care dispensing at the time of the assessment based on qualifying criteria

- No patient copayment for standard stock devices (this will require Local Health Integration Network [LHIN] copayment or a creative funding model) but rather direct billing for reimbursement of the device from the hospital or community organization

- Fitting and application completed by qualified healthcare professionals only

- Ability of the LHIN or other organization to fund alternatives to the above devices (TCC/RWC) if patients have contraindications (e.g., unsteady balance, heel ulcers, ischemia, deep infection)

- A MOHLTC policy to provide direction to hospitals and community organizations (in order to gain their support and understanding of the process for patients to be able to access the offloading device at the point-of-care)

NEXT STEPS

The coalition remains committed to working with other provincial organizations and key stakeholders to address the gaps in care and policy in the area of diabetes-related foot ulcers, as well as ensuring that we reduce the growing numbers of preventable diabetes-related amputations across Canada. The work has started across Canadian provinces.

This case study was a description of a strategic and planned policy advocacy initiative that did not take place overnight but required strong vision focused on improving patient outcomes, collaborations between organizations, persistence, and outstanding leadership.

We need to reiterate that clinical excellence and the use of best evidence in practice, related specifically to care for persons with diabetes and actual or potential foot ulcers, while absolutely necessary, is not enough. We need to work with governments to ensure organizational policy to support foot assessments of all patients with diabetes on a regular basis and preventative care and management. These interventions do cost money, but they are a far cry from the cost of an amputation in terms of quality of life, loss of productivity, and healthcare dollars. The Narayan public health principles have indicated that the identification of the high-risk diabetic foot is both cost-saving to healthcare systems and improves patient outcomes (Venkat Narayan et al., 2006). See Figure 18.6.

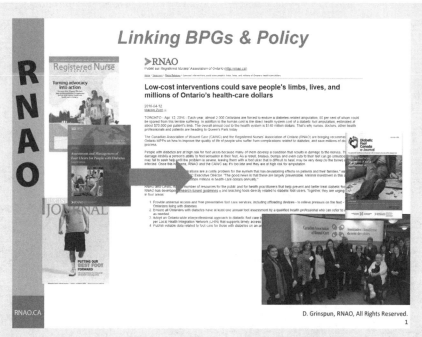

FIGURE 18.6   Linking BPGs and policy—funding for offloading devices.

CONCLUSION

As you can see from these two case studies, RNAO has taken a leadership role in organizing the nursing community and collaboratively supporting others in advancing healthy public policy. Evidence—and especially clinical evidence—is a necessary component of the multipronged strategy to advance healthy public policy. However, as this chapter highlights and the two case studies prove, evidence alone does not suffice to make macro policy changes. As a nursing collective, we can throw up our hands in frustration, or we can chose to join together using our clinical expertise and our collective influence as a body politic, truly speaking truth to power (Grinspun, 2016c).

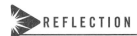 **REFLECTION**

Based on your review of the cases above, do you think there is a role for direct-care nurses or nursing students in policy advocacy? If so, what is it? If not, why not?

Activism on broader health and social issues does not preclude continued activism on professional issues related to nursing practice. Indeed, stage 4 in Cohen and colleagues' (1996) framework for nursing political development does not rule out pursuit of self-interests; it merely does so within a context that emphasizes the larger public good. According to the authors, pursuit of stage 4 can be enhanced by: 1) building coalitions and constituencies around health and social issues; 2) developing leaders and supporting visionaries and risk-takers; 3) mobilizing nursing for campaigns; 4) integrating health policy into curricula; 5) developing public media expertise; and 6) gaining increased sophistication in policy analysis and related research. RNAO's experience, described in this chapter, shows achieving stage 4 following this type of approach is both doable and thrilling to attain.

Improving the health outcomes of the world's people and the effectiveness of our health systems requires the ongoing and persistent engagement of nursing as a collective in the political process. This engagement must be multipartisan to enrich our democracy and grow the respect we have achieved from the public, the politicians, and the media (Grinspun, 2006a, 2012, 2015). By targeting specific policies aimed at closing the gap between what the public needs and what nursing can offer, we can improve our contributions to health for all.

As described in Chapter 1, governments and health service organizations worldwide are seeking to improve healthcare, lower or contain costs, and optimize health outcomes. A large focus is on ensuring appropriateness of clinical interventions, including reducing those interventions that have proven to be unnecessary or ineffective and demanding that clinical care be based on evidence. However, the evidence of clinical care is not always supported by the broad policies and funding that are needed to deliver appropriate interventions. This was the case with both supervised injection services and off-loading devices in the province of Ontario. This reality brings opportunities to nursing and nurses as a knowledge- and solution-oriented profession.

Augmenting the narrative of evidence-based clinical practice with one of demanding evidence-based policies is urgent and achievable. As this book attests, nursing and nurses already have remarkable clinical expertise with proven health and system outcomes. With a nursing collective that also leads the way in policy, we can set endless agendas that, if purposefully guided, can and will benefit the public at large. Moreover, nurses' natural orientation toward upstream approaches to health and healthcare, as well as the profession's strong focus on health promotion and disease prevention, position us as key players in solving the health and healthcare imperatives facing the public both as funders and users of health services.

KEY MESSAGES

- Nursing, as a profession, has a responsibility to assume its role as a body politic to advance healthy public policy. This will ensure the public fully benefits from nurses' contribution as evidence-based experts.

- Nurses and nursing organizations can and should provide political leadership on broader policy issues that speak to the public's interests.

- Evidence-based policy proposals are only one of two vital pillars required to drive healthy public policy at the macro health system level; in addition to the "evidence" pillar, a second pillar of effective "advocacy action" is required to achieve change.

- An advocacy campaign should be strategic, multipronged, adaptive, and nimble, entailing a number of domains of action: knowledge mobilization; communication and grassroots mobilization; coalition building; use of mass social and alternative media; as well as direct engagement with politicians, civil servants, and other opinion leaders. Nurses should educate themselves in all these domains of action.

- Successful advocacy requires building a grassroots movement, ready to mobilize in a concerted fashion and apply maximum pressure at all levels, from the "bottom," from the "sides," and from "above" at the local, state, and federal levels.

REFERENCES

Alinsky, S. D. (1989). *Rules for radicals: A pragmatic primer for realistic radicals.* New York, NY: Vintage.

Amela, V. M. (2012, April 2). "A country with good nurses will be happier." (Spanish). La Vanguardia. Retrieved from http://www.lavanguardia.com/lacontra/20120402/54279639102/doris-grinspun-un-pais-con-buenas-enfermeras-sera-mas-feliz.html

Artuso, A. (2016, April 12). Preventative foot care sought for diabetics. *Toronto Sun.* Retrieved from http://www.torontosun.com/2016/04/12/preventative-foot-care-sought-for-diabetics

Bayoumi, A., Strike, C., Jairam, J., Watson, T., Enns, E., Kolla, G., . . . Brandeau, M. (2012). Report of the Toronto and Ottawa Supervised Consumption Study, 2012. Toronto: St. Michael's Hospital and the Dalla Lana School of Public Health, University of Toronto. Retrieved from http://www.catie.ca/sites/default/files/TOSCA%20report%202012.pdf

Burkoski, V. (2015, March/April). MPPs know nurses' voices will not remain silent. President's View with Vanessa Burkoski. *Registered Nurse Journal.* Retrieved from http://rnao.ca/sites/rnao-ca/files/RNJ-MarchApril2015-PresidentsView.pdf

Canadian Diabetes Association Clinical Practice Guidelines Expert Committee. (2013). Canadian Diabetes Association 2013 clinical practice guidelines for the prevention and management of Diabetes in Canada. Can J Diabetes, 37(1), S1-S212.

Chapman, L., & Grinspun, D. (2016, March 27). Chapman: Learning from the tragic death of a brother. *Ottawa Citizen.* Retrieved from http://ottawacitizen.com/opinion/columnists/chapman-learning-from-the-tragic-death-of-a-brother

Cohen, S. S., Mason, D. J., Kovner, C., Leavitt, J. K., Pulcini, J., & Sochalski, J. (1996). Stages of nursing's political development: Where we've been and where we ought to go. *Nursing Outlook, 44*(6), 259–266.

The Council of the Federation, Health Care Innovation Working Group. (2012, 20 July). *From innovation to action: The first report of the health care innovation working group.* Retrieved from https://www.canadaspremiers.ca/wp-content/uploads/2017/09/health_innovation_report-e-web.pdf

Davidson, T. (2016, March 17). Toronto VIPs give support to safe injection sites. *Toronto Sun.* Retrieved from http://www.torontosun.com/2016/03/17/toronto-vips-give-support-to-safe-injection-sites

Davis, C. L. (2011, May 18). *Chronic disease prevention and management in First Nations and Inuit communities: Care model, current status and next steps.* [Presentation]. First Nations and Inuit Health Home and Community Care Program National Regional Coordinators & Partners Meeting, Port Alberni, BC.

Edwards, N., Rowan, M., Marck, P., & Grinspun, D. (2011). Understanding whole systems change in health care: The case of the nurse practitioners in Canada. *Policy, Politics, & Nursing, 12*(1), 4–17.

Ellenbecker, C. H., Fawcett, J., Jones, E.J., Mahoney, D., Rowlands, B., & Waddell, A. (2017). A staged approach to educating nurses in health policy. *Policy, Politics & Nursing Practice, 18*(1), 44–56.

Elliott, J. (2015). Advocating for the diabetic foot. *Diabetic Foot Canada, 3*(1).

Factor Hispano. (2006, January). Nursing shortage: "A global problem that needs local solutions" (Spanish).

Gardner, D. (2010). A passion for improving health care: An interview with Doris Grinspun. *Nursing Economics, 28*(2), 126–129.

Glauser, W. (2014). Medicare advocates decry medical tourism. *CMAJ, 186*(13), 977.

Gomes, T., Greaves, S., Martins, D., Bandola, D., Tadrous, M., Singh, S., . . . Quercia, J. (2017, April). *Latest trends in opioid-related deaths in Ontario: 1991 to 2015*. Toronto, ON: Ontario Drug Policy Research Network. Retrieved from http://odprn.ca/wp-content/uploads/2017/04/ODPRN-Report_Latest-trends-in-opioid-related-deaths.pdf

Grinspun, D. (2006a, May/June). Political engagement: An integral part of nursing. Executive Director's Dispatch with Doris Grinspun. *Registered Nurse Journal, 18*(3), 7.

Grinspun, D. (2006b, Nov/Dec). Using evidence, politics, communication and media to shape healthy public policy. Executive Director's Dispatch with Doris Grinspun. *Registered Nurse Journal, 18*(6), 7.

Grinspun, D. (2007a, May/June). Communication and media: Key advocacy tools for nurses. Executive Director's Dispatch with Doris Grinspun. *Registered Nurse Journal, 19*(3), 6.

Grinspun, D. (2007b, November). *Using evidence, politics, communications and media to shape health policy: A framework for action* [PowerPoint slides]. Oral presentation at University of Ottawa, master's level nursing course, Policy, Political Action, and Change. Ottawa, ON.

Grinspun, D. (2012. Sept/Oct). Registered nurses shape whole-system change. (Part 3/3), Chief Executive Officer's Dispatch with Doris Grinspun. *Registered Nurse Journal, 24*(5), 6.

Grinspun, D. (2013. Nov/Dec). Expanding our grassroots power. CEO Dispatch with Doris Grinspun. *Registered Nurse Journal, 25*(6), 6.

Grinspun, D. (2014, May/June). Medical tourism: The beginning of the end of Medicare. CEO Dispatch with Doris Grinspun. *Registered Nurse Journal, 26*(3), 6.

Grinspun, D. (2015, Sept/Oct). A platform, members and social media: RNAO's winning recipe. CEO Dispatch with Doris Grinspun. *Registered Nurse Journal, 27*(5), 6.

Grinspun, D. (2016a). Health policy in changing environments. In E. Staples, S. Ray, & R. Hannon (Eds.). *Canadian perspectives on advanced nursing practice: Clinical practice, research, leadership, consultation and collaboration* (1st Canadian ed.) (pp. 285–300). Toronto, ON: Canadian Scholar's Press.

Grinspun, D. (2016b, Sept/Oct). SIS: Keep the conversation going. CEO Dispatch with Doris Grinspun. *Registered Nurse Journal, 28*(5), 6.

Grinspun, D. (2016c, July/August). Speaking truth to power: A moral duty for every nurse. CEO Dispatch with Doris Grinspun. *Registered Nurse Journal, 28*(4), 6.

Grinspun, D. (2017, Jan/Feb). Values. Evidence. Courage. CEO Dispatch with Doris Grinspun. *Registered Nurse Journal, 29*(1), 6.

Howlett, K. (2016, December 6). Powerful opioid carfentanil detected in Ontario for first time. *The Globe and Mail.* Retrieved from https://www.theglobeandmail.com/news/national/powerful-opioid-carfentanil-detected-in-ontario-for-first-time/article33227681/

Howlett, K., Giovannetti, J., Vanderklippe, N., & Perreaux, L. (2017, June 1). How Canada got addicted to fentanyl. *The Globe and Mail.* Retrieved from https://www.theglobeandmail.com/news/investigations/a-killer-high-how-canada-got-addicted-tofentanyl/article29570025/

International Diabetes Federation (IDF). (2012). IDF Diabetes Atlas. Retrieved from http://www.indiaenvironmentportal.org.in/files/file/diabetes%20atlas%202012.pdf

International Diabetes Federation (IDF). (2017) IDF Clinical Practice Recommendations on the Diabetic Foot— 2017. Retrieved from https://www.idf.org/e-library/guidelines/119-idf-clinical-practice-recommendations-on-diabetic-foot-2017.html

International Diabetes Federation & International Working Group on the Diabetic Foot. (2005). *Diabetes and foot care: Time to act.* Retrieved from https://www.worlddiabetesfoundation.org/sites/default/files/Diabetes%20and%20Foot%20care_Time%20to%20act.pdf

Jordan, Z. (2005, Oct/Dec). Turning challenges into opportunities. *PACEsetterS, 2*(4), 6–11.

Lakoff, G. (2004). *Don't think of an elephant! How democrats and progressives can win: Know your values and frame the debate: The essential guide for progressives.* White River Junction, VT: Chelsea Green Publishing.

Marti, G. (2014, May 28). Nursing will be one of the most requested professions (Spanish). *La Vanguardia.* Retrieved from https://www.pressreader.com/spain/la-vanguardia/20140528/282389807526965

McCombs, M. (2014). *Setting the agenda: Mass media and public opinion* (2nd ed.). Cambridge, UK: Polity Press.

McNeil, D. (2012, Jan/Feb). Personal experience informs my perspective on challenges in the north. President's View with David McNeil. *Registered Nurse Journal*. Retrieved from http://rnao.ca/sites/rnao-ca/files/Jan-Feb_2012-3_President-s_View.pdf

Ministry of Health and Long-Term Care (MOHLTC). (2017, May 24). *Joint statement on opioid data* (News release). Retrieved from https://news.ontario.ca/mohltc/en/2017/05/joint-statement-on-opioid-data.html

National Post. (2016, March 17). Re: Toronto needs supervised injection sites. Retrieved from http://nationalpost.com/g00/opinion/letters/letters-who-represents-muslims/wcm/9011ec91-3b4a-4f43-ad49-17ca37c727d3?i10c.referrer=http%3A%2F%2Fnationalpost.com%2Fg00%2Fopinion%2Fletters%2Fletters-who-represents-muslims%2Fwcm%2F9011ec91-3b4a-4f43-ad49-17ca37c727d3%3Fi10c.referrer%3Dhttp%253A%252F%252Frnao.ca%252Fcontent%252Fletter-supervised-injection-sites

Pantaleoni, A. (2014, April 30). "If the health system is privatized, we will lose everything" [Spanish]. *El País*. Retrieved from https://elpais.com/sociedad/2014/04/30/actualidad/1398876710_608236.html

Pearson, C., Janz, T., & Ali, J. (2013). Mental and substance use disorders in Canada. *Health at a Glance*. Ottawa: Statistics Canada. Retrieved from http://www.statcan.gc.ca/pub/82-624-x/2013001/article/11855-eng.pdf

Public Health Agency of Canada. (2017, June 5). *National report: Apparent opioid-related deaths (2016)*. Retrieved from https://www.canada.ca/en/health-canada/services/substance-abuse/prescription-drug-abuse/opioids/national-report-apparent-opioid-related-deaths.html#limits

Registered Nurses' Association of Ontario (RNAO). (n.d.-a). *Nurses speak out for harm reduction*. Retrieved from http://rnao.ca/about/public-impact/harm-reduction

Registered Nurses' Association of Ontario (RNAO). (n.d.-b). *Queen's Park on the Road*. Retrieved from http://qpor.rnao.ca/

Registered Nurses' Association of Ontario (RNAO). (n.d.-c). *Take Your MPP to Work*. Retrieved from http://rnao.ca/policy/political-action/take-your-mpp-work

Registered Nurses' Association of Ontario (RNAO). (2003, May). *Survey of casual and part-time registered nurses in Ontario*. Toronto, ON: Registered Nurses' Association of Ontario.

Registered Nurses' Association of Ontario (RNAO). (2005, June). *The 70 per cent solution: A progress report on increasing full-time employment for Ontario RNs*. Toronto, ON: Registered Nurses' Association of Ontario.

Registered Nurses' Association of Ontario (RNAO). (2009). *Supporting clients on methadone maintenance treatment*. Toronto, ON: Registered Nurses' Association of Ontario.

Registered Nurses' Association of Ontario (RNAO). (2010, May 10). *Nurses launch public awareness campaign to promote the profession*. Retrieved from http://rnao.ca/news/media-releases/Nurses-launch-public-awareness-campaign-to-promote-the-profession

Registered Nurses' Association of Ontario (RNAO). (2011a, February 4). *FAQ About Registered Nurses' Association of Ontario (RNAO), Canadian Nurses Association (CNA), and Association of Registered Nurses of British Columbia (ARNBC) Application for Intervener Status in Supreme Court of Canada hearing on Insite*. Retrieved from http://rnao.ca/sites/rnao-ca/files/7297_Backgrounder_HR_panel_Feb_2011_0.pdf

Registered Nurses' Association of Ontario (RNAO). (2011b, March/April). The Fix: RNs offer harm reduction services as the first line of defence against a life of addiction. *Registered Nurse Journal*. Retrieved from http://rnao.ca/sites/rnao-ca/files/7298_RNAO_RNJ_The_Fix_RNs_offer_harm_reduction_services_March_April_2011_0.pdf

Registered Nurses' Association of Ontario (RNAO). (2011c, September 30). *Nurses praise Supreme Court ruling: Insite saves lives and improves health*. Retrieved from http://rnao.ca/news/media-releases/2011/09/30/nurses-praise-supreme-court-ruling-insite-saves-lives-and-improves-health

Registered Nurses' Association of Ontario (RNAO). (2011d, May 11). *Nursing groups to present arguments on Insite case before Supreme Court of Canada*. Retrieved from http://rnao.ca/news/media-releases/Media-Advisory-Nursing-groups-to-present-arguments-on-Insite-case-before-Supreme-Court-of-Canada

Registered Nurses' Association of Ontario (RNAO). (2012, October). *Enhancing community care for Ontarians (ECCO) 1.0*. Toronto, ON: Registered Nurses' Association of Ontario.

Registered Nurses' Association of Ontario (RNAO). (2013a, July 10). *Deputation to Toronto Board of Health in support of supervised injection services*. Retrieved from http://rnao.ca/policy/speaking-notes/support-supervised-injection-services-toronto

Registered Nurses' Association of Ontario (RNAO). (2013b, July 2). *Open letter: Registered nurses urge provincial funding for supervised injection services*. Retrieved from http://rnao.ca/sites/rnao-ca/files/RNAO_Letter_to_Minister_Matthews_SIS_July_2013_final.pdf

Registered Nurses' Association of Ontario (RNAO). (2013c, July 3). *Support life-saving supervised injection services*. Retrieved from http://rnao.ca/policy/action-alerts/action-alert-support-life-saving-supervised-injection-services

Registered Nurses' Association of Ontario (RNAO). (2014, April). *Enhancing community care for Ontarians (ECCO) 2.0*. Toronto, ON: Registered Nurses' Association of Ontario.

Registered Nurses' Association of Ontario (RNAO). (2015a). *Engaging clients who use substances*. Toronto, ON: Registered Nurses' Association of Ontario.

Registered Nurses' Association of Ontario (RNAO). (2015b, October 29). *Preventing drug-related deaths in Ontario.* Retrieved from http://rnao.ca/policy/letters/preventing-drug-related-deaths-ontario

Registered Nurses' Association of Ontario (RNAO). (2015c, April). *Taking action: A toolkit for becoming politically involved.* Retrieved from http://rnao.ca/policy/political-action/political-action-information-kit

Registered Nurses' Association of Ontario (RNAO). (2016a, April 12). *Low-cost interventions could save people's limbs, lives and millions of Ontario's health-care dollars.* Retrieved from http://rnao.ca/news/media-releases/2016/04/12/low-cost-interventions-could-save-peoples-limbs-lives-and-millions

Registered Nurses' Association of Ontario (RNAO). (2016b, July 5). *Nurses praise Toronto Board of Health move on supervised injection services.* Retrieved from http://rnao.ca/news/media-releases/2016/07/05/nurses-praise-toronto-board-health-move-supervised-injection-services

Registered Nurses' Association of Ontario (RNAO). (2016c, March 17). *Nurses support supervised injection services to save lives and build healthier communities.* Retrieved from http://rnao.ca/news/media-releases/2016/03/17/nurses-support-supervised-injection-services-save-lives-and-build-hea

Registered Nurses' Association of Ontario (RNAO). (2016d, August 5). *Provincial support and funding for Supervised Injection Services* (Letter). Retrieved from http://rnao.ca/policy/submissions/funding-supervised-injection-services

Registered Nurses' Association of Ontario (RNAO). (2016f, July 14). *RNAO celebrates approval of supervised injection services by launching Best Practice Guideline.* http://rnao.ca/news/media-releases/2016/07/14/rnao-celebrates-approval-supervised-injection-services-launching-best

Registered Nurses' Association of Ontario (RNAO). (2016g). *Supervised Injection Services (SIS): We need your help, please take action.* Retrieved from http://rnao.ca/content/supervised-injection-services-sis-we-need-your-help-please-take-action

Registered Nurses' Association of Ontario (RNAO). (2017a, April 4). *Ask Queen's Park to provide immediate funding for supervised injection services (SIS).* Retrieved from http://rnao.ca/policy/action-alerts/ask-queens-park-provide-immediate-funding-supervised-injection-services-sis

Registered Nurses' Association of Ontario (RNAO). (2017b, January 19). *Ontario pre-budget 2017: Nurses call for an upstream strategy.* Retrieved from http://rnao.ca/policy/submissions/ontario-pre-budget-2017

Registered Nurses' Association of Ontario (RNAO). (2017c, April 27). *RNAO hails progressive budget.* Retrieved from http://rnao.ca/news/media-releases/2017/04/27/rnao-hails-progressive-budget

Registered Nurses' Association of Ontario (RNAO). (2017d, February 21). *RNAO urges upstream and effective use of health resources at annual Queen's Park Day.* Retrieved from http://rnao.ca/news/media-releases/2017/02/21/queens-park-day

Registered Nurses' Association of Ontario. (in press). *Implementing Supervised Injection Services: A Health Equity BPG.* Toronto, ON: Registered Nurses' Association of Ontario.

Singh, N., Armstrong, D. G., & Lipsky, B. A. (2005). Preventing foot ulcers in patients with diabetes. *JAMA, 293*(2), 217–228.

Single, E., Rehm, J., Robson, L., & Truong, M. V. (2000). The relative risks and etiological fractions of different causes of deaths and disease attributable to alcohol, tobacco and illicit drug use in Canada. *Canadian Medical Association Journal, 162*(12), 1669–1675.

Social Sciences and Humanities Research Council (SSHRC). (2017, May 1). *Guidelines for effective knowledge mobilization.* Ottawa, ON: Social Sciences and Humanities Research Council. Retrieved from http://www.sshrc-crsh.gc.ca/funding-financement/policies-politiques/knowledge_mobilisation-mobilisation_des_connaissances-eng.aspx

Somerville, R., & Nagpal, S. (2015). *Impact of offloading devices on the cost of diabetic foot ulcers in Ontario* (prepared for the Canadian Diabetes Association). Retrieved from https://www.diabetes.ca/getmedia/5109456e-8c0b-458f-b949-a5ac-cd41513a/impact-of-offloading-devices-ontario.pdf.aspx

Stachowiak, S. (2013). *Pathways for change: 10 theories to inform advocacy and policy change efforts.* Washington, DC: Center for Evaluation Innovation.

Toronto Drug Strategy Implementation Panel. (2013, June). *Supervised injection services toolkit.* Retrieved from http://www.toronto.ca/legdocs/mmis/2013/hl/bgrd/backgroundfile-59914.pdf

Toronto Public Health. (2013, July 2). *Supervised injection services in Toronto.* Retrieved from http://wx.toronto.ca/inter/it/newsrel.nsf/9a3dd5e2596d27af85256de400452b9b/691f7dfbf808db1885257b9c0059e10f?OpenDocument

Toronto Star. (2016, March 17). *Safe injection sites worth supporting.* Retrieved from https://www.thestar.com/opinion/letters_to_the_editors/2016/03/17/safe-injection-sites-worth-supporting.html

Venkat Narayan, K. M., Zhang, P., Kanaya, A. M., Williams, D. E., Engelgau, M. M., Imperatore, G., & Ramachandran, A. (2006). Diabetes: The pandemic and potential solutions. In D. T. Jamison, J. G. Breman, A. R. Measham, G. Alleyne, M. Claeson, D. B. Evans, . . . P. Musgrove (Eds.) *Disease control priorities in developing countries* (2nd ed.) (Chapter 30). Washington, DC: The International Bank for Reconstruction and Development/The World Bank; New York, NY: Oxford University Press.

Weible, C. M., & Sabatier, P. A. (2006). A guide to the advocacy coalition framework. In F. Fischer & G. J. Miller (Eds.), *Handbook of public policy analysis: Theory, politics, and methods* (pp. 123–136). Boca Raton, FL: CRC Press.

Woo, A. (2017, January 18). B.C. asks Ottawa to declare public health emergency as death toll from overdoses continues to surge. *The Globe and Mail.* Retrieved from https://www.theglobeandmail.com/news/british-columbia/more-than-900-fatal-overdoses-in-bc-in-2016-deadliest-year-record/article33659321/

INDEX